Temporomandibular Joint Disorders

Darpan Bhargava
Editor

Temporomandibular Joint Disorders

Principles and Current Practice

Springer

Editor
Darpan Bhargava
Clinical Director
TMJ Consultancy Services
Bhopal, Madhya Pradesh
India

Associate Professor, Oral and Maxillofacial Surgery
People's College of Dental Sciences and Research Centre, People's University
Bhopal, Madhya Pradesh
India

ISBN 978-981-16-2753-8 ISBN 978-981-16-2754-5 (eBook)
https://doi.org/10.1007/978-981-16-2754-5

This Springer imprint is published by the registered company Springer Nature Singapore Pte Ltd.
The registered company address is: 152 Beach Road, #21-01/04 Gateway East, Singapore 189721, Singapore

To My Grandparents,
Harishankar Bhargava-Gopi Bhargava
Dr. P.N. Sharma-Ramakanti Sharma

Foreword

It gives me great pleasure to provide this foreword to this new textbook defining problems around the temporomandibular joint. It is concise, well laid out, and simplifies this complex topic in a logical manner and as such, it is a very meaningful addition to the literature. Problems around the temporomandibular joint are, unfortunately, still very common and they remain something of an enigma. The temporomandibular joint is unusual in the human body in that it is one of only three joints with a meniscus, the only joint which has to move when its opposite number moves, the only joint that is consistently forced into a position that may not be optimal when the teeth come into occlusion, and remains the only joint whose problems are not routinely managed by the speciality of orthopaedic surgery. However, the philosophy on the diagnosis and management of temporomandibular joint problems has evolved over the years and the problems are now not considered to be primarily concerned with the occlusion (the art of gnathology) but more a biological problem aligned to problems occurring in and around other joints in the body. Consequently, the management of temporomandibular joint issues has aligned itself more closely with the management of other joint problems. In general, this divides itself into intraarticular problems that are within the joint itself and myofascial problems which are in the muscles and ligaments around the joint. In general, the latter are not managed surgically but are managed by a number of nonsurgical techniques, while surgery still has a part to play in the management of intraarticular issues. This volume logically discusses all of these problems and also the recent additions to our surgical armamentarium including arthroscopic surgery and alloplastic joint replacement. I wish this new textbook well.

May 27, 2021

M. Anthony (Tony) Pogrel

Department of Oral and Maxillofacial Surgery
University of California,
San Francisco, CA, USA

Preface

सरस्वति नमस्तुभ्यं वरदे कामरूपिणि ।
विद्यारम्भं करिष्यामि सिद्धिर्भवतु मे सदा ॥

Salutations Mother Saraswati, giver of boons, fulfiller of desires;
Bless me, I shall begin my studies, may there be accomplishments.

I wish all the accomplishments for the readers of this text. The text is the compilation of my experiences with the evidenced-based literature available for the treatment of temporomandibular joint disorders. The book contains to the point and concise theoretical text with explanations on clinically oriented management skills. An in-depth understanding of how to appropriately diagnose jaw joint disorders remains a vital aspect, even before knowing or executing the interventions required. I would like to quote my modification of this famous saying here "What the mind does not know, the eyes do not see!" For many, who do not understand the pathogenesis of temporomandibular joint disorders and are not up-to-date with the available treatments and interventions, they still have a simplified diagnosis of "pain in the joint" that requires only analgesics and muscle relaxants for most of the joint-related complaints. Most of the available text on temporomandibular joint disorders is more of a research-oriented content directed at researchers, as this is an evolving science, with very limited established protocols, currently. This fact leaves a clinician in a dilemma of what has to be actually followed for a specific case scenario, which he or she encounters on a day-to-day basis. My patients who entrusted me with my interventions on them and my inquisitive students who managed to learn tips and tricks from my work inspired me to compile a text that aims to help many of my fellow colleagues to get an insight on how to manage some complex problems of the temporomandibular joint. I wish this text helps many more practitioners of medicine and dentistry to get the same satisfaction which I get from relieving the pain and agony of the patients suffering from problems associated with the jaw joint. This book is not complete if I do not acknowledge the numerous people who got involved with me to realize the importance of this topic and its dispersion to the masses in the form of this compilation. First and foremost, the omnipresent blessings of my parents Ragini Bhargava and Dr. Madan Mohan Bhargava, who entrust me with my endeavors at all times. I am indebted for all the sacrifices rendered by them toward my success. This project would not have been complete without the support and love from my wife Dr. Preeti and my little son Darsh who were ready for any help I needed, apart from being considerate for the time which I stole from them and diverted for this project. The editorial director for books on medicine and life sciences for Asia, Springer Nature, Dr. Naren Aggarwal, did realize the importance of this compilation and my evidence-based clinical approach for temporomandibular joint disorders and extended all the guidance and help I needed to publish this book. The project coordinator from Springer Nature Ms. Saanthi Shankhararaman made the journey for this Herculean task smooth, with her promptness and ready solutions to all the issues we encountered with enough flexibility throughout. I am thankful to Ms. Hashwini Vytheswaran, project manager at Straive, for handling the production of the book. I take this opportunity to thank all my colleagues and friends who trust me with my diagnostic and treatment decisions.

As the editor-in-chief of the project, it was not easy to get all 48 contributing authors to a consensus on what should be included in the text from what may not be necessary, to impart clear thoughts to the treating clinicians rather than data on ongoing research.

This aggregation of facts does not intend to teach all the skills to everyone, but to know and diagnose the problems related to the joint aptly and have the knowledge of the available options handy, for an appropriate referral. I wish this compilation help its readers in treating problems associated with the temporomandibular joint in a more refined manner with an augmented approach backed by established protocols discussed in the text.

"Maxillofacial surgery needs dedication and dedication has no shortcuts"

Bhopal, Madhya Pradesh, India Darpan Bhargava

Contents

List of Contributors

Nikita Agrawal Department of Pediatric Dentistry, People's College of Dental Sciences and Research Centre, Bhopal, Madhya Pradesh, India

Rajkumar Ahirwal Department of Anaesthesiology and Critical Care, Gandhi Medical College and Associated Hospitals, Bhopal, Madhya Pradesh, India

P. Anantanarayanan Anantan Dental and Facial Surgery, Chennai, Tamil Nadu, India

Oral and Maxillofacial Surgery, Meenakshi Ammal Dental College and Hospital, Chennai, Tamil Nadu, India

M. Anthony (Tony) Pogrel Department of Oral and Maxillofacial Surgery, University of California, San Francisco, CA, USA

Vishal Bansal Department of Oral and Maxillofacial Surgery, Swami Vivekanand Subharti University, Meerut, Uttar Pradesh, India

Ajay Bhambal Department of Public Health Dentistry, People's College of Dental Sciences and Research Centre, People's University, Bhopal, Madhya Pradesh, India

Mimansa Bhoj Department of Oral and Maxillofacial Surgery, ITS CDSR, Muradnagar (Ghaziabad), Uttar Pradesh, India

Ramesh Chowdhary Branemark Osseointegration Centre, Bengaluru, Karnataka, India

Department of Prosthodontics, Rajarajeswari Dental College and Hospital, Bengaluru, Karnataka, India

Aashna Dhingra Nationwide Quality of Care Network (NQOCN), Delhi, India

George Dimitroulis Maxillofacial Surgery Unit, Department of Surgery, St. Vincent's Hospital Melbourne, The University of Melbourne, Melbourne, Australia

Epworth-Freemasons Hospital, East Melbourne, VIC, Australia

A. Einstein Oral Pathology and Microbiology, Thai Moogambigai Dental College and Hospital, Dr. MGR Educational and Research Institute, Chennai, Tamil Nadu, India

P. Elavenil Anantan Dental and Facial Surgery, Chennai, Tamil Nadu, India

Oral and Maxillofacial Surgery, SRM Dental College and Hospital (Ramapuram Campus), Chennai, Tamil Nadu, India

Suhani Ghai Dharamshila Narayana Superspeciality Hospital, New Delhi, India

Himanta Ghritlahare Oral Pathology and Microbiology, Government Dental College, Raipur, Chhattisgarh, India

Saloni Gupta Department of Oral and Maxillofacial Surgery, Swami Vivekanand Subharti University, Meerut, Uttar Pradesh, India

Preeti Gurjar Oral and Maxillofacial Surgery, TMJ Consultancy Services, Bhopal, Madhya Pradesh, India

Shoomali Hassan Oral Pathology and Microbiology, Bhabha College of Dental Sciences, Bhopal, Madhya Pradesh, India

Rahul Hegde D Y Patil College of Dental Sciences, Pune, Maharashtra, India

Prashant Prakash Jaju Oral Medicine and Radiology, Rishiraj College of Dental Sciences and Research Centre, Bhopal, Madhya Pradesh, India

Sushma Prashant Jaju Conservative Dentistry and Endodontics, Rishiraj College of Dental Sciences and Research Centre, Bhopal, Madhya Pradesh, India

S. Karthiga Kannan Oral Medicine and Radiology, Dental Education Department, College of Dentistry, Majmaah University, Al Majma'ah, Saudi Arabia

Ankit Kapoor Department of Oral and Maxillofacial Surgery, Swami Vivekanand Subharti University, Meerut, Uttar Pradesh, India

Ganesh Koneru Department of Oral and Maxillofacial Surgery, Sibar Institute of Dental Sciences, Guntur, Andhra Pradesh, India

Shail Kumari CHC, Kalyanpur, Kanpur, Uttar Pradesh, India

Vaishnavi Devi Majeti Department of Oral and Maxillofacial Surgery, Lenora Institute of Dental Sciences, Rajahmundry, Andhra Pradesh, India

R. Manikandhan Department of Oral and Maxillofacial Surgery, Meenakshi Ammal Dental College and Hospital, Chennai, Tamil Nadu, India

Craniofacial Surgery, Meenakshi Ammal Dental College and Hospital, Chennai, Tamil Nadu, India

Shubhangi Mhaske Oral Pathology and Microbiology, People's College of Dental Sciences and Research Centre, People's University, Bhopal, Madhya Pradesh, India

Louis G. Mercuri Department of Orthopaedic Surgery, Rush University Medical Center, Chicago, IL, USA

Sunil Kumar Mishra Department of Prosthodontics, Rama Dental College, Hospital and Research Centre, Kanpur, Uttar Pradesh, India

Kishore Moturi Department of Oral and Maxillofacial Surgery, Vishnu Dental College, Bhimavaram, Andhra Pradesh, India

R. S. Neelakandan Meenakshi Academy of Higher Education and Research (Meenakshi University), Chennai, Tamil Nadu, India

Department of Oral and Maxillofacial Surgery, Meenakshi Ammal Dental College and Hospital, Chennai, Tamil Nadu, India

Daniel Oren Oral and Maxillofacial Surgery, Oral Medicine and Dentistry Institute, Galilee Medical Center, Nahariya, Israel

The Azrieli Faculty of Medicine, Bar-Ilan University, Zefat, Israel

Abhay Kumar Pandey NCD, Sadar Hospital, Govt of Jharkhand, Ranchi, Jharkhand, India

Ankit Pandey Amrit Dental and TMJ Centre, Bhopal, Madhya Pradesh, India

Prateeksha Pawar Oral and Maxillofacial Surgery, TMJ Consultancy Services, Bhopal, Madhya Pradesh, India

Kanak Pushkarna Rishiraj College of Dental Sciences and Research Centre, Bhopal, Madhya Pradesh, India

Rahul Rochani Sparkle Dental Hub and Centre for Excellence in Orthodontics, Bhopal, Madhya Pradesh, India

M. Fatih Şentürk Oral and Maxillofacial Surgery, Ankara Yıldırım Beyazıt University Faculty of Dentistry, Ankara, Turkey

Ratna Sharma Department of Psychology, The Sanskaar Valley School, Bhopal, Madhya Pradesh, India

Yogesh Sharma Department of Dentistry, Netaji Subhash Chandra Bose Medical College, Jabalpur, Madhya Pradesh, India

Sudeep Shrivastava Fellow, OM Multispeciality Head and Neck Surgery Centre, Ahmedabad, Gujarat, India

Trilok Shrivastava Department of Orthodontics, People's College of Dental Sciences and Research Centre, People's University, Bhopal, Madhya Pradesh, India

Vankudoth Dal Singh Department of Oral and Maxillofacial Surgery, Lenora Institute of Dental Sciences, Rajahmundry, Andhra Pradesh, India

Beena Sivakumar Department of Oral and Maxillofacial Surgery, Meenakshi Ammal Dental College and Hospital, Chennai, Tamil Nadu, India

Surabhi Somkuwar Department of Dentistry, All India Institute of Medical Sciences, Raipur, Chhattisgarh, India

Samer Srouji Oral and Maxillofacial Surgery, Oral Medicine and Dentistry Institute, Galilee Medical Center, Nahariya, Israel

Galilee College of Dental Sciences, Galilee Medical Center, Nahariya, Israel

The Azrieli Faculty of Medicine, Bar-Ilan University, Zefat, Israel

Bone Regeneration Lab, Galilee Medical Center, Nahariya, Israel

Shaji Thomas Department of Oral and Maxillofacial Surgery, People's College of Dental Sciences and Research Centre, People's University, Bhopal, Madhya Pradesh, India

Parimala Tyagi Department of Pediatric Dentistry, People's College of Dental Sciences and Research Centre, Bhopal, Madhya Pradesh, India

About the Editor

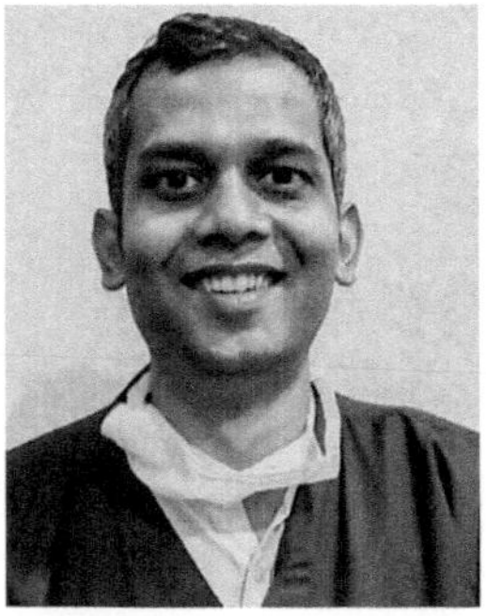

Dr. Darpan Bhargava has completed his bachelors and masters of dental surgery (Oral and Maxillofacial Surgery) from Meenakshi Ammal Dental College and Hospital, Chennai. He was a distinction holder and a gold medalist from The Tamil Nadu Dr. MGR Medical University (Undergraduation) and Meenakshi Academy of Higher Education and Research, Chennai (Post-graduation). He has successfully completed the Diploma of Membership in Oral and Maxillofacial Surgery from the Royal College of Physicians and Surgeons, Glasgow. He holds postgraduate diploma in Hospital Management and Clinical Research. He is credited with the introduction of twin-mix nerve blocks for mandibular anaesthesia. Currently, he is serving as an associate professor and a clinical consultant in the Department of Oral and Maxillofacial Surgery at People's College of Dental Sciences and Research Centre, People's University, Bhopal, Madhya Pradesh, India. He has over 80 national and international scientific publications to his credit. He holds first ever Indian patent and a copyrighted surgical technique for the temporomandibular joint prosthesis. He has been awarded Ph.D. from Meenakshi University, Chennai for his acclaimed research on "Predictability and Feasibility of Total Alloplastic Temporomandibular Joint Reconstruction Using DARSN TM Joint Prosthesis for Patients in Indian subcontinent".

Temporomandibular Joint from the Pyramids to Total Joint Replacement and Beyond

1

Louis G. Mercuri

Medicine, like all knowledge, has a past as well as a present and a future...in that past is the indispensable soil out of which improvement must grow.

Alfred Stille, 1813–1900

Those who cannot remember the past are condemned to repeat it

George Santayana, 1863–1952

The nonsurgical and surgical management of painful temporomandibular joint (TMJ) disorders has evolved over the centuries. Unfortunately, etiologic sophisms and often unproven mechanistic treatment philosophies still survive. Reviewing the history of the management of TMJ disorders not only addresses the complexity of the problem, but also demonstrates the importance of being aware of the prior pitfalls so that as the science of diagnosis and management unfold, we as clinicians and researchers do not continue to fall into or repeat the shortcomings of the past in the future.

Writings dating from the ancient Egyptians, Hippocrates, Vesalius described reduction of the dislocated mandible [1].Thereafter, surgery dominated the earliest management of TMJ disorders. The earliest report involved the concept of *internal derangement* of the TMJ articular disc. This mechanical concept was first described relative to the TMJ disc in 1826 by Astley Paston Cooper [2].Then, in 1887, Thomas Annandale discussed internal derangement of the TMJ and reported the repair of a torn TMJ disc with horse hair in a woman with persistent TMJ pain [3]. In subsequent decades, reports followed related to the use of discectomy in the management of displaced TMJ discs [4–6].However, inclusion and exclusion criteria, standards for successful outcomes, and follow-up were not reported.

Mid-twentieth century, reports surfaced concerning the use of discectomy to manage the anteriorly dislocated TMJ disc associated with degenerative joint disease [7–9].In 1951, Ireland [10] discussed the use of condylectomy to treat anterior dislocation of the disc; and in 1957, Henny and Baldridge [11] presented a series of cases in which arthroplasty was used to treat painful TMJ dysfunction.

Temporomandibular joint surgery lost popularity in the 1960s as clinicians turned to nonsurgical options for the management of TMJ disorders. Surgery was relegated to clinical and

L. G. Mercuri (✉)
Department of Orthopaedic Surgery, Rush University Medical Center, Chicago, IL, USA
e-mail: louis_g_mercuri@rush.edu

D. Bhargava (ed.), *Temporomandibular Joint Disorders*,
https://doi.org/10.1007/978-981-16-2754-5_1

radiographically obvious pathology, such as ankylosis and neoplasia.

The move toward nonsurgical management has been linked to another mechanically based theory. Costen [12] resurrected the old notion that tooth loss resulted in posterior and superior displacement of the mandibular condyle with resultant impingement of the condyle on the auditory canal causing pain in both the TMJ and the ear [13–17]. This concept was anatomically discredited by Sicher [18] and Zimmerman [19].

With the discrediting of Costen's mandibular overclosure theory, hypotheses related to occlusal disharmony and malocclusion arose and became influential. These mechanically oriented, gnathological theories suggested that during mandibular closure occlusal interferences cause mandibular condyle displacement leading to pressure on the highly innervated, vascular retrodiscal TMJ tissue resulting in pain and bony degeneration due to loss of blood supply to joint structures [20–23]. It has since been well-documented that there is an absence of a disease-specific association between malocclusion and TMJ disorders. Therefore, presently there are no grounds for further hypothesizing the role of dental occlusion or malocclusion in the pathophysiology of TMJ disorders. Clinicians are encouraged to abandon this old gnathological paradigm [24].

Schwartz [1] was the first to demonstrate that masticatory muscle tension patterns could be seen in a majority of patients with TMJ pain tested. He related this muscle tension to emotional stress and suggested the term "Temporomandibular joint Pain-Dysfunction Syndrome." Then Laskin, based on extensive clinical and laboratory research, formulated the Myofascial Pain-Dysfunction (MPD) Syndrome theory which like Schwartz stressed emotional rather than mechanical factors leading to masticatory muscle pain and TMJ dysfunction [25].

Over the following decades, the field underwent many taxonomic and conceptual changes. Currently the most popular theories regarding the nonsurgical management of muscle related TMJ pain are based on the biopsychosocial model, which involves a combination of biological, psychological, and social factors [26, 27]. As a result, domains related to orthopedic principles, neurophysiological aspects of pain, neuroanatomic regions of pain processing, molecular, genetic, and cellular pathophysiology of muscle and joints and behavioral aspects of chronic pain are presently being investigated [28].

In the early 1970s, despite the successful management of many muscle related TMJ pain and dysfunction patients using the tenets of the biopsychosocial model, there remained a group of intractable chronic TMJ pain patients. Farrar and Wilkes rediscovered and resurrected the concept of *internal derangement*. They related chronic TMJ pain, headache, ear pain, and mandibular dysfunction, along with other craniofacial pains, to an uncoordinated function of the disc, condyle, articular eminence, and superior head of the lateral pterygoid muscle. Armed with this concept, surgeons started managing chronic TMJ pain and dysfunction as internal derangement which involved open TMJ surgery disc repositioning [29–33] or discectomy [34].

Arthroscopy, and later arthrocentesis, emerged as bridges between nonsurgical [35] and surgical management of TMJ internal derangement. Ohnishi and Murakami were the first to apply arthroscopying patients with internal derangement and arthrosis [36, 37]. Holmlund and Hellsing [38], McCain [39] and Sanders [40] provided studies related to TMJ arthroscopic lysis and lavage. Yang [41] and McCain [42] developed arthroscopic TMJ disc repositioning procedures.

TMJ arthroscopy and magnetic resonance imaging (MRI) [43] provided much more detailed information about not only the disc, but also the pathobiology of TMJ disorders in general as well as paving the way for minimally invasive TMJ arthrocentesis [44].

In 1982 the United States Food and Drug Administration (FDA) authorized the sale of the Proplast-Teflon Interpositional TMJ Implant and total TMJ implants by Vitek, Inc. (Houston, TX) [45].After implantation with these devices, many patients presented with irreversible and life altering signs and symptoms. Reports surfaced that both were causally related to the hard and soft tissue damage created by failure of the Proplast-Teflon TMJ devices and the foreign body giant cell reaction that developed. Therefore, in January 1991, the FDA ordered Vitek to remove its implants from the market [46].

Since Proplast Teflon caused so much bony destruction and consequent significant glenoid fossa architectural variation from the normal, it was extremely difficult to align properly and stabilize the available stock TMJ replacement device [47] components to reconstruct those patients. This led to the development of a computer assisted design/computer assisted manufactured (CAD/CAM) custom patient fitted total TMJ replacement device in 1989 to directly deal with these anatomical discrepancies and issues of device component and fixation long-term stability.

In 1990, Mercuri and Techmedica (Camarillo, CA) developed a prospective multicenter CAD/CAM custom patient fitted total TMJ replacement device clinical trials study [48]. Using mechanical and clinical outcomes data from that publication, in 1999 the TMJ Concepts (Ventura, CA) Patient Fitted TMJ Reconstruction Prosthesis was FDA approved as safe and effective for implantation.

From 1995 to 2005, a clinical trial was conducted by Zimmer Biomet (Jacksonville, FL) using the stock Biomet Microfixation Walter Lorenz Total TMJ Replacement System developed in consultation with Quinn [49]. This device was FDA approved in 2005 for implantation.

Long-term follow-up data for both these devices [50, 51] has demonstrated safety and effectiveness for the management of end-stage TMJ disease [52].

Ellege et al. [53] reported that 15 countries have since developed, or are in the process of developing, 27 TMJ replacement systems. 21 are custom designed and some are 3D printed. The authors found that at publication all of the TMJ systems they found were not equal in terms of design, material composition, preclinical laboratory testing, manufacturing methods, regulatory status, and reporting of clinical outcomes. Those important elements varied widely among the emerging systems. All of these are important issues that must be addressed in the future to assure these merging TMJ replacement devices are truly safe and effective.

Polley et al. [54] concluded that utilization of extended alloplastic TMJ and mandibular replacement in severe grades of craniofacial anomaly patients demonstrated consistently excellent functional and esthetic results in a series of skeletally mature patients. Therefore, the authors felt that these devices offered the best solution for salvage of craniofacial anomaly patients who have had failed autogenous reconstructions.

Hawkins et al. [55] demonstrated that 95% of experienced TMJ surgeons surveyed preferred alloplastic TMJ replacement to autogenous costochondral grafting because of fewer postoperative complications and more predictable outcomes.

In light of increased utilization of extended alloplastic TMJ and mandibular replacements, to assure meaningful clinical outcomes reporting and analysis, Ellege et al. have proposed a classification system [56].

In conclusion, in the pursuit of understanding the etiology, pathophysiology and management of muscle related extra-articular and joint pathology related intra-articular TMJ disorders will be improved as long as both basic science and clinical researchers pursue scientific methodology and evidence-based management founded on well-documented orthopedic joint related principles, rather than the sophisms and mechanical schemes of the past.

Among the many questions future TMJ researchers and clinicians must ponder are: What part does a patient's genetic profile play in TMJ pain and dysfunction? Its etiology, pathophysiology, and management? Are there synovial biomarkers that are indicative of TMJ pathology? Will improved joint replacement device designs and materials improve their performance and longevity?

> The arrogance of success is to think that what you did yesterday will be sufficient for tomorrow.
> C. William Pollard

References

1. Schwartz LL. Disorders of the temporomandibular joint. Philadelphia: WB Saunders; 1959.
2. Ashhurst J Jr, editor. The international encyclopedia of surgery. New York: William Wood and Company; 1889.
3. Annandale T. On displacement of the intra-articular cartilage of the lower jaw and its treatment by operation. Lancet. 1887;1:411–2.
4. Lanz W. Discitis Mandibularis. Zentralbl Chir. 1901;36:289–90.
5. Pringle J. Displacement of the mandibular meniscus and its treatment. Br J Surg. 1918;6:385–92.
6. Wakeley C. The causation and treatment of displaced mandibular cartilage. Lancet. 1929;2:543–4.
7. Dingman RO, Moorman WC. Meniscectomy in treatment of lesions of the temporomandibular joint. J Oral Surg. 1951;9:214–20.
8. Kiehn CTL. Meniscectomy for internal derangement of the temporomandibular joint. Am J Surg. 1952;83:364–8.
9. Silver CM, Simon SD. Meniscus injuries of the temporomandibular joint. J Bone Surg. 1956;38-A:541–52.
10. Ireland VE. The problem of the clicking jaw. Proc R Soc Med. 1951;44:363–72.
11. Henny FA, Baldridge OL. Condylectomy for the persistently painful temporomandibular joint. J Oral Surg. 1957;15:24–9.
12. Costen JB. Syndrome of ear and sinus symptoms dependent upon disturbed function of the temporomandibular joint. Ann Otol Rhinol and Laryngol. 1934;43:1–15.
13. Prentiss HJ. A preliminary report upon the temporomandibular joint articulation in the human types. Dent Cosmos. 1918;60:505–14.
14. Monson GS. Occlusion applied to crown and bridgework. J Nat Dent Assoc. 1920;7:399–413.
15. Wright WH. Deafness as influenced by malposition of the jaws. J Nat Dent Assoc. 1920;7:979–90.
16. Decker JC. Traumatic deafness as the result of retrusion of the condyles of the mandible. Ann Otol Rhinol and Laryngol. 1925;34:519–27.
17. Goodfriend DJ. Symptomatology and treatment of abnormalities of the mandibular articulation. Dent Cosmos. 1933;75:844–52.
18. Sicher H. Temporomandibular joint articulation in mandibular overclosure. JADA. 1948;36:131–9.
19. Zimmerman AA. An evaluation of Costen's syndrome from a dynamic point of view. In: Sarnat BG, editor. The temporomandibular joint. Springfield, IL: Charles C. Thomas Company; 1951. p. 82–110.
20. Christensen G. The modern concept of disturbances of the temporomandibular joint. Austral Dent J. 1956;1:249–57.
21. Davidson AS. Hemodynamic theory of pain production in temporomandibular joint syndrome. J Oral Surg Anes and Hosp Dent Serv. 1964;22:135–8.
22. Granger ER. Occlusion in temporomandibular joint pain. JADA. 1958;56:659–64.
23. Hankey GT. Temporomandibular joint arthrosis. Analysis of 150 cases. Br Dent J. 1954;97:249–70.
24. Manfredini D, et al. Temporomandibular disorders, and dental occlusion. A systematic review of association studies: end of an era? J Oral Rehabil. 2017;44:908–23.
25. Laskin DM. Etiology of the pain dysfunction syndrome. JADA. 1969;79:147–53.
26. Dworkin SF, Massoth DL. Temporomandibular disorders and chronic pain: disease or illness? J Prosthet Dent. 1994;72:29–38.
27. Engel GL. The need for a new medical model: a challenge for biomedicine. Science. 1977;196:129–36.
28. Maixner W, Diatchenko L, Dubner R, Fillingim RB, Greenspan JD, Knott C, Ohrbach R, Weir B, Slade GD. Orofacial pain prospective evaluation and risk assessment study--the OPPERA study. J Pain. 2011;12(11 Suppl):T4–11.e1-2.
29. Farrar W. Differentiation of Temporomandibular.Joint dysfunction to simplify treatment. J Prosthet Dent. 1972;28:629–34.
30. Farrar W. Characteristics of condylar path in internal derangements of the TMJ. J Prosthet Dent. 1978;39:319–23.
31. Wilkes CH. Structural and functional alterations of the temporomandibular joint. NW Dent. 1978;57:287–94.
32. Wilkes CH. Arthrography of the temporomandibular joint. Minn Med. 1978;67:645–52.
33. Mehra P, Wolford LM. The Mitek mini anchor for TMJ disc repositioning: surgical technique and results. Int J Oral Maxillofac Surg. 2001;30:497–503.
34. Miloro M, McKnight M, Han MD, Markiewicz MR. Discectomy without replacement improves function in patients with internal derangement of the temporomandibular joint. J Craniomaxillofac Surg. 2017;45:1425–31.
35. Indresano A, Alpha C. Nonsurgical management of temporomandibular joint disorders. In: Fonseca RJ, Marciani RD, Turvey TA, editors. Oral and maxillofacial surgery. 2nd ed. St. Louis, MO: Saunders/Elsevier; 2009. p. 881–97.
36. Ohnishi M. Arthroscopy of the temporomandibular joint. J Jpn Stomatol Soc. 1975;42:207–13.
37. Murakami K, Matsuki M, Iizuka T. Diagnostic arthroscopy of the TMJ: differential diagnoses in patients with limited jaw opening. J Craniomandib Pract. 1986;4:118–23.
38. Hellsing G, Holmlund A, Nordenram A. Arthroscopy of the temporomandibular joint. Examination of 2 patients with suspected disk derangement. Int J Oral Surg. 1984;13:69–74.
39. McCain JP. Arthroscopy of the human temporomandibular joint. J Oral Maxillofac Surg. 1988;46:648–55.
40. Sanders B. Arthroscopic surgery of the temporomandibular joint: treatment of internal derangement with persistent closed lock. Oral Surg Oral Med Oral Pathol Oral Radiol Endod. 1986;62:361–72.

41. Yang C, Cai XY, Chen MJ, Zhang SY. New arthroscopic disc repositioning and suturing technique for treating an anteriorly displaced disc of the temporomandibular joint: part I—technique introduction. Int J Oral Maxillofac Surg. 2012;41:1058–63.
42. McCain J, Hossameldin RH, Srouji S, Maher A. Arthroscopic Discopexy is effective in managing temporomandibular joint internal derangement in patients with Wilkes Stage II and III. J Oral Maxillofac Surg. 2015;73:391–401.
43. Katzberg RW, Bessette RW, Tallents RH, Plewes DB, Manzione JV, Schenck JF, Foster TH, Hart HR. Normal and abnormal temporomandibular joint: MR imaging with surface coil. Radiology. 1986;1581:183–9.
44. Nitzan DW, Dolwick MF, Martinez GA. Temporomandibular joint arthrocentesis: a simplified treatment for severe, limited mouth opening. J Oral Maxillofac Surg. 1991;49:1163–7.
45. Grushka K. Propast-Teflon jaw implants and FDA review standards for medical device: a case study. Food and Drug Law Fall. 2006;5:1–27.
46. Mercuri LG. History of TMJ TJR. In: Mercuri LG, editor. Temporomandibular joint Total joint replacement – TMJ TJR – a comprehensive reference for researchers, material scientists and surgeons. New York: Springer; 2016. p. 44–52.
47. Christensen RW. Arthroplastic implantation of the TMJ. In: Oral Implantology. Springfield, IL: Charles C. Thomas; 1970. p. 284–98.
48. Mercuri LG, Sanders B, White RD, Wolford LR, Hurder A, Henderson W. Custom CAD/CAM Total temporomandibular joint reconstruction system: preliminary multicenter report. J Oral Maxillofac Surg. 1995;53:106–15.
49. Quinn PD. Lorenz Prosthesis. In: Donlon WC, editor. Oral and maxillofacial surgery clinics of North America. Total temporomandibular joint reconstruction. Philadelphia: Saunders; 2009. p. 93–104.
50. Wolford LM, Mercuri LG, Schneiderman ED, Movahed R, Allen W. Twenty-year follow-up study on a patient-fitted temporomandibular joint prosthesis: the Techmedica/TMJ concepts device. J Oral Maxillofac Surg. 2015;73:952–60.
51. Giannakopoulos HE, Sinn DP, Quinn PD. Biomet microfixation temporomandibular joint replacement system: a 3-year follow-up study of patients treated during 1995 to 2005. J Oral Maxillofac Surg. 2012;70:787–94.
52. Mercuri LG, End-Stage TMD. TMJ reconstruction. In: Miloro M, Ghali G, Larsen P, Waite P, editors. Peterson's principles of oral & maxillofacial surgery. 3rd ed. Shelton, CT: PMPH, USA Ltd.; 2012. p. 1173–86.
53. Ellege ROC, Mercuri LG, Attard A, Green J, Speculand B. Review of emerging temporomandibular joint total joint replacement systems. Br J Oral Maxillofac Surg. 2019;57:722–8.
54. Polley JW, Girotto JA, Fahrenkopf MP, Dietze-Fiedler ML, Kelley JP, Taylor JC, Lazarou SA, Demetriades NC. Salvage or solution: alloplastic reconstruction in Hemifacial Microsomia. Cleft Palate Craniofac J. 2019;56:896–901.
55. Hawkins A, Mercuri LG, Miloro M. Are rib grafts still used for temporomandibular joint reconstruction? J Oral Maxillofac Surg. 2020;78:195–202.
56. Elledge R, Mercuri LG, Speculand B. Extended total temporomandibular joint replacements: a classification system. Br J Oral Maxillofac Surg. 2018;56:578–81.

2 Importance of Identification of Temporomandibular Joint Disorders and Appropriate Referral

R. S. Neelakandan and Darpan Bhargava

Temporomandibular joint (TMJ) is a unique joint having a fibrous avascular disc. It is a diarthrodial ginglymoid joint having an articular surface which includes two distinct condyles of the mandibular bone fitting into reciprocally concave surfaces in the temporal bone just in front of the ear. They permit movement both in transverse axis and a vertical axis. Bilateral joints work synchronously with the dentition and occlusal loading along with the various masticatory muscles together contributing to the healthy stomatognathic system. Any interference in one of the components of this system can adversely affect the TMJ. The peculiarities of the temporomandibular joint are summarized in Table 2.1.

Table 2.1 Peculiarities of the temporomandibular joint

1. Acts as a growth centre and demonstrates structural changes in the joint per se with age.
2. It has bilateral synovial articulation between the mandible and temporal bone which work in synchrony.
3. Ginglymoarthrodial joint—Only joint in the body that has rotation and translatory movements.
4. Presence of an avascular intervening disc.
5. The fibrocartilaginous disc is dynamic with its movements controlled by lateral pterygoid muscle on joint movement.
6. TMJ is influenced by the stomatognathic system (occlusion, surrounding muscles) and requires harmony for its function.
7. Important joint for vital functions like speech, mastication.
8. Local surgical anatomy for surgical access to the TMJ involves vital structures like facial nerve, which require special training in order to perform open joint surgeries.
9. Harmony in function between the intervening disc, osseous joint, and the muscles controlling the movement.

Temporomandibular disorders (TMDs) can often be confused with oro-facial pain of varied origin, otalgic pain or pain originating from the cervical region as the joint is closely associated with these anatomic structures. The clinicians may face difficulty at times in diagnosing TMDs. Patients present with wide range of symptoms such as pain while chewing, pain in the ear or in front of the ear, or with nonspecific referred pain to the forehead and the neck. Most patients report to the general physicians or the dentists, some of them may further be referred to an otolaryngologist or an ear nose throat (ENT) specialist without an appropriate recognition of the TMD. Few

R. S. Neelakandan
Meenakshi Academy of Higher Education and Research (Meenakshi University), Chennai, Tamil Nadu, India

Department of Oral and Maxillofacial Surgery, Meenakshi Ammal Dental College and Hospital, Chennai, Tamil Nadu, India

D. Bhargava (✉)
TMJ Consultancy Services, Bhopal, Madhya Pradesh, India

Oral and Maxillofacial Surgery, People's College of Dental Sciences and Research Centre, People's University, Bhopal, Madhya Pradesh, India
e-mail: drdarpanbhargava@gmail.com

D. Bhargava (ed.), *Temporomandibular Joint Disorders*,
https://doi.org/10.1007/978-981-16-2754-5_2

patients consult with an orthopaedic specialist considering the fact that a recognized problem is present in the joint and a neurologist may come into play when there is a referred pain on the face from the joint.

Most treating clinicians may not be involved in treating the problems of the temporomandibular joint routinely and may find it difficult to diagnose and treat temporomandibular disorders with precision. The fact that the medical or dental graduates and specialists are less aware about the various treatments performed by a specialist trained to treat TMDs, is in itself a proof that they refer such cases with pain in the ear or in the preauricular region directly to an otolaryngologist without considering a potential possibility of a TMD.

It is essential for a clinician dealing with the TMJ and its disorders to understand the influence of the para-functional habits, status of the dentition and influence of the muscles associated with the TMJ. Understanding the synchrony of the joint movement with the other components of the stomatognathic system along with the balance in the joint movement and movement of the disc, is also vital. Any interference in one of the above-mentioned components can significantly affect the form and function of the temporomandibular joint. An appropriate training and experience is mandated to deal with the problems associated with this joint [1, 2].

This book gives a detailed insight into the various temporomandibular joint disorders, clinical and radiographic evaluation methods and management of various conditions affecting the joint. This is a complete book proving a detailed practically achievable clinical care required for the patients diagnosed with TMDs.

References

1. Dimitroulis G. Temporomandibular disorders: a clinical update. BMJ. 1998;317(7152):190–4.
2. Dimitroulis G. Management of temporomandibular joint disorders: a surgeon's perspective. Aust Dent J. 2018;63(Suppl 1):S79–90.

Anatomy and Basic Biomechanics of the Temporomandibular Joint

3

Darpan Bhargava and Preeti Gurjar

3.1 Introduction

The anatomy of the temporomandibular joint (TMJ) is an inimitable considering it has a complex structural architecture with its associated muscles, cartilage, ligaments, vessels and the neural supply to the joint.

3.2 Embryology of Temporomandibular Joint

Jaw joint is derived from the first pharyngeal arch developing as a primitive joint inside the Merkel's cartilage to perform the jaw movements which are noted at eighth week post-conception, much before the definitive development of the TMJ. The pharyngeal arch consists of mesoderm forming the muscles and vessels. The mesenchyme derived from neural crest cells contributes to the development of bone and cartilage. Definitive TMJ develops secondarily on evolutionary as well as embryological basis as an entirely new and separate mechanism in three stages summarized in Table 3.1. Development of the TMJ differs from other synovial joints, as initial cavity for other synovial joints is completed by seventh week post-conception during which the TMJ does not even exist. It develops between temporal blastema which arises from the otic capsule and the condylar blastema arising from the secondary condylar cartilage of the mandible which grows towards each other. Ossification begins first in the

Table 3.1 Stages involved in the formation of definitive TMJ

Stage	Stage nomenclature	Features
I	Blastemic stage	Around seventh week, formation of glenoid fossa and condylar blastema
II	Cavitation stage	Between ninth to tenth weeks, the lower joint space begins to appear. The blastemis initiate to differentiate into multiple layers forming lower synovial layer which is the future joint disc
III	Maturation stage	Beginning of upper joint space formation at around 11th week of gestation Formation of joint capsules is at around 17 weeks Around 19 to 20 weeks the development of the cartilage inside the capsule can be recognized TMJ continues to develop until and after the baby is born

D. Bhargava (✉)
TMJ Consultancy Services,
Bhopal, Madhya Pradesh, India

Oral and Maxillofacial Surgery, People's College of Dental Sciences and Research Centre,
People's University, Bhopal, Madhya Pradesh, India
e-mail: drdarpanbhargava@gmail.com

P. Gurjar
Oral and Maxillofacial Surgery, TMJ Consultancy Services, Bhopal, Madhya Pradesh, India

D. Bhargava (ed.), *Temporomandibular Joint Disorders*,
https://doi.org/10.1007/978-981-16-2754-5_3

temporal blastema. Fibrous cartilage develops on the articular surface rather than a hyaline cartilage. Meckel's cartilage plays no role in definitive TMJ development (Table 3.2). The morphology of the condyle and the glenoid fossa is influenced by several mechanical forces from the surrounding musculature, effects from the teeth and chewing. At birth, child has a flatter glenoid fossa and a loose capsule with absence of cartilage; instead, a fibrous connective tissue will be present. As the child grows, between 5 and 10 years of age, the condyles develop in a posterior, lateral and upward direction proceeding to form a morphologically and histologically adult joint architecture (Fig. 3.1) [1, 2].

3.3 Anatomy of TMJ

TMJ is a bi-condylar, synovial, diarthrodial joint which functions synchronously. It is classified as ginglymus or ginglymoarthrodial joint as it performs both hinge and sliding movements (Table 3.3) (Figs. 3.2, 3.3, and 3.4). This joint forms an articulation between the mandibular condyle inferiorly and the fossa in the temporal bone superiorly. The articular surface is lined by fibrocartilage/white fibrous tissue and not hyaline cartilage unlike most other joints of the body (Figs. 3.5 and 3.6).

Table 3.2 Events in development of TMJ and its surrounding structures

Development in week(s) post-conception	Embryonic development
6th week	First appearance of membranous bone formation lateral to Meckel's cartilage which forms the initial mandibular body and ramus
6th to 7th week	First sign of the temporal muscle primordium
7 and half weeks	• Appearance of a biconcave articular disc suggestive of genetic determination and not by functional shaping • It is sub-divided into superior, intermediate and inferior laminae • The disc is continuous ventrally with the tendon of lateral pterygoid • The dorsal aspect sub-divides its attachments into the superior lamina which follows the outline of squamous temporal bone, inserts in the region of the petro-squamous fissure • Intermediate lamina continues into the middle ear through the petrotympanic fissure where it inserts into the malleus and anterior ligament of malleus (disco-malleolar ligament) • Inferior lamina curves caudally and inserts into the dorsal aspect of the mandibular condyle.
8th weeks	• Development of lateral pterygoid muscle medial to the future condylar area. • Development of masseter muscle
10th week	• Development of two clefts form the two joint cavities and thereby defining the intervening articular disc • Mesenchyme between the superior and inferior TMJ spaces condenses to the TMJ disc • The inferior compartment forms first, separating the future disc from the developing condyle • At this stage, there is first appearance of condylar cartilage • Identification of upper/lower parts of lateral pterygoid muscle
11th week	• Appearance of joint capsule made up of fibrous tissue forms the lateral TMJ ligament.
11 and half weeks	• Initial appearance of the upper joint compartment • Cavitation is caused by degradation rather than by enzymic liquefaction/cell death
Requisites for joint cavitations (at 11 and a half weeks)	1. *Synovial-membrane invasion* • Synovial fluid production lubricates movements in the joint 2. *Muscle movement* • Connective tissues separating the discrete small spaces should be ruptured for the spaces to coalesce forming the functional cavities • Functional pressures add to the contouring of the articulating surfaces
10th to 12th week	• Accessory condylar cartilage develops as initial blastema • The temporal articular fossa progressively assumes its definitive concave shape • The initially wide intervening mesenchyme is narrowed by condylar growth and differentiates into layers of fibrous tissue
By 12th week	• Endochondral ossification and cartilaginous growth

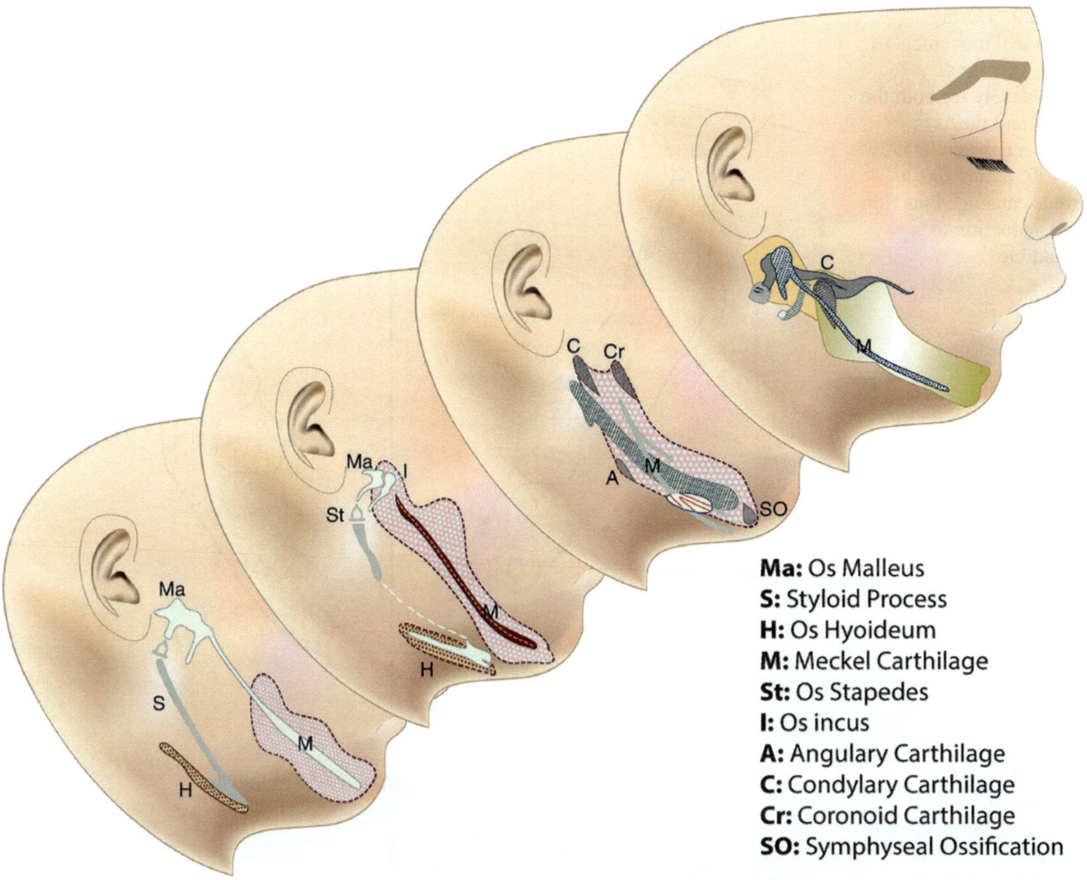

Fig. 3.1 Lateral view of the head and face of embryologic development stages. [Reprinted/adapted by permission from I. Rozylo-Kalinowska, K. Orhan (eds.), Imaging of the Temporomandibular Joint, https://doi.org/10.1007/978-3-319-99468-0_3]

Table 3.3 Classification of the temporomandibular joint

Anatomically	Functionally
Diarthrodial joint (discontinuous articulation of two bones permitting freedom of movement that is dictated by the associated muscles and limited by the ligaments)	Compound joint (composed of four articulating surfaces: the articular facets of the temporal bone and of the mandibular condyle and the superior and inferior surfaces of the articular disc)

3.4 Articular (Bone) Surfaces

1. Mandibular fossa (glenoid fossa) is a depression in the squamous part of the temporal bone with its anterior limit defined by the articular tubercle (eminence). Posteriorly, external auditory canal lies just behind the mandibular fossa. (Fig. 3.5)
2. Head of the mandibular condyle when viewed from above is roughly ovoid in outline. It is 15 to 20 mm from side to side (width) and 8 to 10 mm from front to back (anteroposterior) with the fact that a great variation is seen in the size and shape [3, 4]. (Figs. 3.2 and 3.5)

The articular disc divides the jaw joint into two compartments, superior and inferior joint space. The superior/upper compartment allows sliding or translatory motion and is called arthro-

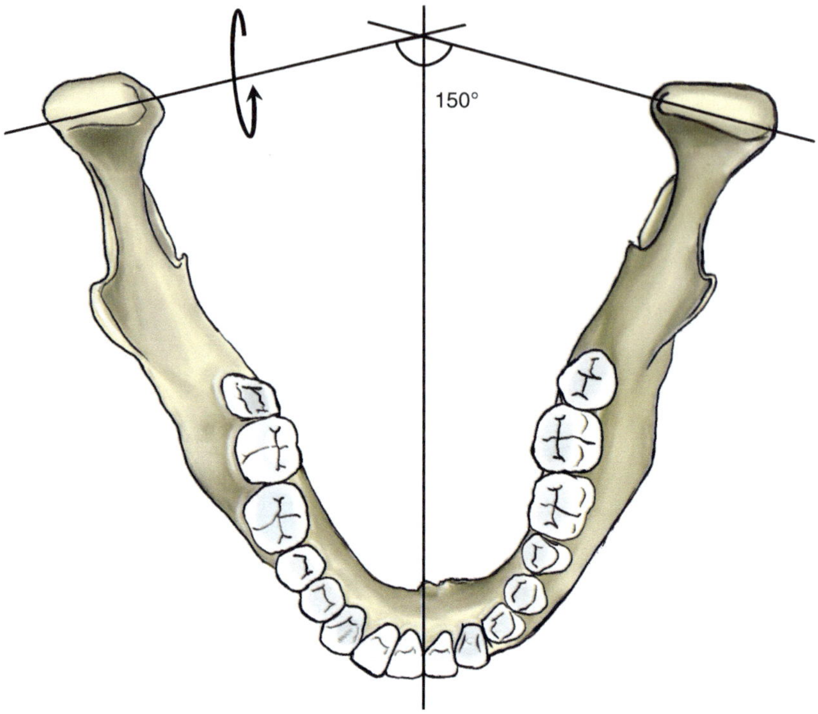

Fig. 3.2 During rotational movement of TMJ, axis runs transversely for both the joints and the axes intersect approximately at 150° acting like a hinge causing abduction and adduction of mandible

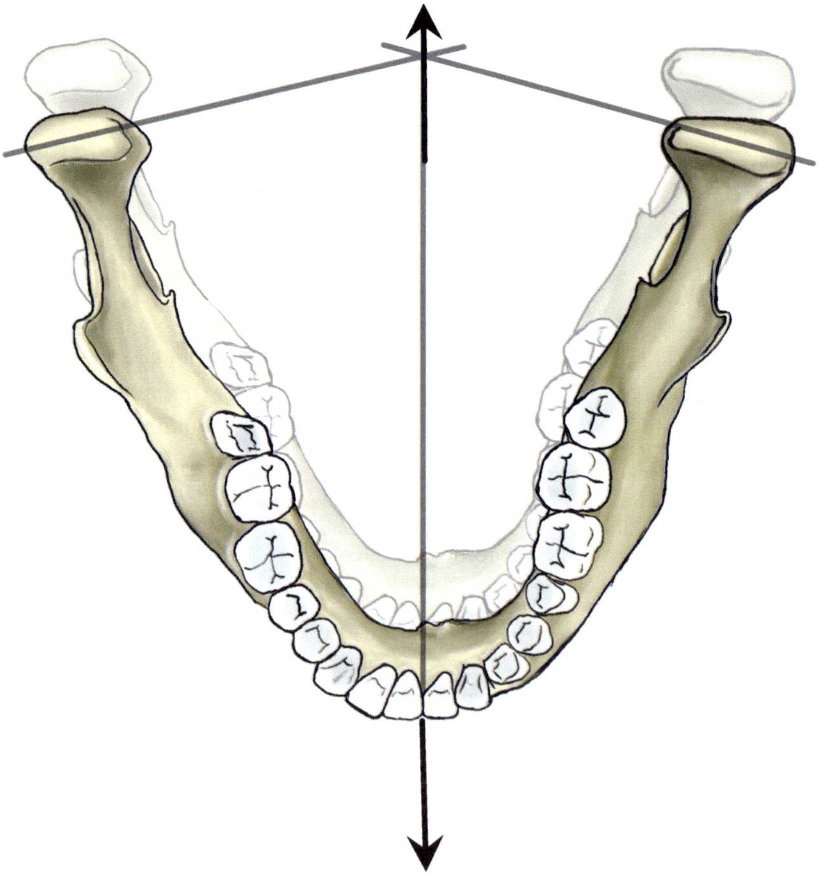

Fig. 3.3 During translation, there is simultaneous protrusion and retrusion of the mandible where the axes are parallel to the median axis via the mid-point of mandible

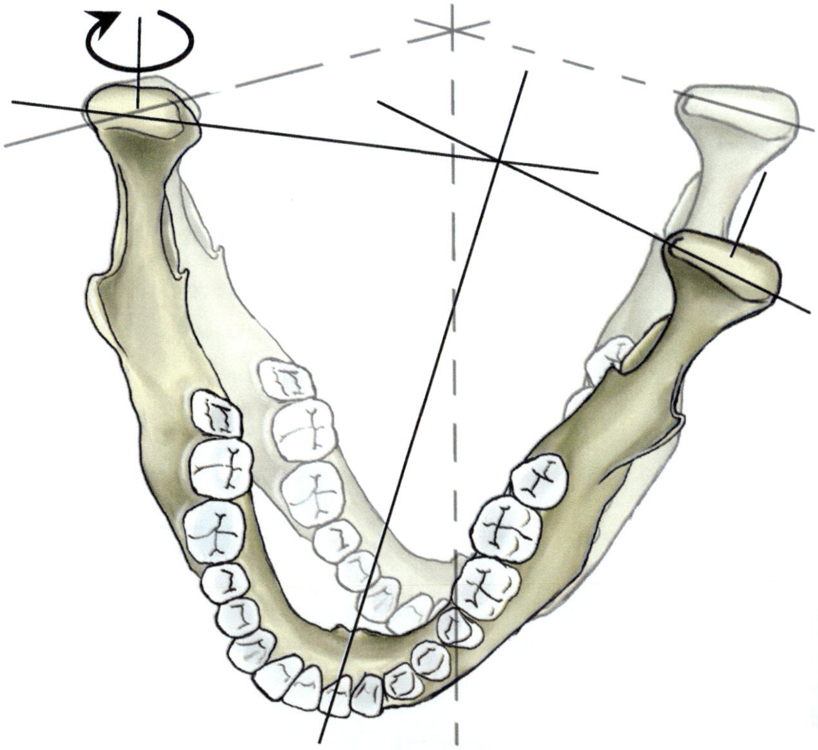

Fig. 3.4 Grinding movement of the right TMJ (which is the working side as shown in this figure) where the condyle rotates on a vertical axis during which the contralateral joint moves forward and inward

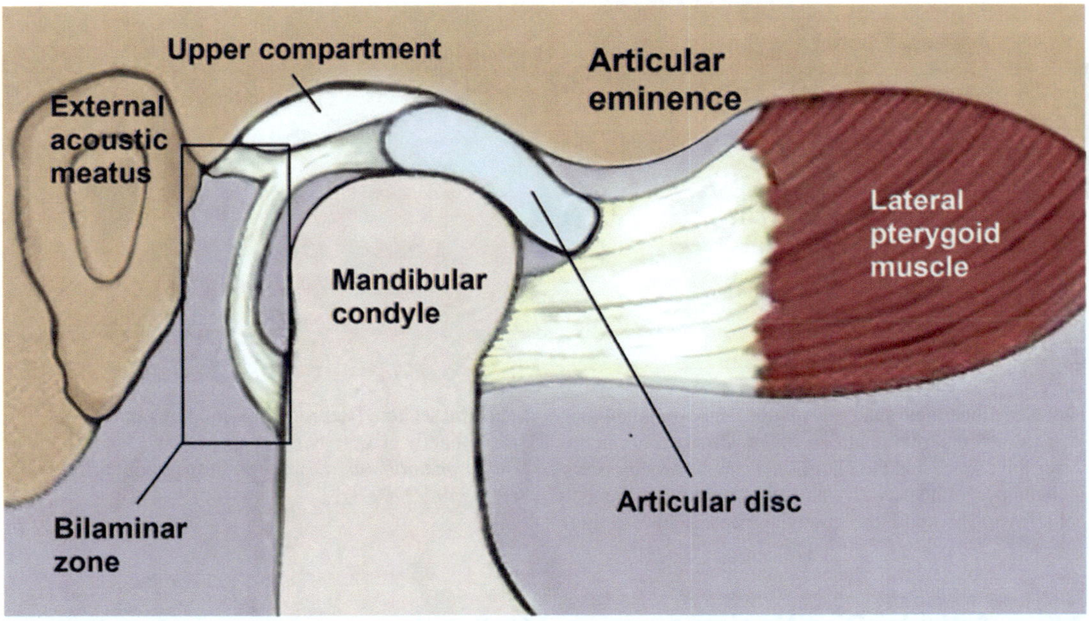

Fig. 3.5 Anatomy of the temporomandibular joint with the jaw closed. [Reprinted by permission from Slusarenko da Silva Y, Borba AM, Naclério-Homem MDG. A clinical-based protocol of diagnosis of temporomandibular joint open lock and treatment with arthrocentesis. Oral Maxillofac Surg. 2020 Jun;24(2):211–215. https://doi.org/10.1007/s10006-020-00844-9]

dial. The inferior/lower compartment allows hinge movement or rotation and is therefore termed ginglymoid. Therefore, the craniomandibular joint is classified as ginglymoarthrodial joint with both rotation and translatory movements in the same joint, bilaterally.

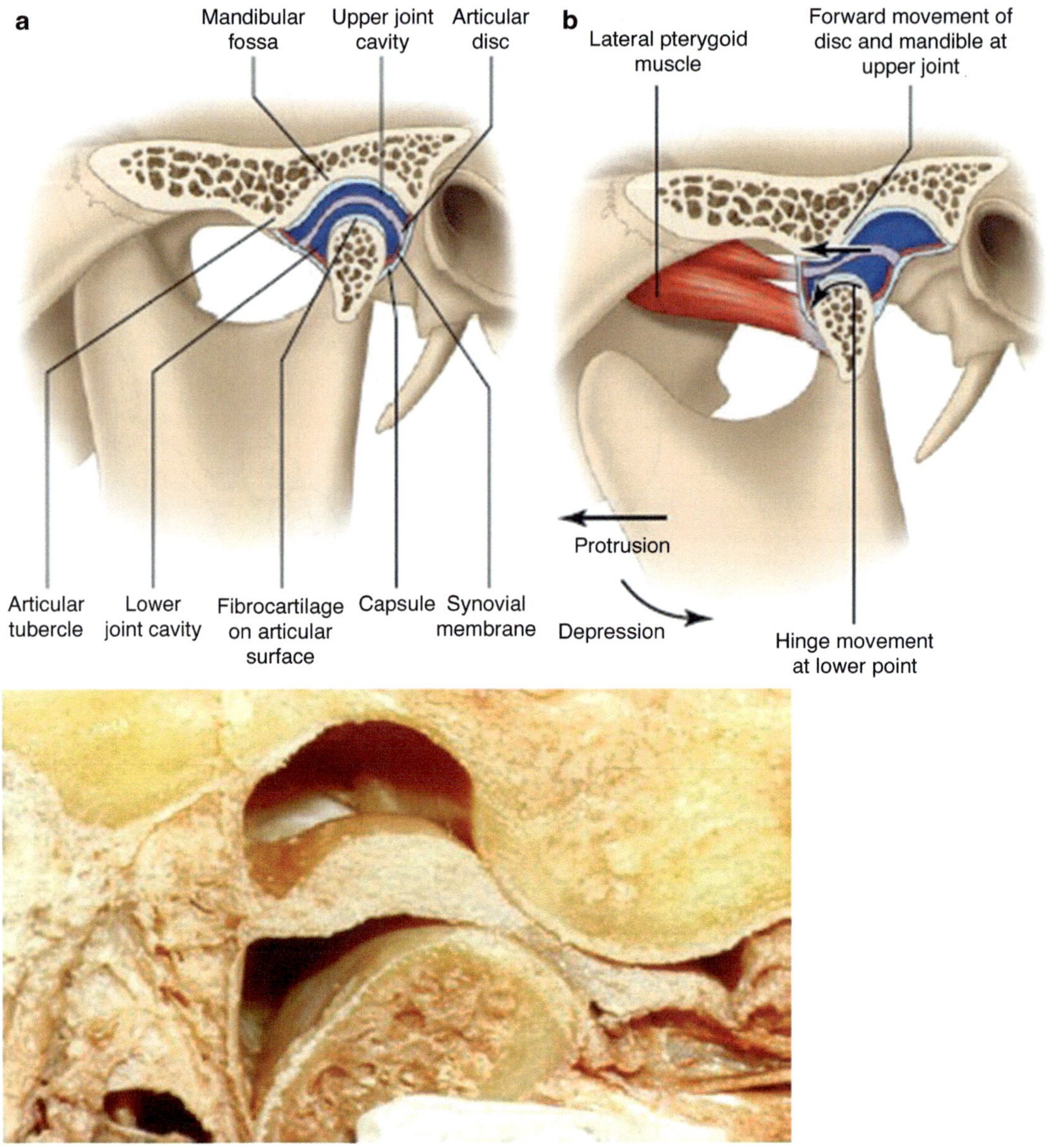

Fig. 3.6 Illustrated anatomy of the temporomandibular joint (**a**) and the rotational movement which occurs in the lower joint space and the gliding movement which occurs in the upper joint space (**b**). Note the anatomy of the glenoid fossa, disc and the condylar head in the sagittal cadaveric section. [Reprinted/adapted by permission from S.T. Connelly et al. (eds.), *Contemporary Management of Temporomandibular Disorders*, https://doi.org/10.1007/978-3-319-99909-8_3]

3.5 Articular Disc/Meniscus

Articular disc is an avascular structure made of fibrous connective tissue which lacks innervation. It is present between the articular surfaces. Its shape is determined by the shape of the condyle and concavity of the mandibular fossa. Medially, it receives attachments from the lateral pterygoid muscle synchronizing the mandibular condyle movements with the disc on function. The periphery of the disc is attached to the capsular ligament.

The disc is a biconcave structure, thick in the anterior and thin in the posterior region. It is attached by the collateral ligaments to the medial and lateral poles of the condyle. The condylar head and the disc move together on translation. The disc splits into two, both anteriorly and posteriorly each aiding in smooth joint function (Table 3.4). The disc is considered to act as a third articular surface providing a movable condylar articulation [4] (Fig. 3.6).

Table 3.4 Anatomical regions in the anterior and posterior to the disc

Anterior part of disc	Superior lamellae	Inferior lamellae
	Attached to anterior edge of articular eminence	Attached to the anterior part of condylar head
	Muscle fibres of lateral pterygoid muscles are attached to the disc in between these lamellae to aid in the unified movement of condyle and disc	
Posterior part of disc	Inferior lamellae	Superior lamellae
	Thin extension of the fibrous disc Runs over the posterior surface of condylar head and fuses with periosteum of condylar neck	A loosely textured tissue present in fibrous disc containing blood vessels and elastic fibres It is contained posteriorly in capsular ligament admixed with the same superiorly. It gets attached to squamotympanic fissure.

3.6 Cartilage, Synovium and the Ligaments

In general, synovial joints are made up of two articulating surfaces covered by hyaline cartilage. The joint is covered by a fibrous capsule which forms the joint cavity. This cavity gets filled by synovial fluid secreted from the synovial membrane which lines the non-articular joint surface. It aids in joint lubrication and movement. In case of the temporomandibular joint, the articulating surfaces are covered with fibrocartilage instead of hyaline cartilage with an outer capsule and an inner synovial membrane, thereby proving that TMJ has all the properties of a synovial joint. The entire TMJ is enclosed in a fibrous joint capsule which is a fibro-elastic sac attached anteriorly to the articular tubercle and posteriorly to the squamous tympanic fissure, with its circumferential attachment to the temporal bone and the mandibular condyle. The inner surface of the joint capsule is lined by synovial membrane which has a smooth and glistening appearance. The lateral ligament of the temporomandibular joint strengthen the lateral aspect of the joint capsule. There are several other ligaments associated with the temporomandibular joint that strengthen, aids in articulation and also

Table 3.5 Ligaments associated with the TMJ (Fig. 3.7)

Ligament	Derivation	Origin	Insertion	Function
Capsular	**Same as joint capsule**	Attached to the margins of the articular surfaces		Resist movement in extreme range of motion (ROM) Contain synovial fluid in superior/inferior joint space
Lateral/temporomandibular	**Same as joint capsule**	Lateral aspect of the TMJ capsule from the articular eminence to the posterior neck of the condyle. Two distinct fibers may be identified: Outer oblique part (**OOP**) Inner horizontal part (**IHP**)		**OOP:** Limits inferior distraction of condyle achieved in translatory and rotational movements **IHP:** Limits posterior condylar movement during pivotal movements
Sphenomandibular	Meckel cartilage residue	Sphenoid spine	Medial wall of TMJ capsule and lingula	Protects the joint from an excessive translation, after 10 degrees of mouth opening

(continued)

Table 3.5 (continued)

Ligament	Derivation	Origin	Insertion	Function
Stylomandibular	First and second branchial arch (through Reichert cartilage)	Styloid process of the temporal bone	Posterior margin of mandibular angle	Limit excessive protrusion of the jaw
Pterygomandibular (antomically a raphe, may be considered a pseudo-check ligament for TMJ)	Mesenchymal connection between first and second branchial arches	Apex of hamulus of the internal pterygoid plate of skull	Posterior area of the retromolar trigone	Limits excessive jaw movements.
Malleolomandibular	Intermediate lamina during disc formation	**First part:** Malleus relative to the anterior ligament in middle ear **Second part:** Extra-tympanic area, in contact with the retro-discal tissues	**Retro-discal region**	**First part:** Manage adequate pressure for middle ear **Second part:** Protects synovial membrane balancing tension from surrounding structures
Collateral/discal	**Same as joint capsule and disc**	Level of intermediate fascia of the articular disc	Medial and lateral poles of condyle	Anchors articular disc to the condyle Restrict movement of disc away from condyle

monitor the excessive joint movements (Table 3.5) (Fig. 3.7) [3, 4].

3.7 Retrodiscal Tissue

The articular disc merges with a vascular and highly innervated structure posteriorly known as the bilaminar zone which is also involved in the production of synovial fluid. The superior retro-discal tissue contains elastic fibres which are instrumental in restraining the disc during extreme translatory movements. Inferior retrodiscal tissue is composed of collagen fibres that serve as a check ligament thereby preventing extreme disc rotation during rotational movements [4].

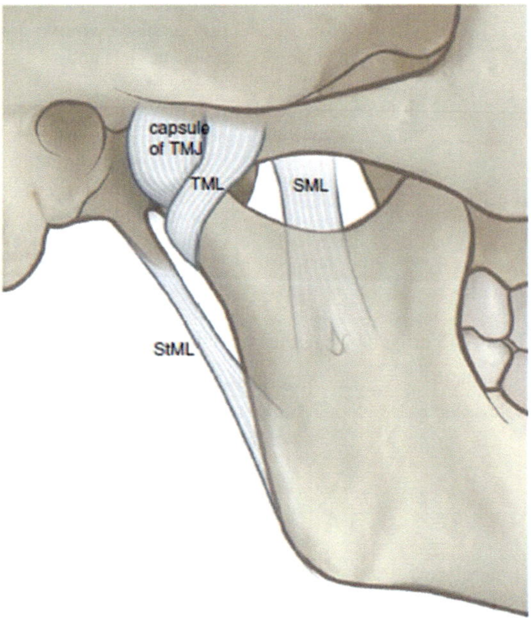

Fig. 3.7 Ligaments associated with the TMJ aids in enhancing the articular process and jaw movements. *SML* sphenomandibular ligament, *StML* stylomandibular ligament, *TMJ* temporomandibular joint, *TML* temporomandibular ligament. [Reprinted/adapted by permission from T. von Arx, S. Lozanoff, Clinical Oral Anatomy, https://doi.org/10.1007/978-3-319-41993-0_25]

3.8 Blood Supply

The main blood supply to the TMJ is by (1) Branches of Superficial temporal, (2) Deep auricular, (3) Anterior tympanic and (4) Ascending

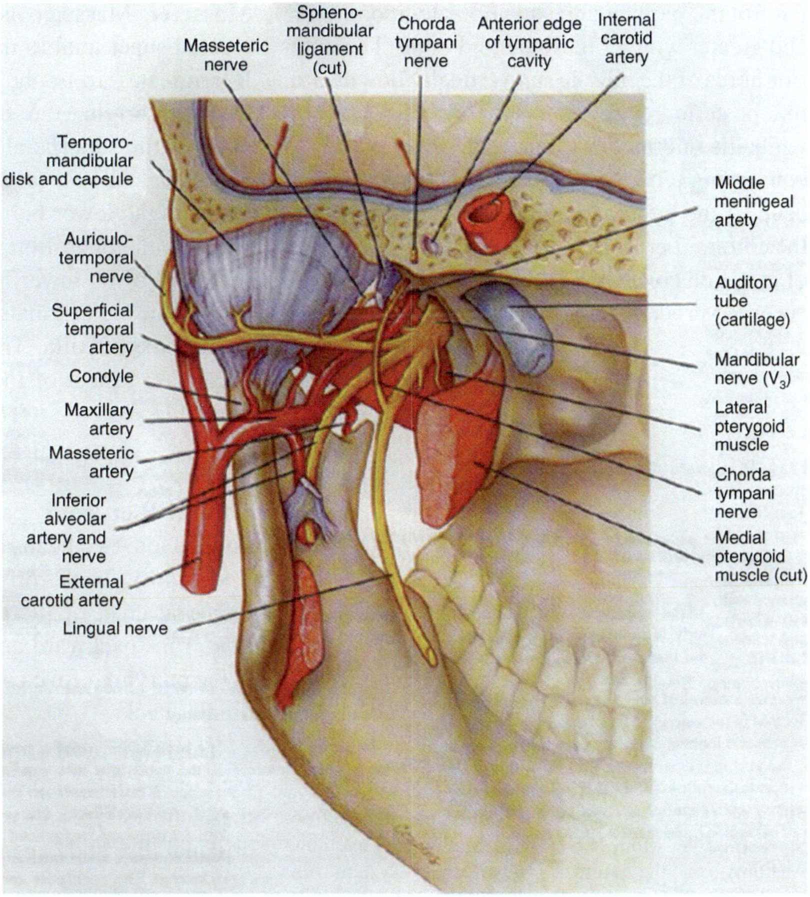

Fig. 3.8 Schematic view of the deep structures around the TMJ viewed from the posterior aspect. Note the nerve innervation to the joint. [Reprinted/adapted by permission from S. T. Connelly et al. (eds.), *Contemporary Management of Temporomandibular Disorders*, https://doi.org/10.1007/978-3-319-99909-8_3]

pharyngeal arteries. They penetrate the joint capsules and provide branches to the disc periphery and posterior joint region. A rich plexus of veins is present in the posterior aspect associated with the retrodiscal tissues (Fig. 3.8) [4, 5].

3.9 Nerve Supply

Nerve supply to the TMJ is from the branches of mandibular division of trigeminal nerve: (1) Auriculotemporal nerve, (2) Masseteric branch and (3) Deep temporal branch. They enter the capsule and disc supplying the joint head, the fossa, innervated portions of the disc and the capsule. Nerve terminals for pain, pressure, touch and temperature are found within the joint cavity and are considered to be vasomotor and vasosensory.

3.10 Musculature

TMJ is associated with different muscles which aid in joint function. The muscles involved to elevate/close the jaw are masseter, temporal is, medial pterygoid. The muscles that depress/open the jaw are lateral pterygoid, geniohyoid, mylohyoid and digastric [4–6].

3.10.1 Masticatory Muscles Controlling the Mandibular Movement (Figs. 3.9, 3.10, and 3.11)

Temporalis The temporalis muscle arises from the temporal fossa on the lateral aspect of the skull bounded above by the temporal lines and below by the zygomatic arch. It embraces parts of the frontal, parietal and squamous temporal bone and greater wing of the sphenoid bone. The anterior fibres of the muscle run vertically downward; the posterior fibres run horizontally forward, while the intermediate fibres run obliquely to the converging tendon inferiorly. This tendon passes deep to the zygomatic arch and is inserted into the coronoid process of the mandible. The region of insertion covers the entire medial aspect of the coronoid process including its apex.

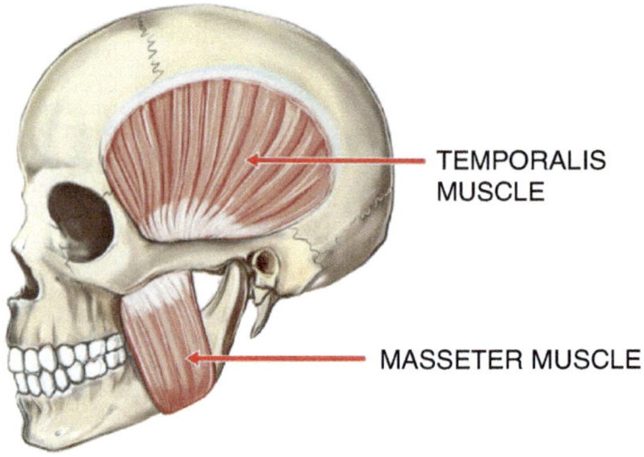

Fig. 3.9 Temporalis and masseter muscle (Adapted from Stockstill J.W., Mohl N.D. (2015) Static and Functional Anatomy of the Human Masticatory System. In: Kandasamy S., Greene C., Rinchuse D., Stockstill J. (eds) TMD and Orthodontics. Springer, Cham. https://doi.org/10.1007/978-3-319-19782-1_1)

Masseter Masseter is a quadrilateral muscle located superficial to the ramus of the mandible. It originates from the zygomatic arch. On the basis of origin, the fibres of this muscle are divided into superficial and deep fibres. The most superficial fibres originate from anterior two thirds of the lower border of the zygomatic arch, whereas the deep fibres arise from the posterior one third of its lower border. The anterior fibres of this muscle originate from the zygomatic process of the maxilla. The muscle is inserted into the lateral aspect of the ramus and angle of the mandible.

Lateral Pterygoid Lateral pterygoid muscle is divided into two heads, the upper and lower head. The upper head originates from the infratemporal crest of the greater wing of the sphenoid, runs backward and laterally to get inserted at the pterygoid fovea on anterior surface of mandibular neck.

The lower head originates from the lateral surface of the lateral pterygoid plate. A portion of these fibres are also inserted into the intra-articular disc and capsule of the TMJ.

Medial Pterygoid Superficial head arises from the tuberosity of maxilla and adjoining bone,

Fig. 3.10 Lateral and medial pterygoid muscles (Adapted from Stockstill J.W., Mohl N.D. (2015) Static and Functional Anatomy of the Human Masticatory System. In: Kandasamy S., Greene C., Rinchuse D., Stockstill J. (eds) TMD and Orthodontics. Springer, Cham. https://doi.org/10.1007/978-3-319-19782-1_1)

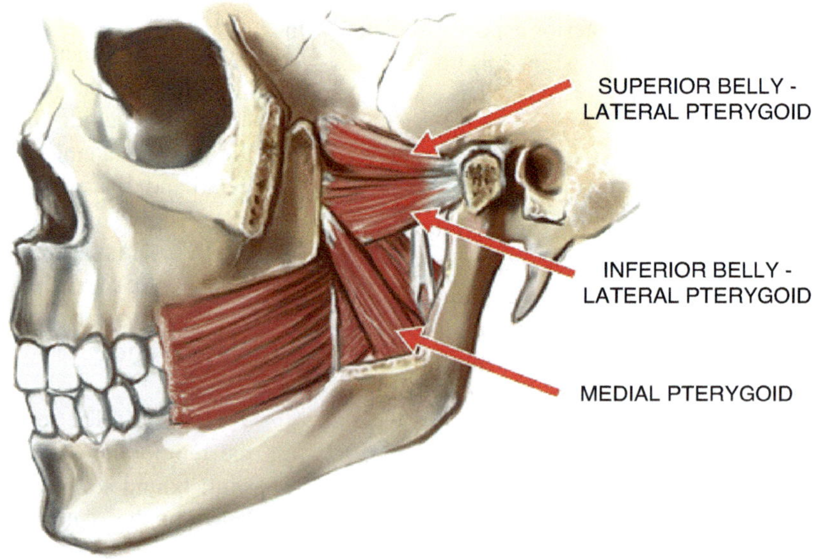

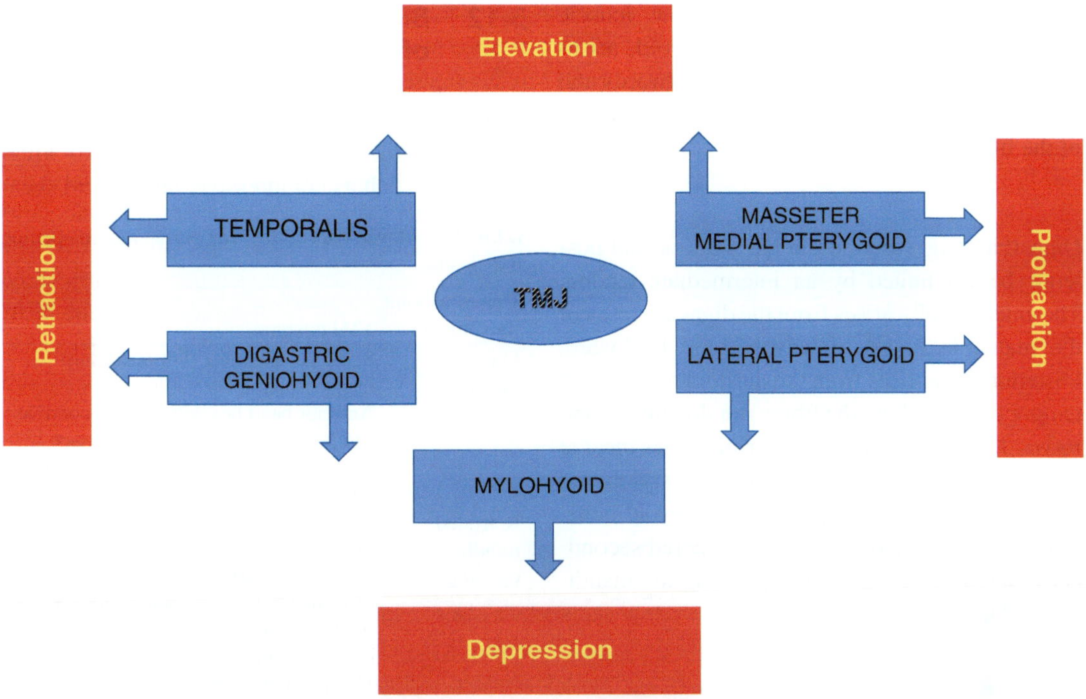

Fig. 3.11 Muscles associated with the mandible and the TMJ which have significant influences on the jaw movement

whilst the deep head originates from the medial surface of the lateral pterygoid plate and adjoining process of the palatine bone. The muscle fibres run downward, backward and laterally to get inserted into the roughened surface of the medial aspect of the mandibular angle and adjoining ramus, inferior and posterior to the mandibular foramen and mylohyoid muscle.

3.10.2 Supra Hyoid Muscle Group Aiding the Mandibular Movement (Figs. 3.11 and 3.12)

Mylohyoid Mylohyoid is a flat triangular muscle having posterior, middle and anterior fibres. They arise from the floor of the mouth, deep to the anterior belly of digastric (the mylohyoid line of the mandible). The fibres run medially and downwards. The posterior fibres get inserted in the body of hyoid bone. Middle and anterior fibres get attached with the fibers of the opposite side, between mandible and the hyoid bone.

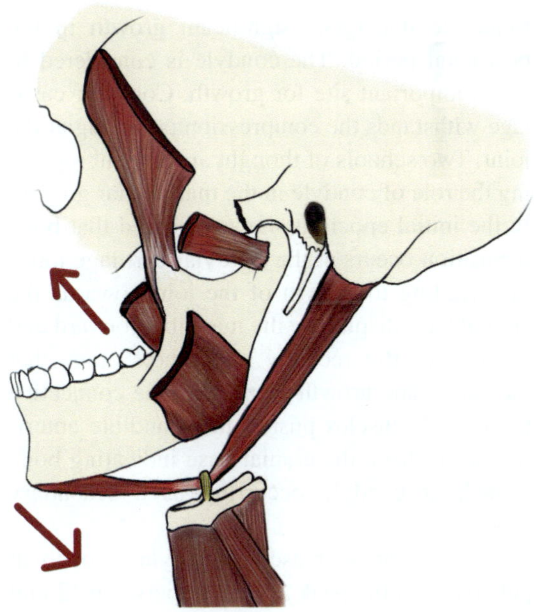

Fig. 3.12 Muscles associated with the mandible and the TMJ which have significant influences on the jaw movement demonstrating vectors of muscle pull (Image courtesy: Dr. Ujjwal Sharma)

Geniohyoid Geniohyoid is a narrow muscle lying at the medial aspect of mylohyoid, arises from the genial tubercles running backwards and downwards to get attached to the anterior surface of the hyoid bone.

Digastric Digastric muscle has anterior and posterior bellies united by an intermediate tendon. The anterior belly arises from the digastric fossa of the mandible to run downward and backward. Posterior belly arises from the mastoid notch in the temporal bone where the fibres run downward and forward. The anterior and posterior bellies meet at the intermediate tendon perforating the stylohyoid and is held by a fibrous pulley to the hyoid bone. Muscle pull of the digastric is considered secondary to lateral pterygoid for depressing the mandible [2–5].

3.11 Post-Natal Growth of Temporomandibular Joint

Mandible undergoes significant growth in the post-natal period. The condyle is considered to be an important site for growth. Condylar cartilage withstands the compression occurring at the joint. Two schools of thought are evident regarding the role of condyle in the mandibular growth. In the initial epoch, it was considered that bone deposition occurs at the condylar-cartilage interface leading to growth of the joint towards the cranial base displacing the mandible forward and downward. But recently researchers opine that the soft tissue growth along with the connective tissue and muscles pushes the mandible anteriorly away from the cranial base indicating bone growth at condyle occurring as a secondary process.

There is an increase in condylar growth at puberty with the peak age range between 12 and 15 years and growth ceases by 20 years of age in an adult (with documented gender differences, earlier in females) [7].

3.12 Biomechanics of Temporomandibular Joint

Mandibular movements cause static and dynamic changes in the TMJ with combinations of stress and strain such as compressive, tensile and shear

Table 3.6 Movements of the TMJ during mouth opening and closing

Phases of joint movement	TMJ position
During occlusion	Static jaw position with maximum inter-cuspation Anterior band lies between the condyle and posterior slope of the eminence Posterior band is present in the deepest region of the fossa
Retruded mouth opening	Condyle moves inferiorly to the intermediate zone by 5–6 mm into the articulating surface Movement of medial pole is antero-superior and lateral pole is postero-inferior in direction. This position is maintained up to 18 mm of mouth opening
Early protrusive mouth opening	Condylar movement occurs in inferior and anterior direction beneath intermediate zone by 6–9 mm stretching of the bilaminar zone. It creates space in the posterior region during condylar translation anteriorly
Late protrusive mouth opening	Condylar movement occurs in an inferior and anterior direction below anterior band. Space is created during rotation posteriorly in the superior compartment followed by inferior compartment. Anterior displacement of the disc is limited during anterior translation of the condyle by exerting a posterior traction of retro-discal tissue
Early mouth closing	Condylar translation occurs for about 6–9 mm in the posterior direction towards the intermediate direction There is a simultaneous reduction of space posteriorly in the superior compartment
Retrusive closing	There is rotation of the condyle which occurs inferior to the posterior band causing reduction of spaces in the inferior compartment while returning near to the occlusal plane

loading on the articulating surfaces. The joint loading and forces are also influenced by the activities of masticatory muscles and occlusal movement. The disc acts as a viscoelastic structure to allow smooth movement of the joint. The normal disc in the posterior band is at 12'o clock position and 1'o clock in the intermediate zone in relation to the mandibular condyle. The joint movements are classified into different phases as summarized in the table (Table 3.6).

The condylar movement occurs either by gliding between the disc and temporal surface or hinge/rotation which occurs between the condylar head and the disc. This dynamic combination aids in mandibular movements for mouth opening, closing, speech and mastication [6, 8–11].

References

1. Sperber GH. Craniofacial embryology. London: Wright; 1989.
2. Bender EM, et al. Development of the pediatric temporomandibular joint. Oral Maxillofac Surg Clin North Am. 2018;30(1):1–9.
3. Bordoni B, Varacallo M. Anatomy, head and neck, temporomandibular joint. Treasure Island (FL): StatPearls Publishing; 2020.
4. Chandra S, et al. Textbook of dental and oral histology with embryology and multiple choice questions. New Delhi: Jaypee Brothers Medical Publishers Ltd.; 2010.
5. Chaurasia BD. Human anatomy, regional and applied dissection. 5th ed. New Delhi: CBS Publishers Ltd.; 2016.
6. Devi VS, editor. Inderbir Singh's textbook of anatomy. 3rd vol: Head & neck and neuroanatomy. 7th ed. New Delhi: Jaypee The Health Sciences; 2019. ISBN 9789389129014.
7. Balaji SI. Textbook. Orthodontics the art and science. 5th ed. New Delhi: Arya Medi Publishing House Ltd.; 2018.
8. Ingawale SM. Biomechanics of the temporomandibular joint. Human Musculoskeletal Biomechanics. 2012. Available from http://www.intechopen.com/books/human-musculoskeletal-biomechanics/biomechanics-of-thetemporomandibular-joint
9. Barbenel JC. The biomechanics of temporomandibular joint: a theoretical study. J Biomech. 1972;5:251–6.
10. Mérida-Velasco JR, et al. Development of the human temporomandibular joint. The Anat Rec. 1999;255:20–33.
11. Peterson LJ. Petersons principles of oral and maxillofacial surgery. Hamilton: PMPH Ltd.; 2012.

Incidence of Temporomandibular Joint Pathology and Disorders

4

Darpan Bhargava, Ajay Bhambal, and Aashna Dhingra

4.1 Introduction

The temporomandibular joint (TMJ) is a ginglymoarthrodial joint, which functions in harmony with various structures that include the bilateral mandibular condyle, meniscus, glenoid fossa, articular ligaments, and the associated musculature [1]. Temporomandibular disorders (TMDs) constitute a group of disorders that cause pain or dysfunction in the jaw joint and muscles that control its movement [2]. It is important to study the epidemiology of TMDs as it comprises of a range of complex etiological factors, age variations, a requirement for multiple diagnostic and therapeutic approaches [3].

D. Bhargava (✉)
TMJ Consultancy Services,
Bhopal, Madhya Pradesh, India

Oral and Maxillofacial Surgery, People's College of Dental Sciences and Research Centre,
People's University, Bhopal, Madhya Pradesh, India
e-mail: drdarpanbhargava@gmail.com

A. Bhambal
Department of Public Health Dentistry,
People's College of Dental Sciences and Research Centre, People's University, Bhopal,
Madhya Pradesh, India

A. Dhingra
Nationwide Quality of Care Network (NQOCN),
Delhi, India

4.2 Epidemiology of TMDs

An incidence of 41% on random sampling in a given study subjects attending a university dental centre was reported to have TMJ disorders of some form or the other and with varying severity [4]. Other epidemiological studies have suggested that approximately 50–75% of the population is affected to some degree and exhibits some sign of TMD. Prevalence of TMDs amongst the general population shows disparity based on varied clinical evaluation methods used (1–75%) or use of pain questionnaires (6–75%) which may not be uniform for various studies conducted and create difficulties in standardizing the pattern for the distribution of the disease. Patients with TMDs present over a broad age range with peak occurrence between 20 and 40 years [4–6]. Studies demonstrate that TMDs are rarely seen in infancy and childhood, but become more prevalent in adolescence and adulthood, gradually increasing with age [7–9].

In a study conducted among adolescents to investigate various aspects of TMDs including the prevalence, diagnosis, and treatment protocol according to the Research Diagnostic Criteria for Temporomandibular Disorders (RDC/TMD) using a questionnaire and clinical examination revealed that TMD pain is more common among girls than in boys in their study population. While evaluating the various factors it was found that stress, somatic complaints, and emotional

D. Bhargava (ed.), *Temporomandibular Joint Disorders*,
https://doi.org/10.1007/978-981-16-2754-5_4

disorders were found to play a significant role in adolescents with TMDs. While evaluating the influence of somatic and emotional stimuli it was observed that adolescents with TMD pain were significantly more sensitive to not only aversive somatic but also pleasant somatic stimuli compared to the control group. This suggests that not only nociceptive but also cognitive processes are implicated in chronic pain states in young TMD subjects [10, 11]. Emotional and psychosocial factors have been correlated and play a key role in initiation and later further progression of TMDs. Studies suggest that the unresolved emotions may obstruct and reduce the peptide flow signals preserving functions at cellular level, thus resulting in dysfunction and pathology. It has also been proposed that the emotional stress leads to clenching and thereby increasing the masticatory muscle activity with alterations in the muscle tone and produce circulatory changes that results in development of TMDs [10, 12]. Females exhibit a marked higher prevalence as compared to the male population, most commonly in the second to fourth decade, during the reproductive period. Few studies claim, that the receptors for female reproductive hormones, the estrogen and progesterone are detected in the intra-articular cartilage in women affected with TMDs. Decreased estrogen levels is potentially associated with TMDs and headaches and can also modulate the effect on the properties of ion channels in neurons of the joint (Yu S, 2009) [7–9, 11, 30].

TMDs are associated with pain and functional limitation, causing masticatory difficulties due to limited mandibular range of motion interfering with normal function. Emotional stress, bruxism, trauma to the orofacial region, occlusal interferences, malposition/loss of teeth, postural changes, dysfunctions of the masticatory musculature, and adjacent structures cause various extrinsic and intrinsic changes on TMJ structure and/or a combination of such factors have been attributed as causative factors leading to TMDs [12]. A clinician, who is involved in primary evaluation of these patient must have a broad knowledge regarding the epidemiology of TMDs which will aid in diagnosing the patient's condition and will guide for further appropriate referral to a TMD specialist, in cases where conservative management is futile. The incidence of commonly encountered TMDs as reported by various authors in there study population is summarized in the table (Table 4.1) [10–18].

Table 4.1 Incidence of common temporomandibular joint disorders as reported by various authors in their study samples

Condition	Incidence
Deviation of the joint [4]	17%
Rheumatoid arthritis [4]	10%
Myofascial Pain Dysfunction Syndrome (MPDS) [13, 14]	1–10% A study reported as less as 0.8% of prevalence in the South Indian population. It was about 10.3% in a Brazilian population
Internal derangement [13, 14]	38% A study reported 78% incidence in the Japanese population.
Disc displacement [14]	8%
TMJ arthralgia [14]	3–4%
Osteoarthritis [13]	14–15%
TMJ tuberculosis [15]	10% extra-pulmonary manifestations of TB
TMJ ankylosis [16]	Ankylosed joint has a higher prevalence in the developing countries, and has a rising incidence in India. Among ankylosis cases, the post-traumatic ankylosis is most common (87%). This condition is more commonly reported in children.

A study was conducted among the Swedish population to determine the incidence and prevalence of craniomandibular disorders in patients having tinnitus using various parameters and it was observed that fatigue/tenderness in the masticatory muscles and frequent headaches were more prevalent in patients having tinnitus than in control group, which co-related with the clinical findings of pain on palpation of masticatory muscles, impaired mandibular mobility, and signs of para-functional habits. Most patients reported an increase in their symptoms on mandibular movements and/or pressure applied to the TMJ or associated pre-auricular region [17]. The patients suffering from sudden sensorineural hearing loss (SSHL) also report statistically significant higher rates of oro-facial pain and tenderness during mandibular movements and on palpation of masticatory muscles along with their aural symptoms when compared with the healthy subjects [18]. A thorough evaluation of ear and stomatognathological system should be performed to differentiate between ear disorders and TMDs as they may have overlap of signs and symptoms [19].

TMJ is also affected in disorders associated with cervical spine. Studies have suggested that treating TMDs effectively improved cervical spine mobility significantly. It is indicated that significant co-relation is found between disorders of the neck and the cervical spine associated with limitations of jaw movements. The documented probable explanation, that the symptoms from the cervical spine region are referred to the stomatognathic system and vice-versa is through the neural overlap and connections at level of the trigemino-cervical nucleus. A thorough evaluation of the head and neck must be carried out to accurately diagnose the condition which should aim at providing an improved overall general quality of life to the patients reporting with TMDs [20–23].

4.3 Incidence for fractures of the TMJ

Incidence of fractures of the mandibular condyle varies with the cause for the injury, with road traffic accidents (RTA) being the leading etiology (68.8%), followed by fall (16.8%), assaults (11.0%) and other miscellaneous causes (3.8%). Males have a higher incidence for condylar fracture (83.27%) than females (16.27%). The most common site for fracture in the mandibular bone is the condylar fracture (29.0%) followed by the anterior mandible (22.0%), as highlighted by Dingman and Natvig. Condyle can be fractured as a result of direct or indirect impact caused by the trauma. The mandibular condyle act as a shock absorber by taking up the force without transmitting them to the cranial fossa leading to a fractured condyle [24–26].

4.4 Incidence for tumors associated with the TMJ

Tumors and pseudo-tumors involving the temporomandibular joint are not uncommon but rare. The reported common benign tumors in the adult includes, chondroblastomas, osteoblastomas, osteochondromas, and osteomas. The metastatic tumors and sarcomas are the common malignant tumors in this region. Conditions reported in pediatric patients include, osteofibroso-hetero-hyperdysplasia, condylar cyst, Langerhans cell histiocytosis and aggressive fibromatosis [27–29]. Benign tumors account for 10.2%, malignant tumors being 18.2% and majority of the cases fall in the category of pseudotumors (71.6%), among all the tumors that affect the tissues of the temporomandibular joint. Pseudotumors, which majorly affects the joint includes, synovial chondromatosis (61.8%), osteochondroma (29.4%), pigmented villonodular synovitis (4.4%) and eosinophillic granuloma (4.4%). The incidence of benign tumors form the next majority followed by pseudotumors, that include chondroblastomas (17.2%), osteoid osteoma (13.8%), chondroma (10.9%), osteoblastoma (10.9%), osteoma (10.9%) and others (37.9%). Malignancy includes scrcomas (53.8%), metastases (32.7%) and other malignant tumors (13.5%) [27].

4.5 Conclusion

TMDs are not an uncommon condition among patients attending the medical or a dental facility. An individual may present with one or more signs and symptoms at the same time and with a variety of causative factors that may be linked to the etiology. Patients especially females between second to fourth decades are the most commonly affected [30]. Deviation on mouth opening may be noted in a significant number of people. TMJ ankylosis in children, MPDS, and internal derangement in adults are commonly encountered by the oral physicians/maxillofacial surgeons. Osteoarthritis is another common disorder, occurring most commonly in females. Other less common disorders but may be encountered in the routine practice include rheumatoid/psoriatic arthritis, malignant or benign tumors involving the condyle, and septic arthritis due to infections including tuberculosis. The understanding of increasing incidence of TMDs and other pathologies of the joint based on the potential risk factors such as age, gender, emotional status and other related factors will provide an appropriate diagnosis for joint diseases and an early intervention may be incorporated in the treatment plan. Also, acknowledging the prevalence of TMDs in adolescents, early interceptive measures can be taken, preventing worsening of the disease progression and improving the quality of life. With the review of recent studies, change in the present epidemiology of TMDs is evident with increase of incidence in joint disorders among the general population due to the modern lifestyle patterns.

References

1. Fehrenbach M, Herring S. Illustrated anatomy of the head and neck. St. Louis, MO: Elsevier; 2012.
2. List T, Jensen RH. Temporomandibular disorders: old ideas and new concepts. Cephalalgia. 2017;37(7): 692–704.
3. Boever JA, Steenks MH. Epidemiology, symptomatology and etiology of craniomandibular dysfunction. In: Steenks MH, de Wijer A, editors. Temporomandibular joint dysfunctions from the point of view of physiotherapy and dentistry. 1st ed. Sao Paulo: Livraria Editora Santos; 1996. p. 35–43.
4. AlShaban KK, Gul Abdul Waheed Z. Prevalence of TMJ disorders among the patients attending the dental Clinic of Ajman University of Science and Technology–Fujairah Campus, UAE. Int J Dent. 2018;2018:1–6.
5. Karthik R, Hafila MF, Saravanan C, Vivek N, Priyadarsini P, Ashwath B. Assessing prevalence of temporomandibular disorders among university students: a questionnaire study. J Int Soc Prev Community Dent. 2017 Jun;7(Suppl 1):S24.
6. Manfredini D, Guarda-Nardini L, Winocur E, Piccotti F, Ahlberg J, Lobbezoo F. Research diagnostic criteria for temporomandibular disorders: a systematic review of axis I epidemiologic findings. Oral Surg Oral Med Oral Pathol Oral Radiol Endod. 2011;112(4): 453–62.
7. Hongxing L, Astrom AN, List T, Nilsson IM, Johansson A. Prevalence of temporomandibular disorder pain in Chinese adolescents compared to an age-matched Swedish population. J Oral Rehabil. 2016;43:241–8. https://doi.org/10.1111/joor.12366. PMID: 26538188
8. Farsi NM. Symptoms and signs of temporomandibular disorders and oral parafunctions among Saudi children. J Oral Rehabil. 2003;30:1200–8. PMID: 14641664
9. Johansson A, Unell L, Carlsson GE, Söderfeldt B, Halling A. Gender difference in symptoms related to temporomandibular disorders in a population of 50-year-old subjects. J Orofac Pain. 2003. Winter;17(1):29–35.
10. Wahlund K. Temporomandibular disorders in adolescents. Epidemiological and methodological studies and a randomized controlled trial. Swed Dent J. 2003;164.):inside front cover(Suppl):2–64.
11. List T, Wahlund K, Wenneberg B, Dworkin SF. TMD in children and adolescents: prevalence of pain, gender differences, and perceived treatment need. J Orofac Pain. 1999 Winter;13(1):9–20.
12. Carlson DS. Growth of the temporomandibular joint. In: Zarb GA, Carlsson GE, Sessle BJ, Mohl ND, editors. Temporomandibular joint and masticatory muscle disorders. 2nd ed. Copenhagen: Munksgaard; 1994. p. 128–50.
13. Muthukrishnan A, Sekar GS. Prevalence of temporomandibular disorders in Chennai population. J Indian Acad Oral Med Radiol. 2015;27(4):508.
14. de Paiva Bertoli FM, Bruzamolin CD, Pizzatto E, Losso EM, Brancher JA, de Souza JF. Prevalence of diagnosed temporomandibular disorders: a cross-sectional study in Brazilian adolescents. PLoS One. 2018;13(2):e0192254.
15. Prasad KC, Sreedharan S, Chakravarthy Y, Prasad SC. Tuberculosis in the head and neck: experience in India. J Laryngol Otol. 2007 Oct;121(10):979–85.
16. Nagori SA, Jose A, Bhutia O, Roychoudhury A. Undiagnosed mandibular condylar fractures causing temporomandibular joint ankylosis: a problem in northern India. Natl Med J India. 2014 Jan 1;27:251–5.
17. Rubinstein B, Axelsson A, Carlsson GE. Prevalence of signs and symptoms of craniomandibular disorders in tinnitus patients. J Craniomandib Disord. 1990 Summer;4(3):186–92.
18. Axelsson R, Tullberg M, Ernberg M, Hedenberg-Magnusson B. Symptoms and signs of temporomandibular disorders in patients with sudden sensorineural hearing loss. Swed Dent J. 2009;33(3):115–23.
19. Kempf HG, Roller R, Mühlbradt L. Correlation between inner ear disorders and temporomandibular joint diseases. HNO. 1993;41(1):7–10. [Article in German]
20. Walczyńska-Dragon K, Baron S, Nitecka-Buchta A, Tkacz E. Correlation between TMD and cervical spine pain and mobility: is the whole body balance TMJ related? Biomed Res Int. 2014;2014:582414. https://doi.org/10.1155/2014/582414.
21. Silveira A, Gadotti IC, Armijo-Olivo S, Biasotto-Gonzalez DA, Magee D. Jaw dysfunction is associated with neck disability and muscle tenderness in subjects with and without chronic temporomandibular disorders. Biomed Res Int. 2015;2015:512792. https://doi.org/10.1155/2015/512792.

22. Kraus S. Temporomandibular disorders, head and orofacial pain: cervical spine considerations. Dent Clin N Am. 2007;51(1):161–93.
23. De Laat A, Meuleman H, Stevens A, Verbeke G. Correlation between cervical spine and temporomandibular disorders. Clin Oral Investig. 1998 Jun;2(2):54–7.
24. Barde D, Mudhol A, Madan R. Prevalence and pattern of mandibular fracture in Central India. Natl J Maxillofac Surg. 2014;5(2):153–6. https://doi.org/10.4103/0975-5950.154818.
25. Morris C, Bebeau NP, Brockhoff H, Tandon R, Tiwana P. Mandibular fractures: an analysis of the epidemiology and patterns of injury in 4,143 fractures. J Oral Maxillofac Surg. 2015;73(5):951.e1–951.
26. Afrooz PN, Bykowski MR, James IB, Daniali LN, Clavijo-Alvarez JA. The epidemiology of mandibular fractures in the United States, part 1: a review of 13,142 cases from the US National Trauma Data Bank. J Oral Maxillofac Surg. 2015 Dec;73(12):2361–6.
27. Wei WB, Chen MJ, Yang C, Qiu Y, Zhou Q. Tumors and pseudotumors at the temporomandibular joint region in pediatric patients. Int J Clin Exp Med. 2015;8(11):21813–7.
28. Yurttutan M, Öncül A, Karasu H. Benign tumors of temporomandibular joint. 2018. https://doi.org/10.5772/intechopen.72302.
29. Stegenga B. Nomenclature and classification of temporomandibular joint disorders. J Oral Rehab. 2010;37:760–5.
30. Warren MP, Fried JL. Temporomandibular disorders and hormones in women. Cells Tissues Organs. 2001;169(3):187–92. https://doi.org/10.1159/000047881.

Understanding Temporomandibular Joint Disorders

5

A. Einstein, Shoomali Hassan, and Himanta Ghritlahare

Temporomandibular disorders (TMDs) refer to a group of musculoskeletal and neuromuscular conditions of the temporomandibular joint (TMJ) along with morphological and functional deformities [1, 2] that include disturbances of intra-articular discal position and/or structure as well as dysfunction of associated musculature [3]. TMDs are considered as a major cause of pain of non-dental origin in the orofacial region.

TMDs usually present as painful joint sounds, restricted or deviating range of motion, and orofacial pain. The TMD diagnosis depends on the nature of these presenting findings and thus TMD patients commonly present with multiple TMD diagnoses, which are ranked relative to their contribution to the patient's complaint, as primary, secondary, tertiary, and so on [4].

Given such inconsistent diagnostic criteria and categories associated with TMDs, the *International RDC/TMD Consortium Network* published validated diagnostic criteria of the assessment of the TMJ [5] that provided a standardized assessment for a limited set of TMDs to generate reliable data for researchers. Later, *American Academy of Orofacial Pain (AAOP)* classified TMDs [4], including a wider group of disorders, finding more widespread clinical acceptance.

A *National Institute for Dental and Craniofacial Research (NIDCR)* funded multisite Validation Project in 2001 highlighted the inadequate criterion and proposed a revised RDC/TMD axis I diagnostic algorithms for the most common TMDs. This was the first public opportunity for the field to contribute to a process that is still ongoing (refer: www.rdc-tmdinternational.org) [6].

A closed workshop held at the 2009 IADR General Session in Miami synthesized the findings of the major studies over the years into a consensus set of criteria for use in the clinical and research settings, referred to as *Diagnostic Criteria for Temporomandibular Disorders (DC/TMD)* [7]. The outcome of these efforts is the evidence-based DC/TMD axis I and axis II diagnostic protocol, which provides a comprehensive assessment of the TMD patient based on the biopsychosocial health model and is appropriate for immediate implementation in clinical and research settings. The AAOP has included the 12 DC/TMD diagnoses in a new revision of their Guidelines manual such that the DC/TMD and the AAOP taxonomic system for TMDs are now consistent.

A. Einstein (✉)
Oral Pathology and Microbiology, Thai Moogambigai Dental College and Hospital, Dr. MGR Educational and Research Institute, Chennai, Tamil Nadu, India

S. Hassan
Oral Pathology and Microbiology, Bhabha College of Dental Sciences, Bhopal, Madhya Pradesh, India

H. Ghritlahare
Oral Pathology and Microbiology, Government Dental College, Raipur, Chhattisgarh, India

D. Bhargava (ed.), *Temporomandibular Joint Disorders*,
https://doi.org/10.1007/978-981-16-2754-5_5

Considering the need to expand the current TMDs classification to develop a consensus-based classification system and associated diagnostic criteria that have clinical and research utility for less common but clinically important disorders, a working group [members of the International RDC/TMD Consortium Network of the International Association for Dental Research (IADR), members of the Orofacial Pain Special Interest Group (SIG) of the International Association for the Study of Pain (IASP), and members from other professional societies] reviewed disorders for inclusion based on clinical significance, the availability of plausible diagnostic criteria, and the ability to operationalize the criteria. The *Expanded TMD classification* presented included 37 TMDs, placed in four categories: temporomandibular joint disorders, masticatory muscle disorders, headache disorders, and disorders affecting associated structures (Table 5.1) [8]. This expanded taxonomy of TMDs for our discussion along with guidelines of DC/TMD and AAOP taxonomic system for TMD form the basis of our discussion.

5.1 Etiology of Temporomandibular Disorders

No single etiologic factor or unique theoretical model can convincingly explain the etiology of TMDs. The following factors, though not causal, have been found to be associated with TMDs:

Table 5.1 Taxonomic classification of temporomandibular disorders [7, 8]

Temporomandibular Joint Disorders
Joint pain
• Arthralgia
• Arthritis
Joint disorders
• Disc disorders
– Disc displacement with reduction
– Disc displacement with reduction with intermittent locking
– Disc displacement without reduction with limited opening
– Disc displacement without reduction without limited opening
• Hypomobility disorders other than disc disorders
– Adhesions/Adherence
– Ankylosis
Fibrous
Osseous
• Hypermobility disorders
– Dislocations
Subluxation
Luxation
Joint diseases
• Degenerative joint disease
– Osteoarthritis
– Osteoarthrosis
• Systemic arthritides
• Condylysis/ Idiopathic condylar resorption
• Osteochondrosis dissecans
• Osteonecrosis
• Neoplasm
• Synovial chondromatosis
Fractures
Congenital/developmental disorders
• Aplasia
• Hypoplasia
• Hyperplasia
Masticatory Muscle Disorders
Muscle pain
• Myalgia
– Local myalgia
– Myofascial pain
– Myofascial pain with referral
• Tendonitis
• Myositis
• Spasm
Contracture
Hypertrophy
Neoplasm
Movement disorders
• Orofacial dyskinesia
• Oromandibular dystonia
Masticatory muscle pain attributed to systemic/central disorders
• Fibromyalgia/widespread pain
Headache Disorders
Headache attributed to TMD
Associated Structures
Coronoid hyperplasia

- *Initiating factors:* That may cause the onset of TMDs.
- *Predisposing factors:* That increase the risk of TMDs.
- *Perpetuating factors:* That interfere with healing or enhance the progression of TMDs.

5.1.1 Trauma

If the force applied to the masticatory structures exceeds that of normal functional loading, then trauma occurs, which can be either macrotrauma (direct and indirect) and/or microtrauma.

Direct Trauma Any sudden and usually isolated blow can result in direct trauma. Direct In TMDs, such trauma includes direct injury to the mandible and/or TMJ resulting in structural failure and loss of function, wide or prolonged mouth opening, self-reported jaw injury due to yawning or prolonged mouth opening, intubation, third molar extractions, and transient and permanent dysfunction of the TMJ after upper airway management procedures [9].

Indirect Trauma A sudden blow without direct contact to the affected structures results in indirect trauma. Indirect trauma concerned with TMDs include acceleration-deceleration (flexion-extension) injury (*whiplash*) with no direct blow to the face (the direct causal relationship is still controversial) [10]. Symptoms of TMDs might result, not owing to the mandibular strain from trauma, but from the pain referred through recognized pathways of heterotopic pain from the cervical area to the trigeminal area [11].

Microtrauma Prolonged, repeated force over time, such as the sustained and repetitious adverse loading of the masticatory system through postural imbalances or from parafunctional habits can result in microtrauma. Postural habits such as forward head position or phone bracing may lead to musculoskeletal pain, including headache, in the TMD patient [12]. The relationship between TMD symptoms and the presence of parafunctional habits is still conflicting.

5.1.2 Anatomical Factors

Skeletal Factors Adverse biomechanical relationships of genetic, developmental, or iatrogenic origin such as severe skeletal malformations, inter-arch and intra-arch discrepancies, and past injuries to the teeth may play a role in TMDs [13], but this role is still not convincing enough.

Occlusal Relationships Occlusal features such as working and nonworking posterior contacts and discrepancies between the retruded contact position (RCP) and intercuspal position (ICP) have been usually identified as predisposing, initiating, and perpetuating factors for TMDs, though recent evidence suggests that this influence of occlusion on the onset and development of TMDs is low [14].

5.1.3 Pathophysiologic Factors

Systemic Factors Include systemic pathophysiology such as degenerative, endocrine, infectious, metabolic, neoplastic, neurologic, rheumatologic, and vascular disorders may influence local TMDs, with the systemic factors acting simultaneously at a central and local (peripheral) level [15]. Such situations should be managed in co-operation with the patient's primary care physician or other medical specialists.

Local (Peripheral) Factors Various local (peripheral) factors that have been implicated in TMDs include masticatory efficiency, masticatory muscle tenderness, cervical muscle activity, pathologic and adaptive responses to disease in the TMJ such as osteoarthritis, cytokine profiles, frictional "sticking" of the disc, intracapsular pressure, female hormones, mechanical breakdown in the articular disc, and accumulation of free radicals following mechanical stress [16, 17].

Genetic Factors Haplotypes of the gene encoding catechol-O-methyltransferase (COMT) were associated with experimental pain sensitivity and were related to the risk of developing myogenous

TMDs [18]. Evidence has been found for genetic associations in several pronociceptive intermediate phenotypes and their contributing role in TMDs. Single-nucleotide polymorphisms (SNPs) representing 358 genes involved in biologic systems associated with pain perception have been identified, supporting that multiple genetic and biologic pathways contribute to the risk for TMDs [19].

5.1.4 Psychosocial Factors

Factors that impact the patient's capacity to function adaptively such as individual, interpersonal, and situational variables constitute the psychosocial factors. Anxiety has been reported more in patients with TMDs than healthy control groups. Also, in some patients, emotional stress may manifest only TMDs or orofacial pain symptoms [20]. Any psychologic impairment in TMD patients may be merely associated with the presence of pain persistence, compared to healthy individuals [21]. As per the Orofacial Pain Prospective Evaluation and Risk Assessment (OPPERA) study group evaluation, TMD cases are different than controls across multiple phenotypic domains including sociodemographic factors, clinical variables, psychologic functioning, pain sensitivity, autonomic responses, and genetic associations [22] (Refer Chap. 8).

5.2 Intra-Articular Disorders of TMJ

5.2.1 Joint Pain

Pain in and around TMJ and associated headache are common presenting complaints in patients with facial pain and are thought to be related to TMJ disorders [23]. It would seem logical that such pain should originate from the articular surfaces when the joint is loaded by the muscles. This is impossible, however, in a healthy joint since there is no innervation of the articular surfaces.

Joint pain can originate only from nociceptors located in the soft tissues surrounding the joint. Three periarticular tissues contain such nociceptors, namely, the discal ligaments, the capsular ligaments, and the retrodiscal tissues. When these ligaments are elongated or the retrodiscal tissues compressed, the nociceptors send out signals and pain is perceived. The person cannot differentiate among the three structures and any nociceptors that are stimulated in any of these structures radiate signals that are perceived as joint pain.

Stimulation of the nociceptors creates inhibitory action in the muscles that move the mandible. Therefore, when pain is suddenly and unexpectedly felt, mandibular movement immediately ceases (*nociceptive reflex*). When chronic pain is felt, movement becomes limited and very deliberate (*protective co-contraction*).

5.2.1.1 Arthralgia

Arthralgia refers to pain of joint origin affected by jaw movement, function, or parafunction [23]. It is the second most common diagnosis for TMD pain (myalgia is the most common) and a common presenting complaint for many patients consulting maxillofacial surgeons, dentists, and otologists. Diagnosis is made on the basis of self-reported history of pain and on the basis of clinical examination. During examination, replication of this pain is done with provocation testing, either during mandibular movement or palpation of the TMJs. Sensitivity is 0.89, and specificity is 0.98.

Etiology Occlusal harmony should be checked for abnormal biting pattern and malocclusion that might increase the condylar pressure in the fossa. High points of restorations and abnormal teeth position causing occlusal interferences while chewing might cause uneven distribution of motion and stress between two joints leading to pain. Also, the development of pain is associated with jaw-clenching habits and nocturnal teeth grinding, as muscular signs of anxiety.

Clinical Findings History is positive for pain in the jaw, temple, in front of the ear, or in the ear with examiner confirmation of pain location in a masticatory structure in the past 30 days and pain altered with jaw movement, function, or parafunction.

Pain in joint is related to motion and thus discomfort may occur on extreme opening of the mouth, while chewing food, with clenching of the jaw, and grinding of teeth (bruxism), and with mandibular movement during talking. It is usually one-sided, but if bilateral, it is worse on one side than on the other [24]. Ear ache may be the patient's initial experience, the common auriculotemporal nerve supply for TMJ, external ear, and tympanic membrane accounting for discomfort in the TMJ being perceived as pain in the ear. Transient and painless clicking or snapping in joints occurs in some patients.

Confirmation of the pain location in the TMJ area includes at least one of the following tests:

- Palpation of the lateral pole (0.5 kg pressure) or around the lateral pole (1.0 kg pressure).
- Maximum unassisted or assisted opening, right or left lateral movements, or protrusive movements.

Examination of the TMJ elicits a report of familiar pain (defined as similar or like the pain the patient has experienced in the masticatory area palpated during the last 30 days). The joint on the affected side is sore, and motion there is restricted. The unaffected side allows its condyle to glide fully in the normal excursion of opening the jaw. The affected side is tethered, and this causes deviation of the chin to the affected side; hence, the grimace is seen when the patient opens the mouth wide [24]. Crepitus within the joint may or may not be found (*Crepitus* is the crunching or snapping sensation beneath the examiner's fingers caused by the grinding of the meniscus within the temporomandibular joint).

Imaging Radiographs of TMJ should be obtained in all cases of arthralgia. Bilateral views are required even though symptoms are one-sided. Examinations of the mouth in open and in closed positions are made, and the diagnostic information is readily obtained regarding condylar form and contour, the presence or absence of an adequate cartilaginous zone between the articular surfaces and the extent of condylar motion [24].

Management Treatment includes medication, occlusal and mechanical correction, and, finally arthroplasty. Useful medication includes drugs that modify the psychic state, specifically the tranquilizers such as meprobamate, chlordiazepoxide hydrochloride, or the antidepressant drugs such as diazepam, prescribed in conjunction with muscle relaxants. Occlusal corrections are done to remove interferences, if any during normal chewing. In addition to bringing about improvement in occlusion, a bite-plane appliance can be used to distract occlusal surfaces, permit mandibular gliding without interference from maxillary dentition, and hence relieve distressing forces in the TMJ. Arthroplasty is reserved for the patient who is not relieved by medication and occlusal balancing.

5.2.1.2 Arthritis

Arthritis is diagnosed when the TMJ is tender to palpation (as with arthralgia), but the TMJ also has clinical characteristics of inflammation or infection, for example, edema, erythema, and/or increased temperature [23]. It may arise in association with trauma. Associated symptoms can include occlusal changes such as ipsilateral posterior open bite if intra-articular swelling is present unilaterally. With this localized condition, there should be no history of systemic inflammatory disease. Sensitivity and specificity have not been established.

Besides a positive history for arthralgia, there is also swelling, redness, and/or increased temperature in front of the ear and dental occlusal changes resulting from articular inflammatory exudate (e.g., posterior open bite). Examination is positive for the same features. Unilateral or bilateral posterior open bite must not be attributable to other causes. The patient is negative for rheumatologic disease, including those in systemic arthritides. The pain is not better accounted for by another pain diagnosis.

Detailed discussion on arthritis and its various types is provided under the topic *"Joint Diseases"*.

5.2.2 Joint Disorders

5.2.2.1 Disc-Condyle Complex Disorders

Disorders of the disc-condyle complex (internal derangement of TMJ represents the very early stages of disc-condyle complex disorder) constitute a majority of TMJ disorders among the general population [4, 25]. Because disc displacement is so common among the general and TMD population, they may be usually considered as just a physiological accommodation without clinical significance. A review of the normal biomechanics of the disc-condyle complex would help to understand better the disc-condyle complex disorders better.

TMJ is capable of both rotational movements in the inferior compartment and translational movements in the superior compartment. During function, the lateral and the medial ligaments allow for free rotational movement of the mandibular condyle on the inferior surface of the interarticular disc, and the disc-condyle complex moves within the fossa and translates unimpeded along the posterior slope of the articular eminence. In addition, limited lateral movements are possible.

During all these normal TMJ movements, the interarticular disc is always positioned between the fossa/eminence and the condyle by the action of the superior lateral pterygoid muscle and by the uppermost elastic properties of the posterior attachment known as the posterior superior retrodiscal lamina of the retrodiscal tissue. Translation of the condyle occurs as a result of the action of the inferior lateral pterygoid muscle, which protrudes the mandible, acting in concert with other mandibular depressors of the infrahyoid and suprahyoid musculature.

Movement of the disc is also controlled by the superior, posterior retrodiscal lamina that acts passively to pull the disc posteriorly during opening as the condyle translates anteriorly. The superior lateral pterygoid muscle contracts eccentrically during closure to stabilize the disc against the distal slope of the articular eminence. Normal disc/condyle/fossa relationships are demonstrated in Fig. 5.1.

Disorders of the disc-condyle complex include anterior disc displacement with and without reduction. For a disc to displace, the retrodiscal tissue and the collateral ligaments must stretch, allowing the disc to move anteriorly [26], as seen in Fig. 5.2. Posteriorly displaced discs are very rare [27]. Once the disc is displaced, the part of the retrodiscal tissue located where the disc used to be is now subjected to repeated loading by the condyle, leading to adaptive changes and thereby providing most of the physical characteristics of the disc; this modified retrodisc is also referred to as *pseudodisc* [28]. The anteriorly displaced disc cannot retract back to its normal disc-condyle relationship, because the stretched ligaments neither shorten nor tighten later.

Wilkes Classification of Internal Derangements Disc-condyle disorders can be staged based on the characteristics of the pain, amount of mouth opening, disc location/condition, and altered joint anatomy, as observed from physical examination, MRI, and arthroscopy (Table 5.2) [29].

Disc Displacement with Reduction (Fig. 5.3)

A diagnosis of disc displacement with reduction is made when the patient presents with a history of a click or pop and it can be felt when the patient moves the mandible [4].

As the patient opens the mouth, the condyle translates forward and moves on to an intermediate zone of the disc (reduced position) that may cause the opening click or pop. As the mouth continues to open, the condyle continues to translate forward with the disc and remains in the

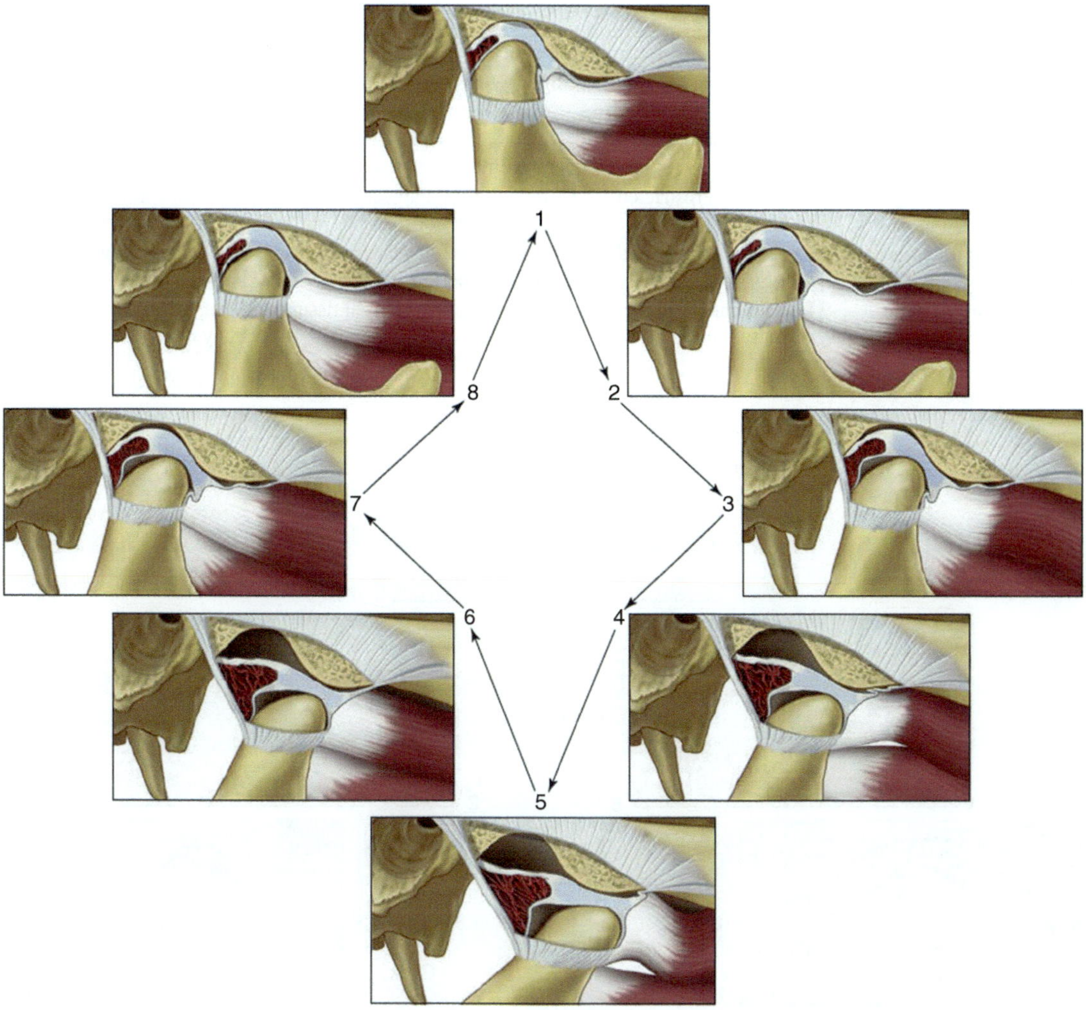

Fig. 5.1 Normal functional movement of the condyle and disc during the full range of opening and closing. Note that the disc is rotated posteriorly on the condyle as the condyle is translated out of the fossa. The closing movement is the exact opposite of opening. *(Reproduced with permission from: Okeson JP. Management of temporomandibular disorders and occlusion, 8th Ed, 2020, p. 19, Fig, 1.31, Copyright Elsevier, St. Louis)*

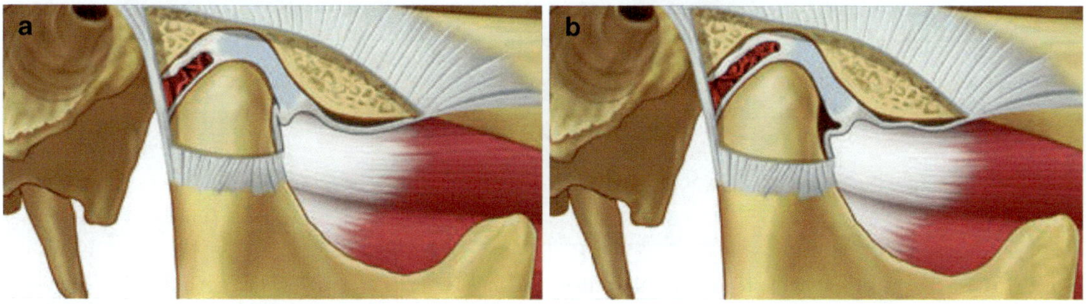

Fig. 5.2 Normal position of the disc on the condyle (**a**) Vs Functional displacement of the disc (**b**). Note that in B, the posterior border of the disc has been thinned and the discal and inferior retrodiscal ligaments are elongated, allowing activity of the superior lateral pterygoid to displace the disc anteriorly (and medially) *(Reproduced with permission from: Okeson JP. Management of temporomandibular disorders and occlusion, 8th Ed, 2020, p. 143, Fig, 8.7, Copyright Elsevier, St. Louis)*

Table 5.2 Staging of disc disorders based on Wilkes classification of internal derangements [29]

	Pain	Opening	Disc location	Anatomy
Stage I	Occasional painless click	No limitation	Slightly forward	Normal
Stage II	Painful click	Intermittent locking	Moderate anterior disc displacement with reduction	Disc deformity
Stage III	Pain during function	Locked and restricted motion	Complete disc displacement without reduction	Disc deformity/no bony or early changes
Stage IV	Continuous pain	Locked and restricted motion	Complete disc displacement without reduction	Moderate degenerative bony changes
Stage V	Severe pain	Locked and severely restricted motion	Perforation of retrodiscal tissue; possible disc perforation	Severe degenerative bony changes

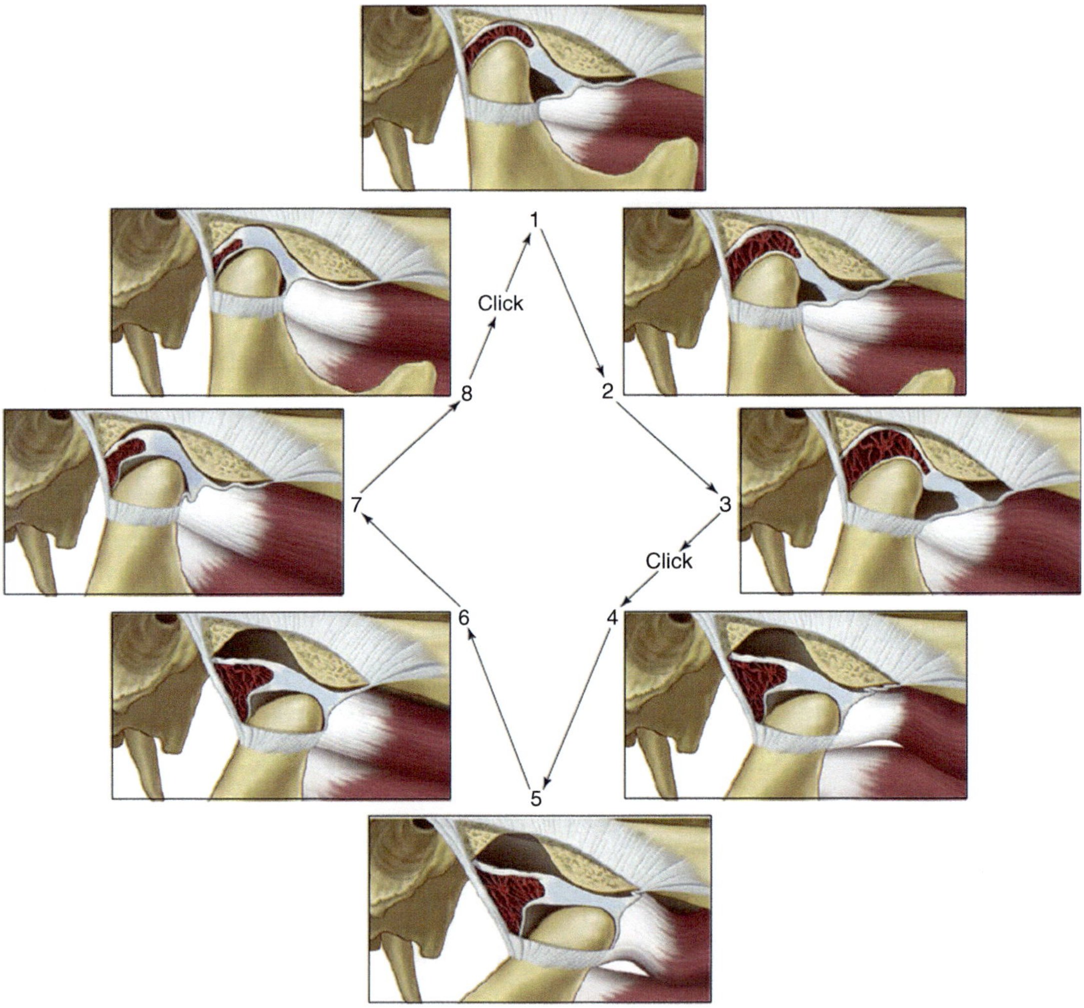

Fig. 5.3 Disc displacement with reduction. Note that during opening, the condyle passes over the posterior border of the disc onto the intermediate area of the disc, thus reducing the anterior displaced disc. This discal movement can lead to momentary mechanical catching or locking. When this is present, the condition is called disc displacement with intermittent locking. *(Reproduced with permission from: Okeson JP. Management of temporomandibular disorders and occlusion, 8th Ed, 2020, p. 148, Fig, 8.13, Copyright Elsevier, St. Louis)*

intermediate zone of the disc. As the patient closes the mouth, the condyle retrudes and moves back under the posterior band onto the retrodiscal tissue, which may again cause the closing click or pop. As the mouth continues to close, the condyle remains on the retrodiscal tissue. If both opening and closing click/pop is present, then the opening click/pop occurs at a wider opening than the closing click/pop.

The meaning of the word *"reduction"* here means "returning to its normal position." In the disc displacement with reduction, the disc-condyle alignment returns to its normal alignment during opening, once the condyle moves under the posterior band and onto the intermediate zone of the disc.

Using MRI as the reference standard, sensitivity is 0.34, and specificity is 0.92. Although not required for this diagnosis and without diagnostic validity, elimination of the opening and closing noise, if present, with protrusion can help corroborate this diagnosis.

History is positive for any noise(s) present with jaw movement or function, or patient report of joint sounds during the examination, in the last 30 days. Examination is positive for at least one of the following: Both an opening and closing clicking, popping, or snapping noise detected with palpation during at least one of three repetitions of jaw opening and closing; either an opening or closing clicking, popping, or snapping noise detected with palpation during at least one of three repetitions of opening and closing and a clicking, popping, and/or snapping noise detected with palpation during at least one of three repetitions of left lateral, right lateral, or protrusive movements.

When this diagnosis needs to be confirmed, then imaging analysis criteria, using TMJ MRI, are positive for both of the following: In the maximum intercuspal position, the posterior band of the disc is located anterior to the 11:30 position, and the intermediate zone of the disc is anterior to the condyle and the articular eminence; on full opening, the intermediate zone of the disc is positioned between the condyle and the articular eminence.

Since the vibration can travel through the mandible and be perceived in the contralateral TMJ and confuse the patient/practitioner as to which TMJ is generating the click/pop, the patient can be asked to start in maximum intercuspation and move laterally to the one side several times and then laterally to the other side several times. The click or pop is generated during the translation phase, and whichever condyle is translating when the noise is generated is generally the source of the noise.

Disc displacement with reduction generally does not progress to disc displacement without reduction unless the patient has pain or intermittent locking [30]. If the noise is the only complaint and is not an issue for the patient, then it is recommended the practitioner provide no therapy beyond education on how the TMJ works and inform the patient that TMJ noise is similar to noises in other joints of the body [31]. If the patient wants treatment for reduction of this TMJ noise, then a stabilization appliance can be advised to be worn at night.

Disc Displacement with Reduction with Intermittent Locking (Fig. 5.3)

A diagnosis of disc displacement with reduction with intermittent locking is made when the patient has a disc displacement with reduction and reports that occasionally the TMJ structure that normally causes the click blocks the condyle's movement, not allowing the mouth to obtain its normal opening. This lock suddenly occurs, may last for seconds to days, and then suddenly releases. When the limited opening occurs, a maneuver may be needed to unlock the TMJ.

History is positive for any noises present with jaw movement or function in the last 30 days or during the examination itself and report of intermittent locking with limited opening in the last 30 days or evidence of intermittent locking during clinical examination.

Examination is positive for disc displacement with reduction as defined above. When this diagnosis needs to be confirmed, the imaging analysis criteria are the same as for disc displacement with reduction. If locking occurs during imaging, then an imaging-based diagnosis of disc displacement without reduction will be rendered, and clinical confirmation of reversion to intermittent locking is needed.

If a click is associated with catching or intermittent locking, out of fear, this may progress to a continuous lock (disc displacement without reduction with limited opening). Traditional TMD therapies should be provided to eliminate the catch or intermittent lock and reduce the potential of it progressing to a continuous lock [30, 31].

Disc Displacement without Reduction with Limited Opening (Fig. 5.4)
A diagnosis of disc displacement without reduction with limited opening (*closed lock*) is made when a patient has a suddenly occurring continuous marked limited opening (less than 40 mm). The patients themselves are usually aware that the TMJ structure that normally caused the click

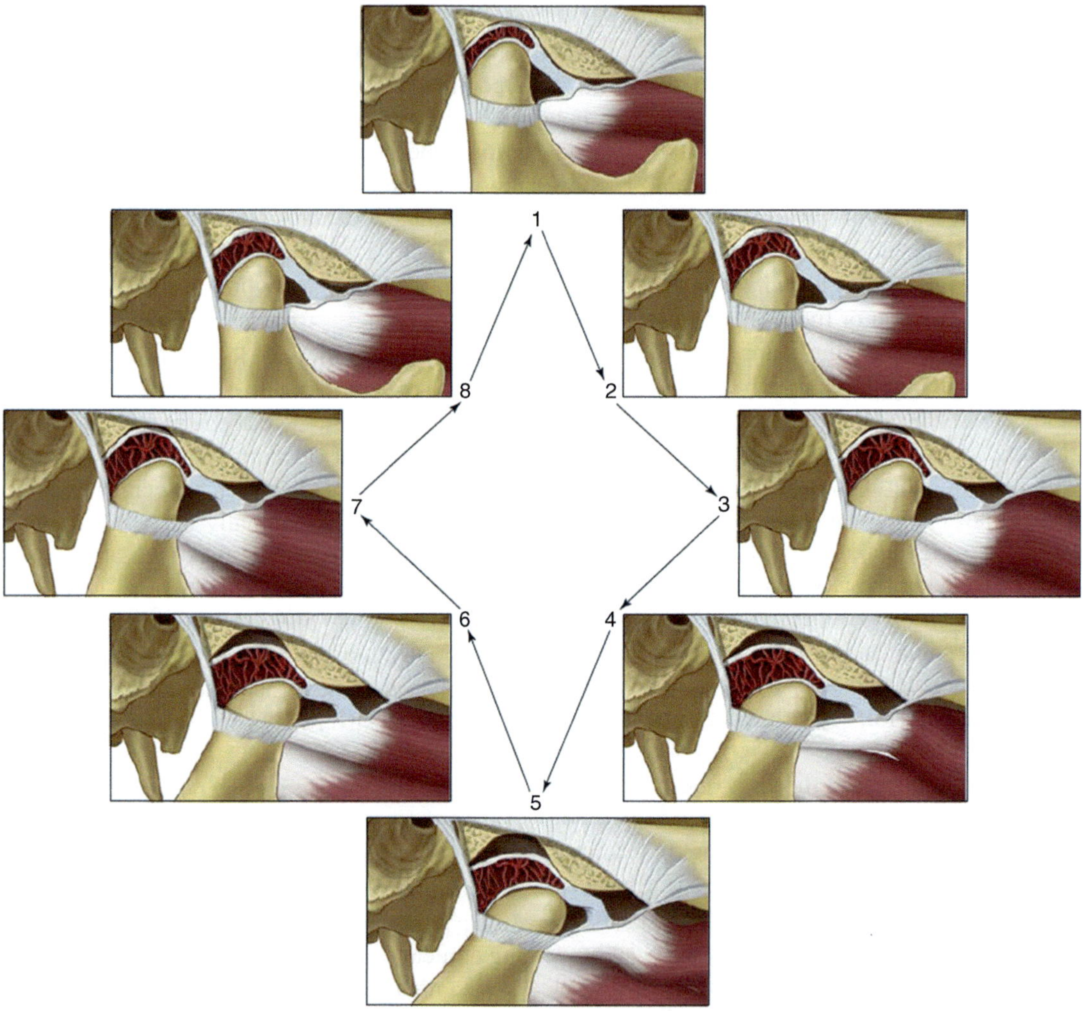

Fig. 5.4 Disc Displacement Without Reduction (*Closed lock*). Note that the condyle never assumes a normal relationship on the disc, but instead causes the disc to be maintained in front of the condyle. This condition limits the distance it can translate forward. *(Reproduced with permission from: Okeson JP. Management of temporomandibular disorders and occlusion, 8th Ed, 2020, p. 149, Fig, 8.14, Copyright Elsevier, St. Louis)*

is now blocking them from obtaining their normal opening. They may also report of their TMJ catching at that location or intermittently having had this problem (lasting seconds to days), which suddenly released and allowed them to regain their normal opening [32].

As the mouth opens, the condyle first rotates and then attempts to translate forward, but the condyle cannot slide under the disc's posterior band to reduce onto the intermediate zone of the disc. The translation is limited by the disc, and typically, the patient is initially able to open only between 20 and 30 mm.

As the patient attempts to open wider, the ipsilateral condylar translation is restricted by the disc while the contralateral condyle translates beyond that point, causing the anterior portion of the mandible to deviate to the affected side. Using MRI as the reference standard, sensitivity is 0.80, and specificity is 0.97.

History is positive for jaw lock or catch so that it will not open all the way and limitation in jaw opening is severe enough to interfere with the ability to eat. Examination reveals maximum assisted opening (passive stretch) < 40 mm including vertical incisal overlap. When this diagnosis needs to be confirmed, then imaging analysis criteria, using TMJ MRI, are positive for both of the following: In the maximum intercuspal position, the posterior band of the disc is located anterior to the 11:30 position, and the intermediate zone of the disc is anterior to the condyle and the articular eminence; on full opening, the intermediate zone of the disc is positioned anterior to the condyle.

Similar marked limited opening can also be seen in a muscle disorder, but the presentation is of gradual onset in the muscle disorder (hours to days). Patients with a lateral pterygoid spasm often present with immediate onset of a limited opening, in which the ipsilateral condyle is restricted in its ability to translate (owing to inability of the lateral pterygoid to contract rather than blocking of condylar translation by the disc), thus mimicking disc displacement without reduction with limited opening. To differentiate these two similar presentations, patients with a disc displacement without reduction with limited opening can generally put their teeth into maximum intercuspation without pain, whereas patients with a lateral pterygoid spasm usually relate that they cannot close or have significant pain when closing into maximum intercuspation.

If the sudden limited opening is due to external trauma, this limited opening may be from a muscle injury, TMJ arthralgia, fractured condyle, or other causes in addition to a disc displacement without reduction with limited opening.

Disc Displacement without Reduction without Limited Opening (Fig. 5.4)

A diagnosis of disc displacement without reduction without limited opening is made when the patient has a history of sudden-onset limited opening that gradually increased to 40 mm or greater. This suggests that the patient had a disc displacement without reduction with limited opening and over time, the retrodiscal tissue stretched and enabled the disc to move forward, thereby allowing the condyle to translate further and permitting the patient to open wider.

Using MRI as the reference standard, sensitivity is 0.54, and specificity is 0.79. History is the same as defined for disc displacement without reduction with limited opening. Examination reveals maximum assisted opening (passive stretch) > 40 mm including vertical incisal overlap. When this diagnosis needs to be confirmed, then imaging analysis criteria are the same as for disc displacement without reduction with limited opening.

Every time the individual attempts to open beyond the restriction, the condyle is pushed against the posterior side of the disc, creating a stretching force on the retrodiscal tissue. Similar repeated bumping of the posterior of the disc will usually sufficiently stretch the retrodiscal tissue over time, allowing the disc to move forward so that the normal translation and opening are eventually regained. This transition can occur immediately or stretch for varying periods of time, like days to years [33]. Some patients can move through this transition without treatment (some with minimal discomfort) whereas the rest seek treatment for opening that is not progressively increasing (Refer Chap. 15).

5.2.2.2 Hypomobility Disorders

Besides disc-condyle complex disorders, few other conditions can also cause restriction of the condyle's ability to translate or rotate, thereby resulting in TMJ not allowing the mandible to the normal range of motion.

Adherence/Adhesions

Adherence refers to a transient sticking of the articular surfaces. However, prolonged periods of adherence may result in true adhesions, wherein fibrous bands of connective tissue form between the articulating surfaces of the condyle or mandibular fossa, the disc, or surrounding tissues.

Adhesions occur secondary to prolonged static loading of the TMJ's surfaces (for example, jaw-clenching during sleep) [31], joint inflammation or hemarthrosis following macrotrauma or surgery of TMJ [31], or systemic conditions such as a polyarthritic disease, and are typically associated with disc disorders [34].

Usually, when the joint is loaded, weeping lubrication is exhausted and boundary lubrication takes over to prevent adhesions. But in case of prolonged static loading of the jaw, the boundary lubrication is not sufficient to compensate for the exhaustion of weeping lubrication, resulting in adherence of the disc either with the upper or lower joint compartment.

The patient presents with history of loss of jaw mobility and no history of TMJ clicking (historically to differentiate from disc displacement without reduction with limited opening).

Examination is positive for limited range of motion on opening, uncorrected deviation of the jaw to the affected side on opening if present unilaterally and marked limited laterotrusion to the contralateral side if unilateral. When this diagnosis needs to be confirmed, arthrography, MRI, or arthroscopy may show the presence of adhesions. Sensitivity and specificity have not been established.

Ankylosis

Ankylosis is the firm restriction of the condyle due to fibrous bands or osseous union within the TMJ, most commonly resulting from trauma to the mandible and/or TMJ. Pain is not usually associated with ankylosis. The involved condyle may not be able to translate and may have limited rotation, causing the patient to have a very limited opening, depending on the type and extent of the ankylosis [35]. Sensitivity and specificity have not been established for these disorders.

Clinical differential diagnosis of ankylosis should include pseudoankylosis of extra-articular pathology occurring in hypomobility of the joint due to coronoid hyperplasia (*Jacob disease*), fibrous adhesions between coronoid and tuberosity of maxilla or zygoma, depressed zygomatic arch fracture, dislocated zygomatic complex fracture, temporalis muscle scarring, or myositis ossificans.

Ankylosis of TMJ has been classified variously (Table 5.3) by Topazian [36]· Sawhney [37], and He et al. [38] based on parameters such as extension of ankylosis, type of ankylosis, and the like.

Etiopathology of Ankylosis

Trauma Most cases of ankylosis result from condylar injuries sustained before 10 years of age. In children, condylar cortical bone is thin with a broad condylar neck and rich subarticular inter-connecting vascular plexus and thus an intracapsular fracture leads to comminution and hemarthrosis of the condylar head, referred to as "*mushroom fracture.*" This results in organization of a fibro-osseous mass in a highly osteogenic environment, the immobility leading to ossification and consolidation of the mass, resulting in ankylosis. Ankylosis may also occur in trauma sustained during forceps delivery. Factors such as age of the patient, type of fracture, damage to the articular disc, and period of immobilization are implicated in the etiology of ankylosis following trauma.

Table 5.3 Classification of ankylosis of TMJ [36–38]

According to tissues involved and extent	• True ankylosis or pseudoankylosis • Extra-articular or intra-articular • Fibrous, bony, or fibro-osseous • Unilateral or bilateral • Partial or complete
Topazian	• **Stage I:** Ankylotic bone limited to condylar process • **Stage II:** Ankylotic bone extending to sigmoid notch • **Stage III:** Ankylotic bone extending to coronoid process
Sawhney	• **Type 1:** Extensive fibrous adhesions around joint, condyle present • **Type 2:** Bony fusion, especially at lateral articular surface, no fusion in the medial joint space • **Type 3:** Bony bridge between ascending ramus of mandible and temporal bone/zygomatic arch • **Type 4:** Joint is replaced by a mass of bone between ramus and skull base
He et al	• **A1:** Fibrous ankylosis without a bony component • **A2:** Bony ankylosis in lateral joint, residual condylar fragment is larger than 50% of contralateral normal condyle • **A3:** Similar to A2 but residual condylar fragment is smaller than 50% of contralateral normal condyle • **A4:** Complete bony ankylosis

Local Infections Otitis media, mastoiditis, osteomyelitis of temporal bone, parotid abscess, infratemporal or sub-masseteric space or parapharyngeal infections, furuncle, and actinomycosis.

Systemic Conditions Tuberculosis, meningitis, pharyngitis, tonsillitis, rubella, varicella, scarlet fever, gonococcal arthritis, and ankylosing spondylitis (the route of spread is hematogenous). The route of infection may either be hematogenous, contiguous, or by direct inoculation. The synovium with its high vascularity and lack of a limiting basement membrane is vulnerable to infection.

Arthritis/Inflammatory Conditions About 50% of cases in juvenile RA (*Still disease*), osteoarthritis, and ankylosing spondylitis.

Neoplasms Sarcoma, osteoma, and chondroma may result in degenerative, destructive, and inflammatory changes in disc followed by repair, leading to ankylosis.

Surgery Post-operative complication of TMJ surgery.

Fibrous Ankylosis

Fibrous ankylosis results when fibrotic tissue forms between the articulating surfaces of the condyle or mandibular fossa, the disc, or surrounding tissues [31]. There are no gross bony changes and no radiographic findings other than absence of ipsilateral condylar translation on opening.

Patient findings include history of progressive loss of jaw mobility; positive findings for severe limited range of motion on opening, uncorrected jaw deviation to the affected side, and marked limited laterotrusion to the contralateral side; and positive CT/CBCT imaging findings of decreased ipsilateral condylar translation on opening and a joint space between ipsilateral condyle and eminence.

Osseous Ankylosis

Bone formation between the condyle and fossa usually results in osseous ankylosis, and the patient has a more restricted opening than with fibrous ankylosis [31] or even complete immobility of the joint. The characteristic findings include radiographic evidence of bone proliferation with marked deflection to the affected side and marked limited laterotrusion to the contralateral side.

Patient findings include history of progressive loss of jaw mobility, positive examination findings such as absence of or severely limited jaw mobility with all movements and CT/CBCT being positive for imaging-based evidence of bone proliferation, with obliteration of part or all of the joint space (Refer Chap. 17).

5.2.2.3 Hypermobility Disorders

Hypermobility disorders include two types of TMJ dislocations in which the condyle is caught in front of the articular eminence, as a result of articular eminence obstructing the posterior movement of the disc-condyle unit, the disc obstructing the posterior movement of the condyle, or a combination of both [39]. Note that the condyle is frequently anterior to the eminence at full mouth opening and thus by itself is not a predictor of hypermobility disorders. The duration of dislocation may be momentary or prolonged. Pain may occur at the time of dislocation with residual pain following the episode.

Subluxation (Partial Dislocation)

This is a condition involving the disc-condyle complex and the articular eminence. A diagnosis of subluxation is made when in the open mouth position, the disc-condyle complex is positioned anterior to the articular eminence and is unable to return to normal closed-mouth position without a manipulative maneuver by the patient. Using history only, sensitivity is 0.98, and specificity is 1.00.

Causes of subluxation include looseness of the joint capsule and ligaments, seen in overextension injury, following dental procedures that require prolonged mouth opening or excessive yawning, extrinsic trauma (intubation, endoscopy), and connective tissue disorders (*Ehlers-Danlos syndrome, Marfan syndrome*).

History is positive for jaw locking or catching in a wide-open mouth position, even for a moment, so the patient could not close from the wide-open position in the last 30 days and for inability to close the mouth from wide opening without a self-maneuver. No examination findings are required.

Luxation (Dislocation, Open Lock)

This is a condition in which the disc-condyle complex is positioned anterior to the articular eminence and is unable to return to the fossa without a specific manipulative maneuver by a clinician. This is also referred to as *open lock.* Sensitivity and specificity have not been established.

Causes of luxation include post-traumatic capsular loosening, prolonged wide mouth opening, chronic subluxation, seizure disorders, Parkinsonism, drug-induced tardive dyskinesia (neuroleptics like phenothiazines), defects in the bony surface (shallow articular eminence), or a genetic predisposition (*Ehlers-Danlos syndrome, Marfan syndrome*).

Patient reports of inability to close from wide opening and that mouth closing can be achieved only with a specific mandibular maneuver by the clinician. Examination is positive for wide open mouth, protruded jaw position, and lateral position to the contralateral side if unilateral.

Types of Dislocation

- *Anterior dislocation*—Condyle moves anterior to the articulating eminence.
- *Anterolateral variant.*
- *Posterior variant*—Head of condyle is displaced posterior to its usual position, usually associated with fracture of base of skull or anterior wall of bony meatus.
- *Lateral dislocation*—Type 1, lateral subluxation, and type 2, a complete dislocation of the condyle if forced laterally and superiorly to the temporal fossa.
- *Superior dislocation*—Dislocation in the middle cranial fossa, associated with fracture of glenoid fossa.

When this diagnosis needs to be confirmed, CT/CBCT or MRI scans reveal that condyle is anterior to the articular eminence with the patient attempting to close the mouth (Refer Chap. 18).

5.2.3 Joint Diseases

5.2.3.1 Arthritides of the Temporomandibular Joint

Arthritis is the most frequent pathology of TMJ, affecting the synovium, cartilage, capsule, bursa, tendons, and condyles [23]. Arthritic diseases of variable etiology affect the TMJ, but present with similar signs and symptoms, and thus, careful history taking, physical examination, and radiographic evaluation are vital to arrive at the exact diagnosis. These TMJ arthritides are broadly divided into low and high inflammatory types (Table 5.4).

Low-inflammatory arthritic conditions begin in the matrix of the articular surface of the joint and further involve the subcondylar bone and capsule. The classic type of low-inflammatory arthritis is a degenerative joint disease like primary osteoarthritis that is due to age-related functional loading or trauma induced. These conditions never require invasive surgical intervention if they are managed appropriately in their early stages. Individuals with the low-inflammatory type have low leukocyte counts in the synovial fluid, laboratory findings are consistent with low-level inflammatory activity, and the affected joint shows focal degeneration on imaging.

High-inflammatory arthritic conditions primarily involve the synovial cells and joint bone. The classic example of high-inflammatory arthritis is rheumatoid arthritis. In all instances, the TMJ can be involved, and surgical intervention may be required to alleviate symptoms and correct associated functional and esthetic problems. Individuals with high-inflammatory-type arthritis have high leukocyte counts in the synovial fluid and show extensive and more diffuse degeneration of the involved joints on imaging.

Table 5.4 Classification of arthritic conditions affecting TMJ [3]

Low inflammatory arthritis	High inflammatory arthritis
• Traumatic arthritis • Degenerative arthritis – *Osteoarthritis* – *Osteoarthrosis*	• Inflammatory arthritis – *Rheumatoid arthritis (RA)* – *Juvenile RA* – *Psoriatic arthritis* – *Ankylosing spondylitis* – *Reiter syndrome* • Infectious arthritis – *Gonococcal arthritis* – *Syphilitic arthritis* – *Tuberculous arthritis* – *Lyme disease–associated arthritis* • Metabolic arthritis – *Gout* – *Pseudogout* • Systemic Arthritides: Associated with connective tissue diseases: *Systemic lupus erythematosus, scleroderma, chronic inflammatory bowel disease, reflex sympathetic dystrophy, and sarcoidosis.*

Traumatic Arthritis

Frequently, arthritis occurs secondary to acute or chronic trauma, most cases reporting history of whiplash injuries in road traffic accidents. Because of the chronic sequelae, careful consideration must be given soon after the injuries in order to grasp the intra-articular pathological condition as well as to avail the therapeutic options.

Traumatic arthritis results from the cascade of events set off by the release of pro-inflammatory cytokines, as an immediate intra-articular response of the joint tissues to single or repetitive episodes of acute trauma. This inflammatory response depends upon the magnitude of the trauma sustained by the joint tissues and the biomechanical pattern of trauma and can vary from edema, synovitis, and hemarthrosis to condylar fractures. The evoked immune response can further result in fibrous adhesion of the condyle to glenoid fossa or can lead to degenerative joint disorders from the persistent inflammation caused by failure of repair mechanisms [40].

- *Minor trauma*—Compression/shearing retrodiscal tissue; dislocation of the disc.
- *Moderate trauma*—Damage to the synovial lining → hemarthrosis + inflammatory response → fibrosis, adhesions, fibrous ankylosis *(Growth abnormalities in children).*
- *Severe trauma*—Damage to articular surfaces/subchondral bone → Degenerative disease.

Clinical Findings Patients present with severe arthralgia, both at rest and during mandibular movements, limited mouth opening (less than 20 mm), tenderness of the joint, and bleeding in the superior joint space. Patients might complain of persistent headache and sometimes pain in the cervical region with or without movement. Prognosis is poor in patients with traumatic arthritis, with the development of post-traumatic syndrome (sometimes psychological), with continuous pain in the joint area accompanied by recurrent headache.

Imaging Edema and swelling can cause an increase in the thickness of the intracapsular and capsular structures, seen radiographically as an increased distance between the roof of the glenoid fossa and the condylar surface in the closed-mouth position. Changes following severe trauma may be observed as bony ankylosis or be similar to changes seen in degenerative joint disease.

Management NSAIDS can be used for patients with post-traumatic syndrome, along with counselling and reassurance to prevent post-traumatic syndrome. Diet restrictions and physiotherapy are implicated as conservative management. Arthroscopic lysis, lavage, synovectomy and debridement of fibrous adhesions are implicated as other treatment modalities [41].

Osteoarthritis

Osteoarthritis (OA), classified as a degenerative joint disease, is a low inflammatory arthritic condition, either primary or secondary to trauma or other acute or chronic overload situations, characterized by deterioration and abrasion of articular tissue that becomes soft or frayed or thinned and resulting in eburnation of subcondylar bone or outgrowths of marginal osteophytes due to overload of the remodelling mechanism. The process accelerates as proteoglycan depletion, collagen fiber network disintegration, and fatty degeneration weaken the functional capacity of the articular cartilage. Most commonly, hips, spine, and knees, the weight bearing joints, are affected. Metabolic, genetic, and systemic causes can also affect the course of disease.

Clinical Findings OA affecting the TMJ is not uncommon and is seen more in females, above 40 years of age. The most common cause for OA of TMJ is overloading of the articular structures, followed by traumatic injury and physical stress. When the precise cause of the osteoarthritis can be identified such as trauma, hypermobility, or internal derangement and is seen in older population, the condition is referred to as *secondary osteoarthritis*. When the cause of the arthritic condition is idiopathic or associated with wear and tear and is seen in younger population, it is referred to as *primary osteoarthritis*.

Osteoarthritis of TMJ is gradual in onset. The patient history is positive for joint noises present with jaw movement or function in the past 30 days duration and for noises reported during the examination. The common presenting complaints include unilateral joint pain that is aggravated by mandibular movement, and worsening in the late afternoon or evening hours. Secondary central excitatory effects are frequently present. Examination is positive for crepitus detected with palpation during at least one of the following—maximum unassisted opening, maximum assisted opening, right or left lateral movements, or protrusive movements. Usual findings also include tenderness over the joint and associated muscles, limited mandibular opening, palpable swelling over the joint, and increase in the pain upon lateral palpation of the condyle or manual loading of the joint.

Imaging TMJ radiographs reveal structural changes in the subarticular bone of the condyle or fossa. There can be flattening and erosive changes on the articular surfaces and osteophytes can be seen. CT scan findings include subchondral sclerosis in mandibular condyle, condylar flattening and marginal lipping, cortical erosion, osteophyte formation, and narrowing of joint space. Another characteristic finding is the presence of subchondral bone cysts (*Ely cysts*), these pseudo cysts representing areas of degeneration, containing fibrous tissue, granulation tissue, and osteoid.

Because a patient may have symptoms for as long as 6 months before there is enough demineralization of bone to show up radiographically, imaging is not helpful in early cases of osteoarthritis. The early changes in the synovial membrane, such as synovial intima hyperplasia, cell hypertrophy with subsequent loss of fibrous material in the intima matrix, and articular cartilage are only detectable with biopsy and arthroscopy.

Management Management depends on its severity. The primary aim is removing the causative factor, so attempt is taken to reduce the functional loading. Positioning appliance therapy can be used to correct condyle-disc relationship and stabilization appliance can be used to correct hyperactive muscles. Parafunctional habits should be taken in consideration and discouraged. The various treatment options include non-invasive modalities (medications), minimally invasive modalities (intra-articular injections, arthrocentesis, arthroscopic surgery), invasive surgical modalities (bone and joint procedures, autogenous/allogenous hemiarthroplasty), and salvage procedures (total joint reconstruction) [42].

Table 5.5 presents the classification of osteoarthritis based on symptoms, signs, and imaging with management options [43, 44].

Osteoarthrosis

Osteoarthrosis is a multifactorial disease associated with TMJ overloading. Though it is synonymous with osteoarthritis in medical orthopedic literature [42], in dental TMJ literature, it has been recently identified as a chronic low inflammatory degenerative disease with progressive loss of articular cartilage in the TMJ resulting from an imbalance between predominantly chondrocyte-controlled reparative and degradative processes.

As with osteoarthritis, the cause of osteoarthrosis is joint overloading. When joint loading is mild, body tries to adapt by bony remodelling. If functional demands exceed adaptability, osteoarthritis begins. Once the adaptive process has caught up to the functional demands, osteoarthrosis remains [45].

Patient generally presents with no symptoms. The past history may reveal a period of time when symptoms were present (osteoarthritis) that can only be confirmed through radiographs. Crepitation is a common finding. In the absence of clinical symptoms like joint pain, treatment of this arthritides is contraindicated. The only treatment that may need to be considered is if the bony changes in the condyle have been significant enough to alter the occlusal condition and, in such cases, dental therapy may need to be considered.

Rheumatoid Arthritis

Rheumatoid arthritis (RA) is a chronic non-suppurative disease of unknown etiology which

Table 5.5 Classification of osteoarthritis [3, 43, 44]

Stage	Symptoms	Signs	Imaging	Management options
I Early disease	Joint/muscle pain Limited function Crepitus	Little or no occlusal or facial aesthetic changes	Mild to moderate erosive changes of condyle/fossa/eminence	Non-invasive (1°) Minimally invasive (2°)
II Arrested disease	Little or no joint pain Muscle pain Some joint dysfunction Crepitus	Class II malocclusion Apertognathia	Flattened condyle/eminence	Bone and joint (1°) Salvage (2°)
III Advanced disease	Joint/muscle pain Loss of function ± Crepitus Progressive retrognathia	High-angle class II malocclusion Apertognathia Developing fibrosis/ankylosis	Gross erosive changes Loss of condyle and eminence height Ankylosis Hypertrophy of coronoid	Salvage (1°)

primarily affects articular structures such as synovial membrane, capsule, tendon, sheath, and ligaments and secondarily involves the articular cartilages and subchondral bone [46]. It is believed that the inflammation of the synovial membranes extends into surrounding connective tissues and articular surfaces (this reactive macrophage laden fibroblastic proliferation from the synovium that extends to the joint surface is called *pannus*), which then become thickened and tender. The cells of the synovial membrane express enzymes that cause destruction of the articular surface, eventually leading to a fibrous ankylosis.

Clinical Findings RA is a polyarticular disease, with a peak onset at 40–60 years of age and a slight female predilection. Systemic weight loss, fever, and fatigue are the first presentation of RA patients, who frequently manifest chronic episodic exacerbations and remissions. To ensure uniformity in investigational and epidemiologic studies, the American College of Rheumatology has developed classification criteria for RA that is presented in Table 5.6 [47].

Clinical TMJ involvement is found in 4–80% of RA patients [48], is usually bilateral in 34% to 75% of those patients, and TMJ may not be the first joint to be affected. The most common clinical symptom of TMJ involvement is deep, dull preauricular pain during function, that may be referred to temporal region and angle of the mandible. Other features include swelling, muscle tenderness with decreased bite force, limited range of motion, crepitation or clicking, and morning joint stiffness. In the later stages, degeneration of the synovial membrane, resorption of condylar bone, and formation of scar tissue between the joint surfaces and within the capsule might lead to severe disability.

Retardation of mandibular growth causing facial deformity and sometimes ankylosis can occur in children. A characteristic feature of advanced RA of TMJ is the development of a progressive class II malocclusion and anterior open bite deformity with impairment of chewing and phonation. This deformity is caused by loss of normal ramus height secondary to destruction of the mandibular condyles.

Table 5.6 Revised criteria for the classification of rheumatoid arthritis, ARA, 1987 [47]

1. Morning stiffness (in/around joints, at least 1 hour before maximal improvement)
2. Arthritis (swelling) of 3 or more joint areas (observed by a physician)
3. Symmetric arthritis (swelling, NOT bony overgrowth)
4. Arthritis of hand joints (wrists, MCPs, or PIPs)
5. Rheumatoid nodules
6. Rheumatoid factor (serum)
7. Radiographic changes (erosions and/or periarticular osteopenia in hand/wrist joints)
Requirements
• ≥ 4 of the above 7 criteria
• Criteria 1–4 must have been present for at least 6 weeks.
Approximately 50% to 75% of patients with rheumatoid arthritis have involvement of the temporomandibular joint during the course of the disease [47]

Imaging/Investigations Early stages show no radiographic changes. With progression of the disease, articular surface of the condyle is destroyed and the joint space is obliterated resulting in anterior open bite. Anteroposterior erosion of the condyle might result in a "*sharpened pencil appearance.*" Other changes observed include subcortical pseudocyst, flattening of the articular eminence, and erosion of glenoid fossa.

Based on the MRI findings, Kretapirom et al. categorized four types of osseous changes in the condyle [46]:

- *Type I:* Abnormal signal intensity of the condylar bone marrow without erosion or resorption.
- *Type II:* Surface erosion of the condylar cortex.
- *Type III:* Bone resorption extending within half of the condylar head.
- *Type IV:* Bone resorption involving more than half of the condylar head.

Laboratory findings include positive rheumatoid factor (RF), antinuclear antibodies (ANA), human leukocyte antigens (HLA) Dw5 and DRw, elevated ESR, decrease in serum albumin, and synovial aspirate revealing cloudy, reduced viscosity, with a white cell blood count >20,000.

Management Disease management through NSAIDs, short-term steroids, soft diet, physical therapy, immunosuppressive drugs (rheumatology referral) and management of structural deformity by TMJ and orthognathic surgery.

Osteoarthritis Vs Rheumatoid Arthritis

Table 5.7 presents the significant differences between osteoarthritis and rheumatoid arthritis affecting the TMJ [49].

Table 5.7 Comparison between osteoarthritis and rheumatoid arthritis [49]

	Osteoarthritis	Rheumatoid Arthritis
Age	Later in life	Anytime in life
Speed of onset	Slow, over years	Relatively rapid, weeks to months
Prevalence of TMJ involvement	8–16%	50%
Joint symptoms	Painful but little or no swelling	Painful, swollen, and stiff
Common joint involvement	Random; single joint involvement common	Symmetric joint involvement; multiple joint involvement common
Morning stiffness	< 1 hour	> 1 hour
Systemic effects	Not present	Present

Juvenile Idiopathic Arthritis

Juvenile idiopathic arthritis (JIA or Juvenile RA or Still disease) is a rheumatic disease of childhood that presents with no symptoms or very mild symptoms in most cases. Thus, it is important to screen for clinical symptoms or signs such as pain at chewing, clicking at TMJ, or the child avoiding chewable food.

JIA starts before 16 years of age, with as high as 87% involvement of TMJ (TMJ may be the only joint involved with JIA) [50]. The initial findings may be limited range of motion and asymmetry of the mandible from abnormal craniofacial growth. Bilateral TMJ involvement may result in progressive Class II malocclusion and apertognathia due to loss of ramal height secondary to condylar destruction (bird face deformity) and ankylosis later. Further, the condition may interfere with proper oral hygiene, leading to dental caries.

Based on the clinical expression at the onset and the first 6 months of the disease, three types have been described: *oligoarticular/pauciarticular* (four or fewer involved joints), *polyarticular* (five or more involved joints), and *systemic* (presence of arthritis and severe systemic involvement).

Imaging reveals condylar cortical bone erosion, disc thinning, loss of ramus height, and increased antegonial notching in late stages. Laboratory findings include positive RF in 20% of patients, ANA in 60–80% of patients, and elevated ESR. Management is similar to rheumatoid arthritis.

Psoriatic Arthritis

Psoriasis is a chronic, often pruritic, skin disease. About 5–10% of the psoriatic population present with psoriatic arthritis (PA), which is diagnosed based on the triad of psoriasis, radiological erosive polyarthritis, and a negative serological test for rheumatoid factor [51]. This distinction from rheumatoid arthritis is further marked by the simultaneous occurrence of both joint and skin manifestations in many instances, by characteristic radiological appearances, and by the absence of subcutaneous nodules. A genetic predisposition and HLA association is also observed.

Clinical Findings PA usually occurs between third and fourth decade of life, with a slight male predilection. Based on the presence of different clinical features, four distinct patterns of PA are recognized [52]:

- Arthritis affecting mostly the distal interphalangeal joints.
- Severe arthritis affecting single or multiple joint, with widespread bone destruction and ankylosis.
- Seronegative polyarthritis that may be difficult to distinguish from seronegative RA.
- Arthritis that is characterized by the presence of spondylitis and peripheral joint involvement and the presence of the HLA-B27 antigen.

PA of TMJ usually has a sudden onset, often following minor trauma. If a patient is likely to have PA of the TMJ, then a careful examination of the nails, scalp, and umbilicus may help in the diagnosis as pitting and oncolysis of nails are evident in many patients. Signs and symptoms of TMJ disease include deviation of the mandible from the midline during opening and closing movements, limitation of opening, subjective stiffness of the joint, joint crepitus on palpation, audible or palpable clicking of the joint detected objectively, subjective joint clicking, pain in the joint itself, referred pain or tenderness of the joint on biting or chewing, tenderness of the joint, joint capsule or muscles of mastication detected by palpation while the patient was performing the full range of mandibular movements, past history of, or presence of, soft-tissue swelling external to the temporomandibular joint, and/or subluxation.

Imaging Radiographic changes include erosion, osteoporosis, and narrowing of joint space, but are nonspecific.

Management The primary goal in management of PA affecting TMJ is to relieve the pain along with counselling and reassurance emphasizing the benign nature of the disease. In the initial stage, rest and use of NSAIDS is recommended. Other treatment modalities include physiotherapy, steroids (topical/systemic) and surgical joint replacement.

Ankylosing Spondylitis

Ankylosing spondylitis (AS, seronegative spondylitis, *Bechterew disease*, *Marie-Strumpell disease*) is a chronic inflammatory disorder affecting predominantly the axial skeleton, although peripheral joint involvement may be a significant feature. The peripheral joints that are affected include the hips, shoulders, knees, hands, wrists, and TMJ (seen in later stages with a frequency of 11% to 35%) [53] AS is nearly 10 times more common in male patients, with an age of onset between the first and fourth decades of life, and is associated with HLA-B27 antigens.

Clinical Findings Flexion deformity of the neck and fixed rigidity of the cervical spine are the most common presentation, with atlantoaxial subluxation seen in few patients. AS causes debilitating postural changes with forward thrusting of the head. When AS affects the vertebral column, the patient complains of back pain and stiffness during morning hours which generally increases during exercise and movements. In the later stages, lumbar lordosis and lumbar kyphosis might occur, with pain in any change in posture. Pain in heel and plantar pain have also been reported [54].

Involvement of TMJ in AS gives rise to few serious symptoms until gross restriction of jaw movement occurs, in contrast to the acute pain and tenderness occurring in rheumatoid arthritis that usually resolves spontaneously and only rarely gives rise to permanent restriction of jaw opening. Asymptomatic or unilateral involvement is seen in nearly half of the patients. Pain, stiffness, and limited mouth opening are the common symptoms of AS in TMJ. Clicking sounds are not common in this disease.

TMJ pathology in AS can be explained by destruction of the capsular/disc attachment, resulting in internal derangement and subsequent degenerative joint disease or by direct breakdown of the articular surfaces due to primary synovitis.

Imaging Non-specific radiographic changes are observed at the later stages of the disease and include joint space narrowing, erosions, reduced mobility, osteophyte formation, excessive sclerosis, and extensive erosion.

AS is negative for Rheumatoid factor and is positive for HLA-B27 antigen. Treatment includes NSAIDs, physical therapy, steroids, disease-modifying drugs.

Reiter Syndrome

Reiter syndrome is a triad of arthritis *(cannot climb)*, conjunctivitis/uveitis *(cannot see)*, and urethritis *(cannot pee)* that occurs as a reactive disease within 2–6 weeks of an episode of genitourinary (chlamydia, gonorrhea) or gastrointestinal infection (*Salmonella, Shigella*).

Clinical Findings Reiter syndrome has a male predominance, is of acute onset, and is associated with inflammatory eye lesions, balanitis, oral ulcers, and keratodermatitis. A classic Reiter syndrome patient presents with a swollen knee or a swollen interphalangeal joint with or without Achilles tendinitis. There may be diffuse swelling of fingers and toes (sausage digits) [55]. There also may be associated low-back pain with involvement of the SI joints, making it difficult to distinguish it at times from ankylosing spondylitis. When TMJ is affected, symptoms like tenderness, erythema, and warmth over the joint are evident which generally have acute onset and asymmetrical presentation.

Imaging In Reiter syndrome, radiologic changes are often absent or minimal. Osteoporosis, periosteal new bone formation, erosive changes at the site of ligamentous insertion, and occasionally a destructive arthropathy may be seen. Sacroiliitis with or without spondylitis may be present. The commonest change is that of plantar spurs at the site of plantar fasciitis.

Treatment Treatment for Reiter syndrome involves anti-inflammatory medications and intra-articular steroid injections as well as physical therapy. Systemic oral steroids have been shown to be of minimal benefit. Topical steroids are used for the skin lesions and also receommended for conjunctivitis.

Septic (Infectious) Arthritis

Septic arthritis of TMJ is an infrequently reported rare disease exclusively seen in adults. A mortality rate of 12% has been reported for cases of septic arthritis in whole body joints, and significant hypofunction of the affected joint is observed in up to 75% of cases. Septic arthritis of TMJ is known to result in significant morbidity if diagnosis is delayed.

Etiopathogenesis Common causative organisms of septic arthritis include *Staphylococcus aureus*, *Neisseria*, *Haemophilus influenzae*, and *Streptococcus*. Predisposing factors for septic arthritis might be local (blunt trauma, burn wounds, drug abuse, iatrogenic causes) or generalized (systemic and autoimmune diseases like rheumatoid arthritis, diabetes, hypogammaglobulinemia or infections like gonorrhea, syphilis, tuberculosis, or actinomycosis). Risk factors can also include prolonged use of systemic steroids and sexually transmitted diseases. AIDS patients are also prone to septic arthritis (usually a bacterial or fungal cause).

The routes of infection and possible pathogenic mechanisms for septic arthritis are presented in Fig. 5.5 [56]. The causative microorganism usually reaches the joint via hematogenous seeding, colonizes the synovial membrane, produces an acute inflammatory response, and reaches the synovial fluid. Pro-inflammatory cytokines are produced in response to the bacterial insult, intensifying the inflammatory response. The by-products of inflammation can rapidly destroy the synovial membrane and collagen matrix, thus inhibiting cartilage synthesis. As the infection progresses, signs of inflammation (such as redness and edema) may appear.

Less commonly, the pathogen enters the joint by local spread, through a skin lesion or from an adjacent osteomyelitis, resulting in compression of intra-articular vessels by the inflammatory infiltrate and reduction of circulation to the cartilage and subchondral bone by the pus. Further, the pressure developed within the joint cavity eventually induces necrosis of the articular structures.

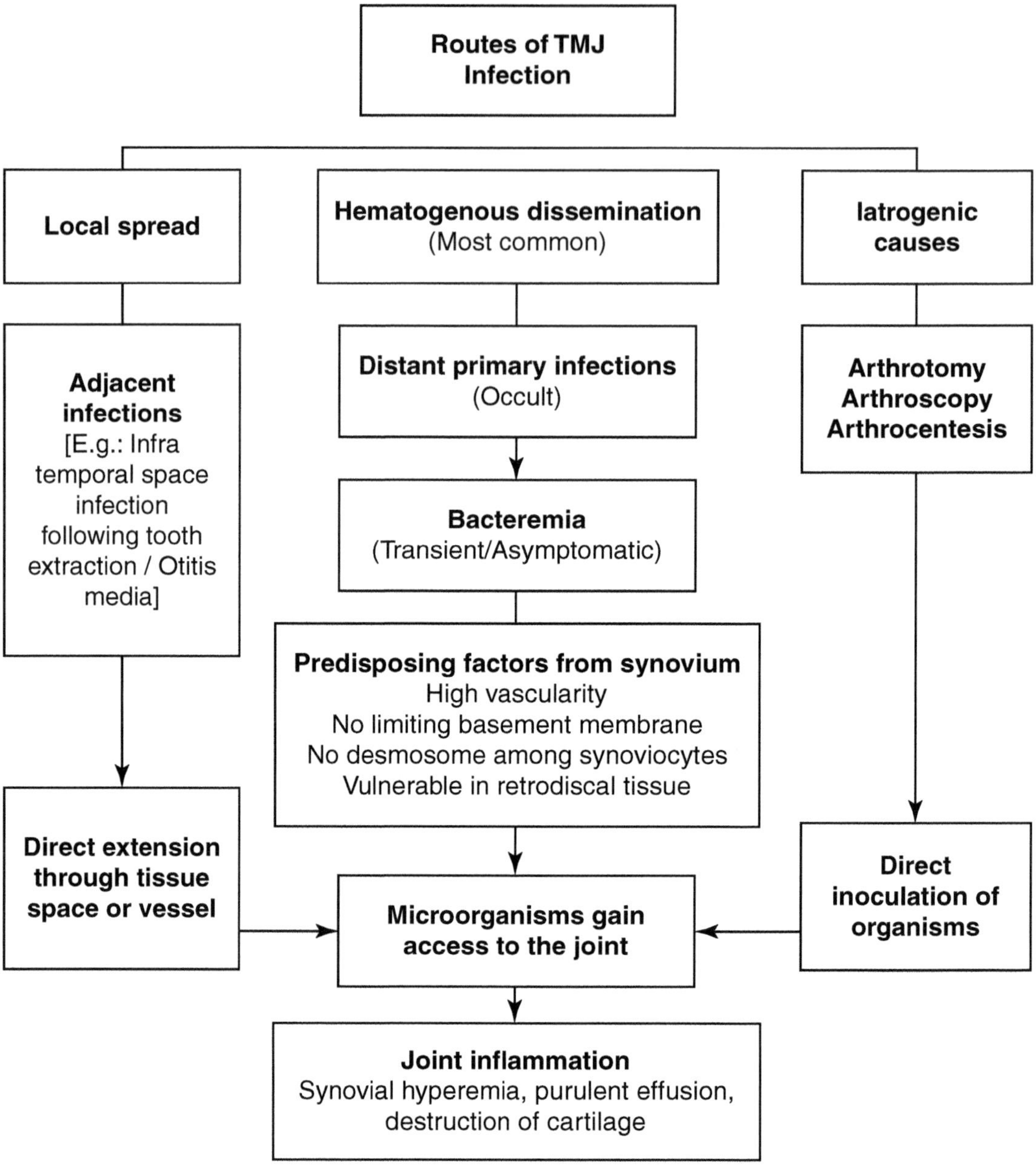

Fig. 5.5 Septic arthritis of TMJ. Routes of infection and possible pathogenic mechanisms *(Adapted from: Cai XY* et al. *Septic arthritis of the temporomandibular joint: a retrospective review of 40 cases. J Oral Maxillofac Surg 2010; 68(4): 731–8)*

Clinical Features Systemic involvement results in fever, rash, malaise, lymphadenopathy, hepatosplenomegaly, pericarditis, pleuritis, and arthritis (intense pain not relieved by rest). The signs and symptoms usually persist for two weeks and may regress thereafter, depending on the virulence of the causative agent and the patient's immune status. The large joints are more often involved, with the knees and hip most commonly affected [57].

In septic arthritis of TMJ, the common clinical manifestations are an erythematous, warm, swollen preauricular region, pain, trismus, regional lymphadenopathy, malocclusion with ipsilateral posterior open bite, limited maximum mouth opening, and contralateral mandible deviation which results from the increased joint fluid presenting as fluctuation in the joint region. In chronic cases, ankylosis of joint may occur resulting in facial asymmetry and might also cause complete destruction of condyle and bone.

Imaging/Investigations OPG can depict joint space widening caused by inflammatory exudates and purulence. However, bony changes do not often occur in the acute phase of infection, and CT scanning is more sensitive in detecting early bony changes [57] such as articular space widening, cellulitis, osteomyelitis, and ankylosis. MRI allows for early detection of increased joint effusion on T2-weighted images and evaluation of the cartilaginous disc and adjacent soft tissues. Technetium-99 phosphate bone scans have low specificity, but high sensitivity for septic arthritis. A negative technetium-99 scan virtually eliminates septic arthritis from the differential diagnosis.

Laboratory findings include increased serum leukocyte count and increased level of C-reactive protein. FNAC should always be performed and gram stain and culture sensitivity test should be done. In 62% of the positive cases of septic arthritis, the isolated organism is *Staphylococcus aureus*.

Management Treatment of TMJ septic arthritis includes irrigation and drainage, antibiotic therapy, and joint rest [58].

- Positive results have been reported from arthrocentesis, for irrigation and drainage of the joint space. In cases where the infection enters the joint by local spread, a conventional submandibular incision is preferable.
- Antibiotic therapy should be initiated immediately after joint fluid aspiration is performed. During the acute phase of the infection, the joint should be rested.
- Joint rest helps to decrease the amount of synovial fluid and inflammatory response and therefore helps minimize proteolytic joint damage. Typically, joint rest consists of a soft diet and restricted range of motion. Joint exercises designed to help the patient open and close the mouth should be started after the acute phase of infection.

Metabolic Arthritis

Two major types of metabolic arthritis affecting the TMJ are gout and pseudogout, two common crystal-induced arthropathies.

Clinical Findings Gout is caused by the deposition of monosodium urate monohydrate crystals in the joints or in soft tissues leading to acute inflammation, with associated pain, impaired movement of the affected joint, and hyperuricemia [59]. Gouty arthritis usually affects men over 40 years of age, with definite genetic predisposition and family prevalence.

The four phases of gout include [60] asymptomatic hyperuricemia (serum urate concentration greater than 416 mmol/l), acute joint arthritis, intercritical gout, and chronic tophaceous gout. Tophaceous deposits of urate crystals commonly occur in the synovium, subchondral bone, and remote subcutaneous and tendinous tissues. Commonly, the small joints of the feet and hands, wrists, elbows and knees are involved. Involvement of the proximal joints is unusual. Only a few cases of isolated TMJ involvement and destruction have been reported. Clinical presentation of TMJ gout includes mild pain, limited joint movements, sometimes warm and tender swelling over the area, and joint sounds.

Pseudogout is caused by calcium pyrophosphate crystals and is more accurately termed calcium pyrophosphate disease and is characterized by pain, stiffness, tenderness, redness, warmth, and swelling in joints. Most commonly affected joints are knees, hips, shoulders, elbow, finger, and ankles and TMJ is rarely affected. Pseudogout can occur in association with diabetes mellitus and hyperthyroidism [61].

Imaging/Investigations Radiographic changes are not characteristic and in the late stages of the disease, TMJ shows enlargement and irregularity of the condylar head. CT scan shows synovial swelling around the TMJ, calcified loose bodies, articular sclerosis, and erosions. Blood investigations and FNAC are recommended. The aspirated fluid is opalescent and contains urate crystals when examined under polarizing microscope. Leukocytosis and elevated ESR are commonly found.

Systemic Arthritides Associated with Connective Tissue Diseases

Systemic Lupus Erythematosus (SLE) SLE is a chronic autoimmune multisystem disease usually affecting the brain and peripheral nervous system, skin, joints, kidneys, lungs, serous membranes, and components of the blood. Symmetric polyarthritis, usually involving the fingers, knees, and wrists is a common feature in SLE patients. Few cases of TMJ involvement in SLE have been reported [62, 63].

Scleroderma Progressive systemic sclerosis is a generalized connective tissue disorder that involves the skin (scleroderma) and organs such as heart, lung, kidneys, and gastrointestinal tract. Besides oral and dental features of systemic sclerosis reported such as limited mouth opening, mucogingival problems, xerostomia, telangiectasia, increased periodontal ligament width, and osseous resorption of the mandible, TMJ dysfunction has also been reported [64].

Mixed Connective Tissue Disease (MCTD) A distinct rheumatoid disease whose features overlap with a number of different connective tissue diseases. Clinical presentation of MTCD includes fatigue, myalgia, arthralgia, and Raynaud phenomenon, with joint pain and stiffness being present in most of the cases. These features of MTCD manifest concurrently with the features of diseases such as SLE, scleroderma, polymyositis, dermatomyositis, and RA. Symptoms and signs of TMDs have been widely reported in MTCD patients [65].

Sjögren Syndrome (SS) A systemic autoimmune disease characterized by xerostomia and dry eyes, resulting from an autoimmune process that often may affect other organs, such as neural systems, skin, mucosa, lungs, and kidneys. SS also can develop as a secondary phenomenon, in which the sicca symptoms are associated with RA, SLE, or scleroderma. SS is sometimes associated with polyarthritis, and thus the TMJ may also be affected [63].

5.2.3.2 Condylysis (Idiopathic Condylar Resorption)

Condylysis is a rare idiopathic osseous degeneration, probably a severe degenerative joint disorder associated with low estrogen levels, leading to the loss of condylar height and a progressive anterior open bite. This condition occurs spontaneously, usually bilateral, in adolescent females, with or without the presence of pain or joint sounds. Dental occlusal changes may be positive, in the early stages. Sensitivity and specificity have not been established.

History is positive for progressive dental occlusal changes. Examination is positive for anterior open bite and progressive dental occlusal changes with either occlusal facets that cannot be approximated or change in sequential occlusal measurement over time based on overbite, overjet, or intercuspal contacts. Imaging includes CT/CBCT evidence of partial or total condylar resorption or change with sequential imaging over time from lateral cephalometric images, which may include clockwise mandibular rotation, increase in mandibular plane angle, or increased A point-nasion-B point. Serologic tests for rheumatologic disease, including systemic arthritides, must be negative.

5.2.3.3 Osteochondrosis Dissecans

Osteochondritis dissecans is a disorder of unclear pathophysiology wherein fragments of articular cartilage and bone freely move within the synovial fluid (*"joint mice"*). It usually occurs in the knee and elbow and is often related to sports. Reports have described this condition in the TMJ but little is known about the signs and symptoms. Sensitivity and specificity have not been established.

History is positive for arthralgia as previously defined and joint noises with mandibular movement or swelling. Examination is positive for similar clinical findings as operationalized for arthralgia, or crepitus detected by the examiner during palpation or reported by patient during mandibular movements or maximum assisted opening plus vertical overlap <40 mm, or swelling around the affected joint. CT/CBCT will provide positive findings for loose osteochondral fragments within the joint. Serologic tests for rheumatologic disease, including systemic arthritides, must be negative.

5.2.3.4 Osteonecrosis

Osteonecrosis (avascular/aseptic necrosis) is a painful condition affecting the epiphyseal or subarticular bone secondary to disrupted blood supply in absence of oxygen. Most commonly heads of femur and hip joint are involved, besides humerus and knees. TMJ is rarely involved [66] and the condition is found in the mandibular condyle on MRI as decreased signal in T1-weighted or proton density images and on T2-weighted images (sclerosis pattern) and can be combined with increased signal on T2 images (edema). The exact cause of the disease is unknown. It can occur as a result of intraluminal or extraluminal obliteration in the bone marrow or trauma leading to direct vascular injury.

Simple imaging in early stages is not useful. To diagnose osteonecrosis, the patient must fulfill criteria for arthralgia as previously defined, and imaging must show a decreased signal in T1-weighted or proton density MR images and can be combined with an increased signal on T2-weighted images. Cancellous bone is more affected than the articular surface. In addition, laboratory testing will confirm negative serologic results for rheumatologic disease. Histological examination reveals subcondylar cyst like change. Sensitivity and specificity have not been established. Treatment options are not validated.

5.2.3.5 Neoplasm

A neoplasm is new, often uncontrolled growth of abnormal tissue, in this case arising or involving the TMJ or supporting structures. Tumors of the TMJ are rare, can be malignant or benign, and present with symptoms similar to intra-articular disorders. Occasionally metastatic tumors have also been reported.

TMJ tumors [67] may originate from the condyle, either the bone or the articular cartilage or from the joint capsule and include osteochondroma, chondroma, chondroblastoma, synovial chondromatosis, osteoma, osteoid osteoma, osteoblastoma, giant cell tumor, hemangioma, lipoma, ossifying fibroma, pigmented villonodular synovitis, and juxta-articular myxoma.

Around 3% of malignancies metastasize to the jaws, extending to the TMJ region, causing pain and dysfunction. These commonly include squamous cell carcinomas of the maxillofacial region, primary nasopharyngeal tumors, and also parotid malignancies like adenoid cystic carcinoma and mucoepidermoid carcinoma.

Presenting symptoms include reduced mouth opening which is progressive, joint pain, malocclusion, swelling in the TMJ region, skin reactions in the TMJ region, lymphadenopathy, and crepitus. If the condyle is involved, there is frequently development of a facial asymmetry with a midline shift as that seen in condylar hyperplasia.

Diagnostic imaging and biopsy are essential when a neoplasm is suspected. Treatment options include surgery, radiotherapy, and chemotherapy. Sensitivity and specificity have not been established.

5.2.3.6 Synovial Chondromatosis

Synovial chondromatosis refers to cartilaginous metaplasia of the mesenchymal remnants of the synovial tissue of the joint, characterized by the formation of cartilaginous nodules that may be pedunculated and/or detached from the synovial membrane and become loose bodies within the joint space. Calcification of the cartilage can also occur (osteochondromatosis) [68].

Primary and secondary forms of synovial chondromatosis have been identified. Primary type is severe than the secondary form and is of unknown etiology. Secondary type is associated with degenerative arthritis or previous trauma or microtrauma to the joint.

Synovial chondromatosis most commonly affects knee and elbow. TMJ is rarely affected. In

such a case, the patient should present history of preauricular swelling or arthralgia as previously defined or progressive limitation in mouth opening or presence of joint noises during the last one month. Examination must confirm at preauricular swelling or arthralgia as previously defined or maximum assisted opening (passive stretch) < 40 mm, including the vertical incisal overlap or crepitus as seen in degenerative joint disorders.
MRI or CT/CBCT is recommended for confirmation and it must be positive for multiple chondroid nodules, joint effusion, and amorphous iso-intensity signal tissues within the joint space and capsule (MRI) or loose calcified bodies in the soft tissues of the TMJ (CT/CBCT). Sensitivity and specificity have not been established.

5.2.4 Fractures

Direct trauma can impact TMJ in the form of fracture, dislocation, contusion, or laceration of articular surfaces, ligaments, and disc, with or without intra-articular hemarthrosis, with sequelae such as adhesions, ankylosis, occlusal abnormalities, or joint degeneration [69, 70].

Examples of fractures of TMJ include closed and open fractures of condylar process and subcondylar process. Subcondylar fractures are the most common among fractures involving the mandible, with the condyle even being dislocated out of the glenoid fossa. It is estimated that of all the mandibular fractures approximately 25–52% involve the condyle.

5.2.4.1 Sources of Condylar Injuries

- Due to kinetic injury imparted to static individual (such as blow to the chin), the fracture of parasymphysis may be seen on the side of trauma along with condylar neck fracture on the contralateral side.
- Due to kinetic injury imparted to moving individual against a static surface (such as in a *"parade ground"* fracture or when an individual falls on the floor in an epileptic fit), the symphyseal fracture may be seen associated with bilateral condylar neck fractures.
- When a moving individual strikes against another moving object (such as in road traffic accidents), a summation of the kinetic energies of the first two varieties occurs leading to bilateral parasymphyseal fracture along with bilateral condylar neck fractures.

5.2.4.2 Classification of Condylar Fractures

Lindahl Classification [71] Divides condylar fractures (Figs. 5.6 and 5.7) based on three parameters as follows. It is mandatory that radiographs be taken in two planes at right angles to each other.

- Based on level of fracture into.
  - Intracapsular head or condylar head fractures.
  - Condylar neck fractures.
  - Subcondylar fractures.
- Based on relationship of the fractured condylar segment to the mandible into.
  - Undisplaced (fissure fracture).
  - Deviated (angulated fractured segment without overlap).

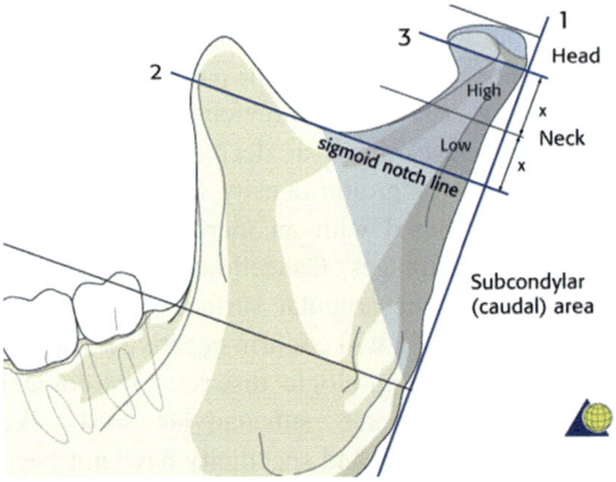

Fig. 5.6 Classification of condylar fractures according to the Comprehensive AOCMF Classification System *(Reproduced with permission from: Al-Moraissi EA* et al. *Does the Surgical Approach for Treating Mandibular Condylar Fractures Affect the Rate of Seventh Cranial Nerve Injuries? A Systematic Review and Meta-Analysis Based on a New Classification for Surgical Approaches. J Craniomaxillofac Surg 2018 Mar; 46(3): 398–412, Copyright Elsevier)*

- Displaced with medial overlap of the fractured segment.
- Displaced with lateral overlap, anterior and posterior overlap.
- Fractured fragment with no contact with the remainder of the mandible.

- Based on the relationship of the condylar head to the glenoid fossa into.
  - No displacement (radiographically the joint space appears normal).
  - Displacement (increased joint space but the mandibular condyle is related to the glenoid fossa.

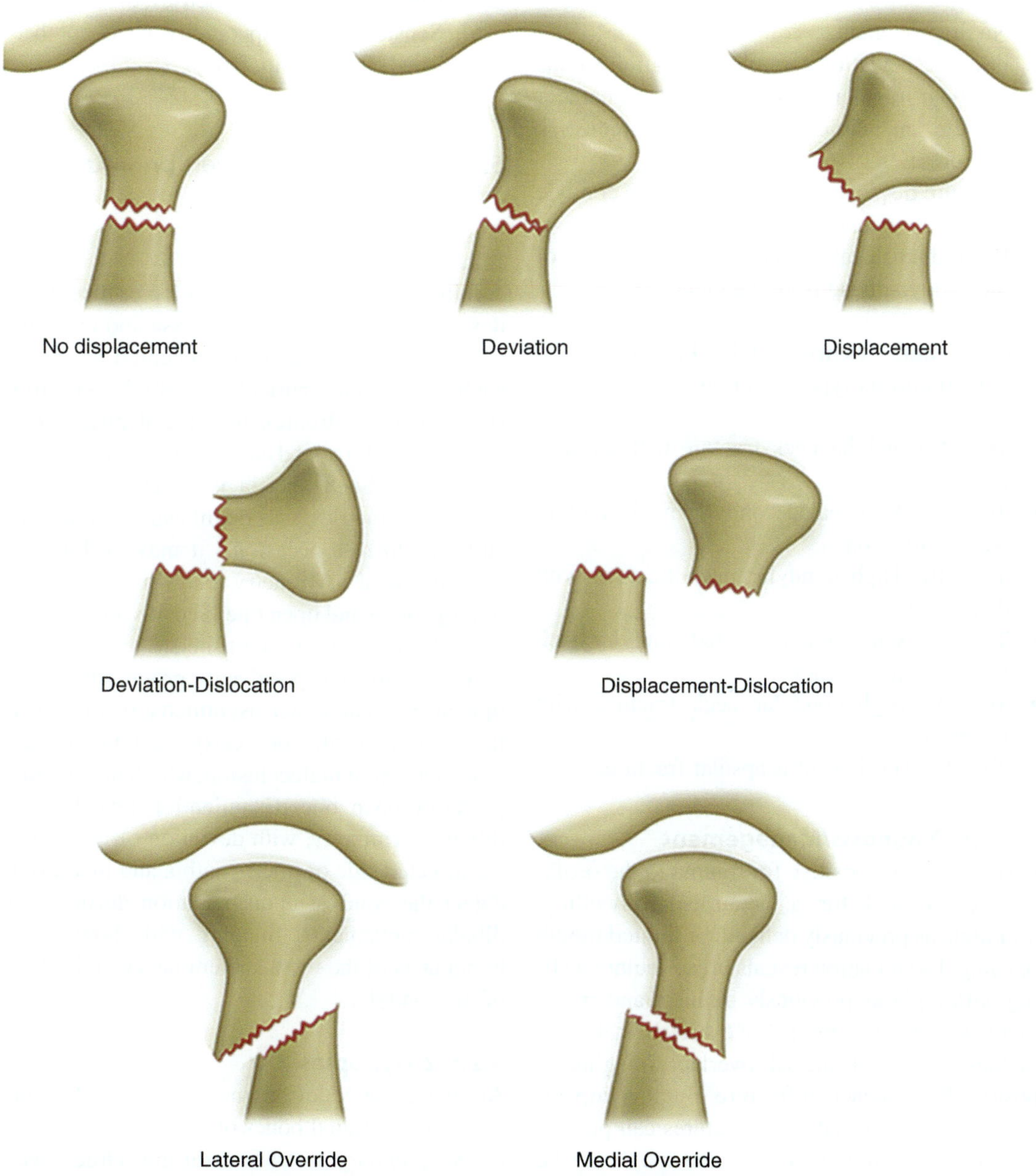

Fig. 5.7 Classification of condylar fractures, based on the relationship of fractured condylar segment to the mandible or glenoid fossa *(Reproduced with permission from: Powers DB. Classification of Mandibular Condylar Fractures. Atlas Oral Maxillofac Surg Clin North Am 2017 Mar; 25(1): 1–10, Copyright Elsevier)*

- Dislocation (condylar fragment is totally out of the glenoid fossa, usually dislocated in an anteromedial direction).

MacLennan Classification [72] Divided condylar fractures into four categories based on the relationship of the fractured condylar fragment to the mandible

- No displacement.
- Fracture deviation (simple angulation of the condylar fragment in relation to the remainder of the mandible as seen in greenstick fractures).
- Fracture displacement (overlap of the condyle and the remainder of the mandible).
- Fracture dislocation (complete disruption of the condylar head from the glenoid fossa).

Spiessl and Schroll Classification [73] Classified into six types as follows:

- Type I: Condylar neck fracture without serious dislocation.
- Type II: Deep seated condylar neck fracture with dislocation.
- Type III: High condylar neck fracture with dislocation.
- Type IV: Synovial deep-seated condylar neck fracture with luxation.
- Type V: High condylar neck fracture with luxation.
- Type VI: Head or intracapsular fracture.

5.2.4.3 Diagnosis/Management

History must be positive for trauma to the orofacial region and for a preauricular swelling, arthralgia as previously defined, or limited mouth opening. Examination reveals preauricular swelling, arthralgia as previously defined, and maximum assisted opening (passive stretch) < 40 mm including vertical incisal overlap. Imaging is positive for evidence of fracture. But it is imperative to remember that TMJ fractures can present with no signs and symptoms and may only be noticed on a routine panoramic radiograph taken for a non-TMD purpose.

Though conservative therapy would do well for most patients with condylar fractures, a higher risk for occlusal changes is associated with bilateral fractures and the condyle being dislocated out of the fossa [74]. Fractures of the condylar process may result in facial asymmetry, with greater skeletal changes when the fracture occurs early in life. Closed treatments have reportedly also resulted in facial asymmetries, even in adults [75]. Sensitivity and specificity have not been established (Refer Chap. 16).

5.2.5 Congenital/Developmental Disorders

5.2.5.1 Aplasia

A failure of the condyle to develop or incomplete development of the articular fossa and eminence is usually associated with congenital anomalies such as oculo-auriculo-vertebral spectrum (Goldenhar syndrome), hemifacial microsomia, and mandibulofacial dysostosis (Treacher Collins syndrome). Such aplasia is unilateral, causing facial asymmetries, and might cause a malocclusion [4]. In rare occasions, it may be bilateral, without facial asymmetry, but with a definitive micrognathia and open bite. Sensitivity and specificity have not been established.

History must be positive for progressive development of mandibular asymmetry or micrognathia from birth or early childhood and development of malocclusion, which may include posterior open bite. Examination reveals mandibular asymmetry, with deviation of the chin to the affected side or micrognathia and inability to detect the condyle upon palpation during mandibular movements. Imaging will show severe hypoplasia of the fossa and eminence and aplasia of the condyle.

5.2.5.2 Hypoplasia

An incomplete development or underdevelopment of the cranial bones or the mandible occurs often secondary to trauma during adolescence, may result in asymmetric growth of the mandible, and may be associated with malocclusion that includes open bite [76]. Sensitivity and specificity have not been established.

History must be positive for progressive development of mandibular asymmetry or micrognathia from birth or early childhood and development of malocclusion, which may include posterior open bite. Examination must confirm this history. Imaging using CT/CBCT will show at least one of the following: hypoplasia of the fossa, hypoplasia of the condyle, or shortened mandibular ramus height.

5.2.5.3 Hyperplasia

Hyperplasia is the overdevelopment of the mandible or cranial bones that occurs unilaterally or bilaterally as a localized enlargement such as condylar hyperplasia or as an overdevelopment of the entire mandible or side of the face. Hyperplasia normally occurs during adolescence, leading to facial asymmetry, mandibular deviation, and a malocclusion [77]. Sensitivity and specificity have not been established.

Facial asymmetry resulting from excessive condylar growth is of two types (Table 5.8):

- Type I: Hemimandibular hyperplasia (HH).
- Type II: Hemimandibular elongation (HE).

To diagnose hyperplasia, the history must be positive for progressive development of mandibular or facial asymmetry, and the examination must confirm this history. Imaging using panoramic radiography and/or CT/CBCT and single-photon emission CT is positive for asymmetry in mandibular ramus height and there is an increased uptake of technetium-99 m hydroxy diphosphonate on bone scintigraphy scan (nuclear imaging).

Table 5.8 Comparison between hemimandibular hyperplasia (HH) and hemimandibular elongation (HE) [49]

	HH	HE
Growth area	Increase in total mandibular mass, bowing of inferior border	Increase only in mandibular length
Cross bite	None or slight	Yes
Open bite	Ipsilateral posterior open bite	Not present
Chin deviation	Moderate	Prominent

5.3 Masticatory Muscle Disorders (Extra-Articular)

The most common reason for TMD patients to seek treatment is for myogenous TMDs or masticatory myalgias that present as pain and dysfunction arising from several well-defined, distinct pathologic and functional processes in the masticatory muscles. These include myofascial pain (myalgia), myositis, muscle spasm, and muscle contracture.

5.3.1 Etiologic Factors for Myogenous TMD [78, 79]

- **Trauma.**
  - Direct microtrauma such as direct blow to the jaw, wider or prolonged opening of mouth during activities such as dental treatment, or yawning or sexual activity.
  - Indirect microtrauma like whiplash-type injury or local infection and trauma (causing myositis and contracture).
- **Repetitive strain.**
  - Repetitive strain activities can result in myalgia or spasm.
  - Sleep disturbances and nocturnal habits can cause myalgia.
  - Psychosocial stressors can play an indirect role.
- **Posture.**
  - Postural strain caused by a forward head posture, increased cervical or lumbar lordosis, some occlusal abnormalities, and poor positioning of the head or tongue.
  - Static postural problems such as unilateral short leg, small hemipelvis, occlusal discrepancies, and scoliosis.
  - Functional postural habits such as forward head, jaw thrust, shoulder phone bracing, and lumbar lifting.

- **Habits.**
  - Oral parafunctional muscle tension produces habits such as teeth clenching, jaw thrust, gum chewing, and jaw tensing.
  - Nocturnal bruxism is often a perpetuating cofactor.

5.3.2 Pathophysiology of Masticatory Myogenous Pain [78, 79]

The mechanisms that produce pain in skeletal muscles are still not conclusively understood, considering the lack of specific anatomic changes in myogenous pain. The various explanations offered to explain the origin and persistence of myogenous pain include the following:

1. **Repetitive strain hypothesis:** Oral parafunctional habits produce repetitive strain that causes localized and progressive increase in oxidative metabolism and depletion of the energy supply, resulting in changes in muscle nociception (*Type 1* muscle fiber—static muscle tone and posture)**.** Locally released noxious substances (kinins potassium, histamine, prostaglandins) may activate *Type III* and *IV* receptors that mediate tenderness and pain in the muscles.
2. **Neurophysiologic hypothesis:** Tonic muscular hyperactivity may be a normal protective adaptation to pain instead of its cause, involving phasic modulation of excitatory and inhibitory interneurons supplied by high threshold sensory afferents.
3. **Central hypothesis** [80]**:** Multiple afferent inputs from muscle and other visceral and somatic structures in the lamina I or V of the dorsal horn converge on the way to the cortex, resulting in perception of local and referred pain.
4. **Central biasing mechanism:** Multiple peripheral and central factors may inhibit or facilitate central input through modulatory influence of the brainstem, explaining the diverse factors that can either exacerbate or alleviate the pain, such as stress, repetitive strain, poor posture, and the like.
5. **Overuse/Ischemia:** Muscle pain from overuse of a muscle or ischemia of a healthy muscle.
6. **Reflexes:** Sympathetic and fusimotor reflexes producing changes in the blood supply and muscle tone [81].
7. Different psychologic and emotional states can alter muscle tone [82].

5.3.3 Muscle Pain Limited to Orofacial Region

5.3.3.1 Myalgia [16, 83]

Myofascial pain or myalgia is the most common muscle disorder [84], characterized by pain and dysfunction that arises from pathologic and functional processes in the masticatory muscles. It is diagnosed when the patient's muscle pain is aggravated by mandibular movement, function, or parafunction and can be reproduced by palpating the painful muscles such as temporalis or masseter.

Trigger points [79, 85]**:** Myalgias are characterized by the presence of tender areas called as trigger points (**TrPs**), which are expressed in taut bands of skeletal muscles, tendons, or ligaments. TrPs are very common and may be *active TrPs* (hypersensitive and display continuous pain in the zone of reference that can be altered with specific palpation) or *latent TrPs* (only hypersensitivity with no continuous pain). TrPs are a reliable indicator of the presence and severity of MFP with both manual palpation and pressure algometers.

Types: Myalgias can be acute or chronic and are of three subtypes:

- Local myalgia.
- Myofascial pain with spreading.
- Myofascial pain with referral.

Of these, local myalgia and myofascial pain with spreading do not have sensitivity and specificity estimates.

History must be positive for pain in the jaw, temple, ear, or in front of the ear in the last

30 days and pain is modified by jaw function or parafunction.

Clinical examination will reveal confirmation of localization of pain in the masticatory muscle structure, confirmed by the examiner, and report of familiar pain during vertical mandibular movements or palpation of the masticatory muscles. The sensitivity and specificity estimates are 0.90 and 0.99, respectively.

Local Myalgia

Local myalgia is diagnosed when the disorder meets the criteria for myalgia, and the report of pain localized only to the site of palpation (immediate site to stimulation). Limitation of mandibular movements secondary to pain may be present. Sensitivity and specificity have not been established. The criterion for this diagnostic group limits the familiar pain to be provoked only with palpation and not with mandibular movement.

Myofascial Pain with Spreading

Myofascial pain with spreading is diagnosed when the disorder meets the criteria for myalgia and the report of pain spreading beyond the location of the palpating fingers but within the boundary of the masticatory muscle being examined. Limitation of mandibular movements secondary to pain may be present. Sensitivity and specificity have not been established.

To diagnose myofascial pain with spreading, the patient must have local myalgia, and the examination of the temporalis or masseter muscle must confirm both of the following:

- Familiar muscle pain with palpation.
- Pain with muscle palpation with spreading of the pain beyond the location of palpation but within the boundary of the palpated muscle.

Other masticatory muscles may be examined as required.

Myofascial Pain with Referral

Myofascial pain with referral is diagnosed when the disorder meets the criteria for myalgia and the referral of pain beyond the boundary of the masticatory muscles being palpated, for example, to the ear, tooth, or eye; spreading may be present. The sensitivity and specificity values are 0.86 and 0.98, respectively.

To diagnose myofascial pain with referral, the patient must have myalgia, and the examination of the temporalis or masseter muscle must confirm both of the following:

- Familiar muscle pain with palpation.
- Pain with muscle palpation beyond the boundary of the muscle.

Other masticatory muscles may be examined as required.

Though it is not significant to differentiate between local myalgia and myofascial pain with spreading, when a patient's pain is due to referred pain from a muscle, it should be diagnosed as myofascial pain with referral.

5.3.3.2 Tendonitis

Tendonitis involves pain of tendon origin aggravated by mandibular movement, function, or parafunction, and it can be reproduced by provocation testing of the painful tendon. Limitation of mandibular movements secondary to pain may be present.

However, it is nearly impossible to know whether the muscle or tendon is being palpated. The only masticatory muscle tendon that can be palpated separately from the muscle is the temporalis muscle tendon, which can be palpated intraorally. Also, the temporalis tendon is a common site of tendonitis with referred pain to the teeth or other structures.

Sensitivity and specificity have not been established. To diagnose tendonitis, the patient must have myalgia as previously defined, and the examination must confirm the diagnosis of myalgia but restricted to the temporalis tendon. This condition could also apply to other masticatory muscle tendons.

5.3.3.3 Myositis

Myositis is diagnosed when the muscle meets the criteria for myalgia and has clinical characteristics of inflammation or infection: edema, erythema, and/or increased temperature. Onset of symptoms is usually acute, related to direct trauma to the muscle or infection of the muscle from orodental causes such as pericoronitis or cellulitis or, or it can occur chronically from an autoimmune disease. In cases of acute overuse, myositis is referred to as *delayed onset muscle soreness*. Limitation of unassisted mandibular movements secondary to pain is often present. Calcification of the muscle can occur (myositis ossificans). Sensitivity and specificity have not been established.

To diagnose myositis, the patient must have local myalgia, and the examination of the temporalis or masseter muscle must confirm both of the following:

- Local myalgia.
- Presence of edema, erythema, and/or increased temperature over the muscle.

In addition, serologic tests may reveal elevated enzyme levels (creatine kinase), markers of inflammation, and the presence of autoimmune diseases. Other masticatory muscles may be examined as required.

If the myositis is due to an infectious cause, the treatment must involve identifying and resolving the infection, along with antibiotic therapy. If the myositis is due to a traumatic cause, the myositis should be treated with NSAIDs, limiting the use of the masticatory muscles (soft diet or avoiding oral habits), and possibly applying ice over the affected area for the first 48 hours after the trauma.

5.3.3.4 Spasm

Spasm refers to the sudden, involuntary, reversible tonic contraction of a muscle that is diagnosed when the muscle meets the criteria for myalgia, the muscle causes a limited range of motion, and the pain and limited range of motion had an immediate onset. Acute malocclusion may be present. Sensitivity and specificity have not been established.

Certain local muscle conditions known to predispose to muscle spasm include muscle fatigue, alteration in local electrolyte balance, and deep pain. Overused muscles or those that have been weakened because of protective splinting more likely undergo a spasm. Certain tranquilizers may also cause masticatory muscle spasm.

Most alarming spasm usually occurs in the inferior lateral pterygoid muscle. Similar to the calf muscle spasm, the individual with a lateral pterygoid spasm has the inferior lateral pterygoid muscle in a painful constant contraction in its midrange position, and there is increased pain when the individual attempts to translate the condyle forward or retrude the mandible so the teeth fit into maximum intercuspation.

The patient usually complains of inability to put the ipsilateral posterior teeth together without excruciating pain (the first tooth contact is in the area of the contralateral canine) and a difficulty in translating the condyle forward leading to a marked limited opening. To diagnose a spasm, the patient must report immediate onset of muscle pain modified by function and parafunction as operationalized in myalgia and immediate report of limited range of jaw motion.

In addition, the examination must confirm myalgia that may include all masticatory muscles and limited range of jaw motion in the direction that elongates the affected muscle (for example, for jaw closers, opening will be limited to <40 mm; for the lateral pterygoid muscle, ipsilateral movement will be limited to <7 mm).

To confirm the diagnosis, laboratory testing will indicate elevated electromyographic activity compared with the contralateral unaffected muscle. Sensitivity and specificity have not been established.

Analgesics can be prescribed. Moist heat fomentation will help in relaxing the muscle. Local anesthetic without vasoconstrictor can be injected into the affected muscle to relieve pain and facilitate speedy recovery. Occlusal bite guards may be given to counteract the effects of parafunctional habits if any.

5.3.4 Contracture

Contracture is a disorder in which fibrosis of tendons, ligaments, and/or muscle fibers does not allow the muscle to stretch to its full length. It is usually not painful unless the muscle is overextended. A history of radiation therapy, trauma, or infection is often present. Sensitivity and specificity have not been established.

Contracture can be myostatic or myofibrotic.

- **Myostatic contracture** occurs when a muscle is kept from fully lengthening (stretching) for a prolonged time because of painful conditions that limit the full functional lengthening of the muscle. Thus, myostatic contracture is often secondary to another disorder.
- **Myofibrotic contracture** occurs as a result of excessive tissue adhesions within the muscle or its sheaths that prevent the muscle fibers from sliding over themselves, disallowing full lengthening of the muscle. This usually happens in myositis or trauma to the muscle tissues.

To diagnose contracture, the patient must have progressive loss of range of motion, and the examination must confirm that unassisted and assisted jaw movements are limited such that maximum assisted opening is <40 mm. It must also be associated with a hardened feel that has been operationalized as having unyielding resistance to assisted movements as felt by the clinician.

5.3.5 Hypertrophy

Hypertrophy is the enlargement of one or more masticatory muscle and is usually not associated with pain. This is usually due to chronic overuse/tensing of the muscle(s), though some cases are familial or genetic in origin. Sensitivity and specificity have not been established.

This is commonly observed as a painless disorder in muscular men who have significant tooth attrition from heavy parafunctional activity. To diagnose hypertrophy, the patient must have enlargement of one or more masticatory muscles as evidenced from photographs or previous records, and the examination must confirm this enlargement. Diagnosis is based on the clinician's assessment of muscle size and requires consideration of craniofacial morphology and ethnicity.

Orthopantomographs may reveal enlarged ramal region and a prominent antegonial notch in masseteric hypertrophy. About 20% of the population may show bone spurs at the mandibular angle in anteroposterior radiographs, caused by periosteal irritation and new bone deposition responding to increased forces exerted by the muscle bundles.

Muscular hypertrophy should be differentiated from conditions such as lipomatosis, vascular tumors, liposarcoma, rhabdomyosarcoma, and infiltrative leukemia and lymphoma. MRI and ultrasound will help in revealing the homogeneous enlargement of the muscles.

5.3.6 Neoplasm

Neoplasms of the masticatory muscles result from tissue proliferation with histologic characteristics and may be benign (myoma), malignant (rhabdomyosarcoma), or metastatic. Reports of TMD symptoms caused by a neoplasm are very rare. They may present with swelling, spasm, pain during function, limited mouth opening, and/or sensory-motor changes (paresthesia). Diagnostic imaging (typically using CT/CBCT and/or MRI) and biopsy are essential when a neoplasm is suspected. Sensitivity and specificity have not been established.

5.3.7 Movement Disorders

Movement disorders include orofacial dyskinesia and oromandibular dystonia that cause involuntary contraction of muscles that move the face, lips, tongue, and/or mandible.

5.3.7.1 Orofacial Dyskinesia [16, 83]

Orofacial dyskinesia is the involuntary, mainly choreatic (dance-like) movements of the face, lips, tongue, and/or mandible that may result in traumatic injury to the oral mucosa or tongue. Reduction or discontinuation of the movement pattern could occur when the mouth or face receives sensory stimulation (sensory trick). Sensitivity and specificity have not been established. Orofacial dyskinesia is more common in older patients, in patients with a history of using neuroleptic medications and/or associated with traumatic brain injury, psychiatric conditions, or other neurologic disorders like Wilson disease.

Different types of orofacial dyskinesia include

- Tremor unspecified.
- Cramp and spasm.
- Fasciculations.
- Ataxia, unspecified.
- Muscular incoordination.
- Subacute, due to drugs *(oral tardive dyskinesia).*

To allocate these diagnoses, the patient must provide a positive history of neurologic diagnosis of dyskinesia in the orofacial region and history components of myalgia and/or arthralgia (diagnostic criteria as previously described) that worsens with episodes of dyskinesia.

Examination will be positive for sensory and/or motor nerve conduction deficit, central and/or peripheral myopathic disease, muscular hyperactivity confirmed by intramuscular electromyography (EMG), and myalgia and/or arthralgia.

5.3.7.2 Oromandibular Dystonia [16, 83]

Oromandibular dystonia involves excessive, involuntary, and sustained muscle contractions of the face, lips, tongue, and/or mandible, which commonly disappear during sleep. The affected muscles are often painful. The condition can make opening and closing the mouth difficult and impair speech, swallowing, and chewing. Sensitivity and specificity have not been established.

Oromandibular dystonia could be components of several central nervous systems disorders, including Parkinson disease and Meige syndrome, and could be an adverse event related to medication usage, notably neuroleptics. Trauma to the brain, head, and neck can trigger the onset of transient or permanent dystonia of the masticatory muscles. The disorder can also be genetically determined.

Two types of orofacial dyskinesia are:

- *Acute*, due to drugs.
- *Deformans, familial, idiopathic, and torsion dystonia.*

To allocate these diagnoses, the patient must provide a positive history of neurologic diagnosis of dystonia in the orofacial region and history components of myalgia and/or arthralgia (diagnostic criteria as previously described) that worsens with episodes of dystonia.

Examination will be positive for sensory and/or motor nerve conduction deficit, central and/or peripheral myopathic disease, dystonia confirmed by intramuscular EMG, and myalgia and/or arthralgia.

5.3.8 Masticatory Muscle Pain Attributed to Systemic/Central Disorders

5.3.8.1 Fibromyalgia

Fibromyalgia involves widespread pain that can contribute to a TMD patient's myalgia, and patients with this disorder do not respond well to TMD therapy. History and examination are positive for both a rheumatologic-based diagnosis of fibromyalgia and myalgia as previously defined. Sensitivity and specificity have not been established.

Historically, in diagnosing fibromyalgia, there needed to be tenderness in at least 11 of 18 specified sites and the presence of widespread pain denoted as axial pain, right and left pain, and upper and lower segment pain. The 18 specified sites for assessing tenderness are:

- **1, 2***(Occiput):* bilateral, at the suboccipital muscle insertions
- **3, 4***(Low cervical):* bilateral, at the anterior aspects of the intertransverse spaces at C5–C7.
- **5, 6***(Trapezius):* bilateral, at the midpoint of the upper border

- **7, 8**(*Supraspinatus*): bilateral, at origins, above the scapula spine near the medial border
- **9, 10**(*Second rib*): *b*ilateral, at the second costochondral junctions, just lateral to the junctions on upper surfaces
- **11, 12** (*Lateral epicondyle*): bilateral, 2 cm distal to the epicondyles
- **13, 14**(*Gluteal*): bilateral, in upper outer quadrants of buttocks in anterior fold of muscle
- **15, 16**(*Greater trochanter*): bilateral, posterior to the trochanteric prominence
- **17, 18**(*Knee*): bilateral, at the medial fat pad proximal to the joint line.

Current criteria eliminate the tender points and focus on a widespread pain index and symptom severity scale [86].

5.3.8.2 Centrally Mediated Myalgia

Centrally mediated myalgia is defined as chronic, continuous muscle pain that is aggravated by function. Intermittent muscle pain conditions may not produce centrally mediated myalgia, while a prolonged and constant period of muscle pain is likely to lead to the condition. The disorder is difficult to delineate from myalgia and may occur in combination with it. Sensitivity and specificity have not been established.

History must be positive for all of the following:

- Prolonged and continuous pain in the jaw, temple, in front of the ear, or in the ear in the past 30 days.
- Regional dull, aching pain at rest.
- Pain is aggravated by function of the affected muscles.
- Presence of at least three nonspecific somatic symptoms, such as sensation of muscle stiffness, weakness, and/or fatigue.
- Sensation of acute dental occlusal changes not verified clinically.
- Ear symptoms (e.g., tinnitus, feeling of fullness, blocked ear), vertigo, dental pain symptoms not attributed to another diagnosis, or headache symptoms not otherwise classifiable by the *International Classification of Headache Disorders* (third Ed, beta version).
- Limited mouth opening (due to pain or myofibrotic contracture).

In addition, the examination must confirm at least two of the following:

- Myalgia.
- Evidence of sensory dysfunction (e.g., allodynia, paresthesia, dental occlusal awareness).
- Muscular atrophy.
- Maximum unassisted opening <40 mm including vertical incisal overlap.

This disorder does not generally resolve as quickly as myalgia. Since neurogenic inflammation releases inflammatory substances into the muscle, it is recommended the patient be prescribed an NSAID in addition to the other therapies recommended for myalgia.

5.4 Headache Disorders

5.4.1 Headache Attributed to TMD

Headache attributed to TMD is a headache located in the temple with a temporal relation to the patient's TMD pain. It worsens with function or parafunctional activities, and it can be reproduced by palpating the temporalis muscle or by its movement.

According to the International Headache Society, this headache is considered present when there is evidence of a pathologic process affecting the TMJ, muscles of mastication, and/or associated structures, together with evidence of a causal relationship with the headache.

Causation is demonstrated when at least two of the following symptoms are present [87]:

- Headache has developed in a temporal relationship to the onset of the TMDs.

- Headache has significantly worsened in parallel with progression of the TMDs, and/or headache has significantly improved or resolved in parallel with improvement in or resolution of the TMDs.
- Headache is produced or exacerbated by active jaw movements, passive jaw movements, and/or provocative maneuvers applied to temporomandibular structures such as palpation pressure.
- When unilateral, headache is ipsilateral to the side of the TMDs.

In the DC/TMD, headache attributed to TMD is included as one of the new diagnostic subtypes. In general, the DC/TMD criteria for this headache closely follow those of the ICHD. An important difference, however, relates to the definition of the TMD subtype that should be present: the DC/TMD specifically links the headache to a pain related TMD diagnosis like myalgia or arthralgia. Sensitivity and specificity values are 0.89 and 0.98, respectively.

To allocate this diagnosis, both of the following criteria must be met:

- History of headaches of any type localized in the temple region during the last 30 days that are modified by jaw movement in function or parafunction.
- During clinical examination, confirmation of the location of the headaches in the temporalis muscle area and report of familiar headache upon palpation of the temporalis muscle or during mandibular movements.

5.5 Associated Structures

5.5.1 Coronoid Hyperplasia

Coronoid hyperplasia is progressive enlargement of the coronoid process that impedes mandibular opening when it is obstructed by the zygomatic process of the maxilla. As the condyle translates, the coronoid process also travels forward. If something (e.g., trauma) caused the coronoid process to enlarge, there may no longer be room for the coronoid process to avoid the zygomatic process as the patient opens.

To diagnose coronoid hyperplasia, the patient must complain of progressive limitation of jaw opening, the examination must confirm the reduction of active and passive maximum jaw opening, and imaging must show an elongated coronoid process that approximates the posterior aspect of the zygomatic process of the maxilla on opening. Sensitivity and specificity have not been established.

References

1. Zarb GA, Carlsson GE. Temporomandibular disorders: osteoarthritis. J Orofac Pain. 1999;13:295–306.
2. Laskin DM, Greenfield W, Gale E. The President's conference on the examination, diagnosis, and management of temporomandibular disorders. Chicago, IL: American Dental Association; 1983.
3. Tanaka E, Detamore MS, Mercuri LG. Degenerative disorders of the temporomandibular joint: etiology, diagnosis, and treatment. J Dent Res. 2008;87:296–307.
4. American Academy of Orofacial Pain. Diagnosis and management of TMDs. In: de Leeuw R, Klasser GD, editors. Orofacial pain: guidelines for assessment, diagnosis and management. 5th ed. Chicago, IL: Quintessence; 2013. p. 137–51.
5. Dworkin SF, LeResche L. Research diagnostic criteria for temporo-mandibular disorders: review, criteria, examinations and specifications, critique. J Craniomandib Disord. 1992;6:301–55.
6. Ohrbach R, Gonzalez Y, List T, Michelotti A, Schiffman E. Diagnostic Criteria for Temporomandibular Disorders (DC/TMD) Clinical Examination Protocol: Version 02 June 2013. www.rdc-tmdinternational.org Accessed on October 20, 2019.
7. Schiffman E, Ohrbach R, Truelove E, et al. Diagnostic criteria for temporomandibular disorders (DC/TMD) for clinical and research applications: recommendations of the international RDC/TMD consortium network and orofacial pain special interest group. J Oral Facial Pain Headache. 2014;28:6–27.
8. Peck CC, Goulet JP, Lobbezoo F, et al. Expanding the taxonomy of the diagnostic criteria for temporomandibular disorders. J Oral Rehabil. 2014;41:2–23.
9. Ohrbach R, Fillingim RB, Mulkey F, et al. Clinical findings and pain symptoms as potential risk factors for chronic TMD: descriptive data and empirically identified domains from the OPPERA case-control study. J Pain. 2011;12(11 suppl):T27–45.
10. Kasch H, Hjorth T, Svensson P, Nyhuus L, Jensen TS. Temporomandibular disorders after whiplash

injury: a controlled, prospective study. J Orofac Pain. 2002;16:118–28.
11. Wright EF. Referred craniofacial pain patterns in patients with temporomandibular disorder. J Am Dent Assoc. 2000;131:1307–15. [erratum 2000; 131: 1553]
12. Simons DG, Travell JG, Simons LS. Apropos of all muscles. In: Travell & Simons' myofascial pain and dysfunction: the trigger point manual, vol. 1. 2nd ed. Baltimore: Lippincott Williams & Wilkins; 1999. p. 94–177.
13. Schellhas KP, Pollei SR, Wilkes CH. Pediatric internal derangements of the temporomandibular joint: effect on facial development. Am J Orthod Dentofac Orthop. 1993;104:51–9.
14. Türp JC, Schindler H. The dental occlusion as a suspected cause for TMDs: epidemiological and etiological considerations. J Oral Rehabil. 2012;39:502–12.
15. Byrd KE, Stein ST. Effects of lesions to the trigeminal motor nucleus on temporomandibular disc morphology. J Oral Rehabil. 1990;17:529–40.
16. Differential diagnosis and management of TMDs. In: de Leeuw R, Klasser GD, editors. Orofacial pain: guidelines for assessment, diagnosis and management. 6th ed., Chicago, IL: Quintessence; 2018. pp. 143–178.
17. Akeel R, Nilner M, Nilner K. Masticatory efficiency in individuals with natural dentition. Swed Dent J. 1992;16:191–8.
18. Diatchenko L, Slade GD, Nackley AG, et al. Genetic basis for individual variations in pain perception and the development of a chronic pain condition. Hum Mol Genet. 2005;14:135–43. 181
19. Smith SB, Mir E, Bair E, et al. Genetic variants associated with development of TMD and its intermediate phenotypes: the genetic architecture of TMD in the OPPERA prospective cohort study. J Pain. 2013;14(12 suppl):T91–T101.
20. List T, Wahlund K, Larsson B. Psychosocial functioning and dental factors in adolescents with temporomandibular disorders: a case-control study. J Orofac Pain. 2001;15:218–27.
21. Magni G, Moreschi C, Rigatti-Luchini S, Merskey H. Prospective study on the relationship between depressive symptoms and chronic musculoskeletal pain. Pain. 1994;56:289–97.
22. Fillingim RB, Slade GD, Diatchenko L, et al. Summary of findings from the OPPERA baseline case-control study: implications and future directions. J Pain. 2011;12(11 suppl):T102–7.
23. Pathology of the temporomandibular joint. In: Carlson ER, Fonseca RJ, Ness GM, editors. Oral and maxillofacial surgery. vol. 2, 3rd ed. St. Louis, MO: Elsevier; 2018. pp. 835-859.
24. Hartwell SW Jr, Siegel BP, Anderson R. Temporomandibular arthralgia. Diagnosis and treatment. Cleve Clin Q. 1967;34(4):235–42.
25. Assessing temporomandibular disorders. In: Carlson ER, Fonseca RJ, Ness GM, editors. Oral and maxillofacial surgery. vol. 2. 3rd ed., St. Louis, MO: Elsevier; 2018. pp. 795-801.
26. Stegenga B. Osteoarthritis of the temporomandibular joint organ and its relationship to disc displacement. J Orofac Pain. 2001;15(3):193–205.
27. Okochi K, Ida M, Honda E, Kobayashi K, Kurabayashi T. MRI and clinical findings of posterior disk displacement in the temporomandibular joint. Oral Surg Oral Med Oral Pathol Oral Radiol Endod. 2008;105(5):644–8.
28. Nitzan DW, Roisentul A. TMJ osteoarthritis. In: Manfredini D, editor. Current concepts on temporomandibular disorders. Chicago, IL: Quintessence; 2010. p. 111–34.
29. Wilkes CH. Internal derangements of the temporomandibular joint. Pathological variations. Arch Otolaryngol Head Neck Surg. 1989;115(4):469–77.
30. Rinchuse DJ, Kandasamy S. Orthodontics and TMD management. In: Manfredini D, editor. Current concepts on temporomandibular disorders. Chicago, IL: Quintessence; 2010. p. 429–45.
31. Okeson JP. Management of Temporomandibular Disorders and Occlusion. 7th ed. St Louis: CV Mosby; 2013. 136, 150, 244–245, 300–303, 362–366, 388
32. Kalaykova SI, Lobbezoo F, Naeije M. Risk factors for anterior disc displacement with reduction and intermittent locking in adolescents. J Orofac Pain. 2011;25(2):153–60.
33. Kalaykova S, Lobbezoo F, Naeije M. Two-year natural course of anterior disc displacement with reduction. J Orofac Pain. 2010;24(4):373–8.
34. Nitzan DW. 'Friction and adhesive forces'–possible underlying causes for temporomandibular joint internal derangement. Cells Tissues Organs. 2003;174:6–16.
35. Zhi K, Ren W, Zhou H, Gao L, Zhao L, Hou C, Zhang Y. Management of temporomandibular joint ankylosis: 11 years' clinical experience. Oral Surg Oral Med Oral Pathol Oral Radiol Endod. 2009;108(5):687–92.
36. Topazian. Etiology of ankylosis of temporomandibular joint: analysis of 44 cases. J Oral Surg Anesth Hosp D Serv. 1964;22:35–41.
37. Sawhney CP. Bony ankylosis of the temporomandibular joint: follow-up of 70 patients treated with arthroplasty and acrylic spacer interposition. Plast Reconstr Surg. 1986;77:29–38.
38. He D, Yang C, Chen M, et al. Traumatic temporomandibular joint ankylosis: our classification and treatment experience. J Oral Maxillofac Surg. 2011;69:1600–7.
39. Okeson JP, de Leeuw R. Differential diagnosis of temporomandibular disorders and other orofacial pain disorders. Dent Clin N Am. 2011;55(1):105–20.
40. De Boever JA, Keersmaekers K. Trauma in patients with temporomandibular disorders: frequency and treatment outcome. J Oral Rehabil. 1996;23(2):91–6.
41. Kaneyama K, Segami N, Nishimura M, Sato J. Traumatic arthritis associated with acute dislocation of the TMJ: a case report. Cranio. 2003;21(3):226–9.

42. Okeson JP. The classification of orofacial pains. Oral Maxillofac Surg Clin North Am. 2008;20(2):133–44.
43. Steinbrocker O, Traeger CH, Batterman RC. Therapeutic criteria in rheumatoid arthritis. J Am Med Assoc. 1949;140(8):659–62.
44. Kent JN, Carlton DM, Zide MF. Rheumatoid disease and related arthropathies. II. Surgical rehabilitation of the temporomandibular joint. Oral Surg Oral Med Oral Pathol. 1986;61(5):423–39.
45. Levorová J, Machoň V, Guha A, Foltán R. Osteoarthrosis of temporomandibular joint related to the defects of posterior dentition: a retrospective study. Prague Med Rep. 2016;117(4):176–84.
46. Ahmad M, Schiffman EL. Temporomandibular joint disorders and orofacial pain. Dent Clin N Am. 2016;60(1):105–24.
47. Arnett FC. The American rheumatism association 1987 revised criteria for the classification of rheumatoid arthritis. Arthritis Rheum. 1988;31(3):315–24.
48. Savtekin G, Şehirli AÖ. Rheumatoid arthritis in temporo-mandibular joint: a review. Niger J Clin Pract. 2018;21:1243–6.
49. Lui DW, Laskin DM. The TMJ. In: Lam D, Laskin DM, editors. Oral and maxillofacial surgery review: a study guide. 1st ed. Hanover Park, IL: Quintessence Publishing Co; 2015. p. 331–57.
50. Chouinard AF, Kaban LB, Peacock ZS. Acquired abnormalities of the temporomandibular joint. Oral Maxillofac Surg Clin North Am. 2018;30(1):83–96.
51. Blair GS. Psoriatic arthritis and the temporomandibular joint. J Dent. 1976;4(3):123–8.
52. Wilson AW, Brown JS, Ord RA. Psoriatic arthropathy of the temporomandibular joint. Oral Surg Oral Med Oral Pathol. 1990;70(5):555–8.
53. Ramos-Remus C, Major P, Gomez-Vargas A, Petrikowski G, Hernandez-Chavez A, Gonzalez-Marin E, Russell AS. Temporomandibular joint osseous morphology in a consecutive sample of ankylosing spondylitis patients. Ann Rheum Dis. 1997;56(2):103–7.
54. Arora P, Amarnath J, Ravindra SV, Rallan M. Temporomandibular joint involvement in ankylosing spondylitis. BMJ Case Rep. 2013. pii: bcr2013009386; https://doi.org/10.1136/bcr-2013-009386.
55. Rowden G, Taylor D. Arthritic, metabolic, and vascular disorders. In: Porter DA, Schon LC, editors. Baxter's the foot and ankle in sport. 2nd ed. Philadelphia, PA: Mosby; 2008. p. 241–9.
56. Cai XY, Yang C, Zhang ZY, Qiu WL, Chen MJ, Zhang SY. Septic arthritis of the temporomandibular joint: a retrospective review of 40 cases. J Oral Maxillofac Surg. 2010;68(4):731–8.
57. Gams K, Freeman P. Temporomandibular joint septic arthritis and mandibular osteomyelitis arising from an odontogenic infection: a case report and review of the literature. J Oral Maxillofac Surg. 2016;74(4):754–63.
58. Sembronio S, Albiero AM, Robiony M, Costa F, Toro C, Politi M. Septic arthritis of the temporomandibular joint successfully treated with arthroscopic lysis and lavage: case report and review of the literature. Oral Surg Oral Med Oral Pathol Oral Radiol Endod. 2007;103(2):e1–6.
59. Oliveira IN, Gomes RC, Dos Santos RR, Oliveira Tde P, Pereira LL, Mainenti P. Gout of the temporomandibular joint: report of a case. Int Arch Otorhinolaryngol. 2014;18(3):316–8.
60. Barthélémy I, Karanas Y, Sannajust JP, Emering C, Mondié JM. Gout of the temporomandibular joint: pitfalls in diagnosis. J Craniomaxillofac Surg. 2001;29(5):307–10.
61. Jacobi AM, Feist E, Rudolph B, Burmester GR. Sinusoidal dilatation: a rare side effect of azathioprine. Ann Rheum Dis. 2004;63(12):1702–3.
62. Jonsson R, Lindvall AM, Nyberg G. Temporomandibular involvement in systemic lupus erythematosus. Arthritis Rheum. 1983;26:1506–10.
63. Könönen M, Wenneberg B. Systemic conditions affecting the TMJ. In: Laskin D, Greene C, Hylander W, editors. TMDs: an evidence based approach to diagnosis and treatment. Chicago, IL: Quintessence; 2006. p. 137–46.
64. Tai CC, Lee P, Wood RE. Progressive systemic sclerosis in a child: case report. Pediatr Dent. 1993;15:275–9.
65. Konttinen YT, Tuominen TS, Piirainen HI, et al. Signs and symptoms in the masticatory system in ten patients with mixed connective tissue disease. Scand J Rheumatol. 1990;19:363–73.
66. Fu KY, Li YW, Zhang ZK, Ma XC. Osteonecrosis of the mandibular condyle as a precursor to osteoarthrosis: a case report. Oral Surg Oral Med Oral Pathol Oral Radiol Endod. 2009;107(1):e34–8.
67. Yurttutan ME, Öncül AT, Karasu HA. Benign tumors of temporomandibular joint. In: Emes Y, Aybar B, Dergin G, editors. Temporomandibular joint pathology. Current approaches and understanding. 1st ed. InTech: Rijeka, Croatia; 2018. p. 99–124.
68. Guarda-Nardini L, Piccotti F, Ferronato G, Manfredini D. Synovial chondromatosis of the temporomandibular joint: a case description with systematic literature review. Int J Oral Maxillofac Surg. 2010;39(8):745–55.
69. Bell WE. Temporomandibular disorders: classification, diagnosis, management, Ed 3. Chicago, IL: Year Book; 1990.
70. Silvennoinen U, Raustia AM, Lindqvist C, Oikarinen K. Occlusal and temporomandibular joint disorders in patients with unilateral condylar fracture. A prospective one-year study. Int J Oral Maxillofac Surg. 1998;27:280–5.
71. Lindahl L. Condylar fractures of the mandible. I. Classification and relation to age, occlusion, and concomitant injuries of teeth and teeth-supporting structures, and fractures of the mandibular body. Int J Oral Surg. 1977;6(1):12–21.
72. MacLennan WD. Fractures of the mandibular condylar process. Br J Oral Surg. 1969;7(1):31–9.
73. Spiessl B, Schroll K. Gelenkfortsatz-und Kieferköpfchenfrakturen. Spezielle Frakturen-

und Luxationslehre. Band I/1: Gesichtsschädel ed. Stuttgart, NY: Georg Thieme Verlag; 1972. p. 136–52.
74. Ellis E 3rd. Method to determine when open treatment of condylar process fractures is not necessary. J Oral Maxillofac Surg. 2009;67(8):1685–90.
75. Ellis E 3rd, Throckmorton G. Facial symmetry after closed and open treatment of fractures of the mandibular condylar process. J Oral Maxillofac Surg. 2000;58:719–28.
76. Nakano M, Fujita T, Ohtani J, Kawata T, Kaku M, Motokawa M, Tsuka N, Hayashi H, Tanne K. Effects of mandibular advancement on growth after condylectomy. J Dent Res. 2009;88(3):261–5.
77. Mehrotra D, Dhasmana S, Kamboj M, Gambhir G. Condylar hyperplasia and facial asymmetry: report of five cases. J Maxillofac Oral Surg. 2011;10(1):50–6.
78. Okeson JP, editor. Orofacial pain: guidelines for assessment, diagnosis, and management. Chicago, IL: Quintessence; 1996.
79. Temporomandibular muscle disorders: diagnostic and management considerations In: Carlson ER, Fonseca RJ, Ness GM, editors. Oral and maxillofacial surgery. vol. 2. 3rd ed., St. Louis, MO: Elsevier; 2018. pp. 962-966.
80. Lund JP, Donga R, Widmer CG, Stohler CS. The pain-adaptation model: a discussion of the relationship between chronic musculoskeletal pain and motor activity. Can J Physiol Pharmacol. 1991;69:683.
81. Mense S. Physiology of nociception in muscles. In: Fricton JR, Awad E, editors. Advances in pain research and therapy. New York: Raven; 1990. p. 67–85.
82. Carlson CR, Okeson JP, Falace DA, Nitz AJ, Curran SL, Anderson D. Comparison of psychologic and physiologic functioning between patients with masticatory muscle pain and matched controls. J Orofac Pain. 1993;7:15–22.
83. TMD diagnostic categories In: Wright EF, editor. Manual of temporomandibular disorders. 3rd ed., Ames, IO: Wiley-Blackwell; 2014. pp. 81-96.
84. Fricton J, Kroening R, Haley D, Siegert R. Myofascial pain syndrome of the head and neck: a review of clinical characteristics of 164 patients. Oral Surg Oral Med Oral Pathol. 1985;60:615.
85. Travell J. Myofascial trigger points: clinical view. In: Bonica JJ, Albe-Fessard DG, et al., editors. Editors: advances in pain research and therapy. New York: Raven Press; 1976.
86. Wolfe F, Clauw DJ, Fitzcharles MA, et al. 2016 revisions to the 2010/2011 fibromyalgia diagnostic criteria. Semin Arthritis Rheum. 2016;46:319–29.
87. Headache Classification Committee of the International Headache Society (IHS). The international classification of headache disorders, 3rd edition (beta version). Cephalalgia. 2013;33:629–808.

Clinical Evaluation of the Temporomandibular Joint

6

Vankudoth Dal Singh and Vaishnavi Devi Majeti

6.1 Introduction

Temporomandibular joint (TMJ) along with the muscles of mastication forms the functional unit primarily responsible for speech, mastication, and deglutition. It is unique since bilateral joints are coupled by a single mandibular bone and move in synchrony with each other. The articular surface is covered with fibro cartilage and not hyaline cartilage like other joints in the body and its movement is guided by the shape of the bones, muscles, ligaments and is also influenced by the occlusion (teeth).

Pain in the TMJ area usually has a local cause; however, it can be referred to other regions. The patient should be questioned about the influence of chewing, yawning, swallowing, or talking. If pain is present during any of these activities, then it is likely to be a temporomandibular joint disorder (TMD). Careful listening/recording the history provided by the patient, inspection, followed by palpation is the sequence to be followed during clinical evaluation to arrive at a provisional diagnosis [1].

V. Dal Singh (✉) · V. D. Majeti
Department of Oral and Maxillofacial Surgery, Lenora Institute of Dental Sciences, Rajahmundry, Andhra Pradesh, India

6.2 Clinical Examination

The clinical examination aims at identifying any abnormalities in the usual health and function of the masticatory system. The examination should start with TMJ, masticatory muscles as well as other non-masticatory structures. Gross examination of the cranial nerves, eyes, ears, parotid gland, and cervical region should be done. Examination of the soft and hard tissues should be performed systematically under the following headings (Table 6.1): inspection, palpation, auscultation, and percussion.

6.2.1 Ergonomics for Patient and Operator

The position in which the patient is seated varies for the examination of various oro-facial structures. History-taking is always carried out with the patient sitting in an upright position. The examination procedure for manual functional analysis for the temporomandibular joint is performed in 12 o'clock patient-operator position (or can be between 11 and 1'o clock position, as per the comfort of the operator/examiner). The patient may be examined in three different ways as summarized in Table 6.2 [1].

D. Bhargava (ed.), *Temporomandibular Joint Disorders*,
https://doi.org/10.1007/978-981-16-2754-5_6

Table 6.1 Examination components for a patient complaining of TMD

Examination	Intra-oral	Extra-oral
Hard tissue	• Dentition/Oral hygiene status **Occlusion:** • Centric/habitual/maximal • Missing/Malposed tooth • Presence of prosthetic appliances/dental implants/restorations	• Facial bones • Temporomandibular joint (TMJ) function **Condylar position:** • Centric/habitual/therapeutic
Soft tissue	• Soft palate • Posterior faucial pillars • Tonsils • Retromandibular region • Hard palate • Buccal mucosa • Alveolar mucosa • Labial mucosa • Tongue	• Facial asymmetry • Facial atrophy • Skin • Lymph nodes examination • Gross ear examination • Masticatory muscles • Other associated muscles • Neck and posture • Any systemic disease process

Table 6.2 Position of patient and operator during TMJ examination

Patient position	Operator position	Advantage	Disadvantage
Semi-reclined position, backrest at 45° angulation (Fig. 6.1)	Upright and behind the patient	Comfortable for a patient who cannot lie in supine position due to general health condition	Nil
Supine	Upright and behind the patient	Ease for operators of short stature	A dental chair cannot be raised for taller clinicians
Supine	Seated (most effective variation)	Most comfortable for tissue-specific examination	Nil

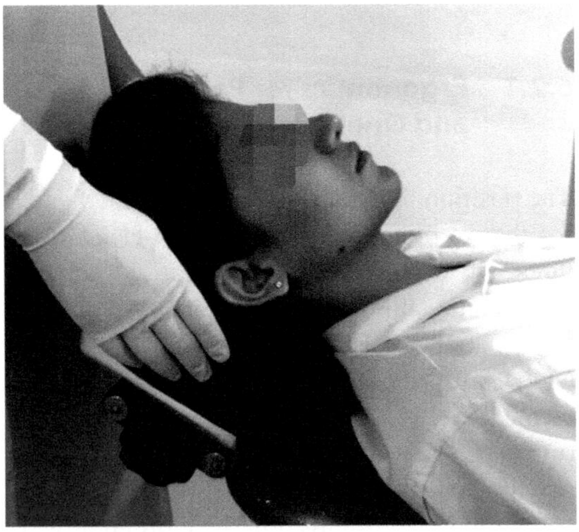

Fig. 6.1 The patient is seated in a semi-reclined position at 45 degrees and examiner standing behind the patient

6.2.2 Stabilization of Head/Cervical Spine

Stabilization of the patient's head in all spatial dimensions is vital for achieving accurate results during the examination. No noticeable head movements must occur when force is applied to the mandible from different directions. Stabilization of the cervical spine in patients having a history of headache/tinnitus is critical, as it can give rise to tinnitus during the examination, which can be misdiagnosed as an arthrogenic cause [2].

6.2.3 Inspection of TMJ

Inspection should begin by observing any noticeable change in the anatomy and skin color in the preauricular region. Inspect for the presence of any swelling, erythema, or deformation. Other parameters to be observed are facial asymmetry, facial atrophy/hypertrophy, deviation of the chin or restricted/reduced mouth opening. The intraoral examination should include occlusion, attrition, inappropriate occlusal contacts due to supra-eruptions and any faulty restorations or prosthesis. Soft tissue abnormalities in the gingival, buccal, palatal, and labial mucosa should also be noted to complete the oral examination [2].

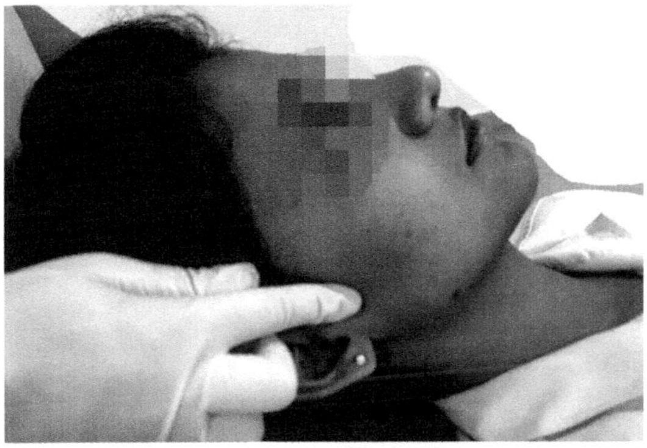

Fig. 6.2 Palpation of the TMJ at the lateral aspect in closed mouth position

6.2.4 Palpation of TMJ

Palpation of the TMJ can be performed by two different methods:

1. **Lateral palpation:** The fingertips of both the hands should be placed over lateral aspects of TMJ bilaterally and palpated for tenderness, click/pop during static and protrusive/lateral mandibular movements.

   The lateral pole of the condyle should be palpated with initial mouth opening to approximately 20 mm. The patient should then be asked to open the mouth as wide as possible to assess the area at the depth of the depression behind the condyles. With fingertip placed in the depression with maximum mouth opening, pull forward to load the posterior aspect of the condyle [2]. (Figs. 6.2, 6.3, and 6.4).
2. **Intra-auricular palpation:**

   While placing the little finger in the external auditory meatus and applying gentle anterior pressure, the patient is instructed to open and close the mouth. This helps to identify pain in the bilaminar zone of the disc and the posterior aspect of the capsule [3]. (Fig. 6.5).

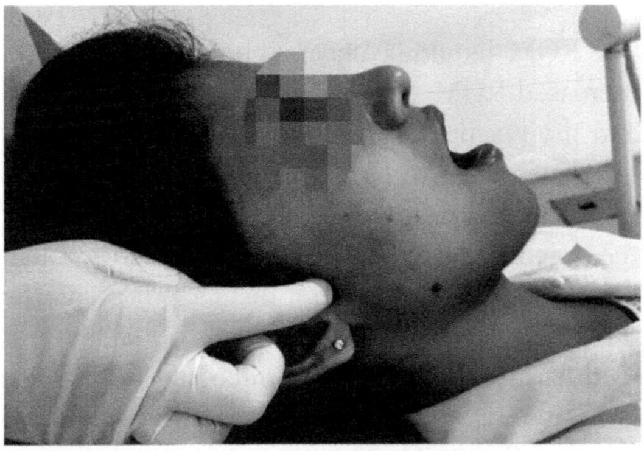

Fig. 6.3 Palpation of the lateral aspect of TMJ (lateral pole of condyle) during open and closed mouth position

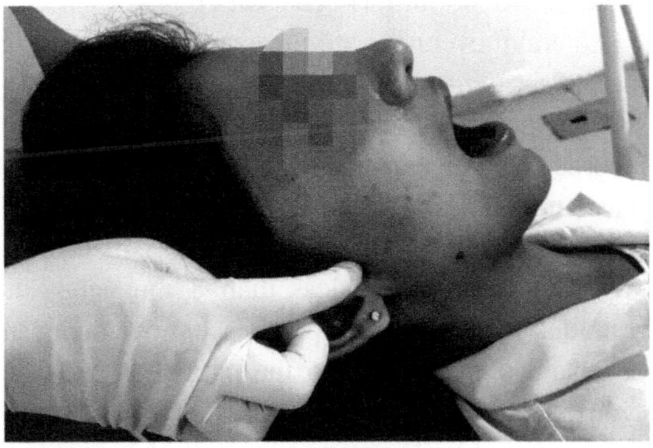

Fig. 6.4 Palpation with mouth fully open at the depression created on the posterior aspect of the condyle

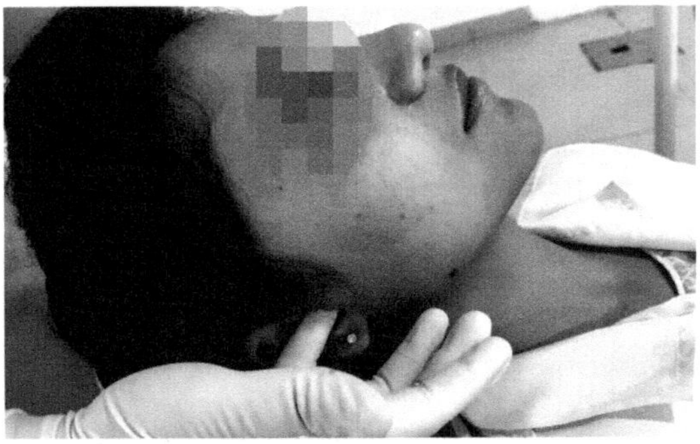

Fig. 6.5 Intra-auricular palpation to palpate the posterior aspect of the TMJ

6.2.5 Range of Motion (ROM)

The ROM should be checked before palpation as increased ROM may aggravate pain in the joint and the masticatory muscles. It is measured by the distance between the incisal edge of maxillary central incisors (CI) to the incisal edge of the mandibular CI. The patient is asked to open the mouth wide till the first instance of pain. The distance between the incisal edges of the anterior teeth is measured, and this inter-incisal distance is known as the maximum comfortable mouth opening (Fig. 6.6). The patient is then asked to further open wide inspite of the pain. This inter-incisal measurement is called the maximum mouth opening (MMO). The normal range of MMO is 40–45 mm. (Fig. 6.7) [4].

Lateral movements are measured by instructing the patient to move his/her mandible as far as possible to one side, and the lateral movements are recorded. For convinence the distance between the fixed maxillary midline and the shift of the mandibular midline on lateral excursion is measured. Any lateral movement less than 8 mm suggests restricted movement. The protrusive movement can be obtained by instructing the patient to close in centric position and slide the lower jaw as far forward as possible. The overjet may also be recorded. Protrusive movements are recorded by adding these two readings. Protrusive movements are considered to be restricted if it is less than 7 mm.

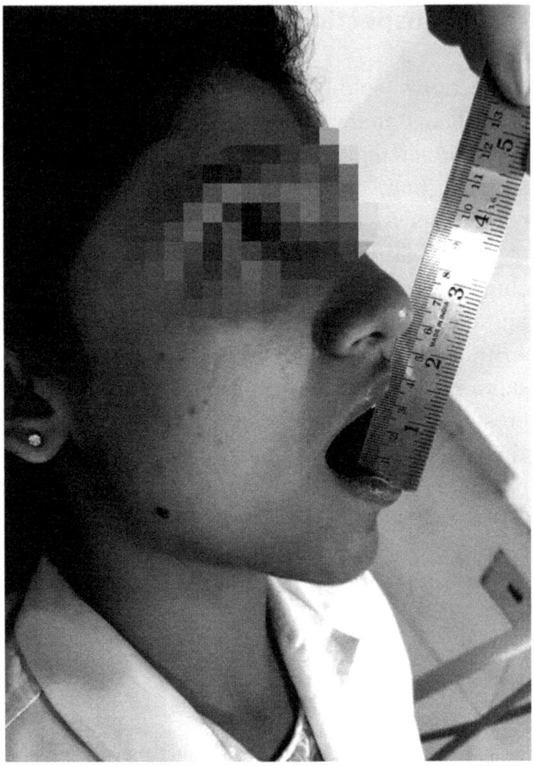

Fig. 6.6 Maximum comfortable mouth opening—Mouth opening until before pain is felt

6.2.6 Mid-Line Shift

The path taken by the mandibular midline during MMO is observed. It should be a linear path during mouth opening, which implies both joints moving synchronously. Two types of alterations in the midline shift may be observed [5].

Deviation: A shift in the midline during mouth opening that disappears with a continued opening is known as deviation, e.g., as in cases with disc displacement with reduction (DDwR). Mandible moving in a straight line in the first phase of movement and deviates laterally at the end of maximum mouth opening, e.g., as in cases with disc displacement without reduction (DDwoR).

Deflection: Deflection from the midline during mouth opening that does not disappear with a maximum opening [5].

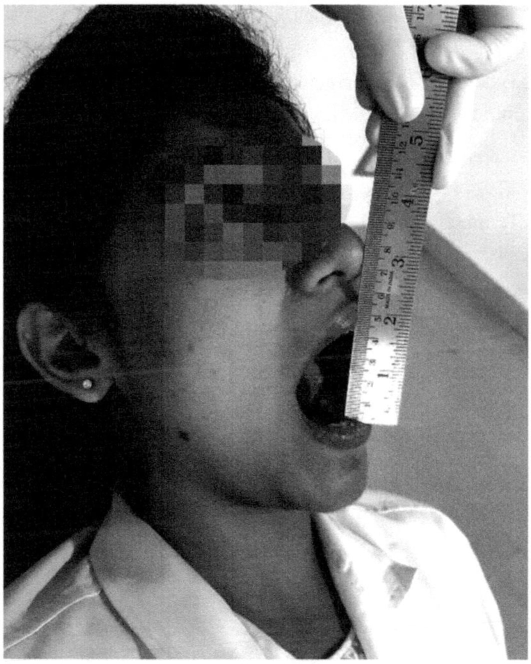

Fig. 6.7 Maximum mouth opening, as wide as possible even with pain

Restricted mouth opening: Limitation of mandibular movement may be caused by two principal factors:

1. Pain in the associated muscles/TMJ—extra- or intra-capsular source.
2. Physical obstruction to movement.

6.2.6.1 Extra-Capsular Source

The spasm of elevator muscles cause restricted mouth opening but not the restriction of the lateral and protrusive movements. In this condition, the patient can open the mouth slowly but with amplified pain. There can be a deflection evident during mouth opening. The location of the muscle that causes the restriction guides the direction of deflection. If the restricting muscle is lateral to the joint (masseter), the deflection will be towards the ipsilateral side. If the muscle spasm is medial to the joint (medial pterygoid), the deflection will be to the contralateral side [2, 5].

6.2.6.2 Intra-Capsular Source

These are associated with disc-derangements. The jaw deflection is towards the affected side. The mouth opening is restricted to 25–30 mm beyond which it is painful and no further mouth opening is possible, not just because of pain but also due to structural interferences [2, 5].

6.2.7 End Feel

To examine this the examiner places the fingers, crossing the thumb and the index finger between the patient's upper and lower incisors and applies gentle force to passively increase the inter-incisal distance. The end feel can have one of the four characteristics—soft, hard, re-bounding or bony (Fig. 6.8) [6]. The "end feel" is felt by the examiner, at the end of a passive movement of the TMJ. It can describe the characteristics of the restricted joint movement. If passive jaw opening causes pain, end feel should not be used as a diagnostic aid to check restricted mouth opening. Non-painful limitations of movement can be differentiated with end feel after passive movement.

6.2.8 Joint Sound

The joint sounds are classified as click/pop and crepitations [5].

Clicking: A 'click' is a single sound of short duration. A louder clicking sound is known as a 'pop'. Clicking and popping are most commonly related to a DDwR. (Table 6.3) [7, 8].

***Crepitation*:** Crepitation is a multiple gravel-like sound (sound produced when a person walks on the gravel), also described as grating. It is commonly related to roughness on the articular surface, which could be secondary to disc perforation, osteoarthritis, chronic DDwoR, or polyarthritides. Crepitation may be felt by placing the fingertips over the lateral aspect of the joint during mandibular movements [9].

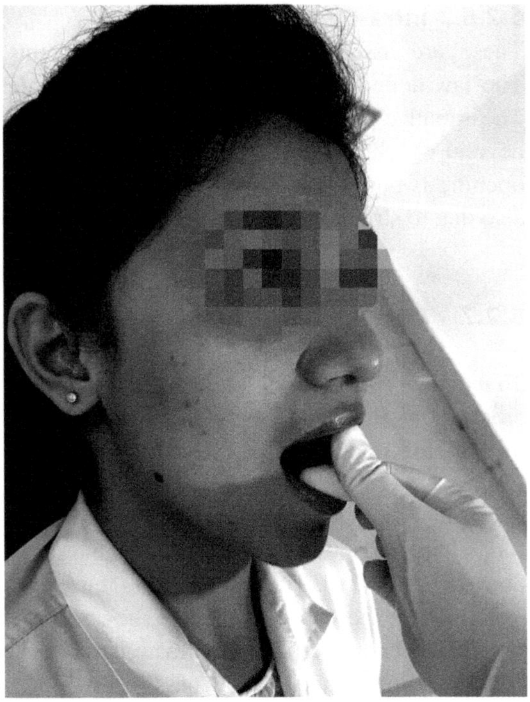

Fig. 6.8 Checking the 'end feel' using index finger and thumb

Table 6.3 Types of click in the TMJ region

Type	Character	Clinical significance
Initial click	The joint clicks just when the mouth opening begins	Indicative of retruded condyle in relation to the disc
Terminal click	The click occurs at the end of the movement when the condyle has moved too far anteriorly in relation to the disc, on maximum jaw opening	Indicative of peripheral irregularity of the articular disc or unevenness of the condylar surface
Intermediate click	All other than the above two sounds are intermediate	Indicative of unevenness of the condylar surfaces and/or of the articular disc/ disturbed synchrony of disc-condyle complex.
Reciprocal click	It occurs during opening and closing due to an incoordination between the condyle and the disc.	Occurs in internal derangement or disc disorders

6.2.9 Examinations when Crepitation is Felt for Clinical Diagnosis

(a) ***Clinical joint surface test:*** For this the examiner should be at 12 o'clock position, placing two fingers over each condyle. The patient is instructed to protrude the jaw and then make a maximal jaw opening from the protruded position. During this movement, grating sounds or pain or both should be noted.

When the crepitus is present during protrusion, it is from temporal joint surfaces; however, when it is felt during jaw opening, it is from condylar surfaces. These two tests are known as active tests. These form the basis for the following tests [2].

(b) ***Dynamic compression test***: Two fingers are placed under the angle of the mandible and a gentle pressure is applied superiorly, while the patient is instructed to protrude the jaw and open the mouth wide.

Under physiologic conditions, neither crepitus nor pain is felt. If it is present during protrusion, it is due to osteoarthritic changes of the temporal part of the joint surface or changes in the condylar surface. An inflammatory stage of joint surface damage such as osteoarthritis can cause crepitus with pain. In the case of osteoarthrosis, there will be a presence of crepitus but with an absence of pain [2].

(c) ***Dynamic translation***:

One hand should stabilize the patient's head by placing it against the neck and the thumb is placed in line with the angle of the mandible. The other hand should brace the forehead from the contralateral side. When a force is applied by the thumb medially toward the contralateral jaw angle, it results in a medial translation of the one condyle and a lateral translation of the other condyle.

The dynamic translation test is repeated with active movements, that is opening the jaw wide and protrusive movements on both right and left sides.

- ***Adaptation (patient's initial response to aberrant joint loading)***: No crepitus or pain during active movements and dynamic tests.
- ***Compensation (absence or a reduction in adaptation capability)***: Crepitus or pain only during the dynamic tests.
- ***Decompensation (inability to compensate, to joint loading during function)***: Crepitus or pain during active movements and during dynamic tests [2].

[Note: The joint sounds can be evaluated best using a stethoscope for auscultating the preauricular region.]

6.2.10 Muscle Examination

Normal function or palpation of a healthy muscle rarely elicits pain. It is experienced in an unhealthy/compromised muscle caused either by trauma or fatigue. Examination of various muscles helps in locating the muscular pain/tenderness. The muscle is examined by digital palpation or by functional manipulation (isometric contractions). Muscles that can be directly palpated are temporalis, masseter, geniohyoid, digastric, sternocleidomastoid, trapezius, posterior cervical muscles. Functional manipulation is preferred for the medial and lateral pterygoids as they are not easily palpable [10].

Palpation is done by using the middle finger's palmar surface, while the index and forefingers are used to test the surrounding areas. Firm pressure should be applied over the region with the fingers compressing the adjacent tissues in a small circular motion. Palpation should be performed perpendicular to the direction of muscle fibers. This technique aids in the detection of lesions in different layers of a muscle. A single firm pressure of approximately 40 N/cm^2 should be applied for 1 or 2 seconds, while palpation and the patient response should be recorded. (Whether it hurts or is just uncomfortable) [2, 5, 11].

Palpation should start with the temporalis, TMJ, masseter, lateral/anterior neck followed by other structures. The operator should stand in front of the patient to observe discomfort during palpation, thereby reducing the patient's discomfort. When a muscle is palpated, the patient's response can be recorded in one of the four categories as summarized in Table 6.4 [12, 13].

Three palpation techniques can be used to provide various stimulation intensities:

1. Non-specific palpation in a predetermined location.
2. Palpation of a trigger point.
3. Firm sustained palpation of the trigger points.

6.2.10.1 Temporalis Muscle

The temporalis is divided into three functional areas, and each area is palpated independently. After palpating the three functional units of the temporalis muscle, the response/trigger point should be identified and noted if present. The examination should be performed from 1'o clock position. The temporalis tendon is palpated with a finger of one hand at the anterior border of the ramus intraorally and a finger of the other hand extra-orally. The intraoral finger should be moved up the anterior border of the ramus until

Table 6.4 Pain score for muscle palpation

Score	Nature of muscular pain
0	No pain/tenderness
1	Slight tenderness/soreness
2	Definite pain/discomfort
3	Exhibit evasive action/eye tearing/verbal information to not to perform the palpation due to pain

the coronoid process and the tendon is palpated. The patient is asked to report any discomfort or pain. This is important as the tendon pain is sometimes referred to the temporalis muscle. (Table 6.5, Figs. 6.9, 6.10, and 6.11) [1, 2, 5].

6.2.10.2 Masseter Muscle

The extent of the masseter muscle can be identified by instructing the patient to clench the teeth, the muscle gets stout and may be easily palpated at the lateral ramal region of the mandible. It is

Table 6.5 Palpation of different functional areas associated with TMJ

Functional area	Area of palpation	The orientation of muscular fibers
Temporalis muscle		**Significance**
Anterior (Fig. 6.9)	Above the zygomatic arch Anterior to the TMJ	Vertical direction
Middle (Fig. 6.10)	Directly above (approximately 2 inches) the TMJ Superior to the zygomatic arch	Oblique direction across the lateral aspect of the skull
Posterior (Fig. 6.11)	Above and behind the ear	Horizontal direction
Digastric muscle		**Significance**
Anterior	Runs from the lingual surface of the chin, near the midline to the hyoid bone.	If tenderness is present, rule out an oral disorder. If the tenderness is not due to an oral disorder, referred pain may be initiated by applying sustained pressure to the tender area.
Posterior	Runs from hyoid sling medial to the sternocleidomastoid muscle Attaches medial to the mastoid process Fingertip placed posterior to the angle of the mandible and medial to the sternocleidomastoid muscle with application of palpation force should direct posteriorly	If the tenderness is noted, referred pain may be generated by applying sustained pressure
Sternocleidomastoid muscle		**Significance**
Palpation of sternocleidomastoid muscles is by squeezing the muscle between the thumb and index finger		If tenderness is present, then holding for 5 seconds may generate referred pain. Clinically, the more superior portions of the muscle are more likely to generate referred pain to the head and face
Medial pterygoid muscle (Internal)		**Significance**
Slide the index finger, slightly posterior to the traditional insertion site for an inferior alveolar injection, until the muscle is felt, and pressed laterally. If the patient gags, the finger is placed too posterior		If the tenderness is noted, referred pain may be generated by applying heavier sustained pressure
Lateral pterygoid muscle (External)		**Significance**
Apply the digital pressure along the lateral side of the maxillary alveolar ridge to the most posterior region of the vestibule. Palpate by pressing in a superior, medial and posterior direction		If the tenderness is noted, a referred pain may be generated by applying heavier sustained pressure
Stylomandibular ligament		
Palpate by placing the fingertip medial to the posterior border of the mandible and 10–15 mm above the angle of the mandible in an anteromedial direction		
Coronoid process		
Place the index finger superiorly along the anteromedial border of the ramus, when the finger approaches the superior extent, palpate the temporalis tendon over the coronoid process		

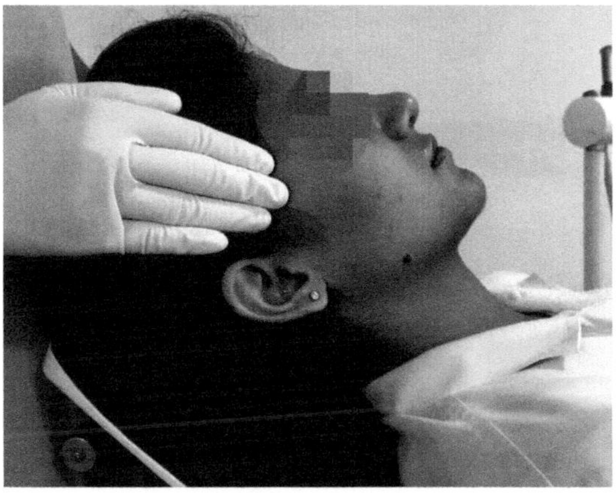

Fig. 6.9 Palpation of anterior part of the temporalis muscle

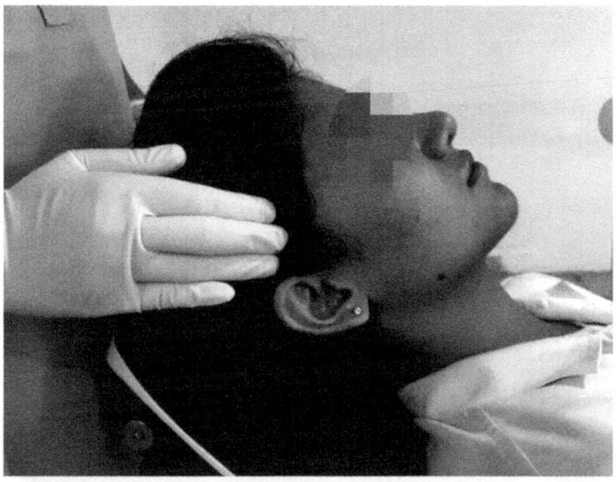

Fig. 6.10 Palpation of middle part of the temporalis muscle

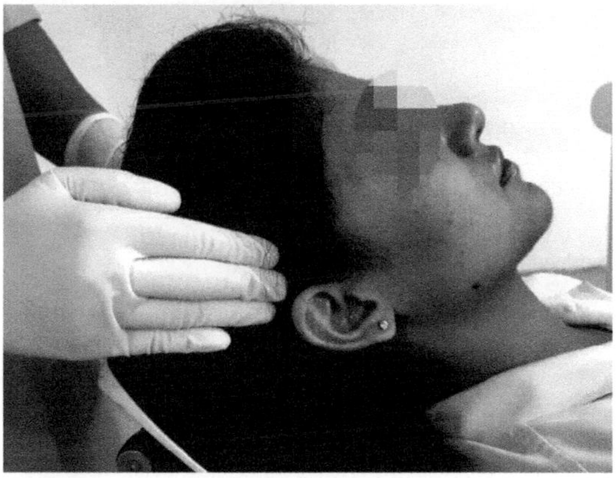

Fig. 6.11 Palpation of posterior part of the temporalis muscle

palpated at its superior and inferior attachments. The fingers should be placed on each zygomatic arch just anterior to the TMJ. This is the deep masseter (superior attachment). The fingers are then passed to the inferior attachment on the inferior border of the ramus (superficial part) [2]. (Figs. 6.12 and 6.13).

6.2.10.3 Geniohyoid Muscle

The index finger of the palpating hand should be placed on the floor of the mouth parallel with the long axis of the geniohyoid muscle with the opposite hand supporting the floor of the mouth extra-orally. Palpation is performed at right angles to the course of the muscle fibers [1, 2]. (Fig. 6.14).

6.2.10.4 Digastric Muscle

(a) ***Anterior belly of digastric***: The palpating index finger should be placed extra-orally parallel to and directly beside the muscle. The finger should make a rolling motion toward the median plane. Swallowing makes it easier to locate the muscle. (Table 6.5) (Fig. 6.15).

(b) ***Posterior belly of digastric***: The posterior belly is palpated by placing the finger behind the angle of the mandible, directly on the muscle. (Table 6.5) [2, 5] (Fig. 6.16).

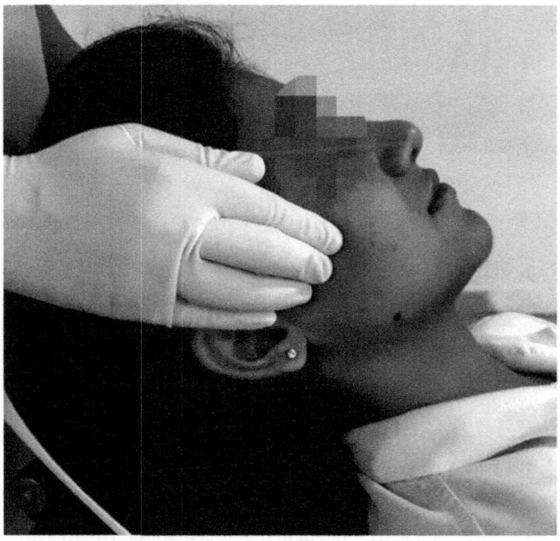

Fig. 6.12 Palpation of the deep part of masseter at the zygomatic arch

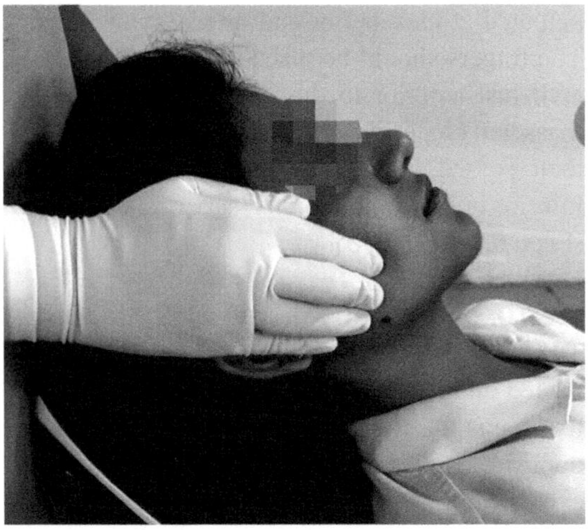

Fig. 6.13 Palpation of the superficial part of masseter at the inferior border of ramus

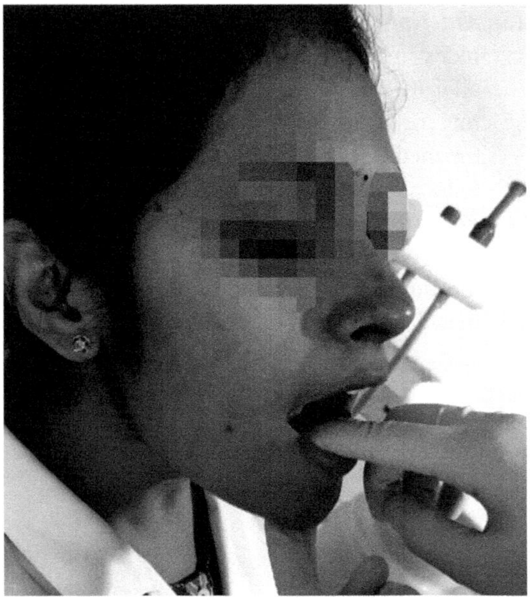

Fig. 6.14 Palpation of the geniohyoid muscle by placing index finger at the floor of the mouth parallel to the long axis of muscle

6.2.10.5 Sternocleidomastoid

This muscle is usually not directly involved as the muscles of mastication and TMJ for the jaw function. Sternocleidomastoid is palpated bilaterally from its insertion on the mastoid, and along its length, to its origin at the clavicle. Any discomfort experienced by the patient during the procedure is noted. The trigger points should be recorded as

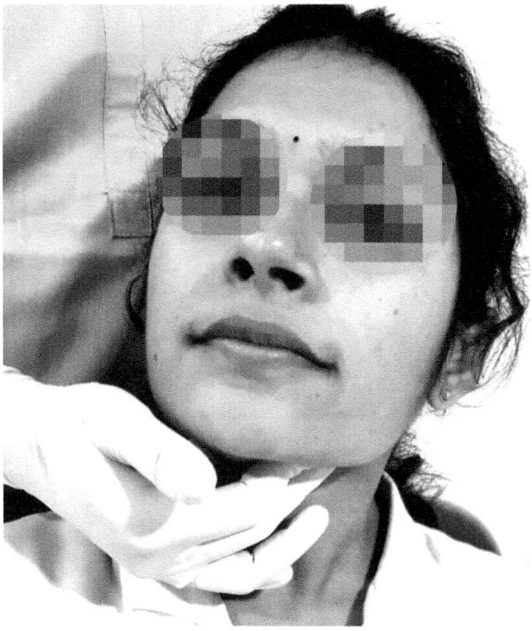

Fig. 6.15 Palpation of anterior belly of digastric muscle

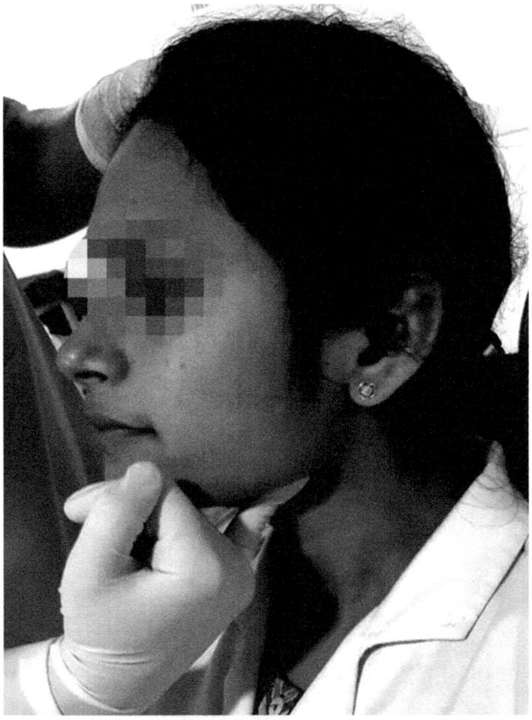

Fig. 6.16 Palpation of posterior belly of digastric muscle

they may cause referred pain to the TMJ region. (Table 6.5) [1, 2] (Figs. 6.17 and 6.18).

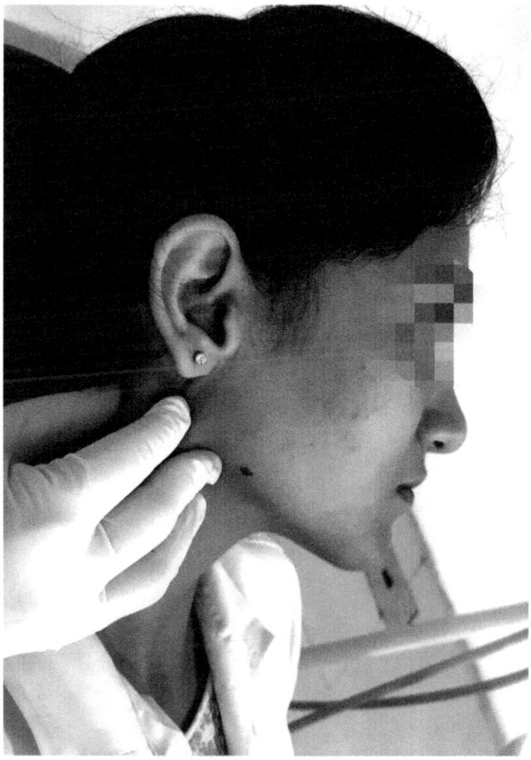

Fig. 6.17 Palpation of sternocleidomastoid muscle at its insertion near the mastoid process

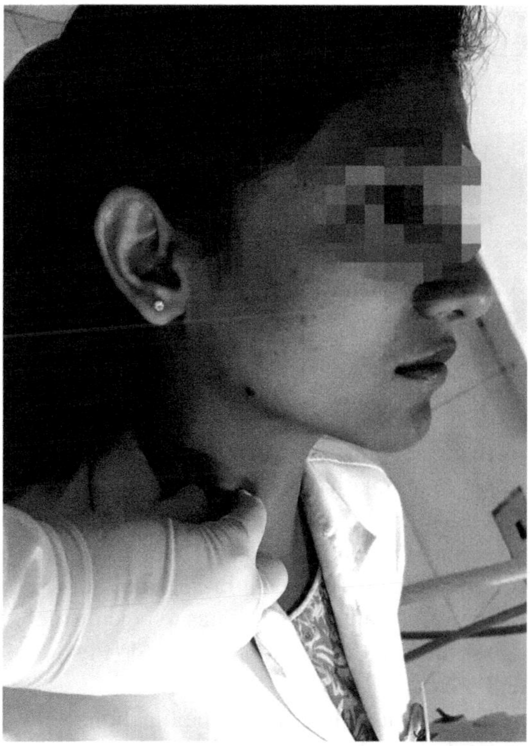

Fig. 6.18 Palpation of sternocleidomastoid muscle at its origin near the clavicle

6.2.10.6 Posterior Cervical Muscles and Other Structures

These muscles are not directly involved functionally but may be symptomatic in TMDs. Palpation should begin bilaterally from the occipital area at the origin of these muscles. The fingers are moved downwards along the length of the muscles to the cervical region. (Table 6.5) [1, 2, 5].

6.2.10.7 Trigger Points

These are nodules of spot tenderness within the muscle and can be active or latent. They are usually localized, firm, hyper-irritable nodules that feel like firm knots (as most patients explain) within the muscle. They are more tender than the surrounding muscle. **Active trigger points** are specific hypersensitive areas within the muscle tissue that elicit pain spontaneously. **Latent trigger points** are palpable, but the pain is not elicited spontaneously during physical examination.

After identification of the trigger points, a gentle sustained pressure should be applied to these sites up to patient's tolerance and sustaining the applied pressure for at least 5 seconds to elicit pain. This will generate intense pain within the muscle that may go beyond the structure and can occasionally cause referred pain to distant locations. This should be mapped and recorded [5, 14].

6.2.10.8 Referred Pain

Pain felt outside the anatomical boundaries of the muscles, triggered during palpation of the muscles of mastication is called referred pain. Three muscles cause referred pain to the teeth. The key to distinguish tooth pain from referred pain is by local provocation of the painful tooth which will not increase the symptoms in referred pain.

- The temporal muscle causes referred pain to the maxillary teeth,
- Masseter refers pain to the maxillary and mandibular posterior teeth,
- The anterior belly of the digastric muscle refer pain to the mandibular anterior teeth [1, 8, 14].

6.2.10.9 Functional Manipulation

The medial and lateral pterygoid muscles can be functionally palpated. The functional palpation is based on the principle that when a muscle becomes fatigued and symptomatic, a further function can elicit pain. During functional manipulation, each muscle is contracted and then stretched. Both activities will increase the pain if the muscle is the source for it. To differentiate between intra-capsular disorder and muscle pain, a fifth test has to be considered as summarized in Table 6.6 [15, 16] (Figs. 6.19 and 6.20).

The four tests to examine the functional activity of the muscle are:

1. Protrusion against resistance.
2. Opening mouth widely.
3. Clenching of teeth.
4. Clenching on separators.

6.2.11 Auscultation of the TMJ

A stethoscope can be used for a better hearing of the click/pop and crepitations. The examination is performed by asking the patient to open and close the jaw into full occlusion. If clicking or crepitation is noted, the patient is instructed to protrude and repeat the opening and closing. Often sounds disappear in protruded position. More sensitive equipment (e.g., Doppler) may also be utilized to verify the TMJ noise [2].

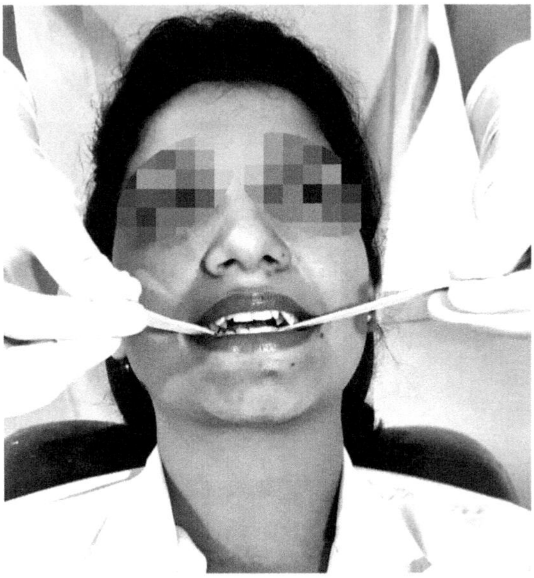

Fig. 6.19 Functional manipulation of the superior lateral pterygoid by instructing the patient to bite the tongue blade bilaterally

Table 6.6 Functional manipulation and pain intensity by activity

Function	Medial pterygoid muscle	Inferior lateral pterygoid	Superior lateral pterygoid	Intracapsular disorder
Opening widely	Pain increases	Pain increase (slightly)	No pain	Pain increases
Protruding against resistance	Pain increase (slightly)	Pain increases	No pain	Pain increases
Clenching on teeth	Pain increases	Pain increases	Pain increases	Pain increases
Clenching on separator (unilaterally)	Pain increases	No pain	Pain increases	No pain (may report pain)
Protruding against resistance with unilateral separator	Pain increase (slightly)	Pain increases	Pain increase (slightly)	No pain (may report pain)

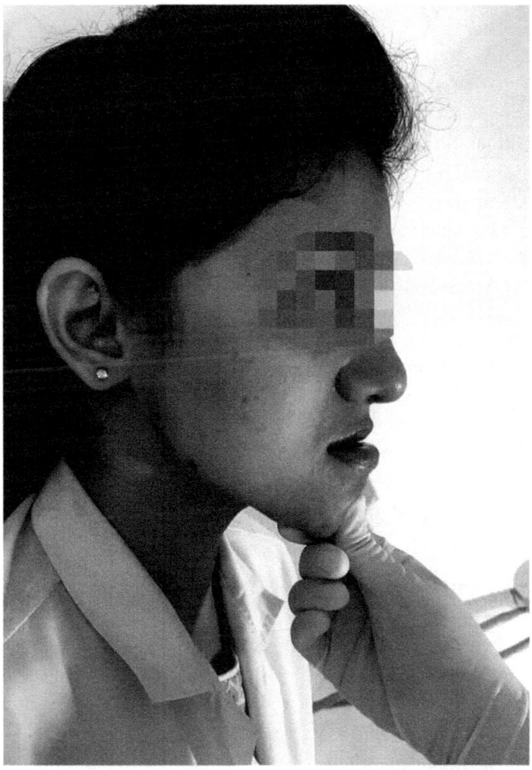

Fig. 6.20 Functional manipulation of the inferior lateral pterygoid by instructing the patient to protrude the mandible against resistance

6.2.12 Percussion for TMJ Examination

The tooth/teeth is/are percussed intraorally using a mouth mirror or probe for tenderness, which can cause a referred pain to the TMJ region.

6.2.13 Intraoral Examination

The most crucial factor to be evaluated is the centric relation and occlusion. A 2 mm shift of the mandible from centric relation to maximum intercuspation is considered to be normal. Evaluation of the dental structure for the presence of any functional disturbance is essential. Presence of high points, faulty restoration/prosthesis or supra-eruption should be noted and corrected.

Mobility of teeth: Mobility can occur because of periodontitis or trauma from occlusion (TFO). Primary TFO can cause massive occlusal forces exceeding the resistance of a healthy periodontium. Secondary TFO leads to regular occlusal forces exceeding the resistance of diseased periodontium.

Tooth wear: Examination of the wear facets on the tooth should be done as the tooth wear is a common cause of functional disturbance in the masticatory system. If the centric relation is near to the maximum intercuspation, it is functional wear. However, if an eccentric position is assumed, the cause is more often due to parafunctional activity. Attrition, scalloping of tongue, and cheek ridging in the occlusal line are the signs noted in patients with parafunctional habits. These features are due to the soft tissues thrust against the teeth during parafunction [1, 2, 5].

6.2.14 Other Methods of Clinical Assessment of TMJ

The *instrumental movement analysis* may be utilized to assess the quantitative characteristics and performance of bilateral condyle. It helps to record the condylar path length to determine the mobility of the joint. It is performed by electronic recording system for recording the mandibular movements based on the (Arcus Digma) ultrasonic measuring device [17]. The T-scan computerized occlusal analysis technology may be utilized to assess occlusal force distribution, where needed. The advanced T-scan III can be linked through software integration with electromyography system along with the assessment of the occlusal forces [18]. These advanced equipments for the analysis may not be universally available.

6.3 Goals of Examination

Clinical examination is the first and foremost vital aspect to diagnose and for managing TMDs. A correct approach to clinical examination and diagnosis is important for achieving a long-term successful treatment outcome.

6.4 Case History Format (For a Temporomandibular Joint Disorder Patient)

Date:	Case Reference No:
Patient Name:	
Age:	Sex:
Contact Number:	
Address:	
Occupation:	
Referring Doctor:	
Chief Complaint:	
History of Presenting Illness:	
Past Medical/Surgical History:	

Personal History

1. History of sub-luxation
2. Restriction in mouth opening due to habits
3. Parafunctional habits: Clenching/Bruxism/Grinding
4. Dietary habits

- **Allergy history:**
- **Drug History:**

General Examination

- **Built/Nourishment:**
- **Gait:**
- **Vitals documentation:**

Systemic Examination

- **Cardiovascular System:**
- **Respiratory System:**
- **Abdomen:**
- **Endocrine System:**
- **Musculoskeletal System:**

Local Examination

Extra-oral examination

- **Face:** Symmetrical/Asymmetrical
- **Ear:**
- **Preauricular region**: Skin/Swelling/Injury
- **Pain score** (10 Point Visual Analog Scale):
- **Range of Motion (ROM)** (In mm):
- Pain free MIO:
- Maximum MIO:
- Protrusive movements:

Other clinical parameters	Right	Left
Lateral movements		
Joint sounds 1. Opening click 2. Closing click 3. Associated pain on mouth opening 4. Crepitus		
Muscle tenderness 1. Temporalis 2. Masseter 3. Sternocleidomastoid 4. Posterior cervical muscles 5. Any other		

Intraoral Examination

- **Dentition**: Primary/Mixed/Permanent
- **Teeth present**:
- **Teeth wear:** Attrition/occlusal facets

Clinical parameters	Right	Left
Occlusion 1. Molar relation 2. Canine relation Status of third molars		

Provisional Diagnosis:
Differential Diagnosis:
Radiographic Evaluation

- Orthopantomogram (OPG):
- TMJ Tomogram (Open/Close):
- CB-CT:
- Ultrasonography:
- CT scan:
- MRI:

Hematological/Biochemical Investigations:
Final Diagnosis:
Treatment Plan

- Patient counselling/Diet modification
- Medical management
- Non-surgical management: Immobilization/Occlusal splints/Physiotherapy
- Minimally invasive management
- Surgical management

References

1. Bumann A, Lotzmann U. TMJ disorders and orofacial pain – the role of dentistry in a multidisciplinary diagnostic approach. 1st ed. New York: Thieme; 2011.
2. Wright EF. Manual of temporomandibular disorders. 2nd ed. Hoboken, NJ: Wiley-Blackwell; 2020.
3. RJM G. Temporomandibular disorders: a problem based approach. 1st ed. Hoboken, NJ: Wiley-Blackwell; 2011. p. 29–46.
4. Agerberg G. Maximal mandibular movement in young men and women. Swed Dent J. 1974;67:81–100.
5. Okeson JP. Management of temporomandibular disorders and occlusion. 5th ed. St. Louis: Elsevier; 2020. p. 245–321.
6. McCarroll RS, Hesse JR, Naeije M, Yoon CK, Hansson TL. Mandibular border positions and their relationships with peripheral joint mobility. J Oral Rehabil. 1987;14:125–31.
7. Yatani H, Sonoyama W, Kuboki T, Matsuka Y, Orsini MG, Yamashita A. The validity of clinical examination for diagnosis of anterior disc displacement with reduction. Oral Surg Oral Med Oral Pathol Oral Radiol Endod. 1998;85:647–53.
8. Rakeshpawar, et al. Examination of temporomandibular joint-a review. J Appl Dent Med Sci. 2016;2:147–51.
9. American Academy of Orofacial Pain. In: de Leeuw R, editor. Orofacial pain: guidelines for assessment, diagnosis and management. 4th ed. Chicago, IL: Quintessence; 2008. p. 145–51.
10. Frost HM. Musculoskeletal pains. In: Alling CC, Mahan PE, editors. Facial pain. Philadelphia: Lea & Febiger; 1977. p. 140–52.
11. Schwartz L, Chayes CM. The history and clinical examination. In: Schwartz L, Chayes CM, editors. Facial pain and mandibular dysfunction. Philadelphia, PA: Saunders; 1969. p. 159–78.
12. Moody PM, Calhoun TC, Okeson JP, Kemper JT. Stress pain relationship in MPD syndrome patients and non MPD syndrome patients. J Prosthet Dent. 1981;45:84–8.
13. Okeson JP, Kemper JT, Moody PM. A study of the use of occlusion splints in the treatment of acute and chronic patients with craniomandibular disorders. J Prosthet Dent. 1982;48:708–12.
14. Simons DG, Travell JG, Simons LS. Travell & Simons' myofascial pain and dysfunction: the trigger point manual. 2nd ed. Baltimore: Lippincott Williams & Wilkins; 1999.
15. Mense S. Nociception from skeletal muscle in relation to clinical muscle pain. Pain. 1993;54:241–89.
16. Svensson P, Arendt-Nielsen L, Nielsen H, Larsen JK. Effect of chronic and experimental jaw muscle pain on pain-pressure thresholds and stimulus-response curves. J Orofac Pain. 1995;9:347–56.
17. Badel T, Laškarin M, Zadravec D, Čimić S, Savić Pavičin I. Subluxation of temporomandibular joint- a clinical view. J Dent Probl Solut. 2018;5(2):029034. https://doi.org/10.17352/2394-8418.000060.
18. Komali G, Ignatius AV, Srivani G S, Anuja K. T-scan system in the management of temporomandibular joint disorders – A review. J Indian Acad Oral Med Radiol. 2019;31:252–6.

7 Temporomandibular Joint Imaging in Health and Disease

Prashant Prakash Jaju, Sushma Prashant Jaju, Kanak Pushkarna, S. Karthiga Kannan, and Darpan Bhargava

7.1 Introduction

Temporomandibular joint disorders (TMDs) are one of the major causes of pain and discomfort affecting the oro-facial region. Imaging of the temporomandibular joint (TMJ) has a significant role in arriving at a definitive diagnosis. Anatomical areas of interest in TMJ imaging cover evaluation of articulating structures: the condyle, the glenoid fossa, articular tubercle, fibrocartilaginous disc, retrodiscal tissue and adjacent soft and osseous structures.

P. P. Jaju
Oral Medicine and Radiology, Rishiraj College of Dental Sciences and Research Centre, Bhopal, Madhya Pradesh, India

S. P. Jaju
Conservative Dentistry and Endodontics, Rishiraj College of Dental Sciences and Research Centre, Bhopal, Madhya Pradesh, India

K. Pushkarna
Rishiraj College of Dental Sciences and Research Centre, Bhopal, Madhya Pradesh, India

S. K. Kannan
Oral Medicine and Radiology, Dental Education Department, College of Dentistry, Majmaah University, Al Majma'ah, Saudi Arabia

D. Bhargava (✉)
TMJ Consultancy Services, Bhopal, Madhya Pradesh, India

Oral and Maxillofacial Surgery, People's College of Dental Sciences and Research Centre, People's University, Bhopal, Madhya Pradesh, India
e-mail: drdarpanbhargava@gmail.com

One of the diagnostic challenges in a patient presenting with facial pain is the selection of an appropriate type of radiographic imaging. It plays a pivotal role in evaluation of the patients with TMDs. The aim of imaging the TMJ is to evaluate the veracity of the joint structures, defining the extent of disease and to monitor the progression and the post treatment changes of related TMDs [1]. The hard and soft tissue components of the TMJ that should be evaluated are summarized in Table 7.1 and the merits and demerits of the various available diagnostic imaging modalities used are listed in Tables 7.2 and 7.3.

The selection of a suitable imaging technique should be based on the value of its image characteristics which could contribute to a valuable information for a comprehensive management of the patient. Selection criteria also include likelihood of hard/soft tissue pathology, availability of imaging equipment, financial factors, quantity of radiation dose, and related physiologic or systemic condition of the patient such as pregnancy, hypersensitivity for intravenous (IV) contrast agents, implanted pacemakers, etc. [1]

Table 7.1 Components of temporomandibular joint (TMJ)

Osseous components	Non-osseous components
Condylar head	Articular disc
Glenoid fossa	Joint capsule
Articular eminence/tubercle	Muscles/ligaments

D. Bhargava (ed.), *Temporomandibular Joint Disorders*,
https://doi.org/10.1007/978-981-16-2754-5_7

Table 7.2 Various imaging for TMJ

Hard tissue imaging		
Two-dimensional (2D)	Three-dimensional (3D)	Soft tissue imaging
1. Orthopantomogram (OPG) 2. TMJ tomogram: open/closed mouth 3. Transpharyngeal view 4. Transorbital view 5. Transcranial view 6. Reverse Townes view	1. Computed tomography (CT) 2. Cone beam computed tomography (CBCT)	1. Ultrasonography 2. Arthrography 3. Magnetic resonance imaging (MRI)

Table 7.3 Advantages and limitations of various imaging techniques of TMJ

Radiographic imaging	Advantages	Limitations
Panoramic imaging (OPG)	1. Ease of availability 2. Common initial screening modality 3. Visualization of bilateral condylar heads	1. Superimpositions 2. Ghost images 3. Insufficient information regarding condylar position 4. Mild osseous change not detected
TMJ tomogram	1. Position of condyle during open and closed mouth is obtained	1. Technique sensitive
Postero-anterior (PA) cephalometric projection	1. Can be advised in general hospital/ casualty set-up when dental radiographic equipment are unavailable	1. Superimpositions
Lateral cephalometric projection	1. Can be advised in general hospital/ casualty set-up when dental radiographic equipment are unavailable	1. Improper/poor image of the contralateral condyle due to superimpositions
Reverse Townes view (open mouth)	1. Excellent bilateral visualisation of condyle displacement in subcondylar fractures	1. Technique sensitive 2. Superimposition of petrous ridge of temporal bone
Oblique lateral view (mandibular body)	1. Uncommonly used to examine the condyle	1. Superimpositions 2. Difficult to examine the condyle
Oblique lateral view (mandibular ramus)	1. Similar to lateral cephalometric projection	1. Improper/poor image of the contralateral condyle due to superimpositions
Submentovertex projection	1. Uncommonly used to examine the condyle 2. Condyle relation to skull base in horizontal plane can be determined 3. Can be used to measure the angle of long axis of condylar heads used for tomography 4. Under-exposed view is used to evaluate zygomatic arch evaluation in trauma	1. Superimpositions 2. Inadequate visualisation of the medial and lateral poles of TMJ
Trans-pharyngeal projection	1. Provides lateral view of the condyle	1. Depicts only the medial aspect of condyle clearly
Trans-cranial view	1. Provides lateral view of the condyle and image can be taken in both open and closed mouth position	1. Only lateral aspect of condyle is visualised clearly
Trans-orbital view	1. Useful to detect condylar neck fractures 2. Image of complete medial-lateral aspect of condyle is obtained in the frontal plane	1. Can be obtained in open/protruded mouth position only

Table 7.3 (continued)

Radiographic imaging	Advantages	Limitations
Conventional tomography	1. Obtains image by blurring the image of structures lying outside the plane of interest	1. Reduced contrast resolution
Computed tomography (CT) scan	1. Fine image of the joint lesions/ disorders/trauma 2. 3D reconstruction allows rapid prototyping	1. Image degradation due to artefacts 2. Contrast media can be toxic in patients with renal disease (if used)
Cone beam computed tomography (CBCT)	1. Rapid prototyping can be done 2. 3D image of the condyle morphology can be obtained	1. Higher radiation dose as compared to conventional radiographs
Ultrasonography	1. Ionising radiation is not used 2. Evaluation of different tissues with its boundaries	1. Interpretation requires sound knowledge for both the radiologist and the maxillofacial surgeon 2. Only lateral side can be visualized adequately
Magnetic resonance imaging (MRI)	1. High quality images of soft tissue in any imaging plane 2. Non-invasive 3. Uses non-ionising radiation	1. Does not provide clear picture of hard tissue changes 2. High cost 3. Long scan time 4. Various metals in imaging field can distort image/injure the patient
Arthrography	1. Permits soft tissue examination	1. Invasive procedure 2. Risk of bleeding/facial nerve injury 3. Allergic reaction to contrast agent 4. High radiation exposure
Single positron emission computed tomography (SPECT)	1. Detects abnormal metabolic bone activity: Condylar hyperplasia/ metastatic lesions	1. Assesses only physiologic changes
Positron emission tomography (PET)	1. Uncommon in TMJ examination	1. Assesses only physiologic changes

7.2 Hard Tissue Imaging of TMJ

Conventional Imaging 2D radiographs, those utilizing plain films, have been well-versed to evaluate TMJ that exemplifies only the mineralized parts of the joint. It does not deliver much information about the nonmineralized components such as the cartilage, soft tissue components and for diagnosing the inflammatory joint effusion. Bony changes in the TMJ are often not detected unless a significant quantity of bone mineral content is lost. Inspite of having ample limitations, several 2D imaging techniques have been utilized for imaging TMJ using various projections which is discussed subsequently in the chapter [1, 2].

7.3 Reverse Towne View (Open Mouth) (Fig. 7.1)

Reverse Towne's projection is a posteroanterior view and is a favoured imaging technique to evaluate bilateral condyles for localization of fractures and anteromedial displacement. Visualization of condylar medial and lateral poles could be achieved by directing the X-ray beam in an open mouth position. This ensures translation and rotation of the condylar head out of the glenoid fossa resulting in a midsagittal image. The relative disadvantages of the technique are superimposition of petrous ridge over base of occipital bone and projection of the condylar heads underneath the articular eminences [3].

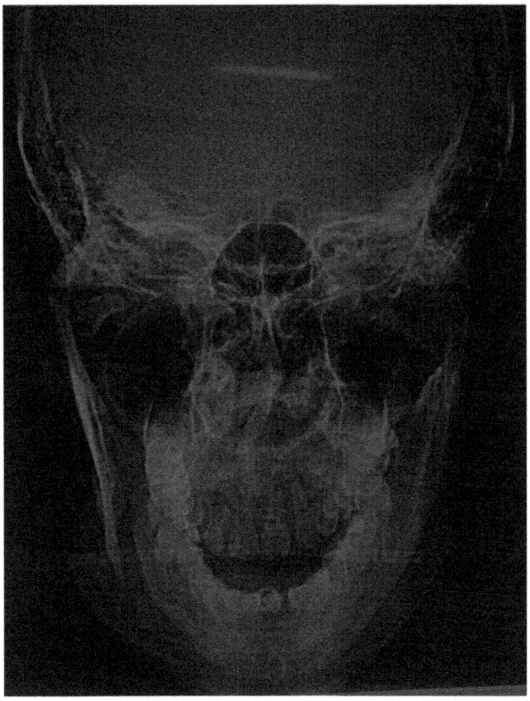

Fig. 7.1 Reverse Towne view—Open mouth projection to visualise bilateral condyle showing mandibular right angle and sub-condylar fracture. (Image courtesy: Dept of Oral Radiology, Rishiraj College of Dental Sciences and Research Centre, Bhopal, India)

7.4 Mandibular Lateral Oblique Projections (Fig. 7.2)

The lateral oblique view targets the mandibular condyle and ramus. It was popularly used before the introduction of panoramic radiography. The ramus projection is obtained by directing the central beam at the midpoint of the ramus. It provides details about the ipsilateral condyle, third molar region and contralateral angle of the mandible. As it provides very less information of TMJ structure and superimposition of the glenoid fossa by overlying anatomical structures, it is least recommended for TMJ evaluation [3].

7.5 Sub-Mentovertex (SMV) Projection

SMV projection has limited applications for the TMJ. In this technique the patient's head is titled back so that the vertex touches the cassette (containing the X-ray film). The midsagittal plane (MSP) is oriented perpendicular to the film/sensor and the radiographic base line (infraorbitomeatal line (IOML)) is parallel to the film/sensor

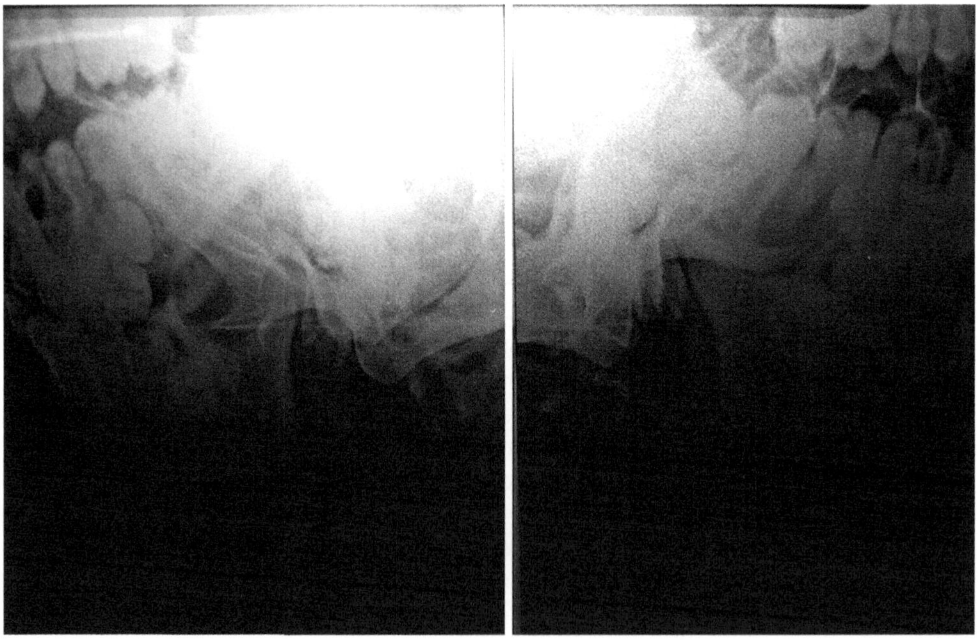

Fig. 7.2 Mandibular lateral oblique projection—body projection. (Image courtesy: Dr. Darpan Bhargava, Oral and Maxillofacial Surgery, TMJ Consultancy, Bhopal, India)

and the primary beam is directed perpendicular to the radiographic film/sensor from beneath the mandible. A similar imaging technique—jug handle view radiograph is used to evaluate the zygomatic arch fracture, where the fragments are displaced or the arch is depressed, restricting the movement of coronoid process and resulting in reduced mouth opening [3].

7.6 Trans-Pharyngeal View (Infra-Cranial/McQueen Dell Technique) (Fig. 7.3)

Trans-pharyngeal view is a lateral projection that gives an overview of the TMJ from the condylar head to the mid-portion of the mandible. This view usually emphasizes on imaging condyle in open and closed mouth position, in order to project the joint in the shadow of air occupied naso-pharyngeal spaces, which increases the contrast of the resultant image of the joint. The X-ray tube should be placed in proximity to the opposite side joint; focussing the beam towards the film placed over the joint to be imaged. As a modification to this technique described by Parma, the tube head is brought closer to the patient producing magnification of the proximal structure reducing superimpositions [2–4].

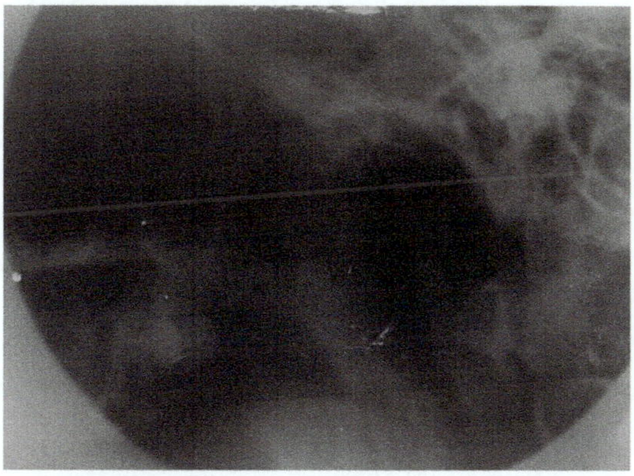

Fig. 7.3 Trans-pharyngeal view of TMJ

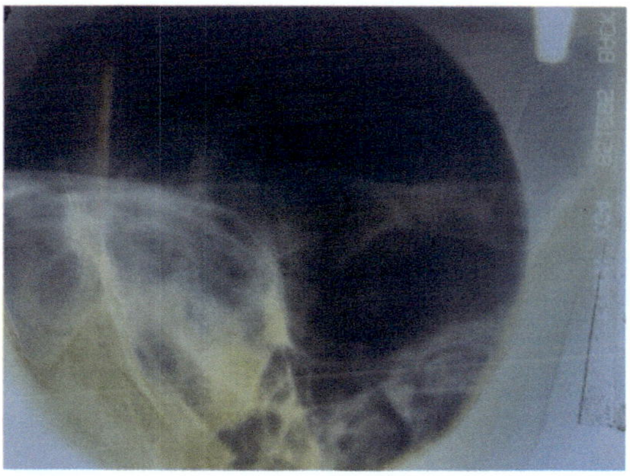

Fig. 7.4 Trans-orbital view of TMJ

7.7 Trans-Orbital View (Zimmer Projection) (Fig. 7.4)

This view depicts a frontal TMJ projection, demonstrating the lateral and medial fronts of the condyle and its articulating surfaces. In this projection the central rays are oriented perpendicular to the condyle. In order to avoid overlapping shadows of the structures of skull base the mandible is placed in a protruded position. It is specified for evaluation of the joint in three dimensions, neoplasms and degenerative joint diseases [2, 3].

7.8 Transcranial View (Fig. 7.5)

Schullerin (1905) introduced transcranial view for visualizing the TMJ. For transcranial lateral oblique projection, the primary beam is focused parallel to the condylar long axis. Using this projection, only the skull bones superimpose over the TM joint but ensuing a relatively sharp image of the osseous components of the joint. This view can be used to evaluate the width of the joint cavity and position or size of the condyle along with its relation to the eminence and the articular fossa [2, 3].

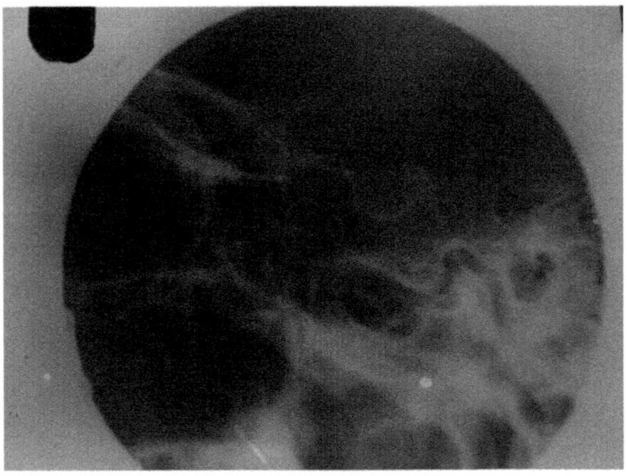

Fig. 7.5 Transcranial view of TMJ

There are three techniques by which transcranial image can be obtained:

(a) **Lindblom or post auricular technique:** The central ray is passed half an inch above the auditory meatus and should be directed posteriorly so that it passes along the long axis of the condyle.
(b) **Grewcock technique:** The central ray passes through a point 2 inches above the external auditory meatus.
(c) **Gills technique:** The central ray is aimed at 25 degrees inferiorly to the horizontal plane across the cranium centring through the TMJ of interest.

7.9 Panoramic Imaging (Orthopantomogram/OPG) (Figs. 7.6 and 7.7)

Panoramic radiographs are more beneficial over plain film radiographs for evaluation of the dentition, jaw bones and TMJ. Lateral view of bilateral condylar heads confined within the focal trough can be visualized in a single projection. Gross anatomical alterations of the head of condyle and the articular fossa are evident. Although this projection has a very limited role in diagnosing TMDs but alteration in the size, shape and integrity of cortical lining of the condyles, flattening of the articular surface and change in joint space can be appraised in these radiographs.

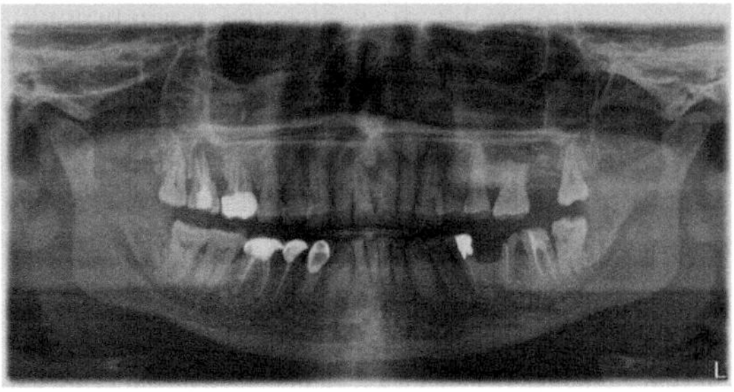

Fig. 7.6 Panoramic image of a dentate maxilla/mandible

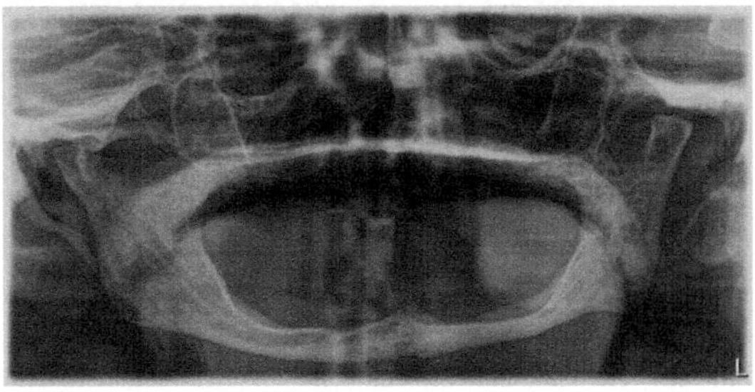

Fig. 7.7 Panoramic image of an edentulous maxilla/mandible

The condyle is placed in an antero-inferior position as the patient's mouth is slightly protruded to engage the panoramic machine. Glenoid fossa can appear as pneumatized by mastoid air cells resulting in a multilocular radiolucency of the articular tubercle and roof of the articular fossa. Peri-condylar soft tissue structures cannot be assessed using this imaging technique [2, 3].

7.10 TMJ Tomogram: Open/Closed Mouth (Fig. 7.8)

TMJ tomogram is referred to as the anteroposterior (AP) view of the mandibular condyle. Changing the configuration of the moving panoramic units and altering the focal trough enables the conventional panoramic radiography to produce localized views of both the joints in a single film in open and closed mouth. During the first exposure, the patient is instructed to keep the mouth in close position and in second exposure, to keep mouth in semi-open position. Superimposition of the cranial vault and cervical spine shadow can be seen. In cases of ankylosis,

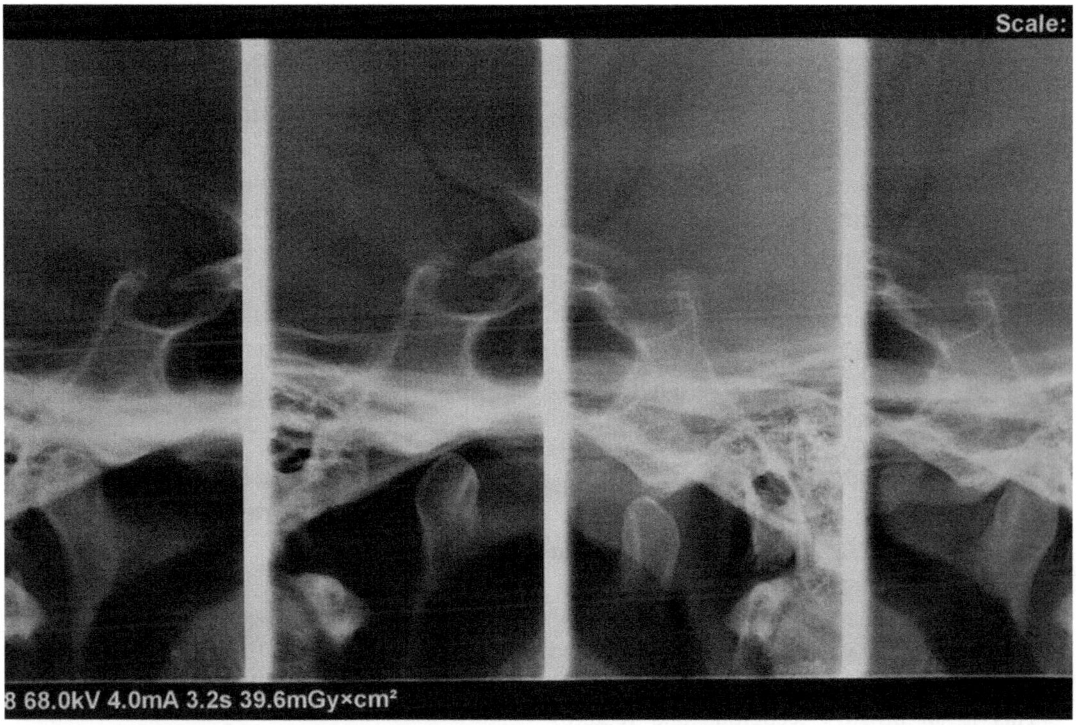

Fig. 7.8 TMJ tomogram (Open/Closed Mouth)

trismus, dislocation (open lock) and subluxation, this technique is beneficial in demonstrating the relation of the condyle to glenoid fossa and articular tubercle at rest and at functional position.

7.11 Conventional Tomography

It is a radiographic technique allowing visualization of osseous structures produced by multiple thin image slices free from super impositions of adjacent structures at right angles to the TM joint showing exact position of the condyle and bony alterations. They produce several images in closed, i.e., centric occlusion and single view in open position. This technique is not in common practice with the advent of advanced imaging modalities [3].

7.12 Cone Beam Computed Tomography (CBCT)

CBCT utilizes X-rays with cone shape centred on a flat panel detector which produces series of 2D images, which are compiled and reconstructed as 3D data. CBCT allows multiplanar reconstruction as in two-dimensional images in sagittal, coronal, axial and oblique sections of the condyle and adjacent structures to analyse morphologic changes in the bone. It can be helpful in detecting degenerative joint disease, abnormalities in the joint morphology and ankylosis. In comparison with basic conventional radiography to advanced computed tomography (CT) imaging modalities, CBCT can provide accurate, area specific submillimetric resolution images in lesser scan time and radiation dose [3].

7.13 Arthrography

Arthrography is an invasive modality for diagnosing TMDs chosen for functional examination of the joint, to envision disc perforation/adherence and loose bodies in the joints. The procedure includes injecting approximately 1.5–2 mL radiopaque high concentration iodine contrast dye into the joint space under the guidance of fluoroscopy to obtain image of the nonmineralized structures of TM joint. Based on the distribution of contrast agents in the joint space, adhesions, disc position and perforations could be analysed during opening/closing jaw positions. A transcranial lateral oblique view of the TM joint can be visualized by vertically positioning the X-ray source in C-arm and patient in lying posture with targeted side facing upwards. Moving the radiation source more caudally, central and medial portions of the joint can be visualized.

This is an invasive technique and requires insertion of a fine needle into the TM joint, therefore complications like bleeding, damage to the disc, facial nerve and introduction of infection could occur. It also poses risk for a hypersensitivity reaction to the contrast media and the increased exposure to radiation. One advantage is as the needle is inserted into the joint under local anaesthesia, any required therapeutic procedures can simultaneously be performed as per the diagnosis including arthrography guided therapeutic injections of corticosteroids and lavage of the joint.

It is rarely used modality for diagnosing TMDs as other imaging modalities reveal excellent soft tissue examination such as ultrasonography (USG) and MRI without a needle insertion. But may be used in patients where an advanced imaging modality (e.g. MRI) is contraindicated [5–7].

7.14 Ultrasonography (USG) (Fig. 7.9)

USG employs high frequency sound waves to create images from the region of interest. While travelling through the human body the sound waves encounter a boundary between various tissue densities. Depending on the density or resistance of the tissue, these sound waves are reflected as echoes back to the ultrasound probe and further returned to the computer that converts these echoes into numerical data assigning grey

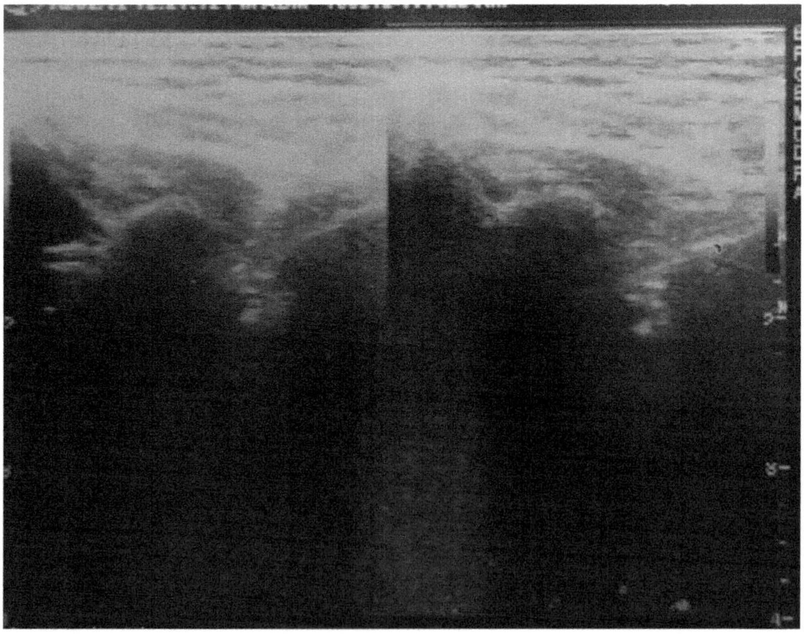

Fig. 7.9 USG of TMJ in open and closed mouth position with hyperechoic condylar head. (Image Courtesy: Dr. Darpan Bhargava, Oral and Maxillofacial Surgery, TMJ Consultancy, Bhopal, India)

Table 7.4 Ultrasonography (USG) interpretation of TMJ and surrounding structure

Type of tissue	Echo pattern	Signal received	Appearance in USG
Joint space Artery/vein Water/fluids	Anechoic	Absent	Black
Internal surface of condyle Articular disc	Hypoechoic	Weak	Grey
Condylar rim Nerve	Hyperechoic	Intense	White/ black
Connective tissue joint capsule, retrodiscal/ muscular tissue	Isoechoic	Intermediate	Grey

values and then into a picture. The TM joint possesses structures of varied nature with different reflective behaviours. Tissues are identified based on the signals they transmit which are classified based on their echo pattern. (Table 7.4).

It is a cost-effective, non-invasive and quick examination technique largely available in most healthcare institutions. A linear probe is used for TMJ, positioned transversely related to the zygomatic arch and adjusted accordingly to obtain images. It can detect degenerative changes and disc dislocations at earlier stages. An important limitation of this modality is that it greatly depends on the operator's skill and experience. Recent advancements in USG include colour doppler to evaluate blood flow and 3D imaging that allows multiplanar reformatting and surface renderings are yet to be explored in the field of maxillofacial region for the temporomandibular joint imaging [3, 8–10].

7.15 Computed Tomography

Computed tomography was first introduced in 1972 by Godfrey Hounsfield. It offers more information regarding the 3D morphology and fine changes of the bony structures, by creating detailed sections of images as small as 0.5 mm; abolishing overlap of superficial and deep structures and providing a factual image of anatomical structure of the condyle. Multi-slice CT provides images in coronal, axial and sagittal planes. It provides details of the surrounding structures unlike a CBCT which only captures the area of interest. Data availability in 3D format has enabled the construction of stereolithographic models which can be used for mock surgeries and as an aid in fabrication of custom-made alloplastic prosthesis for joint reconstructions.

Condylar morphology in an axial plane is depicted as rounded bony projection having an oval, biconcave articular surface of glenoid fossa and the joint space. The anteroposterior dimensions are smaller than the mediolateral dimensions and its terminations are referred to as lateral and medial poles.

This acts as outstanding imaging modality to detect the extent of ankylosis, joint erosions, neoplasms, complex fractures, complications as a consequence of previous surgery, proximity to the middle cranial fossa and also heterotopic osseous growth [1, 3, 11].

7.16 Magnetic Resonance Imaging (MRI)

MRI provides accurate details of the soft tissue structures in the area of interest. The positively charged hydrogen ions within the body such as those found in fat and water align under the influence of the magnetic field. Radio waves are used to alter the alignment of these hydrogen ions which in turn emits a weak radio signal which is received by receiver coil and further amplified by the scanner. Additional magnetic fields can further be employed to manipulate the signals and to aggregate a comprehensive image of the area of interest.

It is proved to be an exceptional technique of choice in the investigation of TM joint dysfunction. Image analysis should be done with T1- and T2-weighted sequences in both in closed/open mouth positions. Recent advancements include the possibility of performing a dynamic study during progressive mouth opening using Cine MRI.

Both bony and soft tissue anatomical structures of joints are better visualized in T1-weighted images, whereas joint inflammation and effusions are well demonstrated in T2-weighted images. MRI is usually not recommended in pregnancy, people with cardiac pacemakers or intracranial aneurysm clips and other implanted metal devices, while MRI can be performed judiciously in patients with titanium dental implants [1, 3, 11–13].

7.17 Imaging in Diseases

7.17.1 Articular Disc Displacement (Fig. 7.10a–d)

Internal derangement of TMJ is a condition in which the fibrocartilaginous biconcave disc between the condyle and the glenoid fossa loses

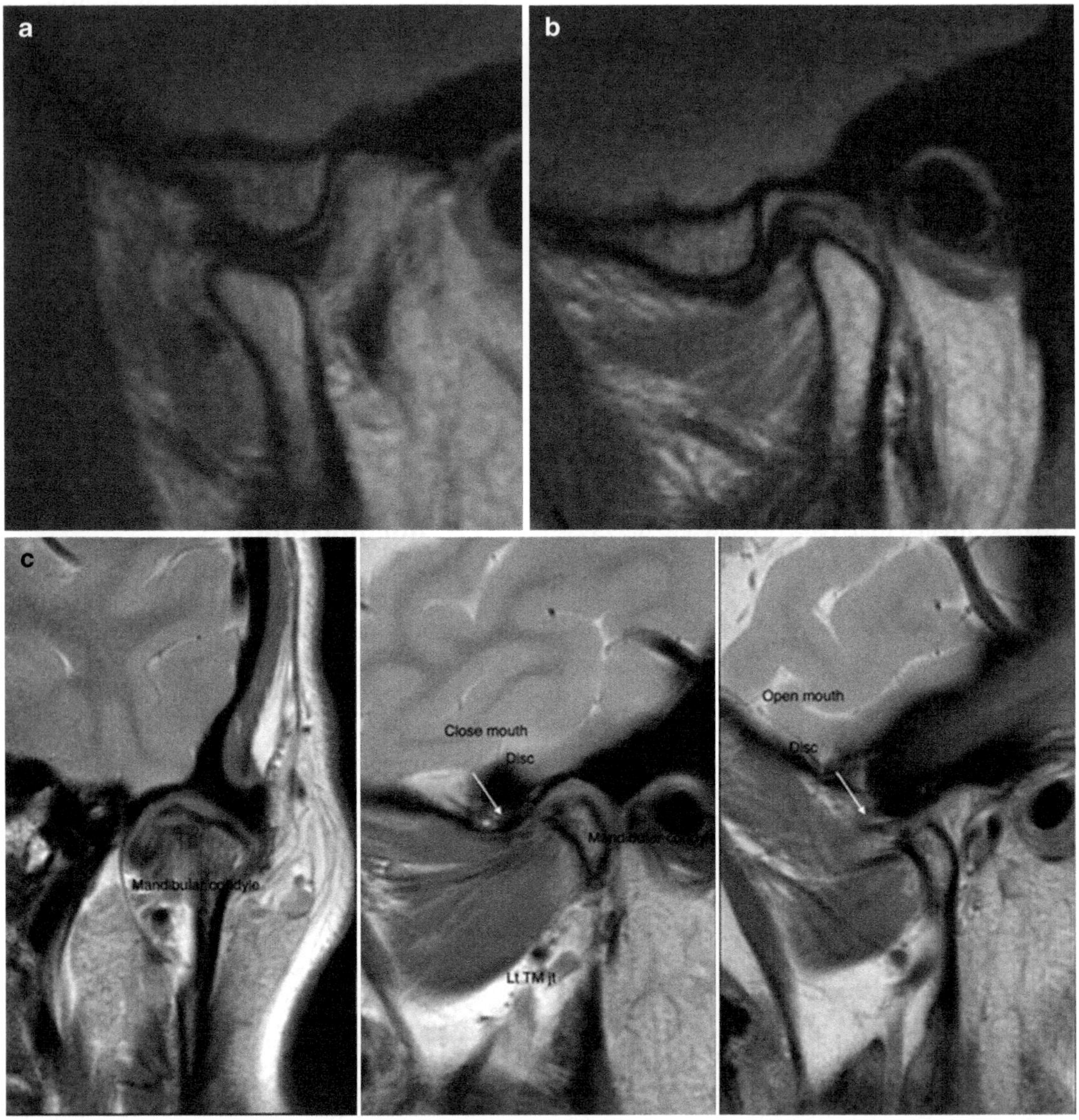

Fig. 7.10 (**a, b**) MRI of joint with internal derangement. Axially-corrected sagittal T1-weighted MRI of the TMJ in the closed (**a**) and open (**b**) mouth position, respectively, exhibits anterior disc displaced with reduction. (Image courtesy: Dr. Dania Tamimi, USA, Diplomate of AAOMR). (**c**) Antero-medial disc location of the left TMJ disc along with osteoarthritic changes. (Image courtesy: Dr. Raashi Khatri Panjabi, MD, Orofacial Pain, Mumbai, India). (**d**) Antero-medial disc location of the TMJ disc along with focal central perforation. (Image courtesy: Dr. Raashi Khatri Panjabi, MD, Orofacial Pain, Mumbai, India)

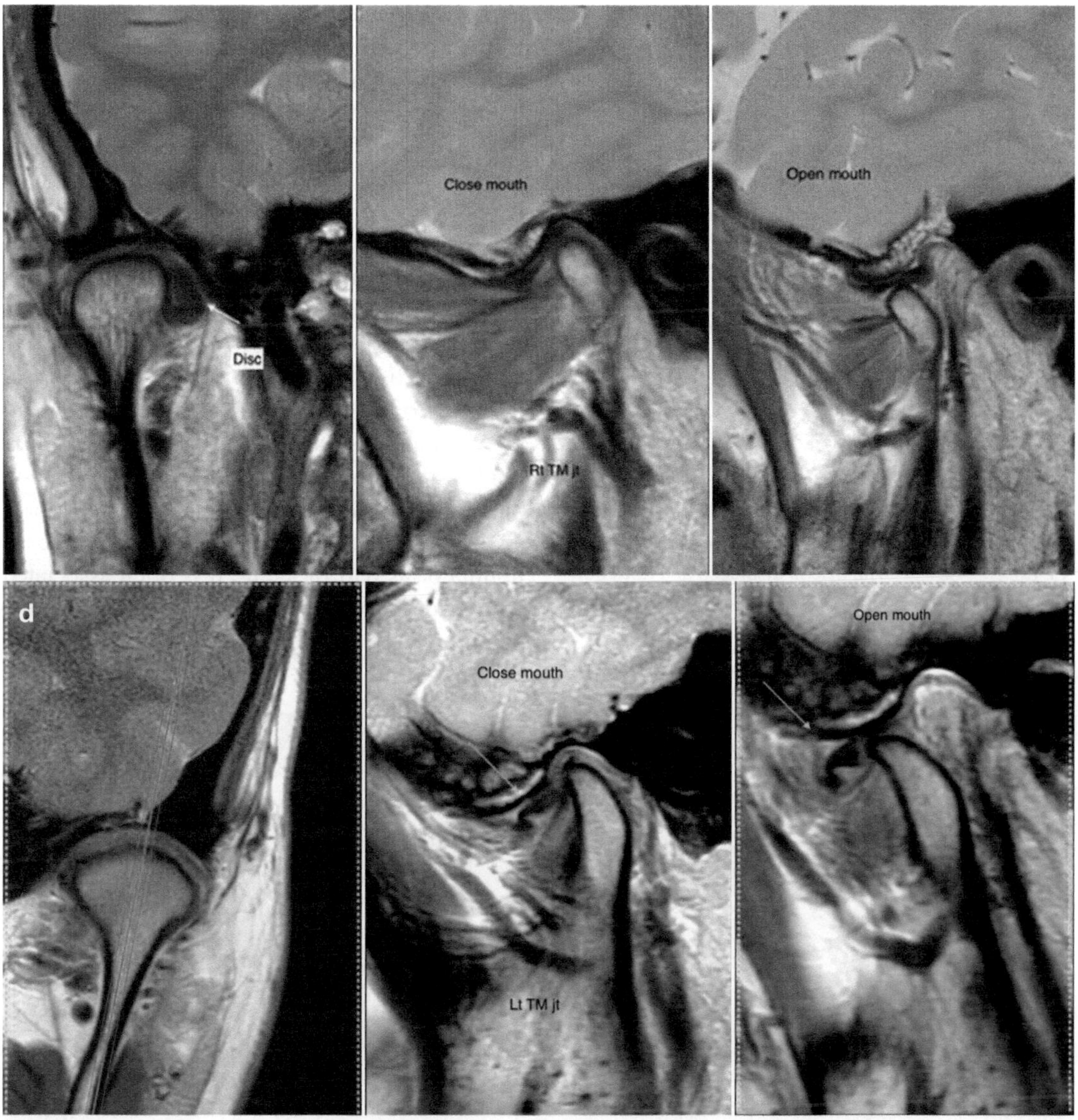

Fig. 7.10 (continued)

its normal relationship because of displacement. There are possibly four clinical stages of disc displacement (Table 7.5). The altered disc and weakened ligaments can cause various displaced positions of the disc like the anterior, anterolateral, anteromedial, lateral, medial and posterior. Proper evaluation of sagittal and coronal images of TM joint in MRI would help the clinician in diagnosing the possible types of internal derangements. MRI could be a valuable tool in imaging TM joint in both closed and open positions for assessing the stage of disc displacement.

In the initial stages of internal derangement, the shape of the disc would be normal. As the disease progresses the displaced articular disc would be altered in shape with thickened posterior band and thin central and anterior band resulting in a biconvex or rounded shaped disc. The features like irregularity, rounding of the shape of articular disc is considered characteristic of a disease process. In the late stages of internal derangement, the articular disc may tear or show perforation.

Table 7.5 Clinical stages of articular disc displacement

Stage	Feature of the articular disc	
	Closed mouth position	Open mouth position
I (disc displacement with reduction)	The articular disc is displaced	Reduces to normal relationship, i.e. the central narrow zone of the disc is in contact with the condylar head and articular eminence
II (disc displacement with reduction with intermittent locking)	The disc is displaced	Intermittent lock
III (disc displacement without reduction)	The disc is displaced	Does not reduce to normal contact (also referred to as closed lock)
IV (disc displacement without reduction)	The disc is displaced and does not reduce with perforation of the disc or posterior attachment tissues	

In inflammatory TM joint disease with a history of trauma fluid effusion within the joint occurs. As effusion fluid produces high signal intensity it could be identified well in T2-weighted images in MRI. (Refer figure in the following sections, Fig. 7.13) [14, 15].

7.17.2 Degenerative Joint Diseases (Fig. 7.11a, b)

Osteoarthritis and osteoarthrosis are the two-disease process discussed under the term degenerative joint diseases (DJD) having the similar clinical findings except for the presence of joint pain in osteoarthritis and absence in osteoarthrosis. The condition could be evolving due to trauma or as part of aging. It is often associated with underlying systemic cause, trauma or the aging process. In temporomandibular joint, 'pri-

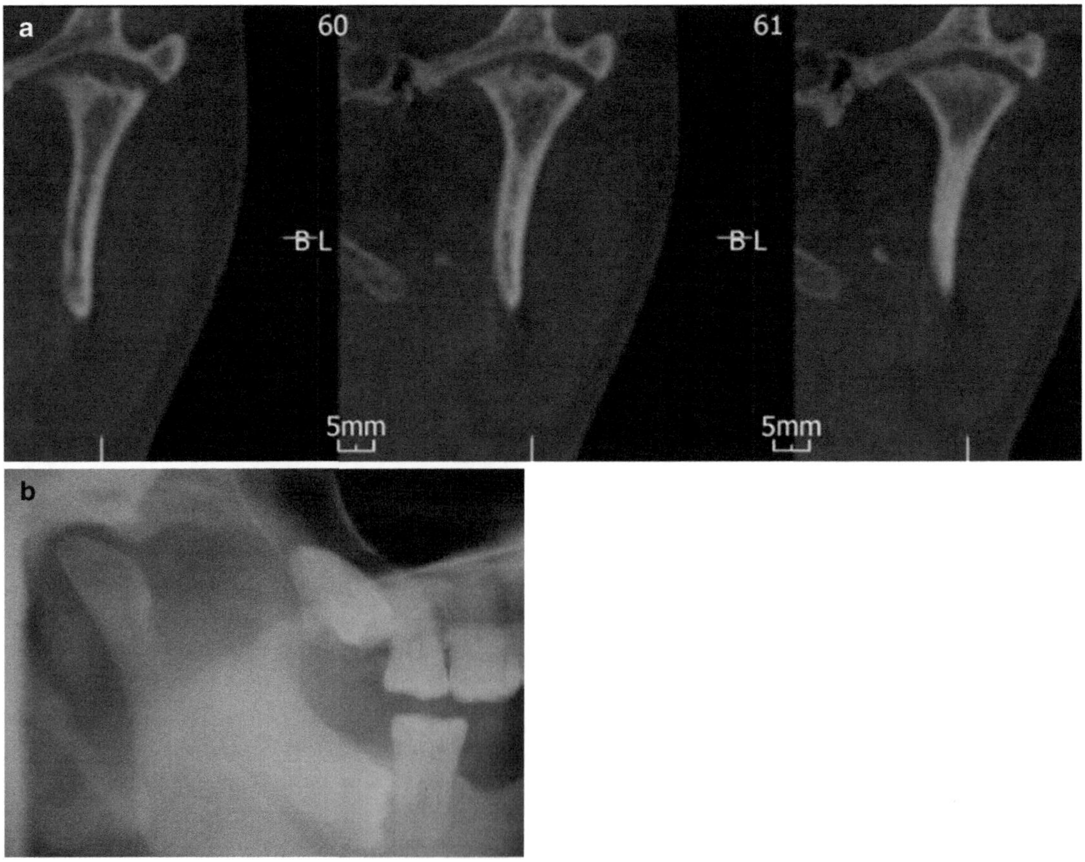

Fig. 7.11 (**a**) Coronal CT images showing alteration in condylar head anatomy and round radiolucent region (Ely's Cyst). (**b**) Articular surface of condyle showing flattening and subcortical sclerosis

mary DJD' is idiopathic by definition. 'Secondary DJD' is assumed to occur after the disc is displaced and bony contact exists between the condyle and articular fossa. Clinical signs and symptoms of DJD are often remarkably absent even when there are severe histologic/radiographic joint changes (i.e., osteoarthrosis). DJD is diagnosed radiographically, as the clinical signs and symptoms are mostly not conclusive.

Three cardinal radiographic features that lead to a diagnosis of DJD are:

1. Bony spurs or osteophyte.
2. Erosion of articular surface.
3. Condylar subcortical pseudocyst.

Other radiographic findings include flattening of the articular surface and also subcortical sclerosis. Additional criterions to diagnose DJD may be used utilizing various imaging modalities that include CT, CBCT and MRI. It may be classified as grade I and II (Table 7.6). Ahmad M et al. adopted two principles for grading DJD. It was suggested that the most advanced changes in all image views should be considered for confirming the diagnosis and two image orientations should have the advanced finding [3, 14].

7.17.3 Rheumatoid Arthritis (RA)

It is a heterogeneous group of chronic inflammatory disorder of autoimmune origin that could involve synovial membrane usually having a poly-articular involvement. Small joints such as hand, wrists, TM joints are involved in a symmetric bilateral fashion. Clinically it may manifest as pain, swelling, stiffness of mouth opening and limited range of motion (ROM). Anterior open bite may be present because of destruction of condylar surfaces bilaterally causing antero-superior positioning of condyle.

There is granulomatous inflammatory reaction of synovial membrane resulting in formation of intra-articular tissue mass known as pannus which evolves as a fibro cartilage/bone releasing some enzymes causing destruction of the articular surface and the bone.

Table 7.6 Classification of degenerative joint disease (DJD)

DJD grade	Radiographic feature	Dimension
I (displays any of the features)	Osteophyte	Greatest length is <2 mm when measured from tip of osteophyte to expected contour of condyle as viewed on the corrected sagittal section
	Erosion	Greatest dimension of the erosion is <2 mm in depth and width The erosion is limited to a single occurrence only
	Sub-cortical pseudocyst	The greatest dimension of the pseudocyst is <2 mm in depth and width The pseudocyst is limited to a single occurrence only
II (displays one or more than one of the features)	Osteophyte	The greatest length is >2 mm measured from tip of osteophyte to expected contour of condyle as viewed on the corrected sagittal section
	Erosion	The greatest dimension of the erosion is >2 mm in depth and width, OR More than 1 erosion of any size
	Sub-cortical pseudocyst	The greatest dimension of the pseudocyst is >2 mm, OR More than 1 pseudocyst of any size
	Two or more imaging signs of grade I DJD	

Radiographically, osteopenia of the condyle may be evident in the initial stage. Erosion occurs in the anterior and posterior surface of condyle resulting in a 'sharpened pencil' appearance. Entire condylar head may be destroyed in some cases. Sub-chondral sclerosis, flattening of articular surfaces, Ely's cyst and osteophyte formation may be evident. Limited ROM depends on duration and severity of the disease.

Using MRI, Kretapirom et al. classified the osseous changes in condyle into four types. Even after severe bony alterations, the articular disc would be in normal position until late stages of RA unlike DJD [3, 14, 15].

7.17.4 Juvenile Rheumatoid Arthritis

It is also known as juvenile chronic arthritis/Still's disease. The mean age of onset is 5 years characterized by chronic, repeated synovial inflammation resulting in effusion causing pain/swollen joints. Earlier onset and severe systemic involvement are differentiating the adult RA from juvenile variant. Rheumatoid factor may be absent in some cases, the preferred term is juvenile arthritis for such cases.

TMJ involvement causes restricted mouth opening and micrognathia with anterior open bite. Mandibular asymmetry can occur if there is unilateral TMJ involvement. Radiographic findings are similar to that of an adult form with an additional feature of impaired mandibular growth. Fibrous ankylosis can occur occasionally. Due to intermittent inflammation in quiescent periods, the cortical bone of the TM joint surface reappears as a flat surface causing anterosuperior positioning of the condyle [3].

7.17.5 Septic Arthritis (Infectious Arthritis) (Fig. 7.12)

It is very rare and may occur as a result of direct spread of infection from hematogenous spread, the cellulitis of nearby tissue, or involvement in presence of systemic/autoimmune disease. It is also reported in paediatric patients after trauma where hyperaemia and damage to the tissues cause hematoma formation. It is a favourable medium for growth of micro-organisms. Osseous ankylosis may occur rarely once the infection subsides warranting a need for careful follow-up. It can mimic DJD/RA but the differentiating feature is this condition is usually unilateral and clinical signs/symptoms of infection are evident [3, 14].

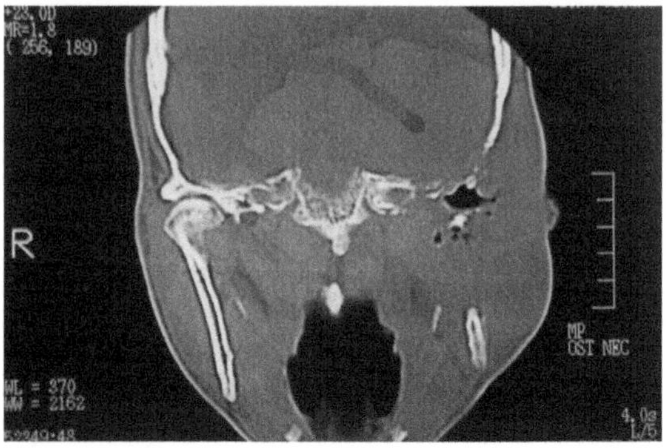

Fig. 7.12 Destructive changes of joint components in infective arthritis of left TMJ

7.18 Articular Loose Bodies

These are radiopaque loose bodies in joint space that occur either inside the joint capsule or in the soft tissue outside the joint capsule. Radiographically, they appear as soft tissue calcifications in and around the TMJ. They may be a part of bone separated from the joint. It can be hyaline cartilage metaplasia where the nodules ossify to form calcifications as in synovial chondromatosis or deposition of calcium pyrophosphate dehydrate crystals in the joint space known as calcinochondrosis/pseudo gout. Studies have reported the use of arthrography in patients diagnosed with synovial chondromatosis. CT can be used to detect the erosions in the glenoid fossa and extension into middle cranial fossa. MRI is required to determine the tissue planes between synovial chondromatosis mass and the surrounding soft tissue [3, 15].

7.19 Injury to the Temporomandibular Joint

Trauma to TM joints can be classified into two major types:

1. Condylar fracture (fracture of the bone).
2. Luxation/subluxation of TMJ (injury to the soft tissues of the joint).

7.19.1 **Effusion** (Fig. 7.13)

Effusion is known as the accumulation of fluid inside the joint either due to trauma (haemorrhage) or from inflammation (exudates) caused by ID, arthritis. MRI is useful in detecting joint effusion. MRI could provide diagnostic information in T2 weighted images as a bright white signal as the evidence for fluid in the peri-capsular space with a widened joint space.

7.19.2 Fracture of TMJ

The classifications of condylar fracture with clinical presentations are discussed in detail as a separate chapter (refer Chap. 16). Condylar fracture is often evaluated using CT because of its superiority in imaging osseous structures and also there are no superimpositions from adjacent structures, with a possibility of evaluating images in different planes with 3D reconstruction. CBCT also provides accurate picture of the fracture. In conventional radiographs, there is an irregular outline/step defect/discontinuity in the cortical border at the fracture site. An undisplaced high condyle fracture may be difficult to detect in conventional radiographs.

7.19.3 Neonatal/Paediatric Condyle Fracture

The anatomy of the condyle is different in paediatric population as compared to the adults. Careful evaluation must be done to assess, manage and follow up such fractures in growing children to prevent growth disturbances [3, 14]. They usually present with a mushroom like intracapsular fracture of the condylar head or a green-stick injury depending on the age of the patient and the type of injury.

7.19.4 **Dislocation (Luxation) of the Condyle** (Fig. 7.14)

Dislocation/luxation of TMJ is the result of excessive anterior movement of condyle to the extent that the condyle comes out of the articular fossa and is positioned in front of the articular tubercle. It is mostly an anterior dislocation.

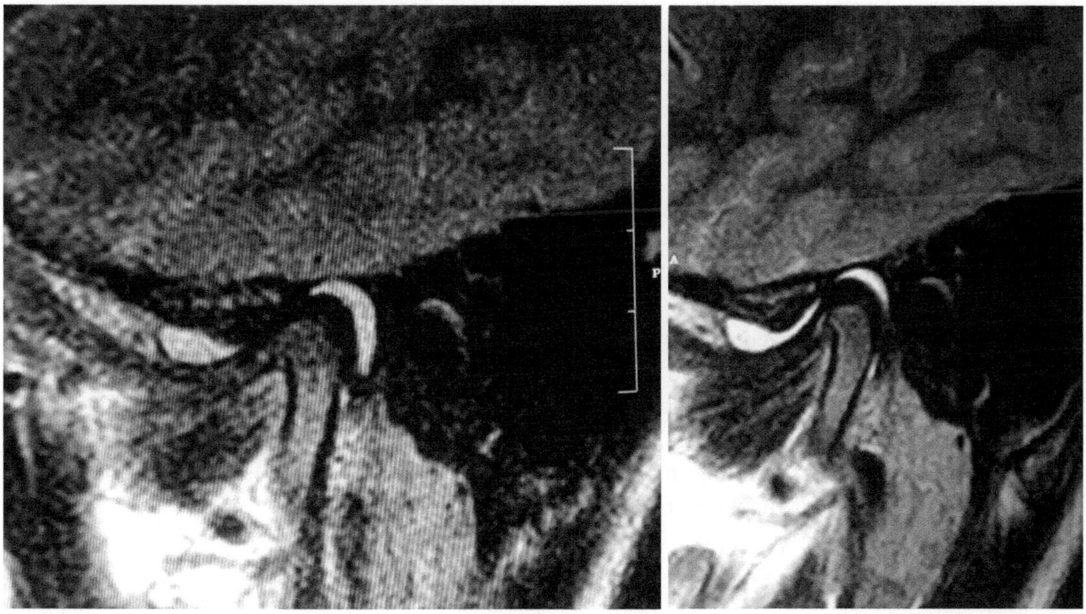

Fig. 7.13 MRI showing effusion in the joint space in a T2 weighted MRI in open and closed mouth position (Image courtesy: Dr. Darpan Bhargava, Private case, Oral and Maxillofacial Surgery, TMJ Consultancy, Bhopal, India)

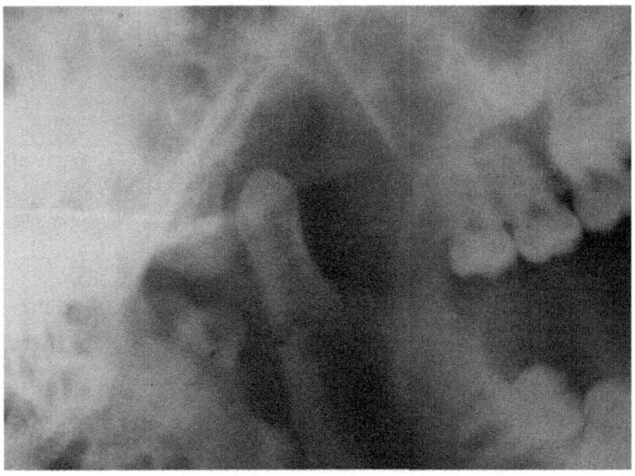

Fig. 7.14 Dislocation of TMJ is characterized by abnormal positioning of condyle out of the glenoid fossa and in front of articular eminence

If the condyle translates anterior and gets locked in front of articular eminence and is not able to bounce back to its normal relation, it would result in an open lock and patient may not be able to close the mouth, the ensuing condition is called luxation or dislocation. A similar condition where the patient would be able to manipulate and self-reduce him/herself, the displaced condyle is referred to as *subluxation or habitual dislocation*. The condyle can be dislocated in anterior/lateral/medial directions. Rarely it penetrates into the cranial fossa. Sometimes the dislocation can be very minimal causing difficulty in identifying it with a conventional radiograph. CT is essential in such cases for proper diagnosis as conventional images may not show the dislocation due to superimpositions [3].

7.20 Ankylosis (Fig. 7.15a–c)

TMJ ankylosis is characterized by the union of articular surface of the condyle of the mandible and glenoid fossa of the temporal bone either with fibrous tissues (fibrous ankylosis) or osseous tissue (bony ankylosis) resulting in partial or complete loss of form and function. The aetiology, clinical features and management of ankylosis are discussed in detail as a separate chapter (Refer Chap. 17).

OPG and other conventional imaging techniques have less significant role in detecting the extent of ankylosis. CT is vital to detect the extent and involvement of the ankylotic mass. 3D reconstruction enables construction of a stereolithographic model to fabricate custom-made alloplastic prosthesis prior to the surgery, where indicated. MRI is essential in case of fibrous ankylosis [3, 14, 16].

7.21 Tumours of TMJ

Tumours of the TMJ are very rare and can be intrinsic or extrinsic. Intrinsic tumours arise from the condyle or the temporal bone and intracapsular soft tissues. Tumours from adjacent region disrupting the morphology of TMJ are classified to be of extrinsic origin. The tumours are broadly classified as benign and malignant. Malignant metastasis to the TMJ have been reported [17–19]. When in doubt, an initial screening radiograph followed by a CT or an MRI is usually the modality of choice [3].

7.22 Developmental Disturbances of TMJ (Figs. 7.16a&b, 7.17, 7.18a&b)

The development of TMJ is not complete at the time of birth. A developmental disturbance can occur before/at the time of/after birth. The clinical features will be suggestive of a definitive disorder in TMJ region in such patients with visible clinical facial disfigurement. The imaging of choice is CT or MRI scan, as per the indication. CBCT may be advised in cases requiring limited area for evaluation [14].

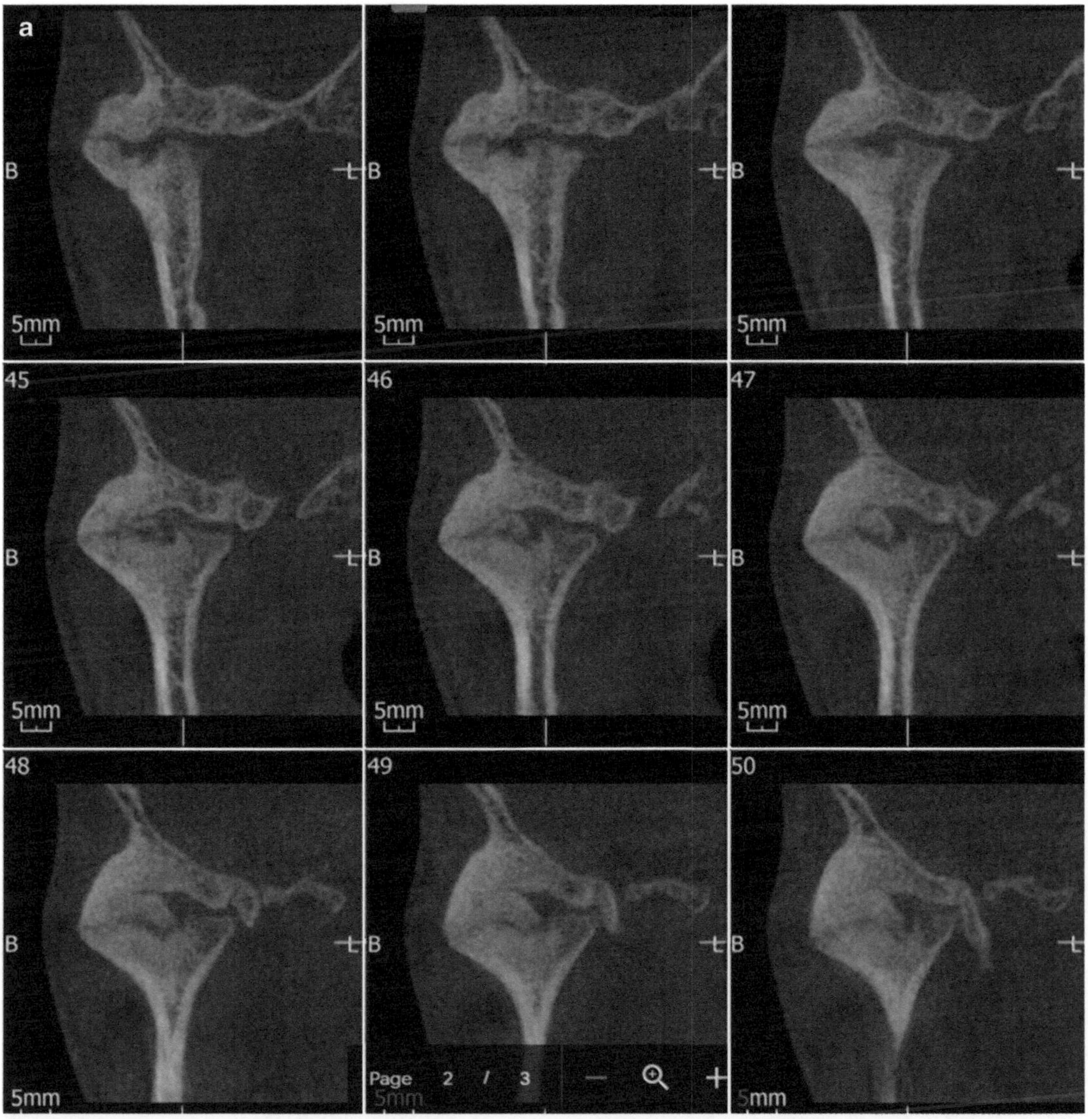

Fig. 7.15 (**a**) Coronal images of true ankylosis (post trauma). (**b**) Coronal CT images of ankylosis, with the evidence of fibrous tissue (radiolucent area) between the ankylosed bones. (**c**) Panoramic imaging of a patient with a long-standing osseous bilateral ankylosis. Note that the extent of ankylosis in the medio-lateral aspect is unclear. (Image courtesy: Department of Oral and Maxillofacial Surgery, People's College of Dental Sciences & Research Center, Bhopal, India)

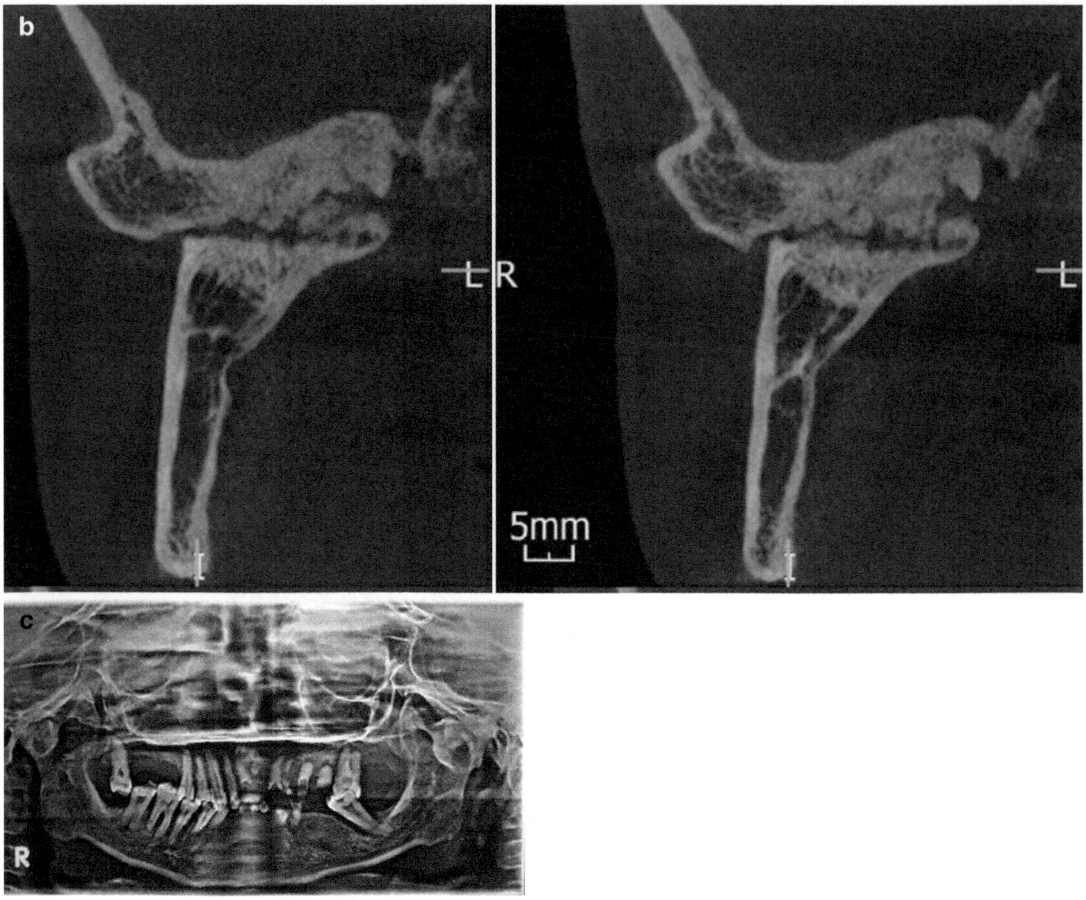

Fig. 7.15 (continued)

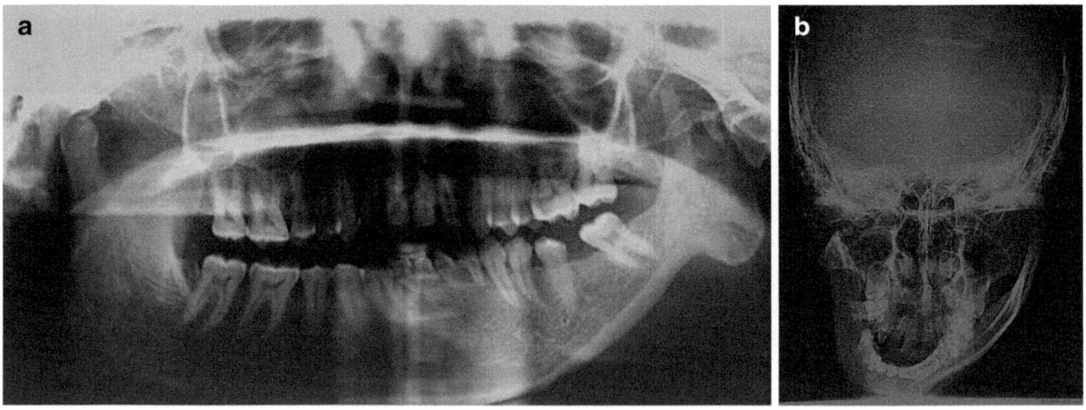

Fig. 7.16 (**a**) Panoramic image of left condyle hypoplasia. Note the prominent anti-gonial notch due to muscular hyper-activity. (Image courtesy: Dept of Oral Radiology, Rishiraj College of Dental Sciences & Research Centre, Bhopal, India). (**b**) Reverse Towne image of left condyle hypoplasia. (Image courtesy: Dept of Oral Radiology, Rishiraj College of Dental Sciences & Research Centre, Bhopal, India)

7.23 Nuclear Medicine Studies (Fig. 7.19)

Conventional radiographs, CT, CBCT, MRI, arthrography and USG are morphologic imaging techniques where it is essential for an anatomic change to occur in order to be visualized in the radiograph by the image receptor. Radionuclide imaging is a type of functional imaging which detects disease by assessing the physiologic changes caused by abnormal biochemical process without any change in the anatomic form. The various nuclear medicine techniques that can be applied to detect the disease in TMJ region are:

1. Radio nucleotide imaging/Scintigraphy.
2. Positron Emission Tomography (PET).
3. Single Photon Emission Computed Tomography (SPECT).

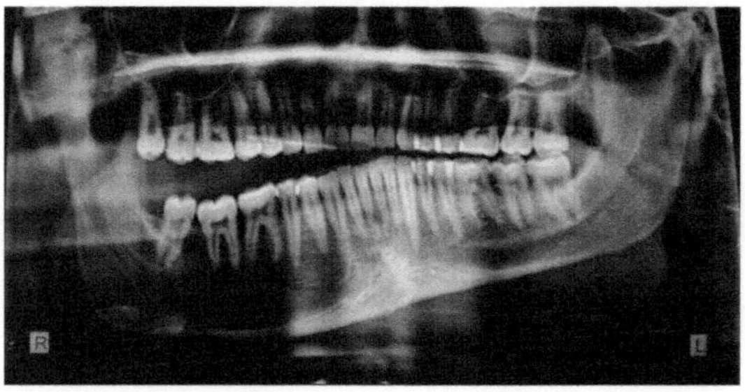

Fig. 7.17 Hyperplasia of right mandibular condyle

Their applications to detect various TMDs have been practised since long and remain controversial as the results vary from each study. It can be inferred that nuclear medicine imaging techniques with other imaging modalities can aid in better understanding of the TMDs than just considering radionuclide imaging alone [3, 20–24].

7.24 Newer Advancements

Few newer technologies are emerging in detecting certain TMDs. One such newer advancement is the digital volumetric tomography (DVT). It was first developed for angiography in 1982, which later found its application in maxillofacial imaging subsequently. Shetty US et al. have reported the use of DVT to assess the condylar changes. Planigraphy is another modality which is similar to panoramic imaging but with specialized options for TMJ [11, 25].

7.25 Goals for Imaging

Selection of an appropriate imaging technique by the clinician must be done after careful considerations of the outcome and possible risks associated with the use of X-rays. Radiographic selection criteria are based on clinical findings of patients for whom a high probability exists that a particular radiographic evaluation could provide

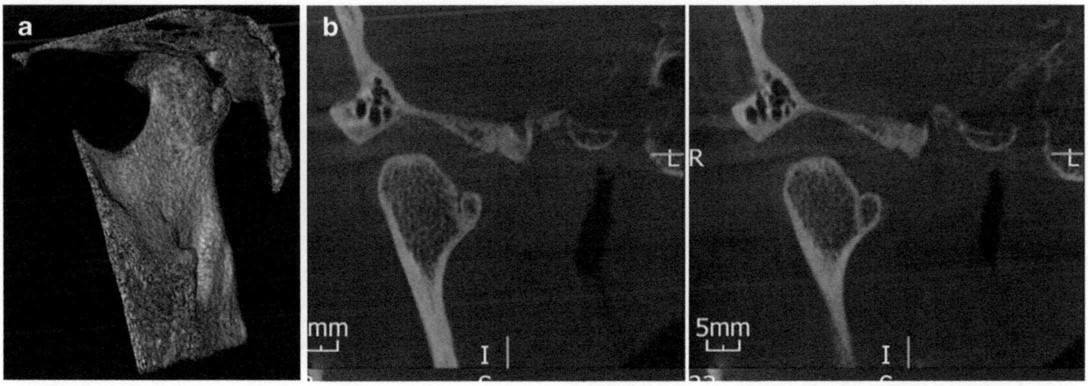

Fig. 7.18 (**a**) 3D reconstructed CT image of Bifid condyle. (**b**) Coronal section of CT images showing bifid condyle

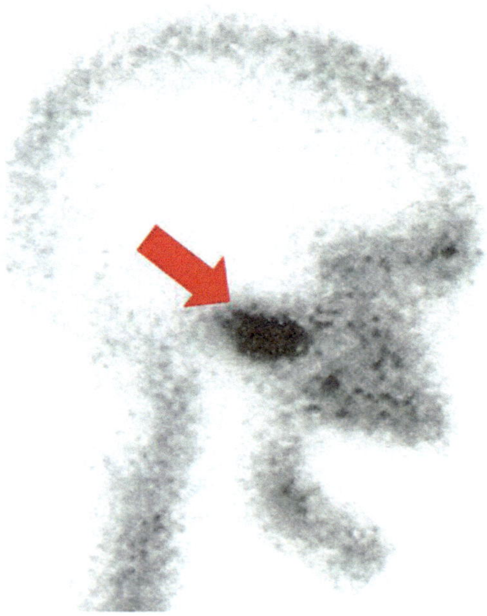

Fig. 7.19 Tc-99 m methylene diphosphonate (MDP) bone scintigraphy with increased tracer concentration in the condyle of the right mandible suggestive of hypermetabolic active bone growth and ossification process (Adapted with permission: Neelakandan RS, Bhargava D. Bifid hyperplastic mandibular condyle. J Maxillofac Oral Surg. 2013 Dec; 12(4): 466-71; Springer)

details in arriving at a definitive diagnosis altering treatment/prognosis. Clear indications should be established to justify any laboratory tests/imaging performed for an individual patient.

Definitions *[1–3]*

1. An osteophyte is a marginal hypertrophy with sclerotic borders and exophyte is an angular formation of osseous tissue arising from the surface.
2. Surface erosion is loss of continuity of articular cortex of the condyle or the fossa.
3. A subcortical pseudocyst is defined as a cavity below the articular surface that deviates from normal marrow pattern. It is not a true cyst but rather the loss of trabeculation.
4. A surface flattening is defined as a loss of rounded contour of the surface of the condyle or the articular eminence. It can be present in normal joints as a variation of normal joint.
5. A subcortical sclerosis is defined as any increased thickness of the cortical plate in the load-bearing areas related to the adjacent non-load-bearing areas.

Appendix

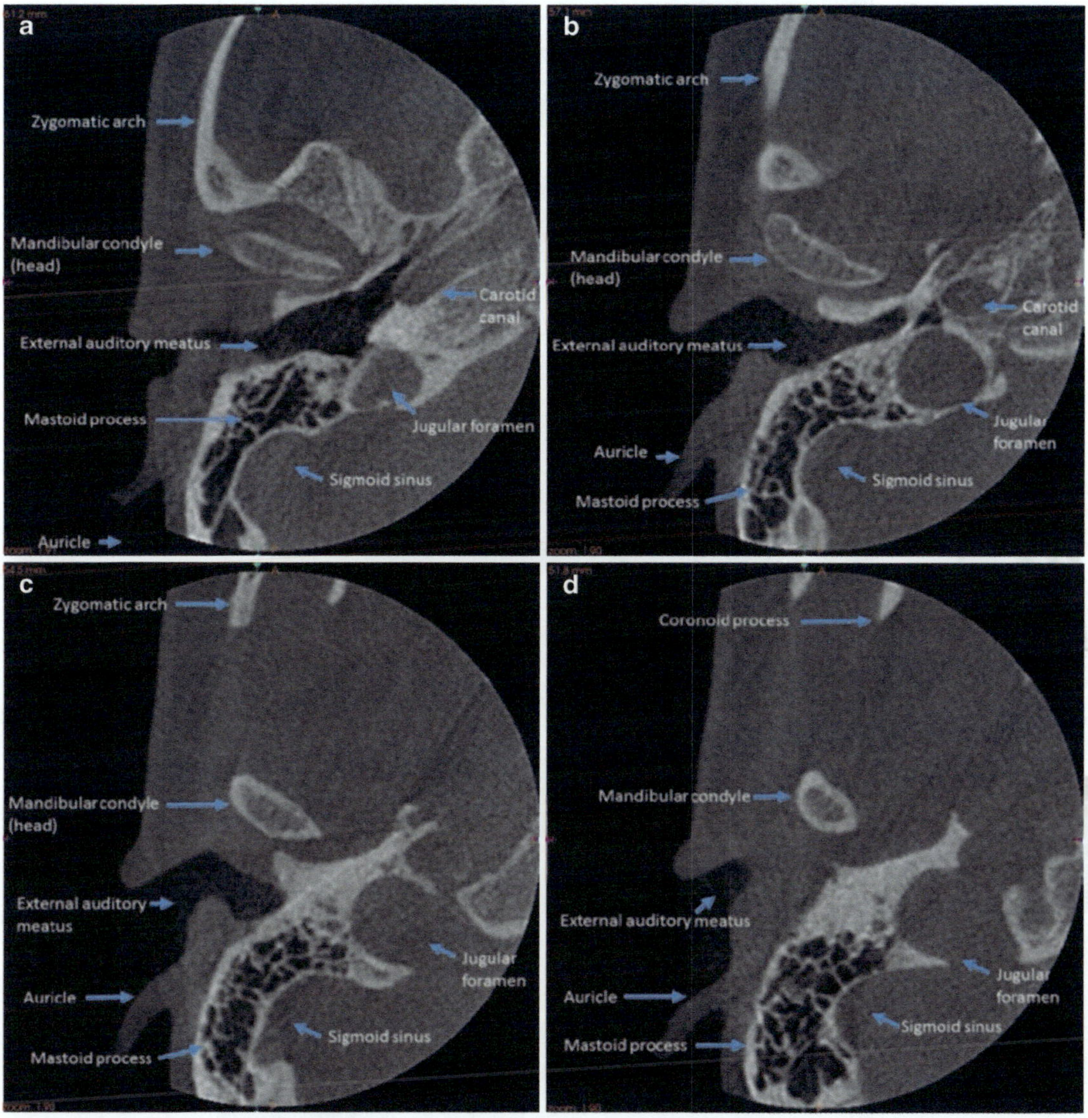

Atlas 7.1 Axial sections (**a**–**d**) radiological anatomy of the TMJ in CBCT. [Reprinted/adapted by permission from I. Rozylo-Kalinowska, K. Orhan (eds.), *Imaging of the TemporomandibularJoint*, https://doi.org/10.1007/978-3-319-99468-0_8]

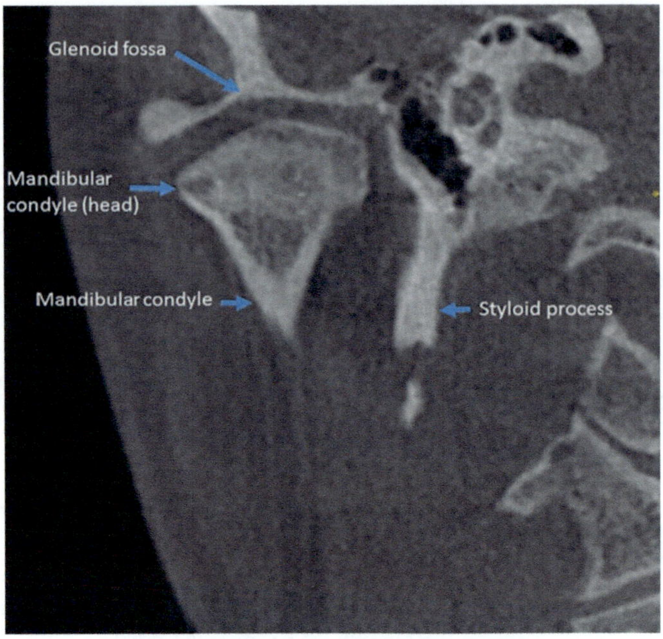

Atlas 7.2 Radiological anatomy of the TMJ in CBCT—image obtained along the long axis of the condyle. [Reprinted/adapted by permission from I. Rozylo-Kalinowska, K. Orhan (eds.), *Imaging of the TemporomandibularJoint*, https://doi.org/10.1007/978-3-319-99468-0_8]

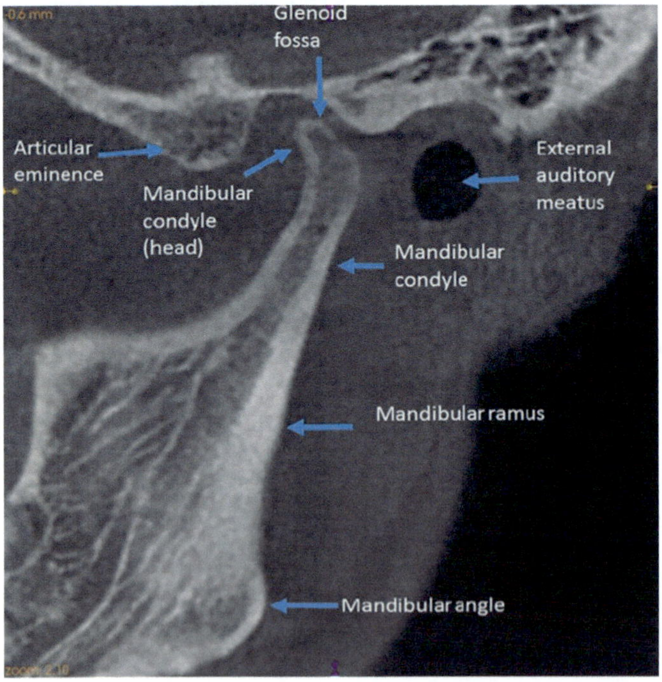

Atlas 7.3 Radiological anatomy of the TMJ in CBCT—image obtained along the short axis of the condyle (para-sagittal). [Reprinted/adapted by permission from I. Rozylo-Kalinowska, K. Orhan (eds.), *Imaging of the TemporomandibularJoint*, https://doi.org/10.1007/978-3-319-99468-0_8]

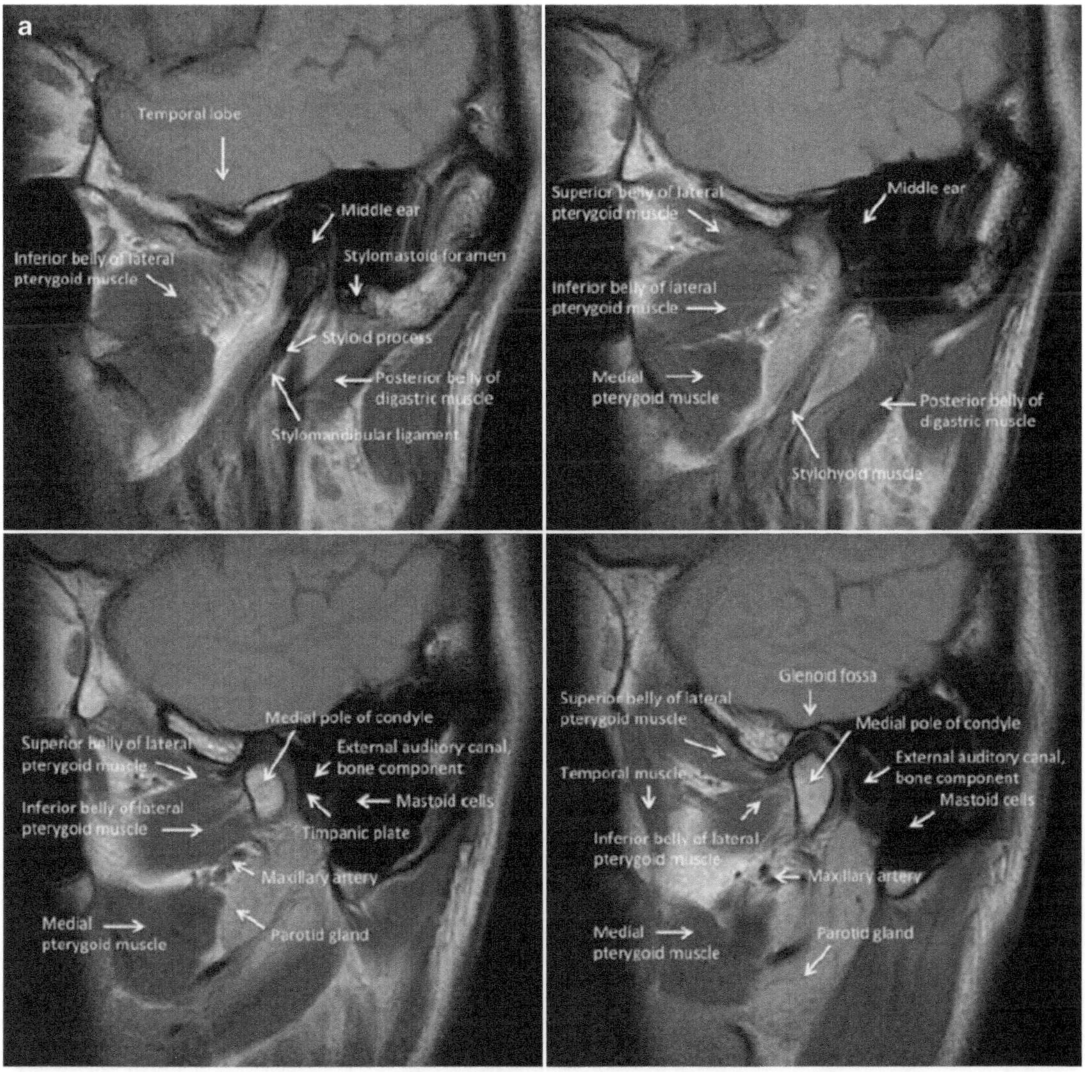

Atlas 7.4 Articular and peri-articular temporomandibular joint anatomy as seen with MRI (**a**–**e**); Sagittal, Coronal and Axial views. [Reprinted/adapted by permission from T. Robba et al. (eds.), *MRI of the Temporomandibular Joint*, https://doi.org/10.1007/978-3-030-25421-6_3]

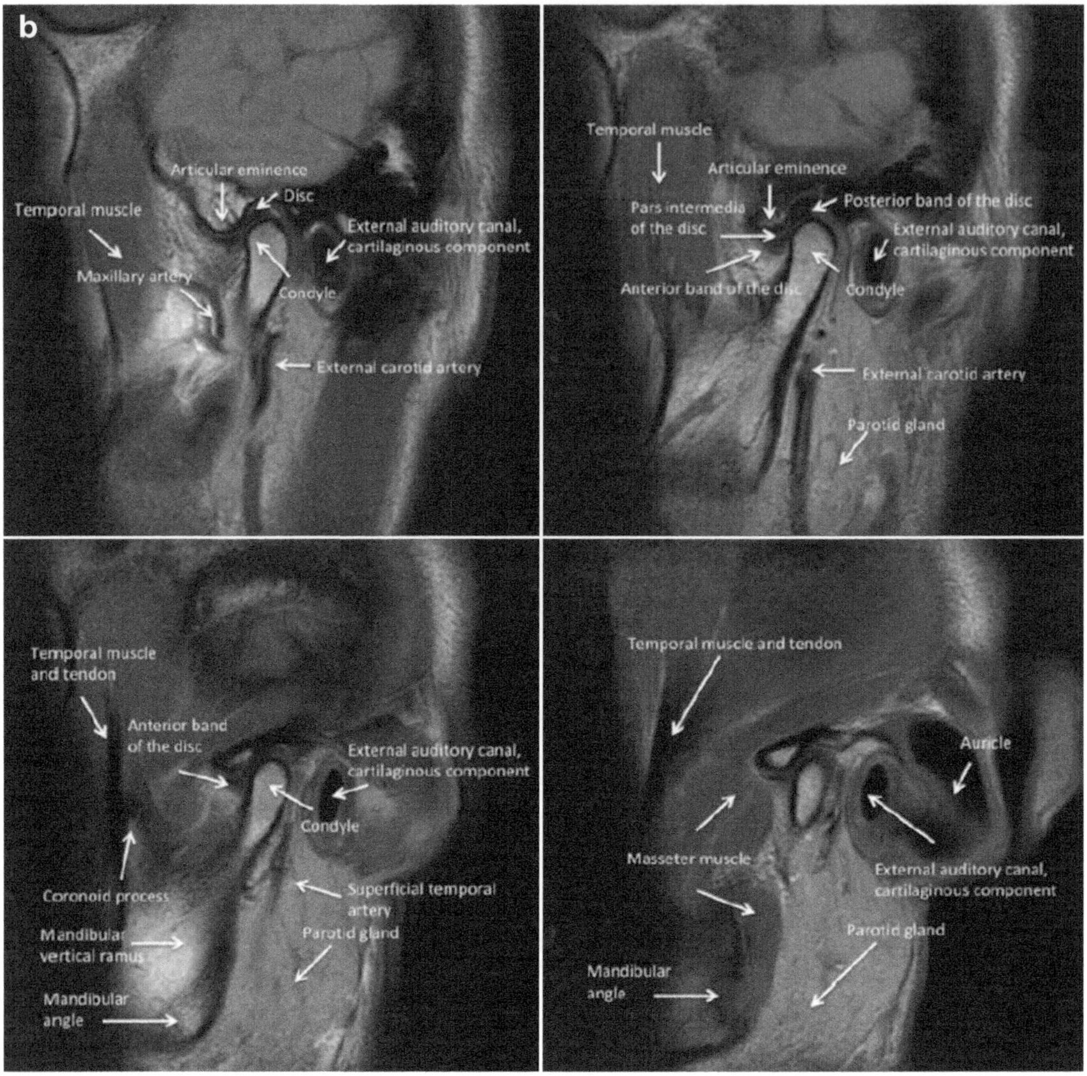

Atlas 7.4 (continued)

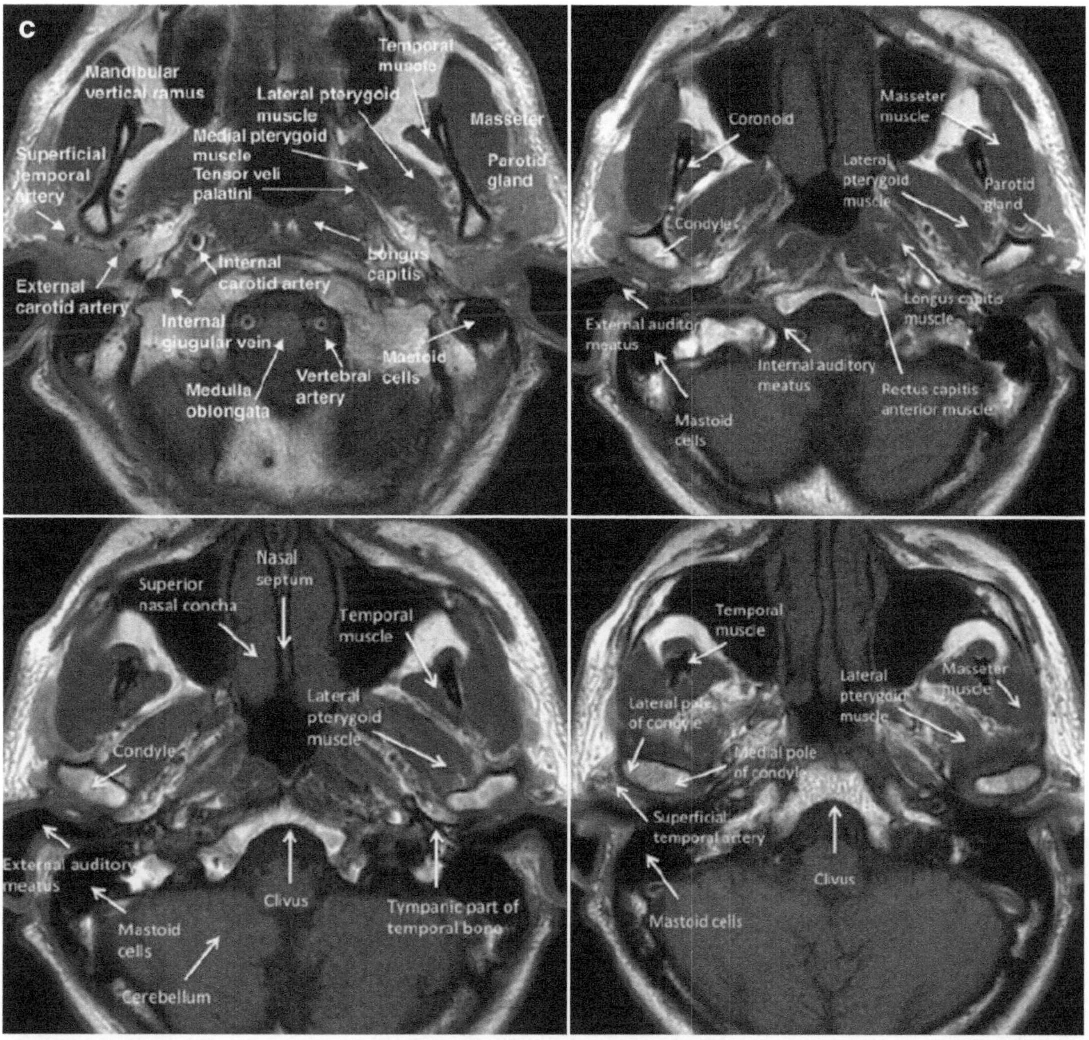

Atlas 7.4 (continued)

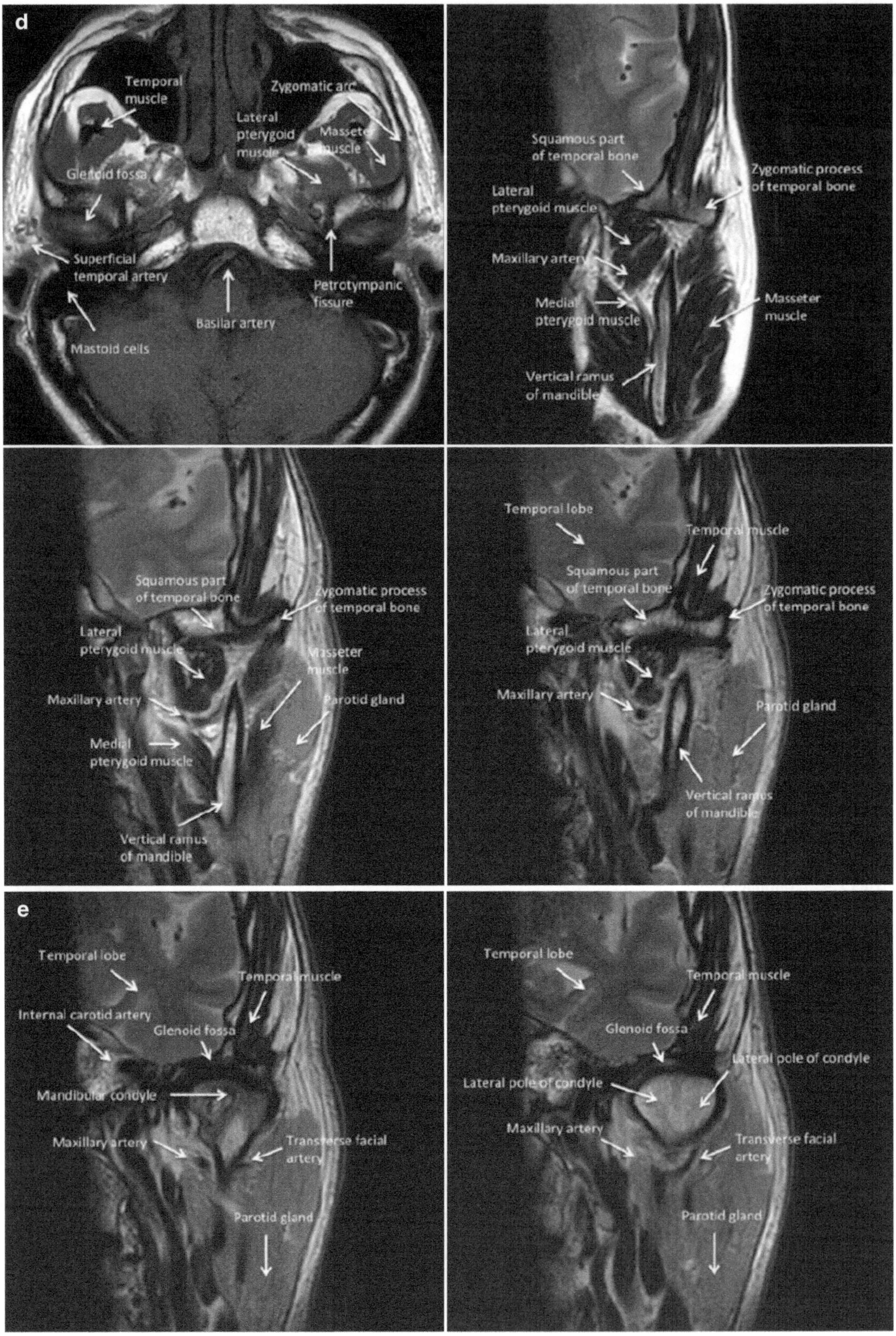

Atlas 7.4 (continued)

References

1. Lewis EL, Dolwick MF, Abramowicz S, Reeder SL. Contemporary imaging of the temporomandibular joint. Dental Clin N Am. 2008;52:875–90.
2. Karjodkar FR. Textbook of dental and maxillofacial radiology. 1st ed. St. Louis: Jaypee Publishers; 2006.
3. White SC, Pharoah MJ. Oral radiology: principles and interpretation. St. Louis, MO: Mosby/Elsevier; 2009.
4. Hansson LG, Petersson A. Radiography of the temporomandibular joint using the transpharyngeal projection. A comparison study of information obtained with different radiographic techniques. Dentomaxillofac Radiol. 1978;7(2):69–78.
5. Doyle T. Arthrography of the temporomandibular joint: a simple technique. Clin Radiol. 1983;34(2):147–51. https://doi.org/10.1016/s0009-9260(83)80294-3.
6. Murphy WA. Arthrography of the temporomandibular joint. Radiol Clin N Am. 1981 Jun;19(2):365–78.
7. Jih CH, Han NT, Lee SK. Arthrographic evaluation of the internal derangement of temporomandibular joint. Gaoxiong Yi Xue Ke Xue Za Zhi. 1991 Jun;7(6):323–8.
8. Ihnatsenka B, Boezaart AP. Ultrasound: basic understanding and learning the language. Int J Shoulder Surg. 2010;4(3):55–62. https://doi.org/10.4103/0973-6042.76960.
9. Bag AK, Gaddikeri S, Singhal A, Hardin S, Tran BD, Medina JA, Curé JK. Imaging of the temporomandibular joint: an update. World J Radiol. 2014 Aug 28;6(8):567–82.
10. Kundu H, Basavaraj P, Kote S, Singla A, Singh S. Assessment of TMJ disorders using ultrasonography as a diagnostic tool: a review. J Clin Diagn Res. 2013;7(12):3116–20. https://doi.org/10.7860/JCDR/2013/6678.3874.
11. Ferreira LA, Grossmann E, Januzzi E, de Paula MVQ, Carvalho ACP. Diagnosis of temporomandibular joint disorders: indication of imaging exams. Braz J Otorhinolaryngol. 2016;82(3):341–52. https://doi.org/10.1016/j.bjorl.2015.06.010.
12. Beer A, Kolk A, Neff A, et al. Cine MRI of the temporomandibular joint in comparison to static MRI and axiography. Rofo. 2004 Apr;176(4):506–12. https://doi.org/10.1055/s-2004-813039.
13. Dorsay TA, et al. Cine MRI diagnosis and posttherapeutic evaluation of an adherent TMJ disc: a case report. J Oral Maxillofac Surg. 2016;52(11):1220–2.
14. Ahmad M, Schiffman EL. Temporomandibular joint disorders and orofacial pain. Dent Clin N Am. 2016;60:105–24.
15. Matsumoto K, Sato T, Iwanari S, et al. The use of arthrography in the diagnosis of temporomandibular joint synovial chondromatosis. Dentomaxillofac Radiol. 2013;42(1):15388284. https://doi.org/10.1259/dmfr/15388284.
16. Thomas X, Pomes J, Berenguer J, Quinto L, Nicolau C, Mercader JM, Castro V. Imaging of temporomandibular joint dysfunction: a pictorial review. Radiographics. 2006;26:765–81.
17. Dodo M, Kumagai M, Kato Y, Hirakawa H, Koseki T. Metastasis in the mandibular condyle: a case report. J Med Case Rep. 2017;11(1):323. https://doi.org/10.1186/s13256-017-1450-9.
18. Kolokythas A, Miloro MB, Olsson AB, Miloro M. Metastatic pancreatic adenocarcinoma to the mandibular condyle: a rare clinical presentation. J Oral Maxillofac Surg. 2014;72(1):83–8. https://doi.org/10.1016/j.joms.2013.06.207.
19. Della Chiesa A, Scherrer B, Kuttenberger JJ. Metastatic breast cancer in the mandibular condyle mimicking temporomandibular joint (TMJ) disease. J Surg Case Rep. 2014;2014(1):rjt130. Published 2014 Jan 27. https://doi.org/10.1093/jscr/rjt130.
20. Katzberg RW, O'Mara RE, Tallents RH, Weber DA. Radionuclide skeletal imaging and single photon emission computed tomography in suspected internal derangements of the temporomandibular joint. J Oral Maxillofac Surg. 1984;42(12):782–7.
21. Oesterreich F-U, Jend-Rossmann I, Jend H-H, Triebel HJ. Semiquantitative SPECT imaging for assessment of bone reactions in internal derangements of the temporomandibular joint. J Oral Maxillofac Surg. 1987;45(12):1022–8. https://doi.org/10.1016/0278-2391(87)90157-1.
22. Hersek N, Canay S, Caner B, Ulutuncel N. Bone SPECT imaging of patients with internal derangement of temporomandibular joint before and after splint therapy. Oral Surg Oral Med Oral Pathol Oral Radiol Endod. 2002 Nov;94(5):576–80.
23. Epstein J, Rea A, Chahal O. The use of bone scintigraphy in temporomandibular joint disorders. Oral Dis. 2002;8(1):47–53. https://doi.org/10.1034/j.1601-0825.2002.10753.x.
24. Park KS, Song HC, Cho SG, et al. Open-mouth bone scintigraphy is better than closed-mouth bone scintigraphy in the diagnosis of temporomandibular osteoarthritis. Nucl Med Mol Imaging. 2016;50(3):213–8. https://doi.org/10.1007/s13139-016-0407-z.
25. Shetty US, Burde KN, Naikmasur VG, Sattur AP. Assessment of condylar changes in patients with temporomandibular joint pain using digital volumetric tomography. Radiol Res Pract. 2014;2014:1–8. https://doi.org/10.1155/2014/106059.

Psychological Assessment for Temporomandibular Joint Disorders

8

Beena Sivakumar, Ratna Sharma, and Darpan Bhargava

8.1 Introduction

Temporomandibular joint disorders (TMDs) are prevalent among population of wide age range. Psychological assessment is essential in these patients as stress and anxiety can significantly contribute to TMDs. They cause chronic pain which can be associated with significant psychological or psychosocial disturbances. These factors, if not identified and appropriately addressed, can often result in poor treatment outcomes. Hence understanding the psychological aspect enhances the feat in treatment outcomes for several TMDs. It is well documented that conditions involving chronic pain such as back ache, tension headache, fibromyalgia and TMDs are known to be associated with transient psychological involvement. They manifest clinically as anxiety, depression, frequent use of pain medication, somatization impacting the patient's lifestyle resulting in diminished productivity at work. A psychological inequity may lead to TMDs and vice-versa [1].

Significant psychological and psychosocial upset is believed to have a negative effect on all forms of treatment, from conservative to surgical modalities. Literature opines that assessment of these factors is an excellent predictor for long-term outcomes of the treatment and is recommended that it should be a routine practice to assess patients diagnosed with TMDs to develop a more rational and comprehensive approach in managing such disorders [1, 2].

8.2 Aetiology

TMDs are associated with complex and heterogenous constellation of problems. The aetiology is usually multi-factorial. Psychological factors like depression, anxiety along with other contributing factors such as central modulation, hypervigilance, stress, sleep disorders are known to be associated with TMDs. They can be managed by proper assessment and combining various management modalities such as biofeedback and cognitive behavioural therapy to eliminate the psychological factors apart from medical and surgical management [2, 3].

B. Sivakumar
Department of Oral and Maxillofacial Surgery, Meenakshi Ammal Dental College and Hospital, Chennai, Tamil Nadu, India

R. Sharma
Department of Psychology, The Sanskaar Valley School, Bhopal, Madhya Pradesh, India

D. Bhargava (✉)
TMJ Consultancy Services, Bhopal, Madhya Pradesh, India

Oral and Maxillofacial Surgery, People's College of Dental Sciences and Research Centre, People's University, Bhopal, Madhya Pradesh, India
e-mail: drdarpanbhargava@gmail.com

D. Bhargava (ed.), *Temporomandibular Joint Disorders*,
https://doi.org/10.1007/978-981-16-2754-5_8

8.3 Diagnostic Criteria

A group of experts on TMDs proposed the Research Diagnostic Criteria for Temporomandibular Disorders (RDC/TMD) in 1992 based on various empirical data and comprehensive literature review. It is a dual axis assessment consisting of Axis I which is a standard diagnostic criterion based on signs and symptoms of TMDs describing the common physical disorders. It is used for screening purpose of intra-articular disorders. Axis II includes psychosocial and behavioural factors describing the aspects of a patient who had the disorder and behavioural factors possibly affecting management of the TMD. It is beneficial to use these criteria for research and clinical comprehensive assessment in TMD patients (Tables 8.1, 8.2 and 8.3). Use of the recommended 'criteria' in clinical practice enhances patients' identification with a wide range of simple to complex TMD manifestations [2].

A thorough history from the patient is essential for assessment of psychological factors such as behaviour, lifestyle and emotional condition. It is generally believed that the clinician often under-recognizes such psychological aspects. Sensitivity measures the instrument's/diagnostic criteria's ability to record a positive response for a positive case. Likewise, specificity measures the instrument's ability to record a negative response for a negative case (Table 8.1). Usually TMDs have an involvement of the associated muscle groups. Physiological parameters exist to access such psycho-physiological parameters caused by stress related and postural jaw muscle function by electromyogram (EMG) [2].

Patil DJ et al. have investigated the prevalence of stress and depression among patient having TMDs with chronic facial pain and compared it to the control group to assess the possible relationships between them. It was observed that anxiety, depression and stress scores were increased in patients diagnosed with myofascial pain. Depression (53.3%) and stress (60%) were more prevalent in the study group patients [4]. They concluded that there was a strong co-relation between depression, stress and TMDs. Initial evaluation should include screening for such behavioural and psychological symptoms for effective cognitive behavioural therapy and enhanced treatment outcomes. The above findings are consistent with several other documentations in the literature emphasizing the strong need for managing such aspects apart from signs and symptoms of TMDs [5].

8.4 Conclusion

Future research should aim at establishing diagnostic protocols based on identification of the aetiology and mechanisms involved in develop-

Table 8.1 Validated Axis I pain-related TMD diagnoses, for RDC/TMD [2]

Validated Axis I pain-related TMD diagnoses		
Disorder	History	Examination findings
Myalgia (sensitivity 90%, specificity 99%)	Pain in masticatory structure modified by jaw movement/function or para-function	Reporting of pain in temporalis or masseter muscles during palpation or during maximum unassisted or assisted opening movements
Myofascial pain along with referral (sensitivity 86%, specificity 98%)	Same as of myalgia	Reporting familiar pain while palpating temporalis or masseter muscles
Arthralgia (sensitivity 89%, specificity 98%)	Same as of myalgia	Reporting familiar pain in TMJ with palpation of joint or maximum unassisted/assisted opening, right or left lateral or protrusive movements
Headache attributed to TMD (sensitivity 89%, specificity 87%)	Headache in temporal area modified by jaw movement, function or para-function	Reporting of similar headache in temple area during palpation of temporalis muscles or during maximum unassisted/assisted opening, right or left lateral or protrusive movements

Table 8.2 Validated Axis I TMJ diagnoses, for RDC/TMD [2]

Validated Axis I TMJ diagnoses		
Disorders	History	Clinical examination findings
DDwR (sensitivity 34%, specificity 92%)	Presence of TMJ noises	Clicking, popping or snapping noises present during opening and closing/opening or closing, and lateral or protrusive movements
DDwR with intermittent locking (sensitivity 38%, specificity 98%)	TMJ noises present Jaw locks with limited opening and then unlocks	Same as DDwR
DDwoR with limited opening (sensitivity 80%, specificity 97%)	TMJ locking with limited opening Limitation severe enough to interfere with the ability to eat is currently present	Maximum assisted opening (passive stretch) <40 mm
DDwoR without limited opening (sensitivity 54%, specificity 79%)	TMJ locking with limited opening Limitation severe enough to cause interfere with ability to eat was present in the past	Maximum assisted opening (passive stretch) ≥40 mm
Degenerative joint disease (sensitivity 55%, specificity 61%)	TMJ noises present	Crepitus present during maximum active opening (crunching, grinding or grating noises)
Subluxation (sensitivity 98%, specificity 100%)	TMJ locking or catching in a wide-open position that resolves with a specific manoeuvre	When disorder is evident, a manoeuvre to unlock the jaw is performed to close mouth.

Table 8.3 Axis II assessment protocol for RDC/TMD [2]

Axis II assessment protocol		
Questionnaire	No. of Items [2]	Usefulness
Graded chronic pain scale	7	**Pain intensity component**: pain amplification and central sensitization **Pain-related disability component**: decreased function caused by pain
Pain drawing	1	Distinguishes among local, regional and widespread pain; assesses for other comorbid pain condition; and may indicate pain amplification, sensitization and central dysregulation
Jaw functional limitation scale	8 or 20	Quantifies effect on jaw mobility, mastication and verbal and emotional expression
Patient health questionnaire-4	4	Identifies psychological distress (depression and anxiety)
Patient health questionnaire-9	9	Identifies depression: contributes to chronicity
Generalized anxiety disorder-7	7	Identifies anxiety: contributes to stress reactivity and to parafunction
Patient health questionnaire-15	15	Measures physical symptoms: assesses for specific comorbid functional disorders
Oral behaviour checklist	21	Measures para-function: contributes to onset and perpetuation of pain prognosis

ing or leading to psychological derangements in TMDs for a more targeted, personalized treatment plans for individual patients. A multidisciplinary approach involving the TMJ specialist and a psychologist is recommended for the initial assessment of the TMD patients, which should aid at planning a tailored treatment remedy, as per the individual patient's requirement.

Acknowledgments Editor would like to thank, Dr. Ratna Sharma, Ph.D, PGDPC, Clinical Psychologist and Counsellor, SkillGapfinder, Bhopal, Madhya Pradesh, India for her special contribution.

References

1. Laskin DM, et al. Temporomandibular disorders: an evidence-based approach to diagnosis and treatment. 1st ed. Chicago, IL: Quintessence Publishing Co; 2006.
2. Schiffman E, Ohrbach R. Executive summary of the diagnostic criteria for temporomandibular disorders for clinical and research applications. J Am Dent Assoc. 2016;147(6):438–45.
3. Rugh JD, Woods BJ, Dahlström L. Temporomandibular disorders: assessment of psychological factors. Advances Dent Res. 1993;7(2):127–36.
4. Patil DJ, Dheer DS, Puri G, Konidena A, Dixit A, Gupta R. Psychological appraisal in temporomandibular disorders: a cross-sectional study. Indian J Pain. 2016;30:13–8.
5. Rollman GB, Gillespie JM. The role of psychosocial factors in temporomandibular disorders. Curr Rev Pain. 2000;4(1):71–81. https://doi.org/10.1007/s11916-000-0012-8.

Non-surgical and Pharmacological Management of the Temporomandibular Joint Disorders

9

S. Karthiga Kannan, Darpan Bhargava, Sudeep Shrivastava, Trilok Shrivastava, and Abhay Kumar Pandey

9.1 Introduction

Diagnosing and treating temporomandibular joint disorders (TMDs) accurately is a complicated and intricate task and demands thorough knowledge, understanding and experience. Usually TMD patients suffer from more than one anarchy which is inter-related, citing a few—joint pain per-se, myalgia, altered muscle tone, occlusal discrepancies, and so on. Therefore, inter-relationship of various problems must be considered for a more appropriate diagnosis and treatment of TMDs. Vast spectrum of treatment modalities are available for the management of TMDs. A logical approach for patient management is to aim at initiating a conservative therapy and reserve surgical treatment when conservative modalities do not show improvement in relieving the symptoms (Fig. 9.1). A conservative non-surgical and pharmacological therapy is readily acceptable by most of the patients in the initial stages of TMDs [1].

TMDs are a collective term that includes manifestations like pain and dysfunction of TMJ, masticator muscles and the associated structures. At most instances, the exact aetiology may remain unidentified, but may be associated with trauma, parafunctional habits, joint overload, malocclusion, psychological factors, arthritis or chronic non-ergonomic positioning of the head and neck (Fig. 9.2). After evaluating and diagnosing the TMD, suitable non-surgical and medical therapy should be initiated in order to achieve reduction in pain/discomfort and functional improvement [2, 3].

Non-surgical and medical therapies resolve symptoms in over eighty percent of the patients with TMDs [4, 20]. The various available conservative therapies can be used alone or in combination with each other. Their goal is to decrease overloading of the masticatory system, pain/dysfunction and promote healing. Most effectual pharmacological agents used in treating TMDs include analgesics, corticosteroids, muscle relaxants, anti-depressants, anxiolytics, benzodiazepines and anticonvulsants

S. K. Kannan
Oral Medicine and Radiology, Dental Education Department, College of Dentistry, Majmaah University, Al Majma'ah, Saudi Arabia

D. Bhargava (✉)
TMJ Consultancy Services, Bhopal, Madhya Pradesh, India

Oral and Maxillofacial Surgery, People's College of Dental Sciences and Research Centre, People's University, Bhopal, Madhya Pradesh, India
e-mail: drdarpanbhargava@gmail.com

S. Shrivastava
Fellow, OM Multispeciality Head and Neck Surgery Centre, Ahmedabad, Gujarat, India

T. Shrivastava
Department of Orthodontics, People's College of Dental Sciences and Research Centre, People's University, Bhopal, Madhya Pradesh, India

A. K. Pandey
NCD, Sadar Hospital, Govt of Jharkhand, Ranchi, Jharkhand, India

D. Bhargava (ed.), *Temporomandibular Joint Disorders*,
https://doi.org/10.1007/978-981-16-2754-5_9

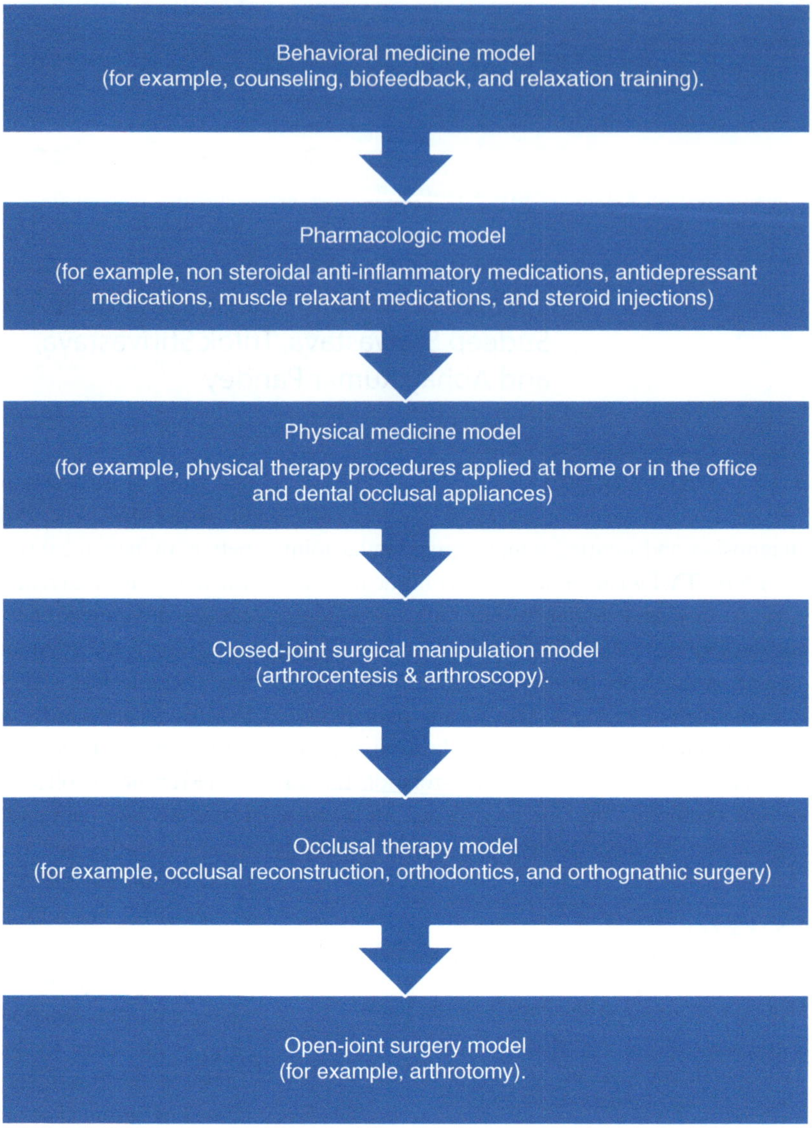

Fig. 9.1 TMD management strategy

[6]. In conjunction to pharmacological therapy patients may be advised for physical exercise, avoid stress, modify habits, and restrict excess jaw function.

9.2 Non-surgical Therapy

The primary goals of the non-surgical therapy include patient education and counselling, diet modification, physical therapy, stress reduction protocols, psychotherapy, appliance therapy and pharmacologic management. One important factor affecting the treatment outcome to such therapy is the fluctuating nature of the TMDs which may undergo remissions and exacerbations independent of the treatment (Fig. 9.3).

9.2.1 Patient Education/Cognitive Awareness Training

Patient education and counselling is the primary step for any treatment plan. The patient should be explained about the co-relation between the emotional stress, muscle hyperactivity, joint over-

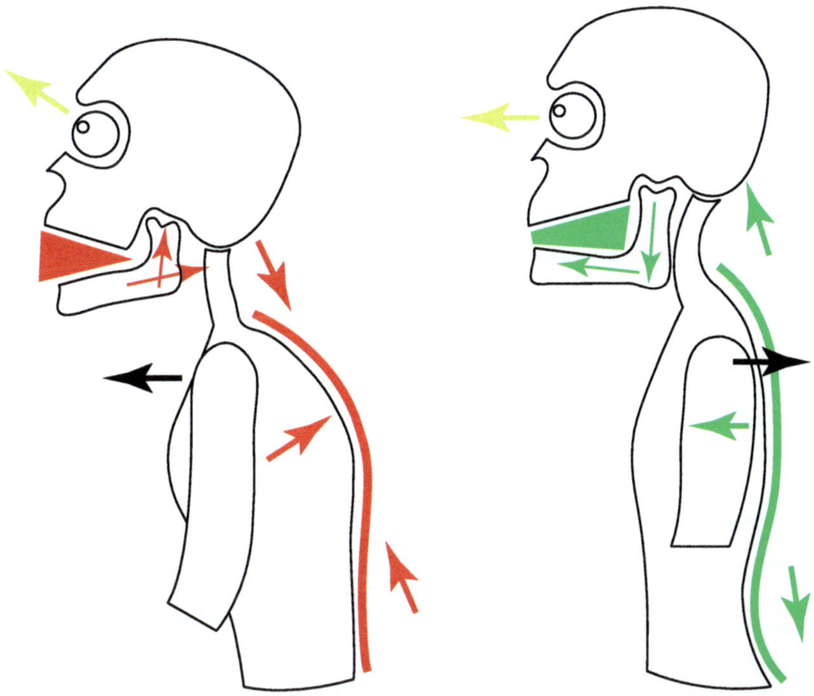

Fig. 9.2 Schematic representation of how a condition of postural imbalance influence mandible position (Adapted with permission from: Sambataro S et al. TMJ Dysfunctions Systemic Implications and Postural Assessments: A Review of Recent Literature. J. Funct. Morphol. Kinesiol. 2019, 4, 58; doi:https://doi.org/10.3390/jfmk4030058)

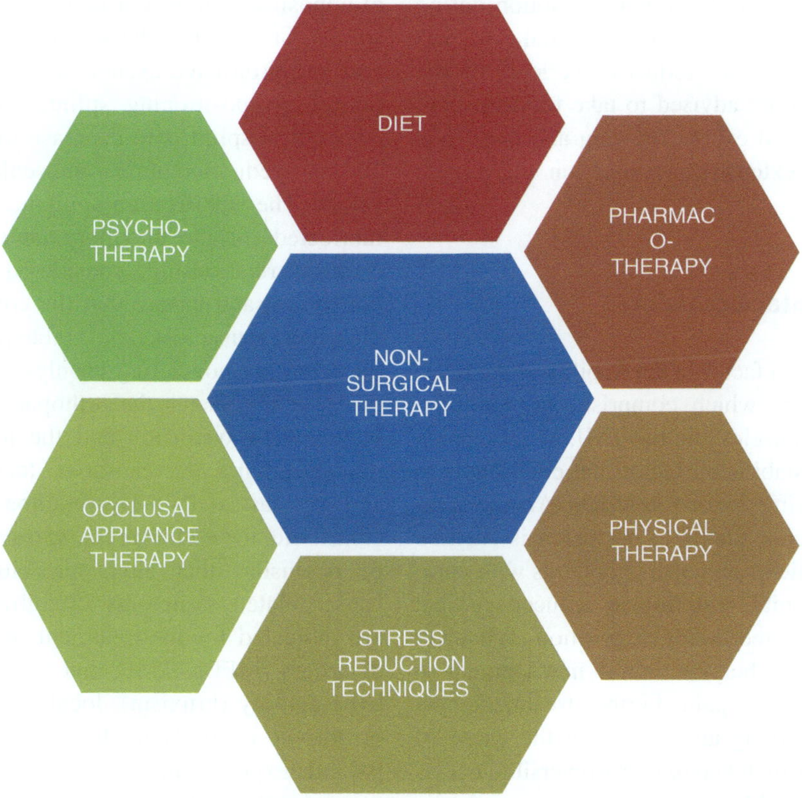

Fig. 9.3 Non-surgical modalities in the management of TMDs

load and interrelation of the same resulting in the disorder of the joint. Patient's understanding of these facts would contribute to an improved patient compliance for various treatment modalities and follow-up. It is essential to explain the cause of the symptoms and probable diagnosis to the patients who are generally unaware of the origin of their pain. This reduces the anxiety which also contributes to pain control to some extent in such patients.

Another important factor is to make the patients aware of any abnormal tooth contact practice other than during physiological rest state of the jaws, chewing, swallowing and speaking to exclude any parafunctional habits that the patients may have.

9.2.2 Diet Modification

Patients may be advised to take a soft diet especially in cases experiencing extreme symptoms. This enables controlled range of motion during the jaw function, decreases muscular hyperactivity and thereby reduces overload of the joint. Patients are advised to take food in small pieces and avoid excess chewing and hard food that requires extensive jaw function and muscle action.

9.2.3 Dental Occlusion

It is an essential factor in the stability of stomatognathic system which comprises of dentition, masticatory muscles and the TMJ. Malocclusion may be a destabilizing factor that contributes to the predisposing factor for TMDs. Another predisposing factor related to occlusion is attrition in elderly patients and also in patients with parafunctional habits, resulting in reduced vertical height and altered condylar position. Whatever the cause may be, the initial management is directed to reduce pain. Further treatment may involve identifying and rectifying the cause of malocclusion by reversible or irreversible occlusal therapy, equilibration procedures, orthodontic correction, prosthodontics and orthognathic surgery to restore form and function [7, 8, 9, 12].

Irreversible occlusal therapy includes selective grinding (reductive) and restorative (additive) procedures which may permanently change the occlusal conditions and should be wisely planned.

9.2.4 Occlusal Appliance Therapy

Splint therapy is the art and science of establishing neuromuscular harmony in the masticatory system and creating a mechanical disadvantage for the parafunctional forces with removable appliances. Occlusal appliance therapy is a form of reversible occlusal intervention that temporarily alters patient's occlusal condition, thereby reducing joint overload. The occlusal bite appliances are removable devices made up of hard acrylic and have custom fit over occlusal surfaces of maxillary/mandibular teeth. Splints are constructed in a way to achieve bilaterally symmetrical occlusal contacts posteriorly with teeth of opposing arch in centric occlusion (flat plane splints) or there may be anterior contacts in lateral and protrusive excursions of the mandible (anterior repositioning splints). Effectiveness of occlusal splint is to decrease loading on the TMJ and reduction of neuromuscular reflex activation. The stabilization appliance is generally fabricated for the maxillary arch. It provides occlusal relationship, considered optimal for the patient and ensure that the condyles are in their most musculoskeletal stable position when the teeth are contacting evenly and simultaneously. It eliminates the orthopaedic instability between the occlusion and the joint position, thus removing the causative factor. Bruxism and Myofascial Pain Dysfunction (MPD) may contribute to a change in vertical dimension of occlusion that alters proprioception and cause related symptoms. Stabilization splints are indicated for the treatment of muscle pain disorders (MPD), TMD that relates to muscle hyperactivity (bruxism), local muscle soreness or chronic centrally mediated myalgia and for patients experiencing retrodiscitis secondary to trauma. This appliance can help minimizing the forces to damaged tissues, thus permitting more efficient healing. Whereas anterior positioning splint is an interocclusal device that encourages the mandible to assume a position more anterior. Its goals are to provide a better condyle–disc relationship in the fossa. So that tissues have a better opportunity to adapt or repair and would eliminate the signs and symptoms associated with **disc derangement disorders**. It is indicated for the treatment of disc derangement disorders, intermittent or chronic locking of the joint and some inflammatory disorders like retrodiscitis are managed with this appliance, especially when a slight anterior positioning of the condyle is more comfortable for the patient (Tables 9.1 and 9.2). Apart from commonly used stabilization/flat plane and anterior repositioning appliances, soft occlusal splints have shown benefit in patients with TMDs. Recently a new type of mouth guard, the Aqualizer has been introduced. The Aqualizer works on the Pascal's Law, producing its effect by evenly distributing the fluid on biting uniformly [5, 8, 9, 19, 69].

Table 9.1 Various types of occlusal appliances/splints

Stabilization appliance	Anterior repositioning appliance
• Hard acrylic flat-plane device • Full coverage maxillary occlusal arch • Worn 24 h/day (± during meals) • Bilateral even distribution of occlusal forces • Provides stabilization of the TMJ apparatus • Relaxation of masticatory muscles	• Hard acrylic device • Maxillary or mandibular occlual coverage splint with anterior inclined plane • During jaw closure, mandible moves anteriorly • Useful for anteriorly displaced disc to change condylar position and recapture disc • Possible need for occlusal equilibration and splint readjustment

Table 9.2 Functions of occlusal appliances/splints

1	To relax the muscles
2	To allow the condyle to seat in centric relation
3	To provide diagnostic information
4	To protect teeth and associated structures from bruxism
5	To mitigate periodontal ligament proprioception
6	To reduce cellular hypoxia levels

9.2.5 Physiotherapy

It is documented that prolonged immobilization of jaws due to TMDs or traumatic injury to the condyle has deleterious effect on TMJ and the facial muscles causing degenerative cartilage and osseous changes in and around the joint surfaces, its surrounding soft tissues, synovial fluid alterations, fibrous tissue contractures, and muscle weakness. Nourishment of the synovium depends upon the normal joint function. Aim of the physical therapy is to put the joint in function in a systematic manner. Physical therapy aids in relaxation of hyperactive muscles, reduces pain, increases range of motion, and helps in improving joint function. Following are the various jaw exercises detailed as under [8, 11, 17].

9.2.5.1 Passive Jaw Exercise

It permits patient to exercise manually (opening using finger stretching) or with a device like jaw openers or activators. It gradually increases the inter-incisal opening and significantly reduces pain, improves jaw mobility as the shortened muscles regain their normal length [11]. It is usually performed as a part of post-operative care after surgical intervention like arthrocentesis, arthroscopy, or open TMJ surgery. It is also effective for patients with muscle-associated trismus, myofascial pain and dysfunction (MPD). It is relatively contraindicated in patients with severe TMJ disc displacement without reduction owing to risk of further damage to the disc and retrodiscal tissue [10, 11, 13, 20].

9.2.5.2 Active/Assisted Jaw Exercises

It is performed by initiating patient's own jaw musculature (as opposed to jaw opening device which allows muscles to be passive). This allows patient to activate suprahyoid musculature (geniohyoid, mylohyoid, digastric, and stylohyoid), and inactivating elevators of jaw (medial pterygoid, masseter, temporalis) causing relaxation of hyperactive masticatory muscles thus facilitating maximal inter-incisal opening. Assisted exercises are helpful post-TMJ surgery, arthroscopy, arthrotomy, and permanent disc dislocation without reduction to achieve improved range of mandibular movements [11].

In this active stretch phase, the patients are advised to keep mouth open for several seconds following relaxation of muscles and are instructed to keep their mouth open till they perceive pain and then hold for several seconds thus, repeating this exercise many times a day with gradual increase in magnitude of mouth opening. The active movements in the form of lateral excursions should be maintained for several seconds, which are then slowly released in order to effect physiologic "stretch" of muscles [12, 13, 15, 18].

9.2.5.3 Isometric Exercises

Patient is advised to place the hand beneath the chin and start the exercise against palm resistance by slowly opening the mouth. Similarly in an open mouth position the patient fingers are placed in the incisal tip of incisors and advise to close the mouth against resistance. Followed by opening mandible in right and left lateral protrusive position against hand resistance, holding for 3 to 5 seconds on each side to activate the muscles isometrically. These exercises benefit young patients with a complain of a painless early clicking. Isometric exercise may be recommended is disc derangements with pain and trismus [11, 14, 16, 18].

9.2.6 Thermal Therapy

Thermal agents can be applied in the form of heat or cold. Heat is frequently used in the form of hot compresses causing vasodilatation thereby increasing the blood flow and reducing pain. Another concept behind thermal therapy is by blocking impulses from c-fibres explained as per gate control theory. Application of hot fomentation using hot moist towel or a hot bottle over a towel applied over the symptomatic area for 10 to 15 minutes not exceeding 30 minutes is beneficial [21, 22].

Coolant therapy reduces transmission of impulse through the nerve endings causing decreased perception of pain and also causes relaxation of muscles. It causes local vasoconstriction and helps in reducing muscle spasm. The use of cold includes fluoro-methane coolant sprays. A simpler method for cold fomentation is using an ice pack for not more than 5 to 7 minutes of application time followed by a warming period before next application not exceeding 20–30 minutes [23, 24].

9.2.7 Ultrasonography

Ultrasonography (USG) is used to deliver deep heat. USG machine operates above frequency of audible sound waves (0.75–1.0 MHz) and converts to heat while travelling through the soft tissues. USG probe is applied over skin using conductive gel and moved slowly over affected area in circular movements. Care must be taken not to keep machine in one area for long which may cause overheating of connective tissue, leading to structural damage. Deep heat is used to increase blood perfusion by vasodilatation, thereby clearing inflammatory mediators. This decreases pain and increase jaw mobility (Fig. 9.4).

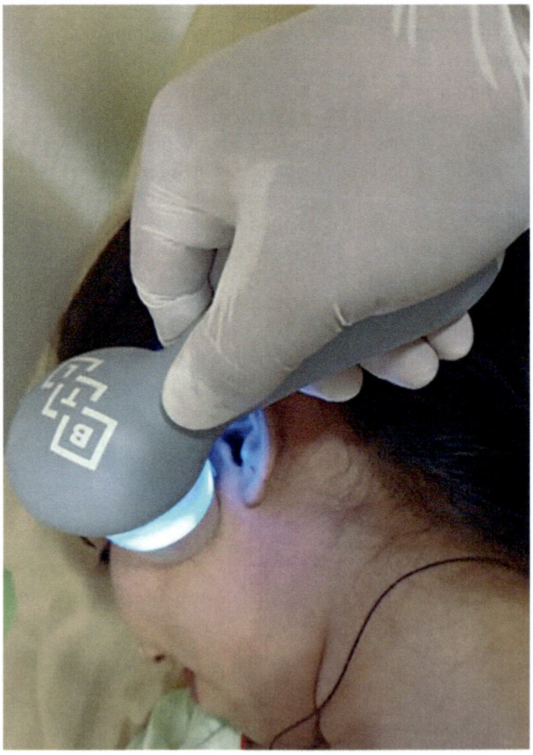

Fig. 9.4 Ultrasound physiotherapy in the TMJ region

Effects include altered permeability of cell membrane, decreased collagen viscosity, intracellular fluid absorption, analgesia and vasodilatation. Beneficial effects include breakdown of local calcium deposits, reduced capsular contracture, decreased hyaluronic acid viscosity of joint synovial fluid and improved mobility. It has advantages in managing tendinitis, muscle spasm, tight/restricted ligaments [25, 26].

9.2.8 Phonophoresis

Phonophoresis is a process of application of ultrasound heat that incorporates pad filled with medicaments like 10% hydrocortisone cream, salicylates or any other topical anaesthetic cream placed over the affected area. When these ultrasound waves are applied, medications perfuse into tissues. Indication for phonophoresis is synovitis with painful jaw hypomobility [27, 28].

9.2.9 Iontophoresis

Iontophoresis is a technique by which certain medicaments can be introduced to the tissues at the target area using low intensity current.

9.2.10 Electrical Stimulation

The mechanism of action of trans-cutaneous electrical nerve stimulation (TENS) is through the gate control theory, counter-irritation, neurohumoral substance release and peripheral blockade mechanisms. It uses low-voltage electrical current designed for sensory stimulation in painful disorders and decreases muscle pain and hyperactivity in neuromuscular disorders. The units of TENS are usually portable; electrodes are placed over specific regions or trigger point sites. Increasing TENS intensity to the point of motor fibres activation cause muscle relaxation (Fig. 9.5) (Table 9.3). It is contraindicated for patients with pacemakers [29, 30].

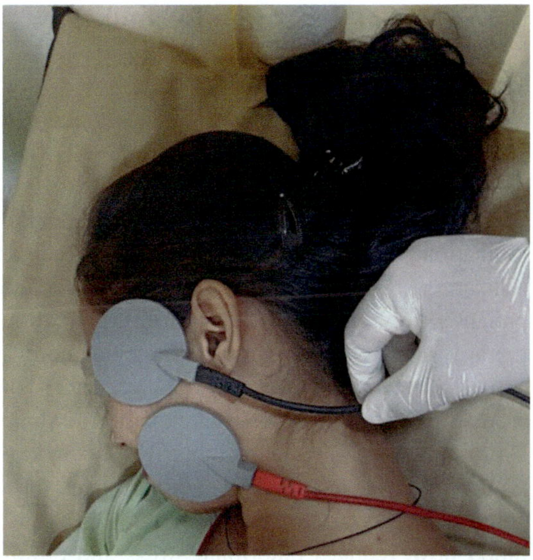

Fig. 9.5 Transcutaneous electric nerve stimulation (TENS) therapy for TMD

Table 9.3 Types of electrical stimulation techniques

Electrical stimulation techniques	TENS
	Iontophoresis: electric current drives drugs into tissues.
	High-volume stimulation (100 V): pumping effects of muscle contraction increase circulation.

9.2.11 Muscle Injection

Trigger point is an area of hyperirritability in tissues when compressed becomes tender and hypersensitive leading to referred pain. It is due to trauma, sustained spasm/contraction or acute muscle strain. Injections of local anaesthesia (LA) enable the clinician to stretch muscles maximally without pain and discomfort to the patient. Injections of LA (2% lidocaine) in trigger point serve two functions. One is to eliminate the local pain, another to diagnose the source of pain. The local anaesthetic blocks the central excitatory effect over the trigger point. Its vasodilator effect improves vascular perfusion to an area allowing metabolites and inflammatory mediators that may induce pain to be readily removed by increased blood flow to the area [31, 32].

9.2.12 Stress Reduction Techniques

Relaxation and Biofeedback

Stress reduction and relaxation techniques can be effective treatment modalities in TMDs. Audiotapes may be used in an attempt to train synchronized breathing patterns and specific relaxation techniques. Substitutive and active relaxation therapies can be used to reduce patient's emotional stress. Substitutive relaxation therapy involves behaviour or lifestyle modification by involving in some hobbies, sports or recreational activities. Active relaxation is done by training the patients to voluntarily relax symptomatic muscles in calm and soothing voice for a couple of sessions by the trainer. This enhances blood flow, reduces emotional stress and eliminates pain [33, 34].

The Biofeedback technique uses electromyography (EMG) and skin temperature to measure patient's physiologic function and response towards treatment. Information obtained is conveyed back to the patient by metre or sound so that patient can gauge level of relaxation, adjust level of relaxation and measure progress. The goal is to achieve psychological self-regulation and to monitor relationship between muscular tension and pain [35, 36].

9.2.13 Acupuncture

Acupuncture is an alternative treatment that can be implemented with other treatment modalities through the course of non-surgical treatment. Proponents claim that it uses relationship between the energy flow through meridians, positive and negative life forces and natural elements. Fine needles are used in order to re-establish energy flow in areas.

First mechanism of action is gate control theory, which states that needle produces painless stimulation, causing neuronal gates to close and prevent signal propagation of pain to spinal cord. Others include release of neuronal opioids (enkephalins and endorphins) flooding the afferent interneurons, blocking pain sensation, promotion of alpha waves and re-balancing electric ion flow pattern, which on disruption, may elicit pain [37, 38].

9.2.14 Psychotherapy

TMDs may present as somatic expression of any underlying psychiatric/psychological disorder like depression. Proper personal/familial history of any psychiatric disease, substance abuse and physical/sexual abuse should be evaluated and obtained. Anxiety disorders occur commonly in patients with the chronic pain syndromes. Once psychiatric component is identified, psychiatric consultation for adjunctive treatment is a must for the contributing factors. It includes cognitive and behavioural therapy, support group involvements and pharmacotherapy [39, 40].

9.2.15 Pharmacotherapy

The pharmacologic management of TMD involves a combination of several drugs to alleviate the signs and symptoms. An analgesic or multimodal methods of analgesia can be used to prescribe several different classes of drugs based on signs and symptoms and the relevant history given by the patient. Various class of drugs that are prescribed include analgesics, corticosteroids, anxiolytics, anti-depressants, muscle relaxants, local anesthetics and anticonvulsants (Fig. 9.6).

9.2.15.1 Analgesics

Analgesics and anti-inflammatory are the drugs that relieve inflammatory conditions like synovitis, myositis, capsulitis, symptomatic disc displacement and osteoarthritis. It includes non-steroidal anti-inflammatory drugs (NSAIDS) and opioids.

NSAIDS are a competitive, reversible; active site inhibitors of enzyme cyclo-oxygenase, thus prevent formation of prostaglandins. Their action is rapid and is generally well tolerated by patients. The spectrum of safety for NSAIDS is higher than opioid analgesics. They cause less dependence/tolerance and can be used to treat mild to moderate pain in TMDs [41, 42].

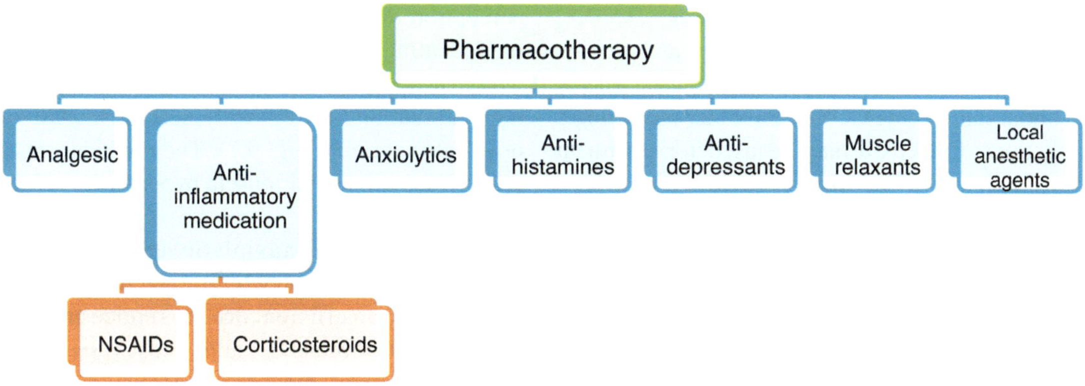

Fig. 9.6 Various pharmacologic agents used in TMDs

Table 9.4 Commonly used analgesics and anti-inflammatory drugs in TMDs

Drugs	Generic name	Average daily dosage in milligrams
NSAIDS	Acetaminophen	325–1000 mg q4h
	Acetylsalicylic (aspirin)	325–650 mg q4h
	Diflunisal	250–500 mg bid
	Ibuprofen	400–800 mg tid
	Ketoprofen	50–100 mg tid
	Naproxen sodium	275–550 mg bid
	Naproxen	250–500 mg bid
	Meloxicam	7.5–15 mg/day
	Diclofenac	25–50 mg tid
	Indomethacin	75 mg/day as sustained release
	Ketorolac tromethamine	10 mg q4–6h
Cyclo-oxygenase 2 inhibitors	Celecoxib	100–200 mg qid/bid
Analgesic combinations	Ibuprofen 400 mg, Acetaminophen 325 mg	1 tablet tid
	Aceclofenac 100 mg, Acetaminophen 325 mg	1 tablet bid
	Diclofenac 50 mg, Acetaminophen 325 mg	1 tablet bid
	Tramadol 37.5 mg, Acetaminophen 325 mg	1 tablet q4–6h
Corticosteroids	Methylprednisolone	4–8 mg/day

bid twice a day, *tid* thrice a day, *q* every, *h* hour

Most commonly used NSAID in TMDs is acetaminophen that has good patient tolerance and minimal side effects. Salicylates to be used include aspirin. Other classes of NSAIDs which are commonly used in TMDs include acetic acid derivatives which include ibuprofen, naproxen, diclofenac, aceclofenac, ketoprofen and indomethacin (indole-acetic acid derivative) [43] (Table 9.4).

There are evidences on the potential adverse effects of NSAIDs when consumed in for a longer period of time in high doses. They cause gastric irritation, allergies, renal disease and adverse cardiovascular events. To evade gastrointestinal irritation being the most common complaint by the patients, they should be asked to take medications immediately after meals. A proton pump inhibitor or H2 antagonist can be added in the regime for patients having good response to NSAIDs in order to prevent the anticipated gastric side effects [44].

9.2.15.2 Selective Cox-2 Inhibitors

COX-2 inhibitors chiefly affect the COX-2 pathway reducing the inflammatory response and it scarcely affects the gastric and renal function. Studies have shown that COX-2 (inflammatory mediator) is present in TMJ synovial fluid and tissues (internal derangement cases). COX-2 inhibitors leads to selective inhibition and provide potent anti-inflammatory and analgesic effects without influencing COX-1 and other physiologic functions. Celecoxib may be used for treatment for chronic TMDs in patients who are unable to tolerate classic NSAIDs [45, 46]. Other COX-2 inhibitors like valdecoxib and rofecoxib have higher incidence of cardiovascular events when taken for longer period (Table 9.4). Naproxen being a dual cyclo-oxygenase inhibitor (COX-1 and COX-2) is considered to be more effective in relieving excruciating pain in TMJ disorders when compared to selective COX-2 inhibitors [47].

9.2.15.3 Corticosteroids

Corticosteroids are potent anti-inflammatory drugs which are either injected directly in the TMJ or topically applied in order to reduce pain and dysfunction associated with TMDs. It acts by the complete blockade of arachidonic acid pathway. These drugs are rarely prescribed for systemic use except in cases of acute polyarthritides. Commonly used oral corticosteroid is methylprednisolone which needs a gradual reduction in dosing until stopped. Long term use in TMJ disorders causes condylar hypoplasia through inhibition of chondroblastic activity and increases calcium loss [48, 49] (Table 9.4).

9.2.15.4 Opioids

Opioids are a group of drugs that acts on specific opiate receptors in central and peripheral nervous system to provide analgesia. But its use remains controversial due to the risk of dependence and substance abuse. Yet it is commonly used by clinicians carefully in selected patients with careful monitoring of the administered dose.

Use of opioids as the first line of drug in TMDs is strongly discouraged. The pain level experienced by the patient and its interference in overall quality of life should be determined before prescribing an opioid. Tramadol and morphine are the most common drugs prescribed in TMDs [43] (Table 9.4).

9.2.15.5 Anxiolytics

Anti-anxiety/anxiolytic drugs can be used as a part of supportive therapy to change patient's perception to emotional stress. These agents are mild Central Nervous System (CNS) depressants which aim to control the symptoms of anxiety without interfering with normal mental or physical functions (Fig. 9.7). They reduce stress, anxiety, insomnia and muscle hyperactivity associated with TMDs.

Commonly used anxiolytic agents are benzodiazepine group of which diazepam is considered to be an efficient drug to reduce anxiety, relax skeletal muscles and causes sedation. A single dose of diazepam consumed (2.5 to 5 mg) at bedtime may often be useful to reduce muscle tonicity and decrease frequency of nocturnal parafunctional activities [50]. Other benzodiazepines that may be effective in treatment of TMDs are clonazepam and alprazolam [51]. Benzodiazepines should not be used for more than a period of 2 weeks because of their potential for dependency. Literature highlights

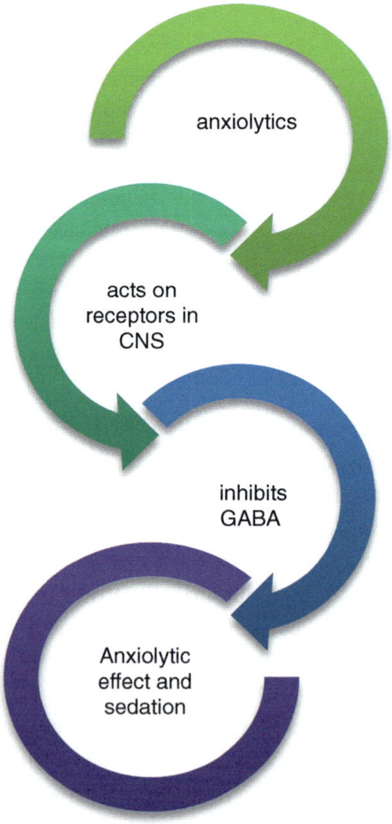

Fig. 9.7 Mechanism of anxiolytic drug in providing sedative effect

that rapid withdrawal after routine consumption for more than 2 weeks can lead to the benzodiazepine withdrawal or rebound syndrome. A large study on patients suffering from fibromyalgia received alprazolam, ibuprofen or combination of both reported enhanced relief in symptoms on palpation after six weeks in the group receiving combination drugs [51, 52] (Table 9.5).

9.2.15.6 Muscle Relaxants

Skeletal muscle relaxants are the drugs that reduce skeletal muscle tone and alleviate increased muscle activity. The muscle relaxants act either by primarily treating spasticity over upper motor neuron syndromes or muscular pain and spasms over peripheral musculoskeletal conditions. They decrease muscle tone without interfering with the motor function by acting centrally to depress polysynaptic reflexes.

Some of the commonly used skeletal muscle relaxants include baclofen, chlorzoxazone and thiocolchicoside. Pre- and post-synaptic GABA β receptors are blocked by baclofen as a result of which excitatory synaptic transmission in the spinal trigeminal nucleus is depressed. Chlorzoxazone is a centrally acting muscle relaxant, which is benzoxazolone derivative. It primarily depresses spinal polysynaptic reflexes over monosynaptic reflexes.

Chlorzoxazone can be used to relax hyperactive muscular activity related to TMDs. It acts as sedative as well. They are usually administered in combination with NSAIDs. Baclofen is a peripheral muscle relaxant used for myofascial pain. It is known for its specificity over severe muscle spasm and neurogenic pain. Cyclobenzaprine is used for chronic musculoskeletal disorders and is very effective in treating pain of lumbar and cervical regions and associated skeletal muscle spasms, may be employed for TMDs [53, 54].

Sedation is a common adverse effect in patients consuming skeletal muscle relaxants. Drug abuse is seen when Carisoprodol is used. Cyclobenzaprine is known to cause xerostomia and tachycardia, as a result of anti-cholinergic activity. It may worsen narrow-angle glaucoma and it should be avoided in such patients. To limit the side effects, it is always recommended that such drugs should always be titrated upward gradually [55, 56] (Table 9.6).

9.2.15.7 Anti-Depressants

Low doses of anti-depressants producing analgesia with no evidence in treatment of depression are useful in the management of chronic pain conditions. The drugs which are mainly administered for TMJ disorders include monoamine oxidase (MAO) inhibitors, tricyclic anti-depressants (TCAs), serotonin reuptake inhibitors (SSRIs).

Table 9.5 Other drugs used in management of chronic TMDs and orofacial pain

Class	Generic name	Average daily dose in milligrams (mg)	Maximum daily dose in milligrams (mg)
Anxiolytics (benzodiazepines)	Diazepam	2.5–5 mg at bedtime	10 mg/day, not more than 14 days
	Clonazepam	0.5 mg at bedtime	4 mg/day not more than 14 days
	Alprazolam	0.25–0.5 mg at bedtime	4 mg/day not more than 14 days
Antidepressants Tricyclic	Amitriptyline	10–20 mg at bedtime	100 mg/day
	Nortriptyline	25–50 mg at bedtime	150 mg/day
	Desipramine	25–50 mg tid	300 mg/day
SSRI	Fluoxetine	20–40 in the morning	60 mg/day
	Paroxetine	20–40 in the morning	60 mg/day
SNRI	Duloxetine	20–60 in the morning	120 mg/day
	Milnacipran	50 mg bid	200 mg/day
Anticonvulsives	Gabapentin	300 mg HS, gradual increase to 1800 mg/day	3600 mg/day
	Pregabalin	75–150 mg bid	300 mg/day

bid twice a day, *tid* thrice a day, *SSRI* Selective Serotonin Re-uptake Inhibitors, *SNRI* Serotonin Nor-epinephrine Re-uptake Inhibitors

Table 9.6 Commonly used muscle relaxants

Generic name	Average daily dose in milligrams (mg)	Maximum daily dose in milligrams (mg)
Cyclobenzaprine	10 mg tid	60 mg/day
Carisoprodol	250 mg tid	1400 mg/day maximum for 2–3 weeks
Baclofen	5 mg tid, dose can be increased gradually	80 mg/day, slow withdrawal
Metaxalone	800 mg tid/qid	2400 mg/day
Methocarbamol	1000 mg qid	8000 mg/day
Thiocolchicoside	4 mg/8 mg bid	16 mg/day
Combination drugs	Chlorzoxazone 500 mg, acetaminophen 325 mg, diclofenac 50 mg (bid)	2 tablet/day
	Ibuprofen 400 mg, acetaminophen 325 mg, Chlorzoxazone 250 mg (bid)	3–4 tablets/day

bid twice a day, *tid* thrice a day, *qid* four times a day

It is advisable to take these drugs for sleep disorders, obsessive compulsive disorders, chronic pain, central mediated pain disorders, etc. [57]. Kinney et al. concluded in their study that 30% of the patients suffering from TMDs present with depression of which 74% with chronic TMDs have faced at least an episode of major depression [58].

MAO inhibitor inhibits the activity of enzyme Monoamine Oxidase, which inhibits the breakdown of monoamine neurotransmitter thereby increasing their availability. They are not prescribed on a regular basis owing to their interactions with food and drugs (which may require a special diet by those who consume them) and side effects such as headache, xerostomia, gastric effects (nausea, vomiting, constipation, etc.), insomnia, dizziness and light headedness [59].

Tricyclic anti-depressants (TCAs) block the reuptake of the monoamine neurotransmitters—including serotonin and nor-epinephrine. The increase in the activity of neurotransmitters in the brain is associated with an alleviation of some symptoms of depression. TCAs help to treat sleep disturbances and nocturnal bruxism during TMDs. It has both serotonergic and noradrenergic effects. The common adverse effects of the drug are constipation, blurred vision, postural hypotension, ventricular arrhythmias (in patients with pre-existing cardiac disease) and urinary retention due to anti-cholinergic activity [60, 61].

Selective serotonin reuptake inhibitors (SSRIs) and serotonin-norepinephrine reuptake inhibitors (SNRIs), the newer generation of anti-depressants may be considered to be efficient over its antidepressant effect in treating fibromyalgia and TMDs in controlling pain and improve quality of life. It inhibits the reuptake of serotonin into the nerve cells in the brain leading to the availability of active serotonin in brain which improves the patient's mood and emotional feelings. Both SSRIs (fluoxetine and paroxetine) and SNRIs (duloxetine and milnacipran) have therapeutic uses in treating fibromyalgia and chronic centrally related myalgia [62]. Common adverse effects of these drugs are low safety margin, hazardous in overdose which can be fatal, frequent anti-cholinergic, cardiovascular and neurological side effects. The only purpose of including these anti-depressants for treating TMDs is for pain control rather than treating depression [63] (Table 9.5).

9.2.15.8 Anti-Histamines

Anti-histamines include conventional and second-generation anti-histamines. Highly sedative promethazine and hydroxyzine are commonly used in TMDs. They antagonize central and peripheral H1 receptors providing sedation and anxiolysis, thus relieving stress induced TMDs. It may also be used for treatment of vertigo and nausea following TMD. The adverse effects are usually mild. Sedation, diminished alertness, light headedness, motor in-coordination, tendency to fall asleep are commonly observed [63].

9.2.15.9 Anticonvulsants

Anticonvulsants are effective in the treatment of oro-facial pain like trigeminal neuralgia and related disorders such as migraine and headache. They also help to reduce central sensitization pain mechanism in fibromyalgia and TMDs. Gabapentin and pregabalin are the two anticonvulsives that may be used to treat chronic pain related to TMDs [64, 65].

The use of N-methyl-D-aspartate (NMDA) receptor antagonists provides great relief from oro-facial pain. Side effects are sedation, dizziness, dissociative effects, nausea and visual disturbances. NMDA are useful when they are combined with opioids as they have synergistic effect in reducing pain and decreases tolerance to opioid [63] (Table 9.5).

9.2.15.10 Injectable Medications

Both diagnostic and definitive management can be done using various injectable medications for TMDs. Local anaesthetics can be used for diagnostic purpose and to differentiate the true source of pain. They can be used as intra-articular, intramuscular injections or nerve blocks. They can be used for therapeutic effects in breaking pain cycle in cases of chronic TMDs. Commonly used local anaesthetic drugs are 2% lidocaine, 3% mepivacaine and 0.5% bupivacaine. Intracapsular injections of hydrocortisone (or betamethasone) may be used for restricted joint movement and pain relief [66].

Botulinum toxin injections, specifically Onabotulinum toxin A have been demonstrated to treat focal dystonias. It is a reversible neurotoxin that causes pre-synaptic blockade of release of acetylcholine at motor end plates, when injected into the muscle. It is injected using 30 gauge short needle (tuberculin syringe) approximately 25 units for a muscle, mostly into the middle body of the muscle and rest is distributed in other parts of muscle [67, 68].

9.3 Summary

A multidisciplinary approach in TMDs should initially begin with conservative and pharmacological management followed by minimally invasive methods. Surgery should be considered as a last resort when all other non-surgical and pharmacologic methods have rendered ineffective. Periodic follow-up for TMD patients helps in assessing patient's signs and symptoms and also the effect of therapy. It also helps in sequencing further treatment plan and assesses patient compliance.

References

1. Miloro M, Ghaji GE, Larsen PE, Waite PD. Peterson's principles of oral and maxillofacial surgery, vol. 6. 3rd ed. London: BC Decker; 2011. p. 1031–68.
2. de Bont LGM, Kijkgraaf LC, Stegenga B. Epidemiology and natural progression of articular temporomandibular disorders. Oral Surg Oral Med Oral Pathol Oral Radiol Endod. 1997;83:72–6.
3. Carlsson GE. Epidemiology and treatment needed for temporomandibular disorders. J Orofac Pain. 1999;13:232–7.
4. Indresano A, Alpha C. Nonsurgical management of temporomandibular joint disorders. In: Oral and maxillofacial surgery. 2nd ed. St. Louis, MO: Saunders/ Elsevier; 2009. p. 881–97.
5. Al-Ani MZ, Davies SJ, Gray RJ, et al. Stabilisation splint therapy for temporomandibular pain dysfunction syndrome. Cochrane Database Syst Rev. 2004;1:0126.
6. Mujakperuo HR, Watson M, Morrison R, Macfarlane TV. Pharmacological interventions for pain in patients with temporomandibular disorders. Cochrane Database Syst Rev. 2010;10:1006.
7. Greene CS. Orthodontics and temporomandibular disorders. Dent Clin N Am. 1988;32:529–38.
8. Clark GT. A critical evaluation of orthopedic interocclusal appliance therapy: design, theory and overall effectiveness. J Am Dent Assoc. 1984;108:359–64.
9. Magnusson T, Syren M. Therapeutic jaw exercises and interocclusal appliance therapy. A comparison between two common treatments of temporomandibular disorders. Swed Dent J. 1999;23(1):27–37.
10. McNeill C, editor. Temporomandibular disorders: guidelines for classification, assessment and management. 2nd ed. Chicago, IL: Quintessence Publishing; 1993.
11. Mejersjo C, Carlsson GE. Long-term results of treatment for temporomandibular pain-dysfunction. J Prosthet Dent. 1983;49:805–15.
12. Cooper BC. Temporomandibular disorders: a position paper of the International College of Cranio-Mandibular Orthopedics (ICCMO). Cranio. 2011;29(3):237–44.
13. Medlicott MS, Harris SR. A systematic review of the effectiveness of exercise, manual therapy, electrotherapy, relaxation training, and biofeedback in the management of temporomandibular disorder. Phys Ther. 2006;86(7):955–73.

14. Kaneyama K, Segami N, Nishimura M, et al. Importance of proinflammatory cytokines in synovial fluid from 121 joints with temporomandibular disorders. Br J Oral Maxillofac Surg. 2002;40:418–23.
15. Israel H, Syrop S. The important role of motion in the rehabilitation of patients with mandibular hypomobility: a review of the literature. J Craniomandib Pract. 1993;II:298–307.
16. Simons DG, Travell JG, Simons LS. Travell & Simons' myofascial pain and dysfunction: a trigger point manual. 2nd ed. Baltimore, MD: Williams & Wilkins; 1999.
17. Karlis V, Andreopoulos N, Kinney L, Glickman R. Effectiveness of supervised calibrated exercise therapy on jaw mobility and temporomandibular dysfunction. J Oral Maxillofac Surg. 1994;52(8 Suppl 2):147.
18. Sebastian MH, Moffet BC. The effect of continuous passive motion on the temporomandibular joint after surgery. Oral Surg Oral Med Oral Pathol. 1989;67:644–53.
19. Maloney G. Effect of a passive jaw motion device on pain and range of motion in TMD patients not responding to flat plane intraoral appliances. J Craniomandib Pract. 2002;20:55–6.
20. Adler RC, Adachi NY. Physical medicine in the management of myofascial pain and dysfunction: medical management of temporomandibular disorders. Oral Maxillofac Surg Clin North Am. 1995;7:99–106.
21. Furlan RM, Giovanardi RS, Britto AT, Oliveira Britto e DB. The use of superficial heat for treatment of temporomandibular disorders: an integrative review. Codas. 2015;27(2):207–12.
22. Nelson SJ, Ash MM Jr. An evaluation of a moist heating pad for the treatment of TMJ/muscle pain dysfunction. Cranio. 1988;6(4):355–9.
23. Schwartz LL. Ethyl chloride treatment of limited painful mandibular movement. J Am Dent Assoc. 1954;48:497–507.
24. Travell J. Ethyl chloride spray for painful muscle spasms. Arch Phys Med Rehabil. 1952;33:291–8.
25. Reid KI, Dionne RA, Sicard-Rosenbaum L, Lord D, Dubner R. Evaluation of iontophoretically applied dexamethasone for painful pathologic temporomandibular joints. Oral Surg Oral Med Oral Pathol. 1994;77:605–9.
26. Srbely JZ, Dickey JP, Lowerison M, et al. Stimulation of myofascial trigger points with ultrasound induces segmental antinociceptive effects: a randomized controlled study. Pain. 2008;139(2):260–6.
27. Kleinkort JA, Wood F. Phonophoresis with 1 percent versus 10 percent hydrocortisone. Phys Ther. 1975;55:1320–4.
28. Cameron MH, Monroe LG. Relative transmission of ultrasound by media customarily used for phonophoresis (see comments). Phys Ther. 1992;72(2):142–8.
29. Rai S, Ranjan V, Misra D, Panjwani S. Management of myofascial pain by therapeutic ultrasound and transcutaneous electrical nerve stimulation: a comparative study. Eur J Dent. 2016;10(1):46–53.
30. Shanavas M, Chatra L, Shenai P, et al. Transcutaneous electrical nerve stimulation therapy: an adjuvant pain controlling modality in TMD patients – a clinical study. Dent Res J (Isfahan). 2014;11(6):676–9.
31. Ernest EA. Temporomandibular joint and craniofacial pain. 2nd ed. Montgomery, AL: Ernest Publications; 1983.
32. Murphy GJ. Physical medicine modalities and trigger point injections in the management of temporomandibular disorders and assessing treatment outcome. Oral Surg Oral Med Oral Pathol Oral Radiol Endod. 1997;83(1):118–22.
33. Moller E, Sheik-Ol-Eslam A, Lous I. Deliberate relaxation of the temporal and masseter muscles in subjects with functional disorders of the chewing apparatus. Scand J Dent Res. 1971;79(7):478–82.
34. Gessel AH, Alderman MM. Management of myofascial pain dysfunction syndrome of the temporomandibular joint by tension control training. Psychosomatics. 1971;12(5):302–9.
35. Flor H, Birbaumer N. Comparison of the efficacy of electromyographic biofeedback, cognitive-behavioral therapy, and conservative medical interventions in the treatment of chronic musculoskeletal pain. J Consult Clin Psychol. 1993;61(4):653–8.
36. Santoro F, Maiorana C, Campiotti A. Neuromuscular relaxation and CCMDP. Biofeedback and TENS. 4. Dent Cadmos. 1989;57(18):88–9.
37. Goldstein L, Gilbert S. Acupuncture: new approach for temporomandibular disorders. Pract Pain Manag. 2017;11(16):1–20.
38. Madani A, Ahrari F, Fallahrastegar A, Daghestani N. A randomized clinical trial comparing the efficacy of low-level laser therapy (LLLT) and laser acupuncture therapy (LAT) in patients with temporomandibular disorders. Lasers Med Sci. 2019 Aug;8:1–12.
39. Katon W, Egan K, Miller D. Chronic pain: lifetime psychiatric diagnoses and family history. Am J Psychiatry. 1985;142:1156–60.
40. Licini F, Nojelli A, Segu M, Collesano V. Role of psychosocial factors in the etiology of temporomandibular disorders: relevance of a biaxial diagnosis. Minerva Stomatol. 2009;58(11–12):557–66.
41. Kuritzky L, Samraj GP. Nonsteroidal anti-inflammatory drugs in the treatment of low back pain. J Pain Res. 2012;5:579–90.
42. Hersh EV, Balasubramaniam R, Pinto A. Pharmacologic management of temporomandibular disorders. Oral Maxillofac Surg Clin North Am. 2008 May;20(2):197–210.
43. Hargreaves KM, Troullos ES, Dionne RA. Pharmacologic rationale for the treatment of acute pain. Dent Clin N Am. 1987;31:675–94.
44. Garcia RLA, Jick H. Risk of upper gastrointestinal bleeding and perforation associated with individual non-steroidal anti-inflammatory drugs. Lancet. 1994;343(8900):769–72.
45. Cicconetti A, Bartoli A, Ripari F, Ripari A. COX-2 selective inhibitors: a literature review of analgesic efficacy

and safety in oralmaxillofacial surgery. Oral Surg Oral Med Oral Pathol Oral Radiol Endod. 2004;97(2):139–46.
46. Zhang J, Ding EL, Song Y. Adverse effects of cyclooxygenase 2 inhibitors on renal and arrhythmia events. JAMA. 2006;296:1619–32.
47. Ta LE, Dionne RA. Treatment of painful temporomandibular joints with a cyclooxygenase-2 inhibitor: a randomized placebo controlled comparison of celecoxib to naproxen. Pain. 2004;111(1–2):13–21.
48. Wright EF, North SL. Management and treatment of temporomandibular disorders: a clinical perspective. J Man Manip Ther. 2009;17(4):247–54.
49. Dionne RA. Pharmacologic treatments for temporomandibular disorders. Oral Surg Oral Med Oral Pathol Oral Radiol Endod. 1997 Jan;83(1):134–42.
50. Turk DC, Rudy TE, Kubinski JA, Zaki HS, Greco CM. Dysfunctional patients with temporomandibular disorders: evaluating the efficacy of a tailored treatment protocol. J Consult Clin Psychol. 1996;64(1):139–46.
51. Harkins S, Linford J, Cohen J, et al. Administration of clonazepam in the treatment of TMD and associated myofascial pain: a double-blind pilot study. Craniomandib Disord. 1991;5(3):179–86.
52. Russell IJ, Fletcher EM, Michalek JE, McBroom PC, Hester GG. Treatment of primary fibrositis/fibromyalgia syndrome with ibuprofen and alprazolam. A double-blind, placebo-controlled study. Arthritis Rheum. 1991 May;34(5):552–60.
53. Stanko JR. Review of oral skeletal muscle relaxants for the craniomandibular disorder (CMD) practitioner. Cranio. 1990;8:234–43.
54. Tseng TC, Wang SC. Locus of action of centrally acting muscle relaxants, diazepam and tybamate. J Pharmacol Exp Ther. 1971;178(2):350–60.
55. Chou R, Peterson K, Helfand M. Comparative efficacy and safety of skeletal muscle relaxants for spasticity and musculoskeletal conditions: a systematic review. J Pain Symptom Manag. 2004;28:140–75.
56. Pal US, Kumar L, Mehta G, et al. Trends in management of myofascial pain. Natl J Maxillofac Surg. 2014;5(2):109–16.
57. Gatchel RJ, Garofalo JP, Ellis E, Holt C. Major psychological disorders in acute and chronic TMD: an initial examination. J Am Dent Assoc. 1996;127(9):1365–70. 1372, 1374
58. Kinney RK, Gatchel RJ, Ellis E, et al. Major psychological disorders in TMD patients: impactions for successful management. J Am Dent Assoc. 1992;123:49–54.
59. Fiedorowicz JG, Swartz KL. The role of monoamine oxidase inhibitors in current psychiatric practice. J Psychiatr Pract. 2004;10(4):239–48.
60. Kinney RK, Gatchel RJ, Ellis E, et al. Major psychological disorders in TMD patients: impaction for successful management. J Am Dent Assoc. 1992;123:49–54.
61. Fiedorowicz J, Swartz K, Brown RS, Bottomley WK. The utilization and mechanism of action of TCA in the treatment of chronic facial pain: a review of the literature. Anesth Prog. 1990;37:223–9.
62. Lee YC, Chen PP. A review of SSRIs and SNRIs in neuropathic pain. Expert Opin Pharmacother. 2010;11(17):2813–25.
63. Syrop SB. Pharmacological therapy. In: Kaplan AS, Assael LA, editors. Temporomandibular disorders-diagnosis and treatment. Philadelphia: WB Saunders; 1991. p. 501–14.
64. Moore RA, Wiffen PJ, Derry S, McQuay HJ. Gabapentin for chronic neuropathic pain and fibromyalgia in adults. Cochrane Database Syst Rev. 2011;3:CD007938.
65. Ifuku M, Iseki M, Hidaka I, et al. Replacement of gabapentin with pregabalin in postherpetic neuralgia therapy. Pain Med. 2011;12(7):1112–6.
66. Poswillo D. Experimental investigation of the effects of intraarticular hydrocortisone and high condylectomy on the mandibular condyle. Oral Surg Oral Med Oral Pathol. 1970;30(2):161–73.
67. Jankovic J, Brin MF. Therapeutic uses of botulinum toxin. N Engl J Med. 1991;324(17):1186–94.
68. Clark GT. The management of oromandibular motor disorders and facial spasms with injections of botulinum toxin. Phys Med Rehabil Clin N Am. 2003;14(4):727–48.
69. Srivastava R, Jyoti B, Devi P. Oral splint for temporomandibular joint disorders with revolutionary fluid system. Dent Res J (Isfahan). 2013;10(3):307–13.

Occlusion and Temporomandibular Joint Disorders

10

Sunil Kumar Mishra, Surabhi Somkuwar, and Ramesh Chowdhary

10.1 Introduction

The term Occlusion belongs to the Latin verb *occludere,* meaning "to close up", "Occludere" in turn comes from the prefix *ob-,* denoting "in the way", and the verb *claudere,* denoting "to close or shut". In dentistry, the term occlusion is used for four separate entities (Table 10.1) [1–3].

As stated by ***Glossary of Prosthodontic Terms*** (GPT) 9, occlusion can be defined as

1. The act or process of closure or of being closed or shut off.
2. The static relationship between the incising or masticating surfaces of the maxillary or mandibular teeth or tooth analogues [4].

The success of any restorative procedure depends solely on the stable occlusal contacts and various components of stomatognathic system. Any discrepancies in the occlusion are identified as a major aetiological factor for the development of temporomandibular joint disorders (TMDs) [1, 3].

Table 10.1 Entities for occlusion in dentistry

1	Angle's classification—For anatomic or orthodontic jaw relation
2	Static contact of the maxillary and mandibular teeth
3	Dynamic contact of maxillary and mandibular teeth in form of canine guided occlusion or group function occlusion
4	Classifications in prosthodontics for the complete dentition or incomplete dentition with fixed or removable prosthetics

10.2 Origin of Occlusion

An initiative to the study of occlusion dates back to the nineteenth century to Orthodontists, who endeavour to decode the concept for arrangement of dentition. Karolyi (1901) discussed the role of occlusion in bruxism, without any evidence and suggested that occlusal interferences are responsible for the atypical temporomandibular joint (TMJ)/masticatory muscle function, periodontal disease and bruxism. In the 1920s Goodfriend dissected cadaver heads with an attempt to correlate the dental occlusion with joint anatomy. He concluded that many factors play an important role in the predisposition and escalation of

S. K. Mishra (✉)
Department of Prosthodontics, Rama Dental College, Hospital and Research Centre, Kanpur, Uttar Pradesh, India

S. Somkuwar
Department of Dentistry, All India Institute of Medical Sciences, Raipur, Chhattisgarh, India

R. Chowdhary
Department of Prosthodontics, Rajarajeswari Dental College and Hospital, Bengaluru, Karnataka, India

D. Bhargava (ed.), *Temporomandibular Joint Disorders*,
https://doi.org/10.1007/978-981-16-2754-5_10

cranio-mandibular disorders like muscle spasms, external injuries, deleterious habits, stressful life style, etc. [5, 6].

Costen reported increase in vertical dimension is responsible for altered pressures on the joint. He assumed that this altered pressure in the joint is responsible for glossopharyngeal neuralgia and disturbed Eustachian tube function. This gave rise to the concept of occlusal pain and dysfunction co-relation. *Travell and Ramjford* reported that occlusal adjustments are beneficial in patients with both intra-capsular and extra-capsular disorders. Contrary to Costen's work, they suggested that the discrepancy between centric relation and centric occlusion is more significant interference rather than changes in vertical dimension [5, 6, 7].

10.3 Various Concepts of Occlusion

10.3.1 Gnathological Concept

The term *gnathology* was coined by Stallard in 1924. In 1926, McCollum formed the Gnathological Society together with Harlan, is credited with the ascertainment of the first conclusive method of locating the transverse horizontal axis. These recordings are transferred to an articulator using a Snow Facebow.

The principles of gnathology include the concept of centric relation, anterior guidance, vertical dimension of occlusion, the inter-cuspal design and the correlation of the anterior and posterior determinants of mandibular movements. According to this theory, condylar guidance is established first then anterior guidance will be designed to deocclude posterior teeth when the anterior teeth come into contact [6, 7].

10.3.2 Schuyler's Concept

The concept of "freedom in centric" was first advocated by Schuyler. This concept states that, "the central fossa exhibits a flat area upon which opposing cusps contact and permits a degree of freedom (0.5–1 mm) in all eccentric movements" [6, 8].

10.3.3 Wiskott and Belser's Concept

According to this concept, rather than three-point contact only one-point occlusal contact is sufficient. Anterior guidance should be followed in order to avoid posterior occlusal interferences during lateral excursive movement. Grossly number of occlusal contacts are diminished. It follows the concept of freedom in centric [6, 7].

Pankey, Mann and Schuylers concept was introduced by Pankey and follows the postulate of occlusion given by Schuyler. It follows the principle of spherical theory of occlusion. The anterior guidance is established according to aesthetics, function and comfort. The main objective is to establish and restore the lower posterior occlusal plane in harmony with the anterior guidance in such a way that it will not impede with condylar guidance. After completion of lower posteriors upper occlusal surfaces are established by following functionally generated path technique. It is based on the principle of long centric and group function in working excursion [9, 10].

10.3.4 Hobo's Twin Table Concept

According to this concept, molar disocclusion is determined by two important factors, namely cusp shape and an angle of hinge rotation. This technique utilizes two incisal tables to achieve molar disocclusion. The first incisal guide table is described as the incisal table without disocclusion. The aim of this table is to fabricate restoration for posterior teeth. The second incisal guide table is described as the incisal table with disocclusion. The aim of this table is to achieve incisal guidance with posterior disocclusion [11, 12].

10.3.5 Hobo's Twin Stage Concept

According to this concept cusp angle is the most reliable determinant of occlusion as it does not deviate. A standard value of cusp angle was determined irrespective of condylar and incisal guidance such that it is possible to establish the standard amount of disocclusion [11, 12].

10.4 Types of Occlusion

10.4.1 Dawson's Classification

This classification system for occlusion links maximal inter-cuspation to the position and condition of the TMJ.

Type I: Maximal inter-cuspation is in harmony with centric relation.

Type IA: Maximal inter-cuspation is in harmony with adapted centric posture.

Type II: For maximum inter-cuspation to occur condyles must displace from a true centric relation.

Type IIA: For maximum inter-cuspation to occur condyles must displace from adapted centric posture.

Type III: Verifying centric relation is difficult.

Type IV: Presence of pathologically unstable TMJs dictates that occlusal relationship is in active stage of progressive disorder [13, 14].

10.4.2 Unilaterally Balanced Occlusion/Group Function

This theory states that, during lateral movement excursive contact occurs between all opposing posterior teeth on the laterotrusive (working) side only. This in turn leads to distribution of load amongst the periodontal support of all posterior teeth on the working side. Disocclusion of posterior teeth occurs during protrusion [13, 14].

10.4.3 Long Centric Occlusion

This theory suggests that there should be some degree of freedom in antero-posterior direction. It is based on presumption that the condyle can translate horizontally in the fossae over a commensurate trajectory before initiating to glide downward. To allow some degree of horizontal movement (0.5–1.5 mm) before posterior disocclusion it is necessary to have a greater horizontal space between maxillary and mandibular anterior teeth [13, 14].

10.4.4 Mutually Protected Occlusion

During the early 1960s, Stuart and Stallard advocated mutually protected occlusion. This theory emphasizes that centric relation coincides with maximum inter-cuspation.

- Uniform occlusal contact of all maxillary and mandibular teeth in centric relation position.
- Posterior tooth contacts should be stable along with vertically directed resultant forces.
- Centric relation must coincide with maximum inter-cuspation.
- During lateral or protrusive movements there should be no contact of posterior teeth.
- Anterior teeth contacts harmonizing with functional jaw movements [13, 14].

10.4.5 Optimum Occlusion

In an ideal occlusal arrangement, there should be optimum load distribution on the dentition. Avoid or minimize horizontal forces on teeth as forces should act predominantly parallel to the long axis of the teeth. The functional cusps tip should be located centrally over the roots. Loading of the teeth occur on the occlusal fossae rather than on the marginal ridges. The contacts of posterior teeth must be avoided during excursive movements [15].

There are various concepts and types of occlusion documented in the literature. Careful assessment of the patient paves way for achieving appropriate contact of the maxillary and mandibular teeth for harmonious function of the stomatognathic system without any adverse effects for the TMJ and other structures in the oro-facial region [15, 16].

10.5 Determinants of Occlusion

Mandibular movements and determinants of occlusion are mainly governed by 3 factors, namely anterior determinants, posterior determinants and others. Anterior determinants include teeth of maxillary and mandibular arches, posterior determinants include right and left TMJ and other determinants include overall neuromuscular system (Table 10.2) [17, 1, 2].

10.6 Aetiology of TMDs

The aetiology for the development of TMDs is multifactorial. It may be biopsychosocial, biomechanical, neurobiological and neuromuscular. The predisposing factors depend on structural, metabolic and/or psychological states. The initiating factors can originate due to recurrent unfavourable loading of the masticatory system or trauma. In addition aggravating factors may include para-functional habits, hormonal changes or psycho social factors [18].

Change in occlusion may be evident in patients undergoing orthodontic, periodontic, prosthodontic or oral surgery procedure(s). Dental procedures like tooth extraction, prosthesis use for missing teeth, correction of malocclusion may change the occlusion in patients. Occasionally the occlusal changes may lead to discomfort in muscles of mastication, with acute pain which later leads to the development of a TMD. The clinical aim of the treating prosthodontist should be to diagnose and manage the occlusal problem initially before the disorder progresses [19].

Several controversies exist regarding the role of occlusion as main aetiological factor for TMDs. Few studies have demonstrated that the occlusion has no role in TMD, unlike others studies where they observed occlusion plays an important role in TMD with the presence of certain features like skeletal anterior open bite, significant over-jet, loss of molar support, extent of lateral deviation of the slide between the retruded contact position and maximal inter-cuspal contact position (RCP-ICP). Severe malocclusion may also be considered as a predisposing factor for degenerative TMJ changes [18, 19].

Table 10.2 Determinants of occlusion

Determinants	Conditions	Effect on cusp height and angulation
Posterior determinants		
During protrusion		
Inclination of articular eminence (Figs. 10.1 and 10.2)	Steep Shallow	More cusp height Less cusp height
During lateral translation		
Morphology of medial wall of glenoid fossa which allows immediate lateral shift	More Less	Less cusp height More cusp height
Inter-condylar distance	More Less	Small angle between working and non-working condylar movement Greater angle between working and non-working condylar movement
Anterior determinants		
Over-jet (Fig. 10.3a, b)	Increased Decreased	Short cusp height More cusp height
Overbite (Fig. 10.4a, b)	Increased Decreased	More cusp height Less cusp height
Others		
Plane of occlusion	More parallel to condylar guidance Less parallel to condylar guidance	Less cusp height More cusp height
Curve of Spee	Radius of curve short Radius of curve large	Less cusp height More cusp height

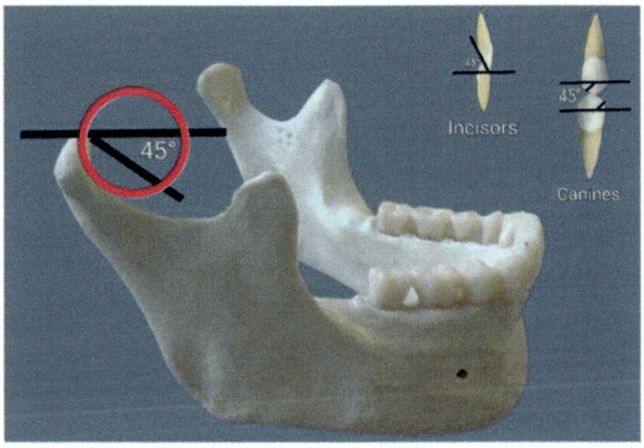

Fig. 10.1 Lesser the angle of articular eminence, lesser the steepness of the cuspal angle and minimum overbite

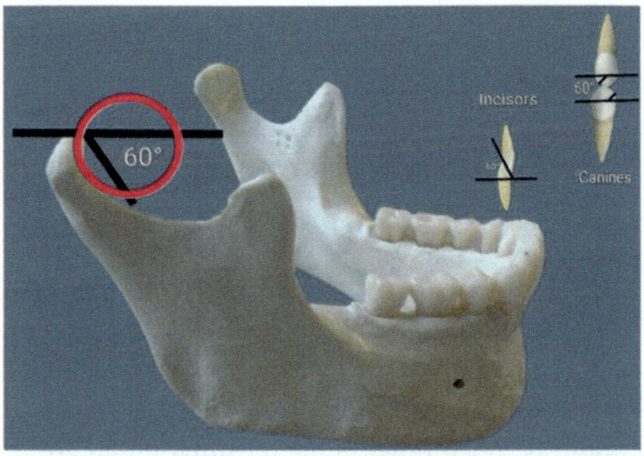

Fig. 10.2 Greater the angle of articular eminence, greater the steepness of cuspal angle and more overbite

Jussila et al. through their research emphasized that occlusal factors exhibited a statistically significant association with development of TMD. The TMD signs were related with unstable occlusion, mainly with the extent of lateral deviation in retruded contact position and inter-cuspal contact position (RCP-ICP) slide, as well as negative over-jet [20].

A typical shift regarding TMDs has occurred recently from the bio-medical model of occlusion to a biopsychosocial model of the disease. In 1977, Engel introduced biopsychosocial model based on a common structure to provide an entire sub-structure in which all the extent of organization relevant to disease and health could be considered. One of the sub-structures of organization in the TMD related to musculoskeletal pain condition is occlusion. The role of occlusion in TMD is not completely assessed and also the effects of the occlusal interferences on TMJ are a subject for exhaustive research [21].

Xie et al. reviewed the association between occlusal interferences and TMDs from insights collected from animal and human experimental analysis and concluded that experimental occlusal alteration can be considered as an interesting topic for occlusion engrossed scientific research. They observed that changes in occlusion leads to

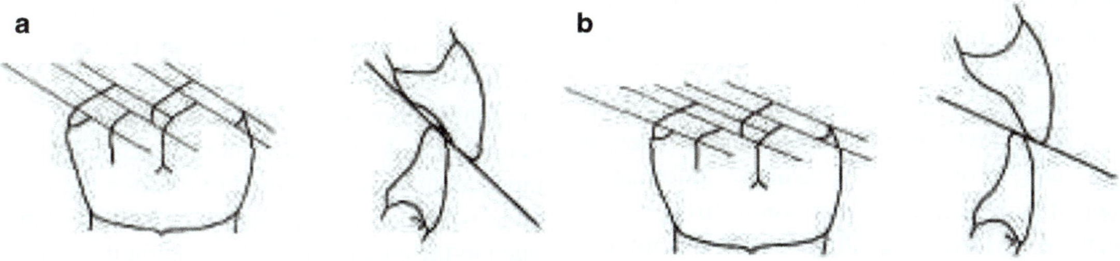

Fig. 10.3 (**a**) Pronounced overbite permits longer posterior cusp. (**b**) Minimum overbite permits short posterior cusp

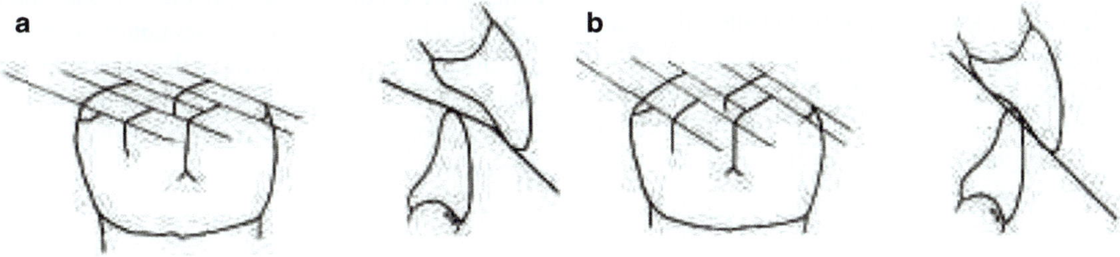

Fig. 10.4 (**a**) Pronounced overjet permits short cusp. (**b**) Minimum overjet permits long cusp

alterations in the masticatory muscles, TMJ and the nervous system in animal models. In human experimental studies, it has been noted that subjects without symptoms of TMD may adapt well to experimental interferences. But patients with a pre-existing symptoms of TMD seem to nominally adapt to the introduced experimental interferences [22].

Many researchers consider occlusal discrepancies as main aetiological factor in the progression of TMJ dysfunction [23, 24]. Zarb and Thompson in their study stated that 61% of the patients had occlusal discrepancy who needed treatment for TMJ dysfunction. The occlusal discrepancies may be in the form of an anterior and/or lateral slide from centric relation (CR) to centric occlusion (CO) or the presence of non-working side contacts and disocclusive contacts distal to the canine on the working side during purposeful lateral side shift of the mandible [23, 25].

10.7 Occlusal Indicators

The main purpose of occlusal indicators is to locate and determine the specific areas of occlusal contact. They may be classified as near contact areas and non-contact areas. Near contact areas are those wherein there is a gap of 0.5 mm between the occluding surfaces, whilst non-contacts are those areas where there is a 0.5–2 mm separation of the teeth.

Presently, a variety of occlusal indicators are available and proper selection of occlusal indicator provides the valuable information regarding refinement of occlusion. Broadly they can be divided as qualitative and quantitative occlusal indicators (Table 10.3). Qualitative indicators are routinely used because of its low cost and ease of use. However, presence of saliva may affect the marking abilities. On the other hand, quantitative indicators mainly identify the time and force of true occlusal contacts. However repeated use of sensor negatively affects the marking characteristics. Every material has its own limitations. The choice of material selection depends upon the clinical condition, clinician's proficiency and sensitivity, economics and comfort [24–28].

Table 10.3 Types of occlusal indicators

Qualitative indicators	Quantitative indicators
Articulating paper	T-scan occlusal analysis system
Articulating silk	Virtual dental patient
Pressure sensitive film	
Metallic shim stock film	
High spot indicator	
Occlusal sprays	
Mylar strips, silk strips	
Polyether rubber impression bites	

10.8 Methods of Occlusal Corrections

10.8.1 Position of the Mandible

McCollum and Stuart had given the centric relation approach and suggested that the condyle should be positioned in the terminal hinge arc of closure. Later, Schuyler, Mann and Pankey suggested that the long centric concept or freedom in centric concept where the terminal hinge position is used as a reference point, with the protrusive movement of mandible in horizontal plane without any change in the vertical dimension. Still, the controversy exists about which position of the mandible is biologically more acceptable. The most common method used to position the mandible is by occlusal splints which will be elaborated in the chapter on occlusal splint therapy.

Enameloplasty/Spot grinding is another technique where only those teeth with heavy occlusal contact were adjusted so that the occlusal load can be re-distributed. Other fewer common methods documented to re-position the mandible are the use of dental, alveolar and skeletal landmarks and by applying external electrical pulses to the pre-auricular region [8, 9].

10.8.2 Canine Protected Occlusion (Group Function Occlusal Scheme)

Nagao, Shaw and D'Amico proposed the theory of canine protected occlusion. It is a type of mutually protected occlusion in which vertical and horizontal overlap of canines disocclude the posterior teeth during excursive movement of the mandible. The protected occlusion is also known as canine disocclusion/canine rise or canine guided occlusion [29]. The most appropriate teeth considered to guide mandibular excursion is canine as

1. It has good crown root ratio.
2. It can tolerate high occlusal forces.
3. It has high proprioceptive response.

The concave nature of the palatal surface of canine makes it suitable for guiding lateral movements. In anterior open bite cases, extreme Angle class II division 1 or class III malocclusion and cross-bite, mandible cannot be guided by anterior teeth and canine guidance cannot be achieved. In order to obtain canine guided occlusion the anterior teeth must be healthy. In cases where healthy canines are present and restoration can re-establish lateral guidance, canine guided occlusion can be given. Cuspid protected occlusion is considered beneficial when posterior teeth have significant bone loss, considerable occlusal wear and in cases of bruxism [30].

10.8.3 Group Function

GPT defines group function as multiple contact relations between maxillary and mandibular teeth in lateral movements on the working side whereby simultaneous contact of several teeth acts as a group to distribute occlusal forces. The group function occlusion was described by Beyron and is commonly known as unilateral balanced occlusion. The group function of the teeth distributes the occlusal load on working side [31].

Group function of working side is indicated in patients with Class I occlusion with extreme over-jet, Class III occlusion with all lower anterior teeth are anterior to the upper arch, end to end and anterior open bite, when the arch relationship is such that it does not allow the anterior guidance to disocclude the teeth on non-working side. Group function is most often seen in elderly population. This occlusal scheme allows achieving harmonious balance of all structures including TMJ and associated musculature.

Furthermore, in a patient with history of bruxism there may be freedom of lateral excursions in group function. Factors such as patient's masticating pattern, craniofacial morphology, type of occlusion, oral hygiene status; para-functional habits might provide the important clue and relevant information about the suitable occlusal scheme for each patient [32].

10.8.4 Tripodal Cusp Contacts

Stuart and Stallard had given tripodal cusp contact theory. It is a posterior tooth-to-tooth contact pattern. Though it is stable in providing occlusion, it is difficult to clinically attain the goals. In this occlusal scheme patient has to function comfortably from a single point centric starting position. Researchers have recommended that "freedom in centric" concept allows cusp tip to fossa or marginal ridge occlusal contact patterns when compared to tripodal concept [33–35].

10.8.5 Occlusal Adjustments to Remove Traumatic Occlusion

Traumatic occlusion should be removed to reduce/eliminate any detrimental effects on the dentition and the TMJ. Traumatic occlusion can produce

1. Cracked/fractured tooth.
2. Initiate pulpitis/pulpal degenerative changes.
3. Leads to tooth mobility.

It is well documented that traumatic occlusion affect the periodontium and can lead to bone loss due to excessive load. It is the responsibility of the clinician to diagnose such discrepancies and deliberately plan the occlusal correction to correct the traumatic occlusion as an early intervention in the course of the treatment [35, 36].

10.8.6 Avoidance/Correction of Occlusal Interferences

An occlusal interference can be defined as any tooth contact that interferes with the remaining occluding surfaces from achieving a balanced and stable occlusal contacts (Table 10.4) [36].

10.8.7 Centric Interference

Centric interference denotes the first tooth contact (FTC) on the arc of rotation enfolding the mandibular movement when maximum inter-cuspation position does not coincide with the centric relation. In this situation the mandible generally avoids this contact and directly closes in to maximum inter-cuspation. During evaluation, the patient is asked to relax and mandible is guided to centric relation. It is the role of the treating prosthodontist to diagnose the problem and adjust occlusal interference by preparation of the involved tooth.

10.8.8 Working Side Interference

Working side interference refers to the side towards which the mandible is moving. The presence of working interference hampers the smooth movement of mandible leading to separation of teeth on working side.

Table 10.4 Types of occlusal interferences

1	Centric interference
2	Working side interference
3	Non-working side interference
4	Protrusive interference

10.8.9 Non-working Side Interference

Non-working side interference occurs between the inner incline of the supporting cusps of antagonist teeth and disocclude other teeth. The tooth involved will act as a pivot shifting the fulcrum from the TMJ and elevates teeth on working side out of contact. This type of occlusal interference may damage the dental structures and TMJ.

10.8.10 Protrusive Interference

Protrusive interference is observed during mandibular protrusion. It is present between the mesial inclines of mandibular posterior teeth and the distal inclines of maxillary posterior teeth. This type of interferences result in disocclusion of the anterior teeth during movement and may predispose to locking of the mandible. During protrusive movements, anterior teeth and TMJ bear majority of the forces of the elevator muscles. In such cases clinician should diagnose the problem and adjust the occlusal interference.

10.9 Occlusal Consideration for Dental Implants

Implant protected occlusion is an elaborate subject and is not covered in the present chapter in total. In brief, few important points to be considered are highlighted. This concept was first put forward by Carl Misch with an aim to reduce the occlusal forces on implant prosthesis. Few important factors should be considered during designing of occlusal pattern. Incisal guidance should be shallow with maximum inter-cuspation and bilateral stability.

The forces on teeth should be evenly distributed with freedom in centric. There should not be either working or non-working side interferences in lateral and protrusive movements. Any occlusal interference between centric relation and maximum inter-cuspal position should be eliminated by giving flat fossae and grooves. There should be reduction of occlusal table by one-third in molar region to eliminate any cantilever effects. A shallow incisal guidance concept permits less loading on the anterior implants by disocclusion of the posterior teeth during lateral and protrusive mandibular movements [14].

10.10 Role of Tekscan (T-Scan) in Occlusion and TMJ Disorders

Tekscan is a computerized system developed in 1984 by Maness et al. which records the intraoral occlusal forces with the help of a pressure mapping sensor. The T-Scan makes it possible to quantify occlusal contact data by registering certain parameters such as the bite length as well as the timing and force of tooth contact and stores the data on a hard drive which can be played incrementally in a time-based video for analysis of data.

T-scan is used to record various functional movements of the mandible. It also records any premature contact in centric relation. Multiple bites can be obtained which helps in identifying the habitual inter-cuspation by the patients. The posterior disocclusion time that occurs during lateral and protrusive-excursive mandibular movements can also be recorded. Any mild painful occlusal contacts which occur during chewing can be easily diagnosed which may not be easily identified utilizing the direct observation or ink ribbon markings.

10.11 Applications of T-Scan in Dentistry

T-Scan finds its clinical applications in various fields of dentistry such as in prosthodontics, implant dentistry, orthodontics, restorative dentistry, oral and maxillofacial surgery and in identifying TMDs related to occlusion. Several studies have highlighted the use of T-scan in identifying occlusal discrepancies causing TMDs in human subjects [37, 38, 39, 40].

10.12 Terminologies [4]

Anterior Guidance: (1). The influence of the contacting surfaces of anterior teeth, limiting mandibular movements; (2). The influence of the contacting surfaces of the guide pin and anterior guide table on articulator movements.

Centric Occlusion/Maximal Inter-cuspal Position: The occlusion of opposing teeth when the mandible is in centric relation. This may or may not coincide with the maximal inter-cuspal position.

Centric Relation: A maxilla-mandibular relationship, independent of tooth contact, in which the condyles articulate in the anterior-superior position against the posterior slopes of the articular eminences; in this position, the mandible is restricted to a purely rotary movement; from this unstrained, physiologic, maxilla-mandibular relationship. The patient can make vertical, lateral or protrusive movements; it is a clinically useful, repeatable reference position.

Condylar Guidance: Mandibular guidance generated by the condyle and articular disc traversing the contour of the articular eminence.

Determinants of Mandibular Movements: Those anatomic structures that dictate or limit the movements of the mandible; the anterior determinant of mandibular movement is the dental articulation; the posterior determinants of mandibular movement are the temporomandibular articulations and their associated structures.

Interference: Any tooth contact that interferes with or hinders harmonious mandibular movement; an undesirable tooth contact.

Lateral Relation: The relation of the mandible to the maxillae when the lower jaw is in a position to either side of centric relation.

Laterodetrusion: Lateral and downward movement of the condyle on the working side.

Laterotrusion: Condylar movement on the working side in the horizontal plane; this term may be used in combination with terms describing condylar movement in other Planes.

Temporomandibular Joint: The articulation of the condylar process of the mandible and the intra-articular disc with the mandibular fossa of the squamous portion of the temporal bone; a diarthrodial, sliding hinge (ginglymus) joint; movement in the upper joint compartment is mostly translational, whereas that in the lower joint compartment is mostly rotational; the joint connects the mandibular condyle to the articular fossa of the temporal bone with the temporomandibular joint articular disc interposed.

Temporomandibular Disorders: A collection of symptoms frequently observed in various combinations first described by Costen (1934, 1937), which he claimed to be reflexes because of irritation of the auriculotemporal and/or chorda tympanic nerves as they emerged from the tympanic plate caused by altered anatomic relations and derangements of the temporomandibular joint associated with loss of occlusal vertical dimension, loss of posterior tooth support and/or other malocclusions; the symptoms can include headache about the vertex and occiput, tinnitus, pain around the ear, impaired hearing and pain around the tongue/jaw.

References

1. Rosensteil SF, Land MF, Fujimoto J. Contemporary fixed prosthodontics. St. Louis, MI: Elsevier; 2006.
2. Shillingburg HT, Hobo S, Whitsett LD, Jacobi R, Brackett SE. Fundamentals of fixed prosthodontics. Chicago, IL: Quintessence Publishing Company; 1997 Jan.
3. Okeson JP, Burch JG. Fundamentals of occlusion and temporomandibular disorders. St. Louis: Mosby; 1985.
4. Academy of Prosthodontics. Glossary of prosthodontic terms: 9th edition. J Prosthet Dent. 2018;117(5S):e1–e105.
5. Pokorny PH, Wiens JP, Litvak H. Occlusion for fixed prosthodontics: a historical perspective of the gnathological influence. J Prosthet Dent. 2008;99(4):299–313.
6. Türp JC, Greene CS, Strub JR. Dental occlusion: a critical reflection on past, present and future concepts. J Oral Rehabil. 2008;35(6):446–53.
7. Levene BF. Basic concepts in occlusal corrections of natural teeth. J Prosthet Dent. 1965;15(4):732–6.
8. Schuyler CH. Factors of occlusion applicable to restorative dentistry. J Prosthet Dent. 1953;3(6):772–82.
9. Mann AW, Pankey LD. Oral rehabilitation: Part I. use of the PM instrument in treatment planning and in restoring the lower posterior teeth. J Prosthet Dent. 1960;10(1):135–50.
10. Pankey LD, Mann AW. Oral rehabilitation: Part II. Reconstruction of the upper teeth using a functionally generated path technique. J Prosthet Dent. 1960;10(1):151–62.
11. Hobo S. Twin-tables technique for occlusal rehabilitation: Part I: mechanism of anterior guidance. J Prosthet Dent. 1991;66(3):299–303.
12. Hobo S. Twin-tables technique for occlusal rehabilitation: Part II-clinical procedures. J Prosthet Dent. 1991;66(4):471–7.
13. Warreth A. Fundamentals of occlusion and restorative dentistry. Part I: basic principles. J Ir Dent Assoc. 2015;61(4):201–8.
14. Warreth A. Fundamentals of occlusion and restorative dentistry. Part II: occlusal contacts, interferences and occlusal considerations in implant patients. J Ir Dent Assoc. 2015;61(5):252–9.
15. Barbosa GA, dos Reis Badaró Filho C, Fonseca RB, Soares CJ, das Neves FD, Neto AJ. The role of occlusion and occlusal adjustment on temporomandibular dysfunction. Braz J Oral Sci. 2016;12:589–94.
16. Dawson PE. Evaluation, diagnosis and treatment of occlusal problems. 2nd ed. St Louis, MO: Mosby. 1989.
17. Glassman B, Malizia D. The curious history of occlusion in dentistry. Dental Town. 2017;1:55–62.
18. de Kanter RJAM, Battistuzzi PGFCM, Truin G. Temporomandibular disorders: "occlusion" matters! Pain Res Manag. 2018;2018:1–13.
19. Suvinen TI, Reade PC, Hanes KR, Kononen M, Kemppainen P. Temporomandibular disorder subtypes according to self-reported physical and psychosocial variables in female patients: a re-evaluation. J Oral Rehabil. 2005;32:166–73.
20. Jussila P, Krooks L, Näpänkangas R, Päkkilä J, Lähdesmäki R, Pirttiniemi P, Raustia A. The role of occlusion in temporomandibular disorders (TMD) in the Northern Finland Birth Cohort (NFBC) 1966. Cranio. 2019;37(4):231–7.
21. McNeill C. Evidence-based TMD guidelines. J Orofac Pain. 1997;11:93.
22. Xie Q, Li X, Xu X. The difficult relationship between occlusal interferences and temporomandibular disorder-insights from animal and human experimental studies. J Oral Rehabil. 2013;40:279–95.
23. Egermark-Eriksson I, Carlsson GE, Magnusson T, et al. A longitudinal study on malocclusion in relation to signs and symptoms of cranio-mandibular disorders in children and adolescents. Eur J Orthod. 1990;12:399–407.
24. McNeill C. Temporomandibular disorders: guidelines for classification, assessment, and management. Quintessence: Chicago, IL; 1993.
25. Zarb GA, Thompson GW. Assessment of clinical treatment of patients with temporomandibular joint dysfunction. J Prosthet Dent. 1970;24:542–54.
26. Panigrahi D, Satpathy A, Patil A, Patel G. Occlusion and occlusal indicating materials. Int J Appl Dent Sci. 2015;1(4):23–6.

27. Millstein P, Maya A. An evaluation of occlusal contact marking indicators: a descriptive quantitative method. JADA. 2001;132(9):1280–6.
28. Caldas W, Conti ACDF, Janson G, Conti PCR. Occlusal changes secondary to temporomandibular joint conditions: a critical review and implications for clinical practice. J Appl Oral Sci. 2016;24(4):411–9.
29. D'Amico A. Origin and development of the balanced occlusion theory. J South Calif Dent Assoc. 1960;28:317–8.
30. D'Amico A. Functional occlusion of the natural teeth of man. J Prosthet Dent. 1961;11:899–915.
31. Sidana V, Pasricha N, Makkar M, Bhasin S. Group function occlusion. Indian J Oral Sci. 2012;3:124–8.
32. Mohan B, Sihivahanan D. Occlusion: the gateway to success. J Interdiscip Dentistry. 2012;2:68–77.
33. Beyron NL. Occlusal changes in adult dentition. JADA. 1954;48(6):674–86.
34. Beyron H. Optimal occlusion. Dent Clin N Am. 1969;13:537–54.
35. Stuart CE, Stallard H. Oral rehabilitation and occlusion. San Francisco, CA: University of California; 1959.
36. Clark GT, Adler RC. A critical evaluation of occlusal therapy: occlusal adjustment procedures. JADA. 1985;110:743–50.
37. Komali G, Ignatius AV, Srivani GS, Anuja K. T-scan system in the management of temporomandibular joint disorders – a review. J Indian Acad Oral Med Radiol. 2019;31:252–6.
38. Kerstein RB. Handbook of research on computerized occlusal analysis technology applications in dental medicine. Hershey, PA: IGI Global Publishers; 2015.
39. Thumati P. The influence of immediate complete anterior guidance development technique on subjective symptoms in myofascial pain patients: verified using digital analysis of occlusion (Tek-scan) for analysing occlusion: a 3 years clinical observation. J Indian Prosthodont Soc. 2015;15:218–23.
40. Dzingute A, Pileicikiene G, Baltrusaityte A, Skirbutis G. Evaluation of the relationship between the occlusion parameters and symptoms of the temporomandibular joint disorder. Acta Medica Lituanica. 2017;24:167–75.

Occlusal Splint Therapy in Temporomandibular Disorders

11

Sunil Kumar Mishra, Ramesh Chowdhary, Rahul Rochani, and Shail Kumari

11.1 Introduction

Temporomandibular joint (TMJ) forms an articulation of the mandible with the skull base. Temporomandibular joint disorders (TMDs) commonly present as clicking, pain, creaking in the jaw joint with difficulty in function. These disorders are sometimes referred to as craniomandibular disorders (CMD) and are one of the most noted causes for facial pain [1–3].

11.2 Definition

According to Glossary of Prosthodontic Terms (GPT), 9th ed., **Splint** is defined as a rigid or flexible device that maintains in position a displaced or movable part. It is also used to keep in place and protect an injured part.

According to GPT (9th ed.), **Occlusal Splint/Occlusal device** is defined as any removable artificial occlusal surface affecting the relationship of mandible to maxillae used for diagnosis or therapy [4].

11.3 Splint Types, Uses, Indications, Contraindications and Theories

There are various types of splints used to relieve TMD symptoms (Table 11.1), with several indications, contra-indications, and uses (Tables 11.2, 11.3, and 11.4). The uses include diagnostic purpose before any substantial intervention, to stabilize the occlusion to treat TMDs, in radiation therapy, for proper occlusal positioning, and to prevent occlusal wear or any damage to prosthesis/restorations which are brittle in nature (Table 11.5). They are termed based on their uses such as occlusal appliance, mouth/bite guard, orthodontic appliance, surgical splint, or stent [4–8]. There are several theories based on which the occlusal splints perform its function in various TMDs (Table 11.6) [9].

S. K. Mishra
Department of Prosthodontics, Rama Dental College, Hospital and Research Centre, Kanpur, Uttar Pradesh, India

R. Chowdhary
Department of Prosthodontics, Rajarajeswari Dental College and Hospital, Bengaluru, Karnataka, India

R. Rochani (✉)
Sparkle Dental Hub and Centre for Excellence in Orthodontics, Bhopal, Madhya Pradesh, India

S. Kumari
CHC, Kalyanpur, Kanpur, Uttar Pradesh, India

D. Bhargava (ed.), *Temporomandibular Joint Disorders*,
https://doi.org/10.1007/978-981-16-2754-5_11

Table 11.1 Classification of occlusal splints

Author	Types	Uses
Okeson	1. Muscle relaxation/ stabilization appliance	Reduce muscle activity in cases of masticatory myalgia and TMJ arthralgia, especially if the pain is worse upon awakening. Used to provide a postural stabilization so as to protect the muscles, TMJ, and teeth. The centric relation splint is generally used to treat muscle hyperactivity in patients with myospasm or myositis Used in case of parafunctional habits
	2. Anterior repositioning/ Orthopaedic repositioning appliance	Cases with disc derangement disorders and jointsounds Cases with inflammatory disorders (retrodiscitis) Cases with intermittent jaw locking and TMJ arthralgia not responsive to other treatment
	3. Soft/resilient appliance	Used by athletes as protective device to prevent trauma to their dental arches In cases of clenching and bruxism In few cases with symptoms of TMDs (joint dysfunction and myalgia) to reduce symptoms In cases of chronic sinusitis to relief the sensitive posterior teeth
	4. Anterior/posterior bite plane	Anterior bite plane acts by dis-occluding the posterior teeth and prevents clenching during parafunctional habits Posterior bite plane is used in severe loss of vertical dimension When there is a need to make major changes in the anterior repositioning of the mandible This appliance produces an ideal maxilla-mandibular relationship
	5. Pivoting appliance	The appliance is used to unload the joint articular surface Used in treating joint sounds and degenerative joint diseases Used for the treatment of symptoms related to osteoarthritis of the TMJs Also used for the treatment of an acute unilateral disc dislocation without reduction
Dawson	1. Muscle deprogrammer or permissive splints	Helps in unlocking the occlusion so as to remove any deviating tooth inclines from contact Helps the condyles return to their correct seated position in centric relation
	2. Directive splints or non-permissive splints	Help in positioning mandible in a specific relationship to maxilla so as to align the condyle-disc assemblies Used in painful joint problems Used in cases of severe trauma which leads to retro-discal oedema and in cases of chronic disc displacement disorders
	3. Pseudo-permissive splints. E.g. soft splints and hydrostatic splints	Indicated in TMJ pain, headache, neck and shoulder pain and stiffness, orthodontic triggered muscle pain during treatment, pre-surgical differential diagnoses, post-surgical pain, and inflammation

Table 11.2 Indications for occlusal splint

Modification of growth during mixed dentition
Limited tipping movements desired for individual tooth malposition and arch expansion
In orthodontic treatment, for retention purpose
As an adjunct to fixed appliance therapy in orthodontics
Prevent/interfere with abnormal oro-facial habits
TMJ disorders
Mandibular fractures in paediatric/edentulous patients

Table 11.3 Contraindications for occlusal splint

Cases with vertical discrepancy
Severe rotation cases where bodily movement is required
Cases with severe skeletal discrepancy
Cases with severe crowding
Cases having very dense bone

Table 11.4 Functions of occlusal splint

Provide diagnostic information in patients
Relaxes the muscles
Positioning/seating of condyle in stable musculoskeletal position
In bruxism patients to protect their teeth and associated structures
To mitigate periodontal ligament proprioception
Cognitive awareness

Table 11.5 Various applications of occlusal splint

Temporomandibular disorders (TMDs)	• Disc displacement disorders of TMJ • Arthritis of TMJ
Pain disorders	• Myofascial pain • Headaches/migraine
Sleep and motor disorders	• Sleep apnoea • Sleep bruxism • Parkinson's disease • Oral tardive dyskinesia
Occlusal rehabilitation	• Loss of vertical dimensions • Excessive tooth wear
Prevention from trauma/abnormal habits	• Fingernail or cheek biting • Lip commissure burn • Sports injury • Diurnal bruxism • Electroconvulsive therapy • Oesophageal reflux • Sinusitis

Table 11.6 Theories based on which occlusal splints work in the oral cavity with associated facial structures

According to Glenn T Clark theories on which occlusal splint work
Restored vertical dimension theory
TMJ reposition theory
Occlusal disengagement theory
Cognitive awareness theory
Maxillo-mandibular aliment theory

11.4 Stabilization Appliance

(Muscle relaxation appliance/Flat plane stabilization appliance/Gnathologic splint/Michigan splint/Superior repositioning splint/Tanner appliance/Fox appliance/Centric relation appliance) (Fig. 11.1).

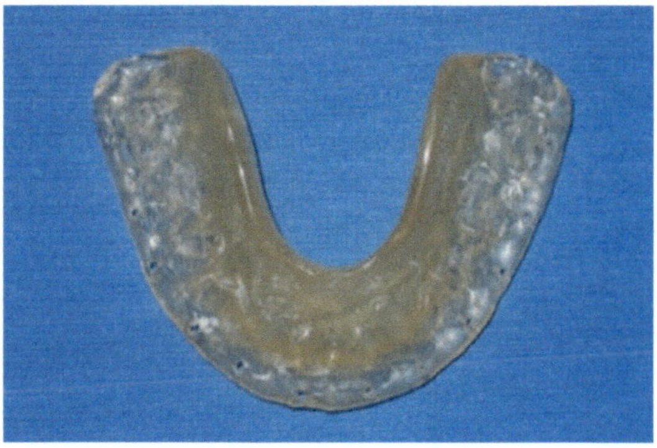

Fig. 11.1 Stabilization appliance

Table 11.7 Occlusal splint decreasing the TMD symptoms by various mechanisms

General features of occlusal splints responsible for decreasing muscle activity and symptoms
Aids in changing the occlusion/condylar position
Helps in increasing the vertical dimension of occlusion
Cognitive awareness
Psychological effect to the patients with TMDs
Increases the peripheral input to the CNS which provides an inhibitory effect to the CNS activity

A stabilization splint is the most commonly used intraoral appliance with full coverage of the teeth and it incorporates a full occlusal scheme with incisal guidance and centric relation occlusion. It helps in elimination of any posterior interference, and provides anterior guidance. It helps in achieving a stable occlusion with uniform contacts of teeth throughout the maxillary and mandibular arch (Table 11.7). Stabilization appliance helps in joint stabilization, protection of teeth with redistribution of occlusal forces. It helps in relaxing the elevator muscles, and thus decreases bruxism in patients. Wearing the appliance helps in increasing the patient's awareness towards jaw habits and thus alters the rest position of the mandible in a more open and relaxed position [7].

The stabilization splint provides a removable and temporary ideal occlusion and comes in category of hard acrylic splint. Splint therapy provides an ideal occlusion and helps in providing a neuromuscular balance by reducing abnormal muscle activity. Splint should be adjusted properly by rebalancing and trimming to the altered jaw position. There should be uniform contact of the occluding surface of the appliance with the opposing dentition and both the condyles should be in their most stable position to allow better lateral and protrusive movements with incisal guidance [8].

11.4.1 Duration for Wearing the Splint

The patient should be reviewed at regular intervals and repeated adjustments for 2–3 months are needed for a successful splint therapy. In case of bruxism the wearing of appliance at night is very essential. For para-discitis, it is advised to wear the appliance most of the time. If the pain is myogenous in origin, then part-time wearing of appliance that to at night is much helpful. In case of any intra-capsular disorders, it is advised to wear the appliance continuously. If there is increase in pain on wearing the appliance, then it is advisable to discontinue the use of appliance and immediate evaluation and correction should be undertaken [8].

The verification of condyle to disc assemblies should be done for normal functioning in the most superior position. The same can be achieved tentatively by evaluation in the following ways

1. Bilateral pressure on the joints for load testing
2. Doppler auscultation
3. Clench testing by clenching on some object to separate the teeth

11.4.2 Review of Literature

The appliance is usually fabricated for maxillary arch for better stability but in some cases where aesthetics and speech are the prime concern it can be given in the mandibular arch. No difference in symptom reduction was found in patients when splint was used either in maxilla or mandible as reported by Turp et al. [10] in their systematic review [11]. The incorporation of canine guided occlusion in splint therapy is not very clear as Manns et al. [12, 13] preferred this occlusion in asymptomatic individuals and found that muscle activity was reduced quite effectively [14, 15]. Borromeo et al. [16] found no differences in muscle activity in healthy subjects and Conti et al. [17] found no difference in TMD symptom reduction by giving canine guided occlusion to the appliance [16].

Kreiner et al. stated that the mechanism of action by which occlusal appliance helps in the treatment of localized myalgia and arthralgia is a behavioural modification of jaw clenching. However, if the behaviour continues unabated, even the best splints will not work. The splint provides conditions for the patient to develop a means to resist the TMDs by means of elimination of several aetiologic factors. Akbulut et al. evaluated whether a stabilization splint with 3 mm thickness has effects on all TMD symptoms. They concluded that therapy with 3 mm splint should be maintained for at least a time period of 6 months to obtain desired results [18, 19].

11.5 Anterior Repositioning Appliance (ARA)/ Orthopaedic Repositioning Appliance

In 1971, Farrar suggested anterior repositioning appliance that helps mandible to attain a more anterior position to that of centric occlusion in an attempt to provide a more favourable condylar position in their fossa. This position helps the condylar head to obtain a more anterior and inferior position that allows the disc to be on top of the condylar head. It helps in unloading the joint and thus increases the mandibular range of motion (ROM), decreases the inflammation in the joint and signs and symptoms of TMJ disorder. It further helps in healing of the retro-discal tissues and regaining a backward pull on the disc [20].

The anterior repositioning appliance can be given in either arch but preferably in maxillary arch. It is a complete-arch hard acrylic appliance with an anterior ramp which engages mandibular anterior teeth during initial closure. The mandib-

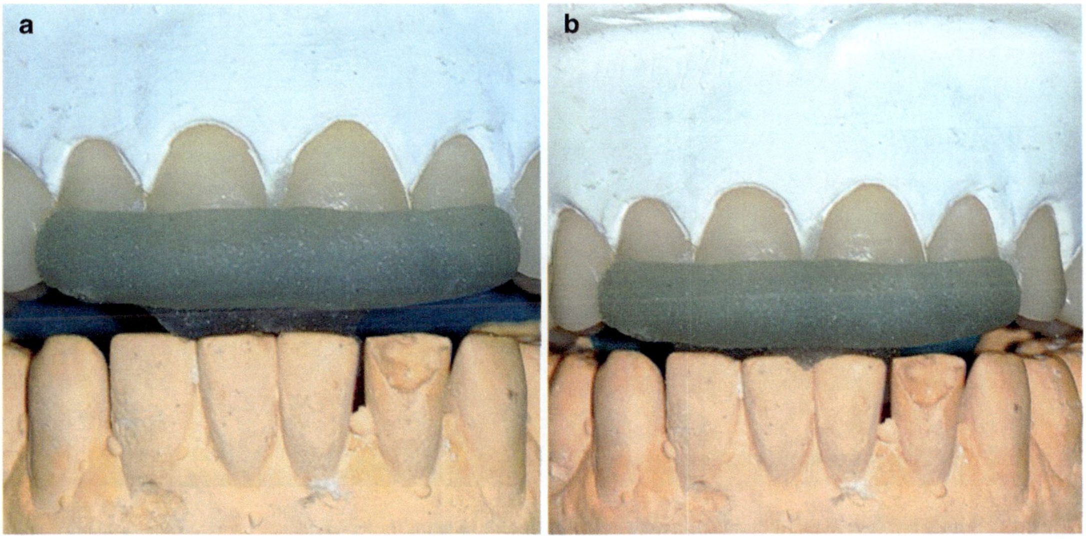

Fig. 11.2 (**a**) Anterior repositioning splint in the maxilla during open mouth position. (**b**) Anterior repositioning splint in contact with the mandible

ular jaw moves forward as the mandibular teeth contact the splint while final closure [21] (Fig. 11.2a, b).

The treatment goal is to alter the mandibular position temporarily to return back the condyle-disc complex function. Once the normal/optimal function is obtained, the splint is eliminated gradually so that patient returns to normal condition. The patient should wear the appliance during night and in day time if needed, depending on the severity of the symptoms to reduce them. Repositioning appliances should be used for short periods of time. It should be restricted primarily for temporary therapeutic measure in patients, to control symptomatic painful internal derangements. It should not be used as a permanent measure as it may lead to permanent change in occlusion [20].

11.5.1 Review of Literature

Therapy with anterior repositioning appliance in TMJ internal derangements is successful in long-term for recapturing of discs in reducing and non-reducing joints. Lundh et al. compared the treatment of TMJ with reciprocal clicking using flat occlusal splint, anterior repositioning splint, and control group without any treatment. They found that anterior repositioning splint decreases the joint pain while rest and also during protrusion and chewing. The flat occlusal splint although decreases the joint tenderness but had no effect on muscle tenderness and clicking. The subjects in control group had clicking with increase in frequency of muscle tenderness. Conti et al. emphasized that if repositioning splints are used partially in a controlled way, it would be beneficial in managing intra-articular dysfunction and pain without any risks of irreversible occlusal changes [21, 22].

11.6 Soft/Resilient Appliance

According to GPT, soft splint is a resilient device covering either the maxillary or mandibular teeth for the purpose of preventing trauma to dentition or acting as a deprogrammer [4]. They are used to prevent bruxism and clenching of teeth and also to reduce the symptoms of joint dysfunction or myalgia. The soft splint is made from a 2–4 mm resilient polyvinyl sheet material adapted to the maxillary arch, which is usually worn only at night and generally produces symptomatic relief within 6 weeks.

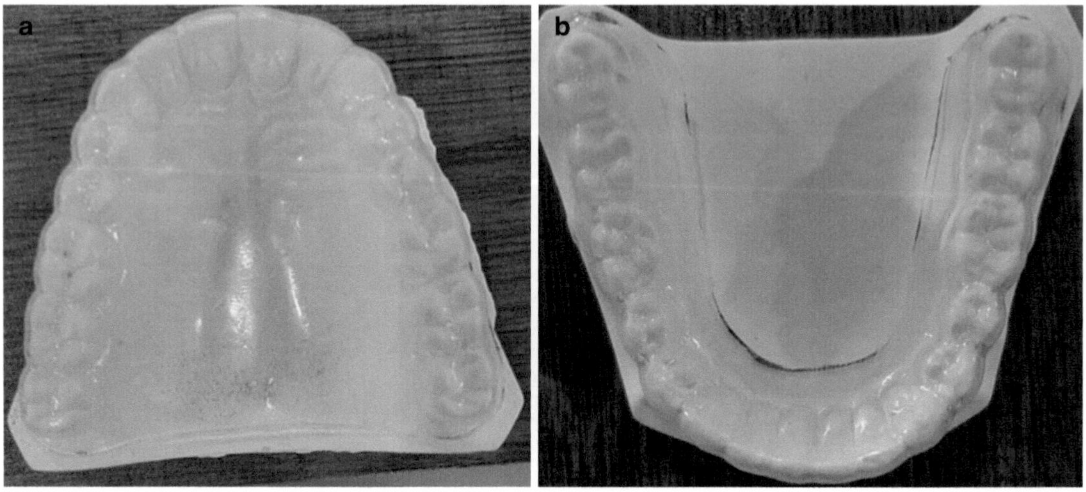

Fig. 11.3 Soft splint (**a**) Adapted on maxillary cast; (**b**) Adapted on mandibular cast

Soft splint less likely causes significant change in occlusion that is occasionally found with hard occlusal splints. The soft appliance loses their resiliency in less time, making it necessary to replace the same after 4 to 6 months of use. These splints are not able to provide a proper balance during premature contacts of posterior teeth and may lead to increase in bruxism in such cases. They have low density and amorphous structure; therefore, they are compressed or worn before the masticatory muscles are stretched beyond their physiologic limits [23, 24] (Fig. 11.3a, b).

11.6.1 Review of Literature

Seifeldin and Elhayes [25] compared hard splint with soft occlusal splint used for internal derangement (ID) of the TMJ with reciprocal clicking or myofascial pain dysfunction (MPD). They found that both the splints had improved the TMJ symptoms of the patients. However, soft splint therapy resulted in better results during 4 months of use. Soni et al. [23] analysed the effectiveness of soft occlusal splint therapy in patients with TMDs with diagnostic category based on Research Diagnostic Criteria for TMDs (RDC/TMD). During follow-up evaluations, a progressive decrease in tenderness and pain was indicated on visual analogue scale scores. There was significant improvement in mouth opening of the subjects with decrease or absence of joint sounds [25].

The soft occlusal splint therapy is a minimal invasive treatment with fewer complications and provides significant clinical benefits to patients with TMDs. Naikmasur et al. evaluated the efficacy of soft occlusal splint therapy and compared it with pharmacotherapy in the management of MPD Syndrome. There was a progressive decrease in TMJ clicking and tenderness with significant increase in mouth opening of the patients with soft occlusal splint therapy compared to patients on pharmacotherapy during follow up [24].

11.7 Anterior/Posterior Bite Plane

Bite plane is a horse shoe shaped appliance with palatal coverage and an occlusal table covering 6 to 8 maxillary anterior teeth. Anterior bite plane is used to treat TMDs by disocclusion of the posterior teeth and preventing clenching during parafunctional habits. The disadvantage of this appliance is that there are chances of overeruption of posterior teeth and overloading of the TMJ. There might be chances of anterior open bite due to intrusion of maxillary anterior teeth which retain the appliance.

Nociceptive Trigeminal Inhibition Tension Suppression System (NTI-tss) is a mini anterior bite appliance engaging 2–4 maxillary incisors. It is made of hard acrylic resin commercially available or can also be fabricated chair side. The appliance needs to be relined in patient's mouth with self-cure acrylic resin while insertion forms a platform which provides contact with the mandibular incisors. This appliance is very effective in TMD's, bruxism, and treatment of tension type headaches and migraine [26] (Fig. 11.4).

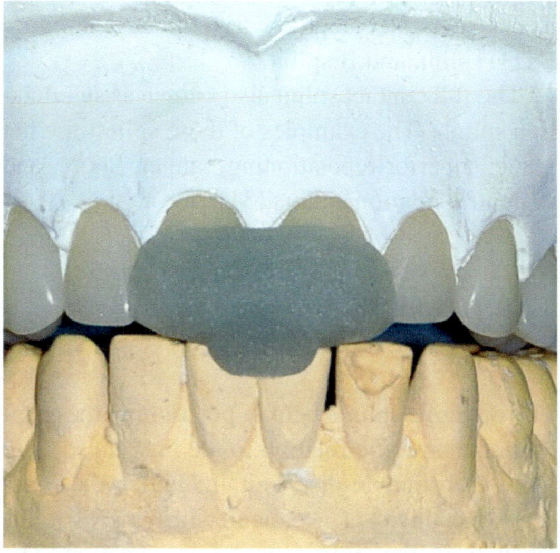

Fig. 11.4 NTI-tss Appliance for the maxillary arch

11.7.1 Review of Literature

Literature evidence suggests successful use of NTI-tss device for the management of TMDs and bruxism. However, patient should be monitored to avoid potential unwanted effects due to appliance during the follow-up appointments. NTI-tss splint should be used in cases where a reduction of jaw closer muscle activity is desired or in patients with acute TMJ pain, as an emergency device. Jokstad et al. compared NTI appliance with a flat plane appliance in TMD patients having headache and found no difference in both appliances in three months follow up [27].

Posterior bite plane (Mandibular orthopaedic repositioning appliance) helps in disocclusion of the anterior teeth. It is fabricated for the mandibular arch with a hard acrylic table over the molars and premolars connected by a lingual metal bar. It produces an ideal maxilla to mandibular relationship. The drawback of the appliance is that, it causes posterior open bite due to intrusion of the posterior teeth of the opposing arch and over-eruption of the anterior teeth [28] (Fig. 11.5a, b).

11.8 Pivoting Appliance (Distraction Splint)

The pivot splint was advocated by Krough-Poulsen for patients with ID and/or osteoarthritis. It is fabricated using hard acrylic resin covering

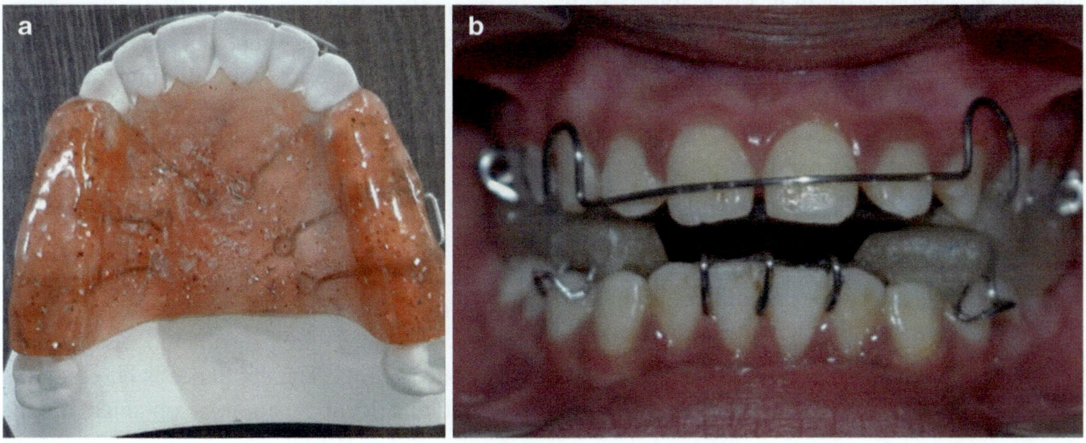

Fig. 11.5 Posterior bite plane appliance (**a**) on maxillary cast; (**b**) In oral cavity

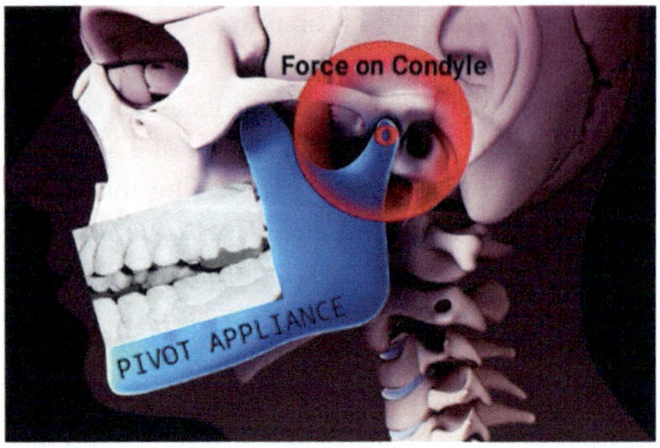

Fig. 11.6 Forces acting on condyle when a pivot appliance is given

either of the arches with a single occlusal contact in each quadrant as far posteriorly as possible. The appliance helps in condylar distraction which leads to unloading of joint and thus there is reduction in intra-articular pressure. The drawback of the appliance is occlusal changes resulting in posterior open bite in the pivot region. It is suggested that whenever the splint is inserted, an elastic bandage should be wrapped encircling the chin to the top of head so that the forces in the joint may be reduced (Fig. 11.6).

11.8.1 Review of Literature

Muhtarogullari et al. evaluated the efficiency of pivot splints in jaw exercises to that of stabilization splints in patients having anterior disc displacement without reduction. Pivot splints were given to patients for jaw exercises and rest of the times stabilization splints were advised. The patients were followed for 2–4 weeks. The pivot splint when used for exercise along with a stabilization splint, pain was eliminated along with establishment of normal mandibular ROM. Seedorf et al. investigated the distractive effect of the posterior occlusal pivots on the TMJ and found no distractive effect of occlusal pivots on TMJ. They stated that it can lead to unnecessary compression of the joint if the design of the appliance prevents protrusion [29, 30].

11.9 Permissive Splints (Muscle Deprogrammers)

Permissive splints help in unlocking the occlusion in order to remove deviating tooth that is inclined from the contact. This process helps in eliminating the cause and effect of the muscle incoordination and condyles return to seated position in centric relation. Permissive splints has two classic designs

1. Anterior midpoint contact splints
2. Full contact splints

Anterior midpoint contact splints: Examples—Lucia jig, Nociceptive trigeminal inhibition (NTI) splint, and B splint.

The full contact splint also known as stabilization splints. The examples of these splints are flat plane, superior repositioning, tanner, Shore, and in-centric relation splints [31].

11.9.1 Non-permissive Splint (Directive Splints)

The directive splints help in positioning the mandible in a specific relation to the maxilla so as to align the condyle-disc unit. It guides the mandibular condyle of a patient with painful joints away from the fully seated joint position. The movement of mandible is limited by giving ramps or indentations in the non-permissive splint [32].

Examples of non-permissive splints: Mandibular orthotic repositioning appliance (MORA) and anterior repositioning appliance (ARA).

11.9.2 Pseudo-permissive Splints

The functions of soft splints and hydrostatic splints (Aqualizer) are different from permissive splints and they are considered as pseudo-permissive splints. The appliance is based on the concept that ideal position is obtained by the mandible itself and the appliance is not directing the jaw position. Lerman has originally designed the hydrostatic splint and later the design was modified. The splint is retained under the upper lip and the fluid chambers are placed in between mandibular and maxillary posterior teeth.

The splint has a bilateral water filled plastic chamber connected with an acrylic palatal appliance. The posterior teeth of the patient occlude with water filled chambers. The drawback of the appliance is that it can increase bruxism due to loss of balance of the appliance leading to premature contacts of the posterior teeth. Aqualizer is the commonly used splint. Macedo and Mello evaluated the effectiveness of the hydrostatic splint Aqualizer, transcutaneous electrical neural stimulation (TENS), and microcurrent electrical nerve stimulation (MENS) treatment in patients with TMD. They found MENS and hydrostatic splints as an effective modality of treatment in TMD than TENS [26].

11.10 Materials Used for Fabrication of Occlusal Splints

Occlusal splint are mainly fabricated using two materials of different consistency and named as hard, soft, or dual laminated splint.

Hard splint is fabricated from self-cured or heat-cured acrylic resin. Soft splint is resilient in nature with flexible, pliable tooth-borne and occlusal surface. Dual laminated splint consists of an occlusal surface with hard acrylic resin and soft material over the tooth-borne surface.

Hard splint can either be fabricated directly on chair side or by indirect fabrication in the laboratory. The soft occlusal splint can be fabricated with vacuum formed technique in the dental clinic or readily available as 'boil and bite' which is boiled in water and adapted intraorally. Hard occlusal splint has an advantage over soft splint, in the maintenance phase in terms of its easy and quick adjustments. It is easily repairable, good accuracy, greater longevity, more colour stable, and has less accumulation of food debris [24, 25]. The clinical outcome with various splints remains variable.

11.11 Mechanism of Action of Occlusal Splint Therapy

The splint therapy helps the patient to close the mandible in a new posture providing muscular and articular balance. It prevents the patient to close in maximum inter-cuspation position. It helps in protection of TMJ as patients with bruxism will not clench his teeth in their previous abnormal occlusion. The occlusal splint triggers the muscle with the help of proprioception received in periodontal ligament from central nervous system which helps in distribution of abnormal forces across the masticatory system and protects the TMJ from masticatory overload.

The splint therapy aids in relaxation of the hyperactive muscles with equal occlusal contacts of all teeth and disocclusion of all the posterior teeth. This helps in relaxing the elevator muscles as well as positioning muscles. When condyle-disc unit is not in normal physiologic position then there is joint overloading leading to TMDs. The splint positions the condyle in centric relation and helps in managing TMDs.

The splint helps in increasing the vertical dimension of occlusion exceeding the physiologic inter-occlusal distance which helps in decreasing the hyperactivity of jaw muscles. Splint has psychological advantage to the patients according to the cognitive awareness theory which makes patients aware about the treatment and helps them in proper jaw positioning [9].

11.11.1 Goals of Treatment

The goals of occlusal splint therapy in patients with TMDs is to relieve any occlusal forces causing uneven joint loading, relaxation of the hyperactive muscles and thus reducing the symptoms. They can be given in the initial stages when surgery is not an option for the patients, selected splints may also be indicated in the post intervention phase. Careful selection of the type of splint and appropriate duration for use should be advocated to achieve satisfactory results.

References

1. Dawson PE. Evaluation, diagnosis and treatment of occlusal problems. 2nd ed. St Louis, MO: Mosby; 1989.
2. Okeson JP. Management of temporomandibular disorders and occlusion. 4th ed. St. Louis, MO: Mosby; 1998. p. 509.
3. Okeson J. Etiology of functional disturbances in the masticatory system. In: 7th, editor. Management of Temporomandibular Disorders and Occlusion. St Louis, MO: Elsevier Mosby Inc; 2013. p. 102–69.
4. Academy of Prosthodontics. The glossary of prosthodontic terms: 9th edition. J Prosthet Dent. 2017;117(5S):e1–e105.
5. Koh H, Robinson PG. Occlusal adjustment for treating and preventing temporomandibular joint disorders. J Oral Rehabil. 2004;31:287–92.
6. McNamara JA Jr, Seligman DA, Okeson JP. Occlusion, orthodontic treatment, and temporomandibular disorders: a review. J Orofac Pain. 1995;9:73–90.
7. De Leeuw R, Pain O. Guidelines for assessment, diagnosis, and management. (5th ed), Quintessence Publishing Co, Inc, Chicago; 2013.
8. Shankland WE. 2nd temporomandibular disorders: standard treatment options. Gen Dent. 2004;52:349–55.
9. Clark GT. A critical evaluation of orthopedic interocclusal appliance therapy: design, theory, and overall effectiveness. JADA. 1984;108:359–64.
10. Türp JC, Komine F, Hugger A. Efficacy of stabilization splints for the management of patients with masticatory muscle pain: a qualitative systematic review. Clin Oral Investig 2004;8:179–95.
11. Dabadie M, Renner RP. Mechanical evaluation of splint therapy in treatment of the edentulous patient. J Prosthet Dent. 1990;63(1):52–5.
12. Manns A, Chan C, Miralles R. Influence of group function and canine guidance on electromyographic activity of elevator muscles. J Prosthet Dent 1987;57:494–501.
13. Manns A, Miralles R, Pena M. The effects of different occlusal splints on the electromyographic activity of elevator muscles: a comparative study. J Gnathol 1988;7:61–73.
14. Manns A, Chan C, Miralles R. Influence of group function and canine guidance on electromyographic activity of elevator muscles. J Prosthet Dent. 1987;57:494–501.
15. Manns A, Miralles R, Pena M. The effects of different occlusal splints on the electromyographic activity of elevator muscles: a comparative study. J Gnathol. 1988;7:61–73.
16. Borromeo G, Suvinen T, Reade P. A comparison of the effects of group function and canine guidance interocclusal device on masseter muscle electromyographic activity in normal subjects. J Prosthet Dent. 1995;74:174–80.
17. Conti PC, dos Santos CN, Kogawa EM, de Castro Ferreira Conti AC, de Araujo Cdos R. The treatment of painful temporomandibular joint clicking with oral splints: a randomized clinical trial. J Am Dent Assoc 2006;137:1108–114.
18. Kreiner M, Betancor E, Clark GT. Occlusal stabilization appliances. Evidence of their efficacy. J Am Dent Assoc. 2001;132(6):770–7.
19. Akbulut N, Altan A, Akbulut S, Atakan C. Evaluation of the 3 mm thickness splint therapy on temporomandibular joint disorders (TMDs). Pain Research and Management. 2018;2018:1–7.
20. Simmons C. Temporomandibular joint orthopedics with anterior repositioning appliance therapy and therapeutic injections. J Calif Dent Assoc. 2014;42(8):537–47.
21. Lundh H, Westesson P, Kopp S, Tillström B. Anterior repositioning splint in the treatment of temporomandibular joints with reciprocal clicking: comparison with a flat occlusal splint and an untreated control group. Oral Surgery, Oral Medicine, Oral Pathology. 1985;60(2):131–6.
22. Conti PCR, Miranda JES, Conti ACCF, Pegoraro LF, de Araújo CDP. Partial time use of anterior repositioning splints in the management of TMJ pain and dysfunction: a one-year controlled study. J Appl Oral Sci. 2005;13(4):345–50.
23. Soni A, Wanjari PV, Warhekar A. Role of soft occlusal splint therapy in the management of temporomandibular disorders: a 6-month follow-up study. J Indian Acad Oral Med Radiol. 2018;30:355–60.
24. Naikmasur V, Bhargava P, Guttal K, Burde K. Soft occlusal splint therapy in the management of myofascial pain dysfunction syndrome: a follow-up study. Indian J Dent Res. 2008;19:196–203.
25. Seifeldin SA, Elhayes KA. Soft versus hard occlusal splint therapy in the management of temporomandibular disorders (TMDs). Saudi Dent J. 2015;27:208–14.
26. Stapelmann H, Türp JC. The NTI-tss device for the therapy of bruxism, temporomandibular disorders, and headache – where do we stand? A qualitative systematic review of the literature. BMC Oral Health. 2008;8:22.
27. Jokstad A, Mo A, Krogstad BS. Clinical comparison between two different splint designs for temporomandibular disorder therapy. Acta Odontol Scand. 2005;63:218–26.
28. Al Quran FA, Kamal MS. Anterior midline point stop device (AMPS) in the treatment of myogenous TMDs: comparison with the stabilization splint and control group. Oral Surg Oral Med Oral Pathol Oral Radiol Endod. 2006;101:741–7.

29. Muhtarogullari M, Avci M, Yuzugullu B. Efficiency of pivot splints as jaw exercise apparatus in combination with stabilization splints in anterior disc displacement without reduction: a retrospective study. Head Face Med. 2014;10:42.
30. Seedorf H, Scholz A, Kirsch I, Fenske C, Jüde HD. Pivot appliances-is there a distractive effect on the temporomandibular joint? J Oral Rehabil. 2007;34(1):34–40.
31. Magnusson T, Adiels AM, Nilsson HL, Helkimo M. Treatment effect on signs and symptoms of temporomandibular disorders-- comparison between stabilisation splint and a new type of splint (NTI) – a pilot study. Swed Dent J. 2003;28:11–20.
32. Macedo JF, Mello EB. Therapeutic of urgency in temporomandibular disorders. Rev ATM service. 2002;2:22–8.

12 Synovial Fluid Analysis for Temporomandibular Joint Disorders

Beena Sivakumar and Darpan Bhargava

12.1 Introduction

Any disease process in the body requires a thorough clinical assessment along with the radiological and pathological examinations. Various laboratory investigations can be advised and used as an adjunct to arrive at a definitive diagnosis. Temporomandibular Joint (TMJ) is no exception to this. Apart from several clinical and radiographic methods, investigations such as synovial fluid analysis can enhance the decision making for treatment plan and diagnosis as the synovial fluid in the joint space contains several enzymes, cytokines, tissue breakdown products which act as diagnostic markers. They can be utilized to identify and aid to arrive at specific diagnosis, monitor disease progression, and response to the treatment is cases of internal derangement, synovitis, chondromalacia, and autoimmune arthritis [1].

B. Sivakumar
Department of Oral and Maxillofacial Surgery, Meenakshi Ammal Dental College and Hospital, Chennai, Tamil Nadu, India

D. Bhargava (✉)
TMJ Consultancy Services, Bhopal, Madhya Pradesh, India

Oral and Maxillofacial Surgery, People's College of Dental Sciences and Research Centre, People's University, Bhopal, Madhya Pradesh, India
e-mail: drdarpanbhargava@gmail.com

12.2 Synovial Fluid

The synovial fluid is produced by type B synovial cells, a dialysate of plasma consisting of various phospholipids, cholesterol, hyaluronic acid, immunoglobulins, glycosaminoglycans, collagenase, cathepsins, cytokines, transforming growth factors (TGF), and other growth factors. Apart from the above-mentioned components, traces of inflammatory cell degradation products and mesenchymal stem cells may be identified. It not only provide nutrients and scavenges waste products but also acts as a lubricant and a medium of stress distribution in the joint. Fluid dynamics in the upper joint compartment of a normal TMJ in a closed and open jaw position is depicted in Fig. 12.1.

Pathological conditions of the temporomandibular joint cause an alteration in synovial fluid composition, viscosity, molecular size of the hyaluronic acid and the cytokine levels. Both qualitative and quantitative analysis of the fluid can be done using various proposed methods. Synovial fluid biomarkers are unique to several disease processes such as osteoarthritis, internal derangement and other diseases affecting the joint. Quantitative analysis can be an indicator and may be co-related with monitoring the disease progression or regression. Synovial fluid from healthy TMJ consists of inflammatory and anti-inflammatory cytokines. The various pro-inflammatory and anti-inflammatory factors are

D. Bhargava (ed.), *Temporomandibular Joint Disorders*,
https://doi.org/10.1007/978-981-16-2754-5_12

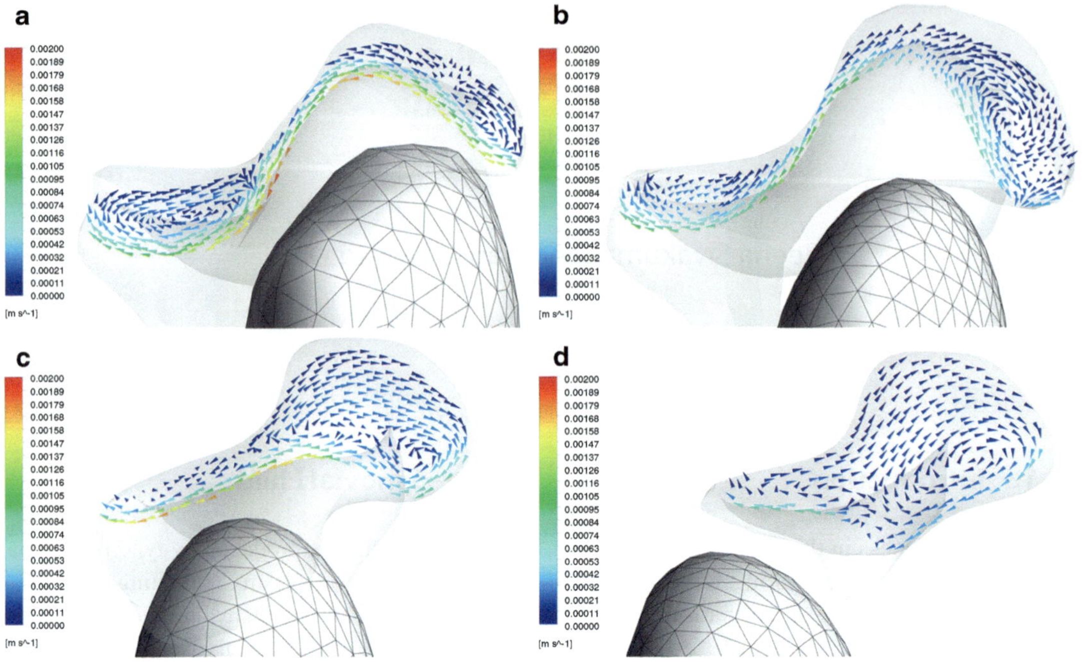

Fig. 12.1 Finite element analysis of the volume fluid dynamic and fluid velocity contours in the upper compartment of a normal TMJ. TMJ (**a**) in a closed-jaw position, and at jaw openings of (**b**) 1 cm, (**c**) 2 cm, and (**d**) 3 cm. Note the overall anticlockwise circulation of synovial fluid and the formation of local vortices at the anterior and posterior parts of the compartment. [Reprinted from Journal of the Formosan Medical Association, Vol.112 Issue 6, Yue Xu et al., Computational synovial dynamics of a normal temporomandibular joint during jaw opening, Pg.349, Copyright (2013), with permission from Elsevier.]

Table 12.1 Various cytokines and growth factors present in the synovial fluid of a healthy temporomandibular joint

Cytokine/Growth factors	Source of the cells	Activity
IL-1α, IL-1β	Inflammatory and synovial cells	Pro-inflammatory
IL-2, IL-4, IL-6sr, IL-12, IL-17, TNF-α, TNF-β, IFN-γ, MMP-3, MMP-7	Inflammatory cells	Pro-inflammatory
IL-1Ra, IL-10, TIMP-1	Inflammatory cells	Anti-inflammatory
VEGF	Most of the cells	Angiogenesis
Osteoprotegerin	Mesenchymal stem cells	Inhibit osteoclasts
RANKL	Most of the cells	Bone turnover and immune regulation
ADAMTS	Most of the cells	Pro-inflammatory
IL-8	Inflammatory cells, endothelial cells, fibroblasts, synovial cells	Pro-inflammatory
IL-11	Endothelial cells, fibroblasts, synovial cells	Pro-inflammatory

(Abbreviations: IL-Interleukins; MMP-Matrix metalloproteinases; IFN-Interferon; RANKL-Receptor activator of nuclear factor; TNF-Tumor necrosis factor; TIMP-Tissue inhibitor of metalloproteinases; VEGF-Vascular endothelial growth factor; ADAMTS-A disintegrin and metalloproteinase with thrombospondin motifs) interleukins (IL), tumour necrosis factor (TNF), and interferon-γ (IFN-γ) [2, 3].

12.3 Synovial Fluid in TMJ Disorders

As documented by various authors, a co-relation exists between the presence of the disease and the levels of cytokines. In healthy subjects, the levels of inflammatory and anti-inflammatory cytokines maintain a balance for homeostasis within the joint for normal functioning and coping with the stresses and strains on function. The key cytokines include IL-1b, IL-6, IL-11, TNF-α, and TGF-β1, among many others summarized in the table (Table 12.1). Mechanical stress is thought to induce and initiate a degenrative process, although the mechanism appears to be complicated. Mechanical stress to the joint is believed to induce a disease process causing tissue destruction caused by production of free radicals and reactive oxygen by neutrophils and macrophages. It is evident by increased viscosity of the synovial fluid, causing further tissue destruction, impaired lubrication and nutrition supply to the disc and articular cartilage [1, 2]. The free radicals and the reactive oxygen present in the joint causes the degradation of proteins and proteoglycans resulting in progressive tissue distruction.

12.4 Sample Collection

Synovial fluid sample collection can be done during arthrocentesis or arthroscopy. It is a technique sensitive procedure as the synovial fluid should not get contaminated with blood. The standard arthrocentesis or arthroscopy needle or the cannula with trochar is inserted in the superior joint space after manipulating the mandible and 1 ml of saline should be injected followed by aspiration of the synovial fluid for analysis. Enzyme-Linked Immunosorbent Assays (ELISA) and Polymerase Chain Reaction (PCR) are used for relative and absolute quantitation. The biotin-labelled based protein array, cytotoxic assays, and enzymography may be utilized for cytokine analysis [2].

12.5 Synovial Fluid Analysis in TMJ Disorders

Internal derangement (ID) is a precursor of osteoarthritis (OA). Cytokine levels are accurate in diagnosing different stages of Wilkes for ID along with the presence or absence of osteoarthritis. There are limitations due to lack of adequate data regarding levels of cytokines in a healthy joint, TMJ affected with ID and OA. Also, there remains a lack of a standard simplified technique for obtaining a chair-side synovial fluid sample. The methods utilized to perform the qualitative and quantitative analysis are not widely available, requires specialized equipments and reagents. Synovial fluid analysis may also be employed for the diagnosis and evaluate progression or treatment outcome in cases of rheumatoid and reactive arthritis apart from OA. Leibur et al. observed from their study that the presence of chondromatosis granules and increased levels of PGE_2 in synovial fluid is indicative of inflammatory pathology in the joint apart from the documented cytokines [1–3]. Cytokines found in the synovial fluid for patients with internal derangements and osteoarthritis are summarized in Table 12.2. In general, in an established osteoarthritic disease process, there is a recruitment of T cells, B cells, and macrophages. Various cytokines as summarized in the Table 12.2, are released, which initiate an inflammatory response proceeding to tissue destruction. In addition, metalloproteinases and disintegrin-metalloproteinase with thrombospondin motifs enzymes are produced, resulting in further degradation of cartilage, bone, synovial proteoglycans, and aggrecan. In the synovial fluid of the patients with rheumatoid arthritis and juvenile idiopathic arthritis, TNF-α is detected in significantly higher levels [2].

12.6 Micro-organisms in Synovial Fluid

The Th1 T-cell response is effective in destroying the intra-cellular pathogens in reactive arthritis caused due to microbial infection of the

Table 12.2 Cytokines found in synovial fluid of patients with internal derangements and osteoarthritis [Reprinted from Oral and Maxillofacial Surgery Clinics of North America, Vol 30/Issue 3, Gary F. Bouloux, The Use of Synovial Fluid Analysis for Diagnosis of Temporomandibular Joint Disorders, Pg No.254, Copyright (2018), with permission from Elsevier]

Author	Cytokines	ID		OA
Fang et al. (1999) [4]	IL-1RA	175.78		187.85
	IL-10	ND		ND
	TGF-β1	47.93		143.61
Fu et al. (1995) [5]	IL-6	>100		–
Fu et al. (1995) [6]	TNF-α	3.86		11.27
Kaneyama et al. (2002) [7]		*Wilkes I, II*	*Wilkes III*	
	IL-1β	0.14	0.12	0.13
	TNF-α	0.03	0.17	0.17
	IL-6	0.2	14	30
	IL-8	16	13	14
Kaneyama et al. (2003) [8]	OCIF/OPG	160		80
	IL-1b	0.08		0.1
	TNF-α	0.4		0.3
Kaneyama et al. (2004) [9]	IL-6	5		25
	IL-11	2		7
Kaneyama et al. (2005) [10]	IL-1β	0.8		0.6
	IL-RA	42		41
	IL-6	5		5
	IL-6SR	343		644
	TNF-α	0.1		0.1
	sTNFR	197		261
Shinoda & Takaku (2000) [11]	IL-1b	0.8		1.7
	IL-6	2.1		8.8
	TIMP-I	25.6		120.3
Takahashi et al. (1998) [12]		*Wilkes I, II*	*Wilkes III*	
	IL-1β	14.5	7.2	56.9
	IL-6	ND	15.9	7.3
	IL-8	138.1	58.0	50.3
	TNF-α	ND	413	193
	IFN-γ	78.8	36.1	91.8
Wakita et al. (2006) [13]		*Wilkes I, II*	*Wilkes III*	
	RANKL	125	100	112.5
	OPG	600	300	200
	RANKL/OPG ratio	0.3	0.4	0.8

joint. TNF-α, IFN-γ, and IL-12 are the key cytokines in a Th1 T-cell response. It is also evident that identification of a Th-2 T cell drived humoral immune response is associated with the presence of bacteria in the joint. This may be detected with increased levels of IL-10, and decrease in TNF-α and IFN-γ levels. PCR remains to be the most sensitive method to detect intra-cellular pathogens followed by immuno-histochemistry. PCR identifies the micro-organisms by amplifying the bacterial DNA.

Chlamydia trachomatis, Chlamydia pneumoniae, Yersinia enterocolitica, Campylobacter species, Mycoplasma genitalium, Mycoplasma fermentans and Ureaplasma urealyticum are some of the few documented micro-organisms isolated from the temporomandibular joint. These micro-organisms are known to thrive in the sub-synovial tissue within the macrophages and monocytes. When suspected, this warrants the requirement of obtaining a biopsy specimen from the retrodiscal tissue to detect the pathology in the joint rather than synovial fluid analysis [2].

12.7 Conclusion and Future Directions

A thorough clinical and physical examination along with an accurate radiographic evaluation is the key to arrive at an appropriate diagnosis in patients with TMDs. Synovial fluid analysis gives an additional information regarding the presence of inflammatory mediators and denuded proteins. Apart from cytokine analysis, proteomics may be utilized for disease identification which explains that each specific disease has its own protein profile [2]. This would enable the way forward to make a specific diagnosis using synovial fluid proteomics with accurate sensitivity and specificity along with monitoring the disease and for evaluation of the response to the treatment. Synovial fluid analysis may serve as an excellent diagnostic tool for cases, otherwise difficult to diagnose and treat. This area has a tremendous scope for research in future.

References

1. Laskin DM, et al. Temporomandibular disorders: an evidence-based approach to diagnosis and treatment. 1st ed. Chicago, IL: Quintessence Publishing Co Inc.; 2006. p. 343–62.
2. Bouloux GF. The use of synovial fluid analysis for diagnosis of temporomandibular joint disorders. Oral Maxillofac Surg Clin N Am. 2018;30(3):251–6. https://doi.org/10.1016/j.coms.2018.03.001.
3. Aghabeigi B, et al. Temporomandibular joint synovial fluid analysis. Br J Oral Maxillofac Surg. 1993;31:15–20.
4. Fang PK, Ma XC, Ma DL, et al. Determination of interleukin-1 receptor antagonist, interleukin-10, and transforming growth factor-beta1 in synovial fluid aspirates of patients with temporomandibular disorders. J Oral Maxillofac Surg. 1999;57:922–8. [discussion: 928–9]
5. Fu K, Ma X, Zhang Z, et al. Interleukin-6 in synovial fluid and HLA-DR expression in synovium from patients with temporomandibular disorders. J Orofac Pain. 1995;9:131–7.
6. Fu K, Ma X, Zhang Z, et al. Tumor necrosis factor in synovial fluid of patients with temporomandibular disorders. J Oral Maxillofac Surg. 1995;53:424–6.
7. Kaneyama K, Segami N, Nishimura M, et al. Importance of proinflammatory cytokines in synovial fluid from 121 joints with temporomandibular disorders. Br J Oral Maxillofac Surg. 2002;40:418–23.
8. Kaneyama K, Segami N, Nishimura M, et al. Osteoclastogenesis inhibitory factor/osteoprotegerin in synovial fluid from patients with temporomandibular disorders. Int J Oral Maxillofac Surg. 2003;32:404–7.
9. Kaneyama K, Segami N, Sato J, et al. Interleukin-6 family of cytokines as biochemical markers of osseous changes in the temporomandibular joint disorders. Br J Oral Maxillofac Surg. 2004;42:246–50.
10. Kaneyama K, Segami N, Sun W, et al. Analysis of tumor necrosis factor-alpha, interleukin-6, interleukin- 1beta, soluble tumor necrosis factor receptors I and II, interleukin-6 soluble receptor, interleukin-1 soluble receptor type II, interleukin-1 receptor antagonist, and protein in the synovial fluid of patients with temporomandibular joint disorders. Oral Surg Oral Med Oral Pathol Oral Radiol Endod. 2005;99:276–84.
11. Shinoda C, Takaku S. Interleukin-1 beta, interleukin- 6, and tissue inhibitor of metalloproteinase-1 in the synovial fluid of the temporomandibular joint with respect to cartilage destruction. Oral Dis. 2000;6:383–90.
12. Takahashi T, Kondoh T, Fukuda M, et al. Proinflammatory cytokines detectable in synovial fluids from patients with temporomandibular disorders. Oral Surg Oral Med Oral Pathol Oral Radiol Endod. 1998;85:135–41.
13. Wakita T, Mogi M, Kurita K, et al. Increase in RANKL: OPG ratio in synovia of patients with temporomandibular joint disorder. J Dent Res. 2006;85:627–32.

Surgical Classification for Temporomandibular Joint Disorders

13

George Dimitroulis

13.1 Introduction

Temporomandibular (TMJ) surgery is highly controversial because the role of surgery is not well defined [1]. Unlike Orthopaedic surgery, the evidence is poor because there is no clinically practical classification of TMJ disorders that allows the direct comparison of standardized data between various TMJ surgical treatment modalities. Non-surgical specialists in Temporomandibular Disorders (TMD) have been proactive in their TMJ classification endeavours, but have come up with a highly complicated and clinically impractical Research Diagnostic Criteria (RDC) which have been largely confined to TMD research in non-surgical TMD treatment strategies [2, 3]. Unfortunately, TMJ surgery is peppered with classifications that apply to specific TMJ disorders such as ankylosis [4], joint dislocations [5], and internal derangement [6], but none that cover the full spectrum of TMJ surgical diseases.

In 2013, Dimitroulis [7] proposed a new classification that covered the full spectrum of TMJ surgery that is slowly gaining traction across the world. To properly define the role of TMJ surgery, hard evidence is required based on clearly defined data derived from universal medical codes which are in turn, collected from appropriately validated classifications. The justification of surgical interventions clinicians undertake to treat TMJ disorders must rely on properly acquired evidence based on a universally accepted classification. The aim of this chapter is to present the essential features of the TMJ surgical classification [7] and to discuss the clinical and research implications of the five categories it describes.

G. Dimitroulis (✉)
Maxillofacial Surgery Unit, Department of Surgery, St. Vincent's Hospital Melbourne, The University of Melbourne, Melbourne, Australia

Epworth-Freemasons Hospital, East Melbourne, VIC, Australia

13.2 The Importance of a Surgical TMJ Classification

Universal medical codes are simply descriptions of diagnosis and treatments which are derived from classifications. Codes are then transformed into data points which are collected and analysed for evidence as to whether TMJ surgery does indeed provide a positive benefit to patients [1]. A surgical classification of TMJ disorders is the vehicle that drives the evidence for TMJ surgery.

At present, there are three main TMD classifications. The most widely used is the Research Diagnostic Criteria or RDC-TMD classification [2] which stresses the psychosocial dysfunction (Axis 2) over physical disorders (Axis 1). Unfortunately, even with its numerous iterations [3], the RDC-TMD has failed to gain traction in everyday clinical practice and remains firmly entrenched in the world of research because of its

D. Bhargava (ed.), *Temporomandibular Joint Disorders*,
https://doi.org/10.1007/978-981-16-2754-5_13

complicated and impractical nature that has little bearing in clinical practice.

Most oral and maxillofacial surgeons who treat TMJ disorders utilize the Wilkes classification system [6] which largely focuses on TMJ internal derangement and osteoarthritis. It is a simple classification that describes five stages of escalating TMJ disease which is why it has gained such widespread acceptance for over 30 years since it was first published [6]. Unfortunately, the Wilkes classification does not include other TMJ disorders such as tumours, trauma, and ankylosis which are, in turn, covered by other sub-classifications [4, 8, 9] that will not be elaborated further in this chapter.

Finally, the American Academy of Orofacial Pain (AAOFP) classification of TMD [10] has encompassed a broader range of articular disorders, not just limited to internal derangement and osteoarthritis, but also includes trauma, ankylosis, and even TMJ development conditions [10]. Extra-articular disorders are also mentioned in this classification as centrally mediated, local, and general which reflects our limited understanding of masticatory muscle disorders. While the AAOFP classification of TMD is an enormous improvement compared to the cumbersome RDC-TMD classification, the data collected is not quantifiable in terms of degree of disability which is why the Wilkes classification has endured for clinical practice.

13.3 Essential Criteria for a Practical Classification (Table 13.1)

Many classifications appear in the literature often, but the ones that are readily adopted are simple to understand, and easy to remember by

Table 13.1 Criteria for a TMJ surgical classification

SIMPLE—Easy to understand and remember
CLEAR—Unambiguous description of each category
FOCUSED —On the TMJ
INCLUSIVE—Of all TMJ specific disorders and diseases
SPECIFIC—So that patient populations can be easily defined and compared
UNIVERSAL—Adopted by all TMD clinicians and researchers

Table 13.2 Surgical classification of TMJ disorders (Dimitroulis 2013)

Category 1
• TMJ Normal
• No surgery required or indicated
Category 2
• TMJ minor changes (all joint components are salvageable)
• TMJ arthrocentesis/arthroscopic lavage
Category 3
• TMJ moderate changes (Most joint components are salvageable)
• TMJ operative arthroscopy/TMJ arthroplasty/modified Condylotomy
Category 4
• TMJ severe changes (few joint components are partly salvageable)
• TMJ discectomy +/− condylar surgery
Category 5
• TMJ catastrophic changes (nothing in the joint is salvageable)
• TMJ resection +/− Total joint replacement

the wider medical community. History has demonstrated that clinically useful classifications are often modifications of existing classifications that have been updated to reflect new findings and knowledge. Like the Wilkes classification [6], the TMJ Surgical classification [7] describes five categories of increasing degrees of joint disease applicable to TMJ surgical practice (Table 13.2). In simple terms, category 1 applies to painful but structurally normal joints and category 5 describes catastrophic structural changes to the TMJ. The obvious advantages of the TMJ surgical classification are not only its simplicity, but it also includes surgical recommendations for each of the five categories of the TMJ disease. The TMJ surgical classification as proposed by Dimitroulis (2013) will be discussed in detail.

13.4 Category 1: TMJ Arthralgia (Table 13.3)

For a category 1 TMJ, the main presentation is pain specifically in and around the TMJ. Furthermore, there are no clinical signs of joint noises or trismus, and no history of difficulty in chewing, dislocation, or locking with the patient exhibiting full range of mandibular

Table 13.3 Category 1: Normal TMJ

Clinical presentation
TMJ pain
No joint noises
No history of locking or dislocation
Full range of jaw movement
Normal chewing
Radiological features
OPG—Normal condyles
MRI—Normal TMJ
Diagnosis
Joint contusion—Acute trauma
Myofascial pain
Ear pathology—Otalgia
Neuropathic
Psychogenic
Treatment
Medication +/− occlusal splint
Surgery has no role

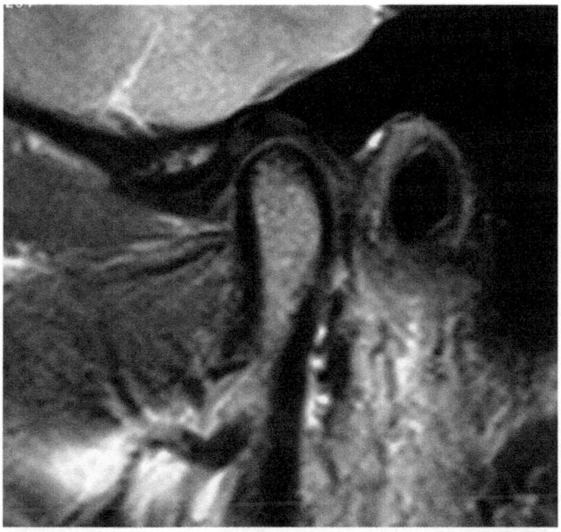

Fig. 13.1 Category 1 normal TMJ—MRI showing anatomically normal disc in the normal position relative to the condyle. Category 1 patients offer researchers the ideal control group with which to compare surgical outcomes in other categories

movement with symmetrical jaw opening. Category 1 joints have no radiological evidence of any structural joint abnormalities on plain x-rays, tomograms, CT scans, and MRI's which all exhibit normal TMJ anatomy (Fig. 13.1). The joint pain experienced by the patient may be acute, such as in cases with traumatic incident related to assault, a fall, whiplash, or sporting contact which has caused contusion within the joint but no obvious structural damage. Alternatively, the arthralgia may be chronic and related to chronic ear disorders, neuralgia, neuropathic or psychosomatic disorders, or simply part of a wider spectrum of myofascial pain and fibromyalgia that may or may not be associated with underlying anxiety or depression. The TMJ pain, or arthralgia, may respond to TMJ arthrocentesis only if there is an inflammatory component causing the joint pain but otherwise, TMJ surgery has no role to play. These patients must be managed non-surgically. It is important to note that patients who have no joint pain or other related joint signs or symptoms cannot be included in this category of the TMJ surgical classification.

13.5 Category 2: TMJ Minor Changes (Table 13.4)

TMJ reducing disc displacement is the most common disorder represented in this category which clinically presents with joint clicking, occasional locking, and intermittent joint pain. Normal condyles are seen on plain x-ray films but MRI's may demonstrate inflammation (Fig. 13.2) (excess joint fluid/effusion) or disc displacement with reduction. While the primary treatment modality remains conservative, i.e., soft diet, jaw rest, physiotherapy, splint therapy, and anti-inflammatory

Table 13.4 Category 2: Minor TMJ changes

Clinical presentation
Intermittent joint pain
Joint clicking
Occasional locking
Radiological features
OPG—Normal condyles
MRI—Disc displacement with reduction
Disc and condyle Normal contour
Diagnosis
Early stage TMJ internal derangement
Joint inflammation/adhesions
Treatment
TMJ arthrocentesis
TMJ arthroscopic lavage and lysis

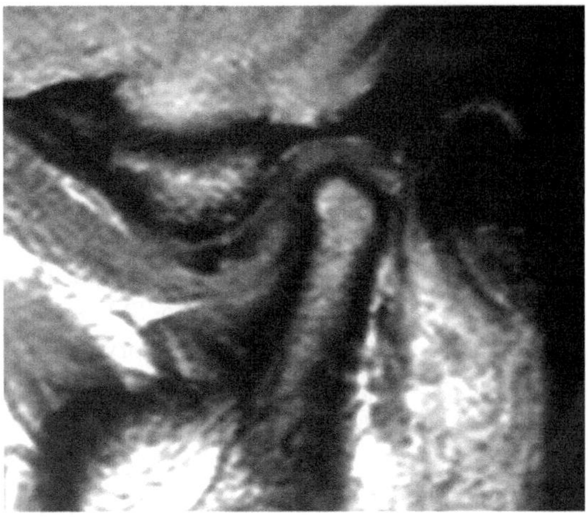

Fig. 13.2 Category 2, Minor TMJ Changes—MRI showing mildly displaced disc which reduces on opening. Condyle is normal. Future studies may look at whether TMJ arthrocentesis/arthroscopy significantly reduce the treatment time span compared to conservative measures alone in category 2 patients

medication, both TMJ arthrocentesis and TMJ arthroscopy may be useful in releasing a stuck or locked disc, particularly in cases of closed lock where the interincisal opening remains below 30 mm for more than 2–3 weeks.

13.6 Category 3: TMJ Moderate Changes (Table 13.5)

TMJ non-reducing disc displacement is the most common disorder in this category. Patients with category 3 disorder may report moderate to severe joint pain which is exacerbated by jaw function with difficulty in chewing. This may be accompanied by joint swelling, painful long-standing closed lock (>2 months), or painful recurrent TMJ dislocation. Jaw deviation to the affected side on mandibular opening may be caused by the pain or locked joint. Joint noises are often absent in those with chronic closed lock of their TMJ. Plain x-rays and CT scans may show normal condyles but the main diagnostic assessment is with a MRI scan which will demonstrate a displaced, non-reducing disc (Fig. 13.3). The displaced articular disc may have normal morphology in the early stages, but may progressively become distorted in long-standing cases.

Table 13.5 Category 3: Moderate TMJ changes

Clinical presentation	
	Painful chronic closed lock
	Recurrent joint swelling
	Painful recurrent dislocation
Radiological features	
	OPG—Normal condyles
	MRI—Disc displacement without reduction
	Disc Normal or mildly deformed contour
	Prominent Eminence
Diagnosis	
	Moderate TMJ internal derangement
	Recurrent TMJ dislocation
	Extracapsular condylar fracture
Treatment	
	TMJ arthroscopy (operative)
	TMJ arthroplasty—Disc plication/repositioning +/– Eminectomy
	Modified Condylotomy
	ORIF fractured condyle

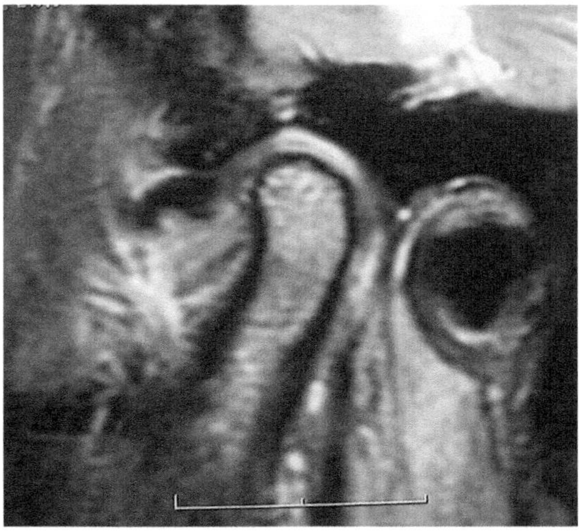

Fig. 13.3 Category 3, Moderate TMJ Changes—MRI showing moderately displaced disc that still has the biconcave appearance suggesting it can be salvaged

Category 3 joints may also include TMJ's with a history of recurrent dislocation or fracture dislocation of the condylar head that has been surgically reduced and resulted in moderate TMJ internal derangement. In category 3 cases, the most appropriate surgical interventions may include TMJ arthroplasty consisting of disc repositioning with or without eminectomy, or operative TMJ arthroscopy [11].

13.7 Category 4: TMJ Severe Changes (Table 13.6)

Constant joint pain with mildly limited mouth opening, painful chewing and yawning with intermittent locking are the hallmarks of a category 4 patient. While plain x-ray films and CT scans may show early degenerative changes in the condylar head, the signs of significant disc pathology are best seen on MRI scans (Fig. 13.4).

Table 13.6 Category 4: Severe TMJ changes

Clinical presentation
Constant joint pain
Painful crepitus
Mildly limited mouth opening
Painful chewing
Radiological features
OPG—Early condylar changes
CT scans—Mild to moderate condylar degeneration
MRI—Severely degenerated, displaced, and deformed disc
Early condylar changes—Osteophytes, flattening
Diagnosis
Advanced TMJ internal derangement
Rare TMJ disorder—Metabolic, inflammatory, or developmental joint disease
Intracapsular condylar fracture
Treatment
TMJ discectomy +/– Condyloplasty/shave
Debridement of glenoid Fossa +/– eminoplasty

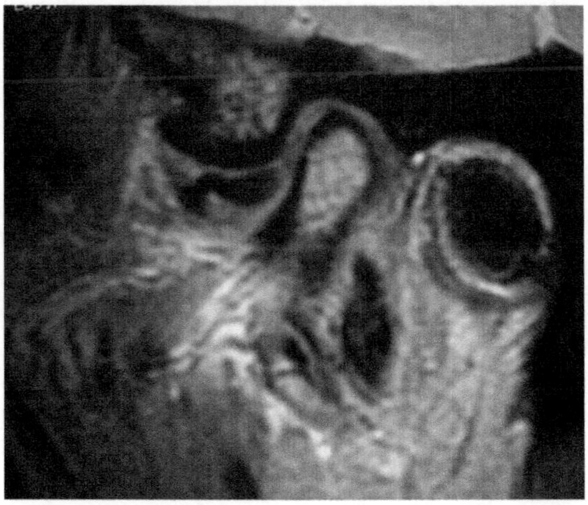

Fig. 13.4 Category 4, Severe TMJ Changes—MRI showing a severely displaced and deformed disc that cannot be salvaged and hence will require discectomy

Occasional tears and perforations are seen on severely displaced, deformed, and degenerate discs. Category 4 TMJ may also include rare developmental disorders, inflammatory or metabolic joint diseases such as gout. TMJ discectomy with or without debridement of surround structures and interpositional grafts is the mainstay in the treatment of category 4 cases [8].

13.8 Category 5: TMJ Catastrophic Changes (Table 13.7)

Finally, category 5 cases are those where none of the joint components can be salvaged because of significant destructive disease affecting the whole joint (Fig. 13.5). Clinically, these patients present with joint crepitus, constant locking, and inability to chew solid food because of intolerable low grade joint pain which is easily exacerbated by jaw function. Obvious degenerative changes of the mandibular condyle, that may also be deformed or dimunitive, are easily seen on plain x-ray films, tomograms, and CT scans. Higher resolution cone-beam CT scans may demonstrate subchondral cysts and irregular articular surfaces that may be flattened and beaked due to osteophytes. Discs are often so degenerate, they are

Table 13.7 Category 5: Catastrophic TMJ changes

Clinical presentation
Intolerable low grade pain
Constant crepitus
Locking
Malocclusion
Unable to chew anything solid
Radiological features
OPG—Obvious degenerative changes to condyle
MRI—Disc destroyed/difficult to see
CT scan—Condyle severely degenerate with subchondral cysts, etc.
Diagnosis
TMJ osteoarthritis
TMJ Condylysis
TMJ Ankylosis
TMJ tumour
Treatment
TMJ resection
TMJ Total joint replacement

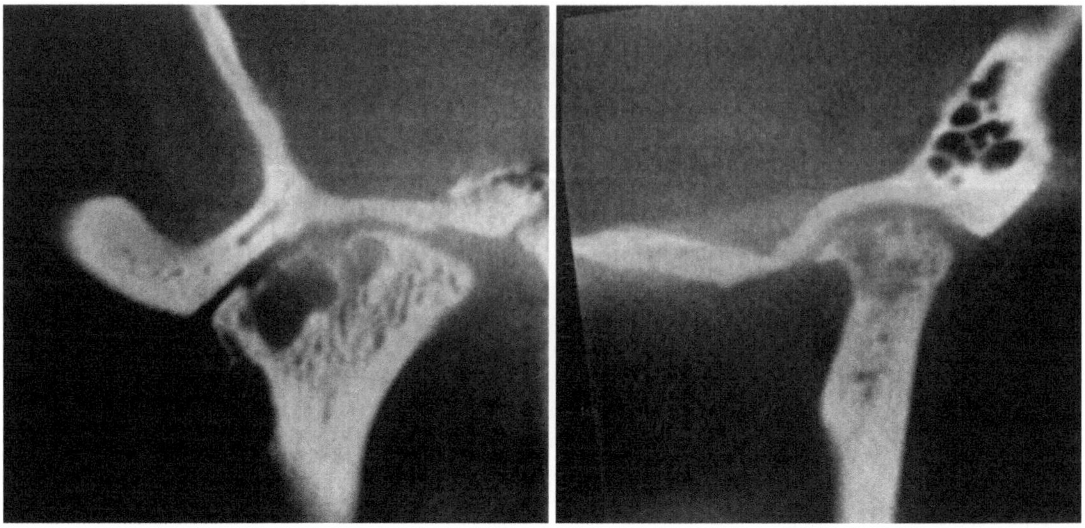

Fig. 13.5 Category 5 Catastrophic TMJ Changes—Cone beam CT scan showing large sub-chondral cyst in the roughened condylar head which is typical of severe degenerative joint disease in which the joint cannot be salvaged

difficult to visualize on MRI scans which also demonstrate low signal intensity from the degenerated condylar head. The most common category 5 joint are those with advanced degenerative joint disease often related to primary (idiopathic) osteoarthritis or secondary to trauma or previous TMJ surgical procedures. In some cases of category 5 joints, joint pain is very low or entirely absent, particularly in patients with TMJ condylysis/resorption, ankylosis, benign tumours, developmental disorders, and even long-standing TMJ osteoarthrosis. Patients with Category 5 joints benefit from discectomy, condylectomy, and, where indicated, total joint replacement since all the structural joint components are beyond salvage [12].

13.9 Discussion

The Wilkes classification has been the standard classification for surgical TMJ disorders throughout the world since it first appeared in the literature some 30 years ago [6]. The five distinct stages of TMJ disease levels first described by Wilkes have been embodied in the Dimitroulis's TMJ surgical classification [7] which has expanded the classification to include other less common TMJ disorders such as ankylosis and TMJ dislocations. A simple scale of 1 to 5 reflecting the increasing severity of the TMJ disorder with each category helps simplify data collection through numerical quantification which not only facilitates research data collection and analysis, but also allows a clear communication between surgeons. For example, a patient with a category 5 TMJ being referred by a TMD specialist clinician to an Oral and Maxillofacial Surgeon will only require the referring clinician to mention "Cat 5 joint" and the receiving surgeon will be in a position to understand that the patient will require a TMJ joint replacement or a similar surgical intervention. Conversely, a referring surgeon may diagnose a "Cat 1 patient" and the recipient clinician would be in a position to understand that the TMJ is structurally sound and the arthralgia needs to be managed non-surgically.

The fundamental purpose of the proposed TMJ surgical classification [7] is to overcome the current dilemma in the literature of trying to compare treatment outcomes on TMJ patients without a standard and specific diagnosis. It is glaringly obvious that there is an acute lack of a definitive method of collecting standardized data that will properly demonstrate the efficacy of the multitude of TMJ surgical procedures published in the literature [1]. This classification aids in surgical treatment planning by not only codifying the diagnosis, but also clearly defining the salvage potential of the structural joint components. When it comes to multicentre clinical trials, TMJ patient populations can be easily compared as they can be better defined using the categories described in the classification. Meta-analysis of treatment options will also be easier to assess and analyse when clinical studies start to focus on specific categories of patients described in this classification. For instance, the studies comparing operative TMJ arthroscopy to open TMJ arthroplasty on category 3 patients are conducted, the researches can compare treatment outcomes on patients with similar levels of disease with comparisons of like with like, the treatment will be the only variable under scrutiny.

Simple and straightforward classifications are essential if we are to make progress in TMJ surgery. A classification that is validated by research and universally accepted by clinicians is what is required to better define the role of TMJ surgery, as scientific evidence is crucial to the widespread acceptance of surgery as an essential treatment option in the management of TMDs.

References

1. Dimitroulis G. The role of surgery in the management of disorders of the temporomandibular joint: a critical review of the literature Part 2. Int J Oral Maxillofac Surg. 2005;34:231–7.
2. Dworkin SF, LeResche L. Research diagnostic criteria for temporomandibular disorders: review, criteria, examinations and specifications, critique. J Craniomandib Disord. 1992;6:301–55.
3. Schiffman E, Ohrbach R, Truelove E, et al. Diagnostic Criteria for Temporomandibular Disorders (DC/TMD) for Clinical and Research Applications: recommendations of the International RDC/TMD Consortium Network and Orofacial Pain Special Interest Group. International RDC/TMD Consortium Network, International association for Dental Research; Orofacial Pain Special Interest Group, International Association for the Study of Pain. J Oral Facial Pain Headache. 2014;28:6–27.
4. Sawhney CP. Bony ankylosis of the temporomandibular joint: follow-up of 70 patients treated with arthroplasty and acrylic spacer interposition. Plast Reconstr Surg. 1986;77:29–40.
5. Akinbami BO. Evaluation of the mechanism and principles of management of temporomandibular joint dislocation review of literature and a proposed new classification of temporomandibular joint dislocation. Head Face Med. 2011;7:10.
6. Wilkes CH. Internal derangements of the temporomandibular joint: pathological variations. Arch Otolaryngol Head Neck Surg. 1989;115:469–77.
7. Dimitroulis G. A new surgical classification for temporomandibular disorders. Int J Oral Maxillofac Surg. 2013;42:218–22.
8. Lindahl L. Condylar fractures of the mandible I. Classification and relation to age, occlusion and concomitant injuries of teeth tooth-supporting structures and fractures of the mandibular body. Int J Oral Surg. 1977;6:12–21.
9. Wolford LM, Movahed R, Dhameja A, Allen WR. Low condylectomy and orthognathic surgery to treat mandibular condylar osteochondroma: a retrospective review of 37 cases. J Oral Maxillofac Surg. 2014;72:1704–28.
10. Klasser GD, Manfredini D, Goulet JP, De Laat A. Oro-facial pain and temporomandibular disorders classification systems: A critical appraisal and future directions. J Oral Rehabil. 2018;45:258–68.
11. Breik O, Devrukhkar V, Dimitroulis G. Temporomandibular joint (TMJ) arthroscopic lysis and lavage: Outcomes and rate of progression to open surgery. J Craniomaxillofac Surg. 2016;44:1988–95.
12. Dimitroulis G. Comparison of the outcomes of three surgical treatments for end-stage temporomandibular joint disease. Int J Oral Maxillofac Surg. 2014;43:980–9.

Surgical Approaches to the Temporomandibular Joint

14

P. Anantanarayanan, P. Elavenil, and Mimansa Bhoj

14.1 Introduction

Surgical approach to the TMJ is indicated in various clinical scenarios such as pathological/developmental changes involving the TMJ as well as peri-joint structures, reconstruction of the joint and trauma. Surgical exposure and access to this joint is challenging because of its close proximity to vital structures such as the facial and auriculotemporal nerves, superficial temporal vessels, parotid gland and EAC. A thorough understanding of the same is essential for a surgeon to ensure a safe dissection and exposure of TMJ. The various approaches employed in reaching the joint along with the advantages and limitations of each are elaborated below. A brief description of the rationale behind choosing the ideal incision for a specific clinical indication is also presented.

P. Anantanarayanan
Anantan Dental and Facial Surgery,
Chennai, Tamil Nadu, India

Oral and Maxillofacial Surgery, Meenakshi Ammal
Dental College and Hospital, Chennai, Tamil Nadu,
India

P. Elavenil (✉)
Anantan Dental and Facial Surgery,
Chennai, Tamil Nadu, India

Oral and Maxillofacial Surgery, SRM Dental College
and Hospital (Ramapuram Campus),
Chennai, Tamil Nadu, India

M. Bhoj
Department of Oral and Maxillofacial Surgery,
ITS CDSR, Muradnagar (Ghaziabad),
Uttar Pradesh, India

14.2 Surgical Anatomy

Anatomical relations of TMJ with structures of surgical significance have been enlisted in Table 14.1.

Table 14.1 Anatomic relations of Temporomandibular Joint

Relation to the TMJ	Anatomic structures
Lateral	Skin Fasciae Parotid gland Temporal branch of facial nerve
Medial	Lateral pterygoid muscle Roots of auriculotemporal nerve Middle meningeal artery Spine of sphenoid Sphenomandibular ligament Chorda tympani nerve
Anterior	Lateral pterygoid muscle Temporalis muscle Masseteric nerve and vessels
Posterior	Parotid gland Superficial temporal vessels Auriculotemporal nerve External auditory meatus
Superior	Floor of middle cranial fossa Middle meningeal vessels
Inferior	Maxillary artery and vein

D. Bhargava (ed.), *Temporomandibular Joint Disorders*,
https://doi.org/10.1007/978-981-16-2754-5_14

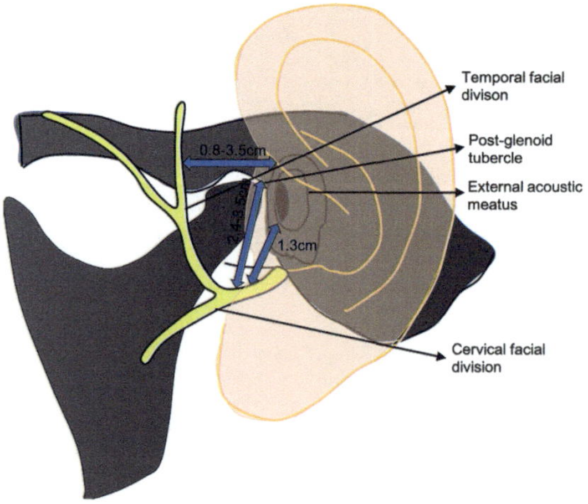

Fig. 14.1 Surgical anatomy of the facial nerve in the pre-auricular region

14.2.1 Facial Nerve (Fig. 14.1)

- Course: The facial nerve enters the parotid gland after exiting the skull through the stylomastoid foramen and divides into two main trunks (cervicofacial and temporofacial)—the branches of which anastomose variably and form a parotid plexus. The terminal branches emerge from parotid and radiate in an anterior direction
- Supply: Muscles of facial expression
- *Surgical Note*:
  - The branch most likely to be damaged during TMJ surgery is *temporal branch* as it crosses the lateral surface of the zygomatic arch lying below the temporoparietal fascia (8–35 mm, mean: 20 mm, anterior to external auditory canal). It can be protected by incising through the superficial layer of temporalis fascia and periosteum of the zygomatic arch not greater than 8 mm anterior to the external auditory canal.
  - Alkayat and Bramley (1979) [1]: Distance of facial nerve bifurcation to lowest concavity of the external auditory canal was 1.5–2.8 cm (mean 2.3 cm) and to the post glenoid tubercle was 2.4–3.5 cm (mean 3 cm).
  - Frontal nerve trajectory follows the "Pitanguy line" which corresponds to a line starting from a point 0.5 cm below the tragus to a point 1 cm above the lateral edge of the eyebrow

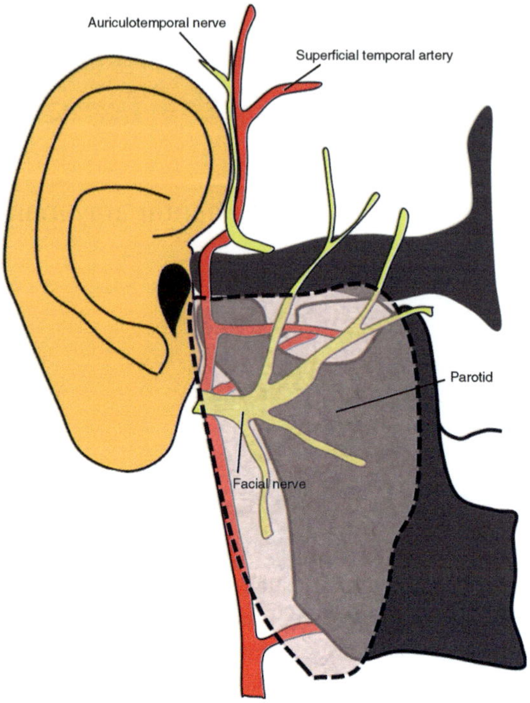

Fig. 14.2 Anatomic structures of importance in the preauricular region. The location of the parotid salivary gland is represented as the black dotted line. Note the relation of the facial nerve and the parotid gland. Also note the auriculotemporal nerve running superiorly from the medial side of posterior neck of condyle to the zygomatic root

14.2.2 Auriculotemporal Nerve (Fig. 14.2)

- Branch of: Mandibular division of Trigeminal Nerve (cutaneous sensory branch)
- Course: runs superiorly from the medial side of posterior neck of condyle to the zygomatic root of temporal bone and divides into its terminal branches in the skin of the temporal area anterior to the auricle.
- Supply: parts of auricle, external acoustic meatus, tympanic membrane and skin in temporal region.
- *Surgical Note:* Terminal branches are prone to injury during the preauricular approach.
  - Minimize damage by placing incision and dissecting in close apposition to the carti-

laginous portion of the external auditory meatus and placing temporal extension of the incision posteriorly (assists in dissecting of main nerve trunk and retracting it in the anterior flap).

14.2.3 Parotid Gland (Fig. 14.2)

The parotid gland lies in close association with the TMJ as the superficial pole of the gland lies directly on the TMJ capsule. The parotid gland itself is enclosed in a capsule (*parotido masseteric fascia*) which is a derivative of the superficial layer of the deep cervical fascia. The surgical approach to the TMJ may involve dissection through the parotid gland to reach the joint, *in such cases special precaution must be taken to dissect parallel to the course of the facial nerve which runs across the gland substrate.*

14.2.4 External Auditory Canal (Figs. 14.2 and 14.3)

The anatomy of human TMJ demonstrates a close embryological, anatomical and functional relationship with the middle ear. The superior stratum of the TMJ is attached posteriorly to the cartilaginous auditory meatus making it prone to injury and subsequent stenosis in incorrectly placed incisions or iatrogenic trauma during surgery. *The direction of the canal is forward and downward and the same should be kept in mind while explor-*

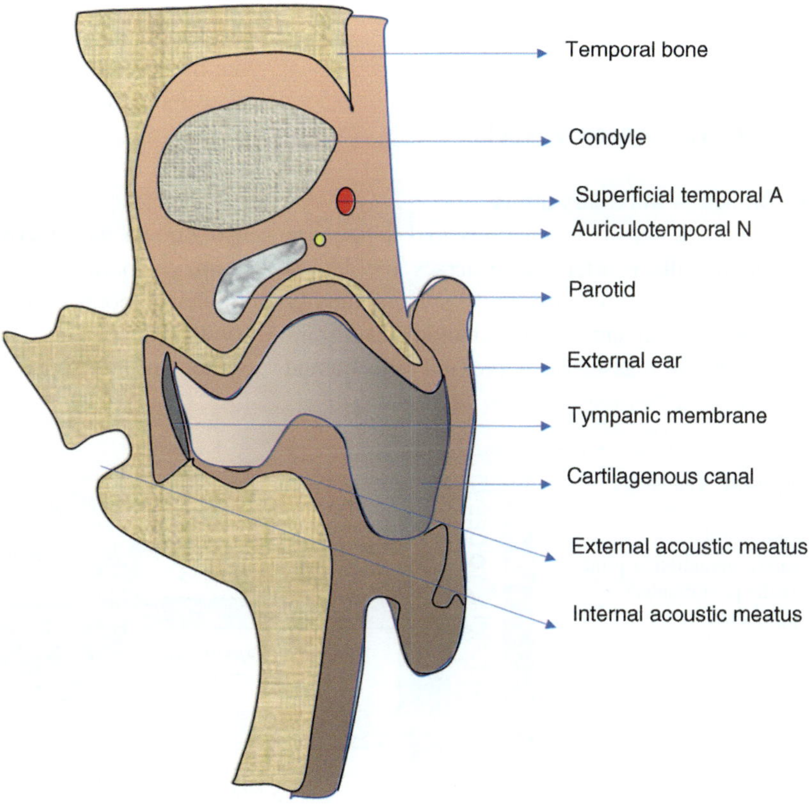

Fig. 14.3 Axial view demonstrating the mandibular condyle and its relation to various anatomic structures

ing the restricted surgical field in TMJ surgeries. High risk of cicatricial stenosis of external auditory meatus in retro auricular approach is one of the biggest disadvantages of the approach.

14.2.5 Superficial Temporal Vessels (Fig. 14.2)

- Terminal branch of External Carotid artery.
- Course: Emerge from the superior aspect of parotid and course along the auriculotemporal nerve (lies posterior to artery). Gives a temporal branch as it crosses the zygomatic arch and a parietal and frontal branch, few centimeters above the arch. The superficial temporal vein lies superficial and posterior to the artery.
- *Surgical Note:* The temporal branch is a common source of bleeding and routinely ligated during preauricular approach to the joint.

14.2.6 Masseteric Vessels

- Branch of Maxillary artery
- Course: It exits from the pterygoid segment of the maxillary artery, transverses the lateral pterygoid muscle between the sphenomandibular ligament and neck of condyle and accompanies the masseteric nerve and vein behind the temporalis tendon and through the sigmoid notch to the deep surface of the masseter.
- *Surgical Note:* The close proximity of the artery to the joint makes it a likely candidate to cause hemorrhage during TMJ surgeries.

The mean distance of the artery was determined in a cadaveric study to the following structures:

- to the anterior-superior aspect of the condylar neck: 10.3 ± 4.4 mm
- to the most inferior aspect of the articular tubercle: 11.47 ± 4.6 mm
- to the most inferior aspect of the sigmoid notch: 3.00 ± 1.2 mm.

14.2.7 Layers of Temporoparietal Region

The layers encountered while accessing the TMJ via the preauricular approach are depicted in Flowchart (Fig. 14.4).

The *temporoparietal fascia* is the lateral extension of galea. It is continuous with superficial musculoaponeurotic system (SMAS) and also known as superficial temporal fascia and suprazygomatic SMAS.

The temporalis Fascia is the fascia of the temporalis muscle. It splits at the level of superior orbital rim into superficial and deep layer attach-

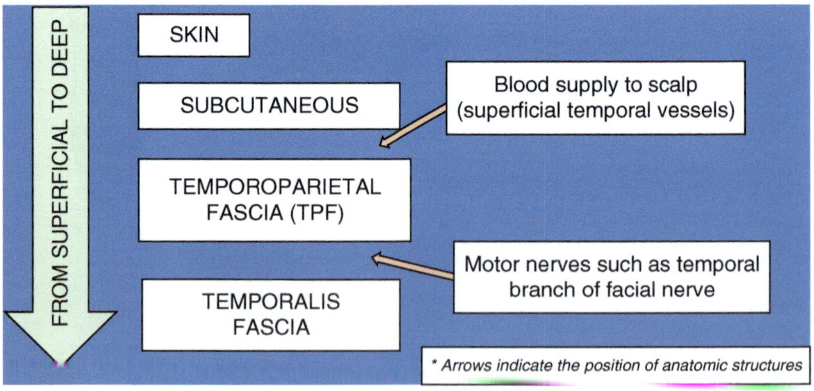

Fig. 14.4 The layers encountered while accessing the temporomandibular joint via the preauricular approach

ing at lateral and medial border of zygomatic arch, respectively, to encompass the superficial temporal fat pad. A large vein is often encountered just deep to the superficial layer of temporalis fascia.

14.3 Classification of Approaches

Any approach to the TMJ must ensure the following objectives; (a) complete visualization of structures, (b) permit easy access to all anatomic structures to perform the required surgical technique, (c) facilitate adequate instrumentation and most importantly (d) eliminate the risk of facial nerve injury.

Approaches may be cutaneous, arthroscopic, endoscopy assisted or intra-oral, based on the route of entry to the joint. Though arthroscopic/endoscopy assisted procedures demonstrate less surgical morbidity, their clinical indications are limited. A thorough knowledge of the various approaches is hence obligatory for effective management of various clinical scenarios.

Approaches to surgery of the TM joint may also be divided based on the exposure achieved;

1. Approach to the joint proper (comprising of the skeletal articulating surfaces, articular disc and the capsule)
2. Capsular incisions
3. Approaches to the peri-joint structures such as articular eminence, zygomatic arch, the temporal region and sub-condylar region.

   The peri-joint structures require exposure for various surgical techniques aimed at restraining the abnormal joint movement or reconstruction purposes.

14.4 Approaches and Incisions

14.4.1 Approach to the Joint Proper

This includes the following incisions; Preauricular, Post auricular, Combination (Preauricular and Post auricular) and Transoral. The detailed description of various incisions is given below.

14.4.1.1 Preauricular

The preauricular is by far the most preferred and commonly followed surgical approach to the TMJ world over. The advantages of the preauricular approach include (1) ease of technique, (2) optimal exposure, (3) flexibility to incorporate minor modifications and (4) minimal complications.

The original description of the approach was given by Risdon (1934) but the technique gained popularity with the work of Rowe and Killey in 1968 and further by Rowe again in 1972 [2]. The various preauricular incisions and their modifications commonly mentioned in literature include the following [3]

- Preauricular incision—standard
- Preauricular with temporal extension
- Preauricular—Alkayat Bramley modification
- Endaural
- Lazy "S" modification of the preauricular approach

14.4.1.2 Preauricular—Blair 1917 [4] (Fig. 14.5a)

The original description of the preauricular incision was shaped like an inverted hockey stick which has the standard preauricular vertical component which gradually curves anterior and forwards to a height 1 cm above the helix of the ear before descending downward to stop 2.5 cm anterior to the attachment of the helix.

14.4.1.3 Preauricular Incision—Thoma (1945) (Fig. 14.5b, b1 and b2)

The modification constitutes an incision along the preauricular crease extending superiorly with a 45 degrees angulation, between the bifurcated superficial temporal vessels [5].

14.4.1.4 Standard Preauricular Incision—Dingman 1946 (Fig. 14.5c)

This incision involves a vertical cutaneous incision in the preauricular crease extending from helix of the ear to the attachment of the lobule along with a gentle curve along the tragal margin.

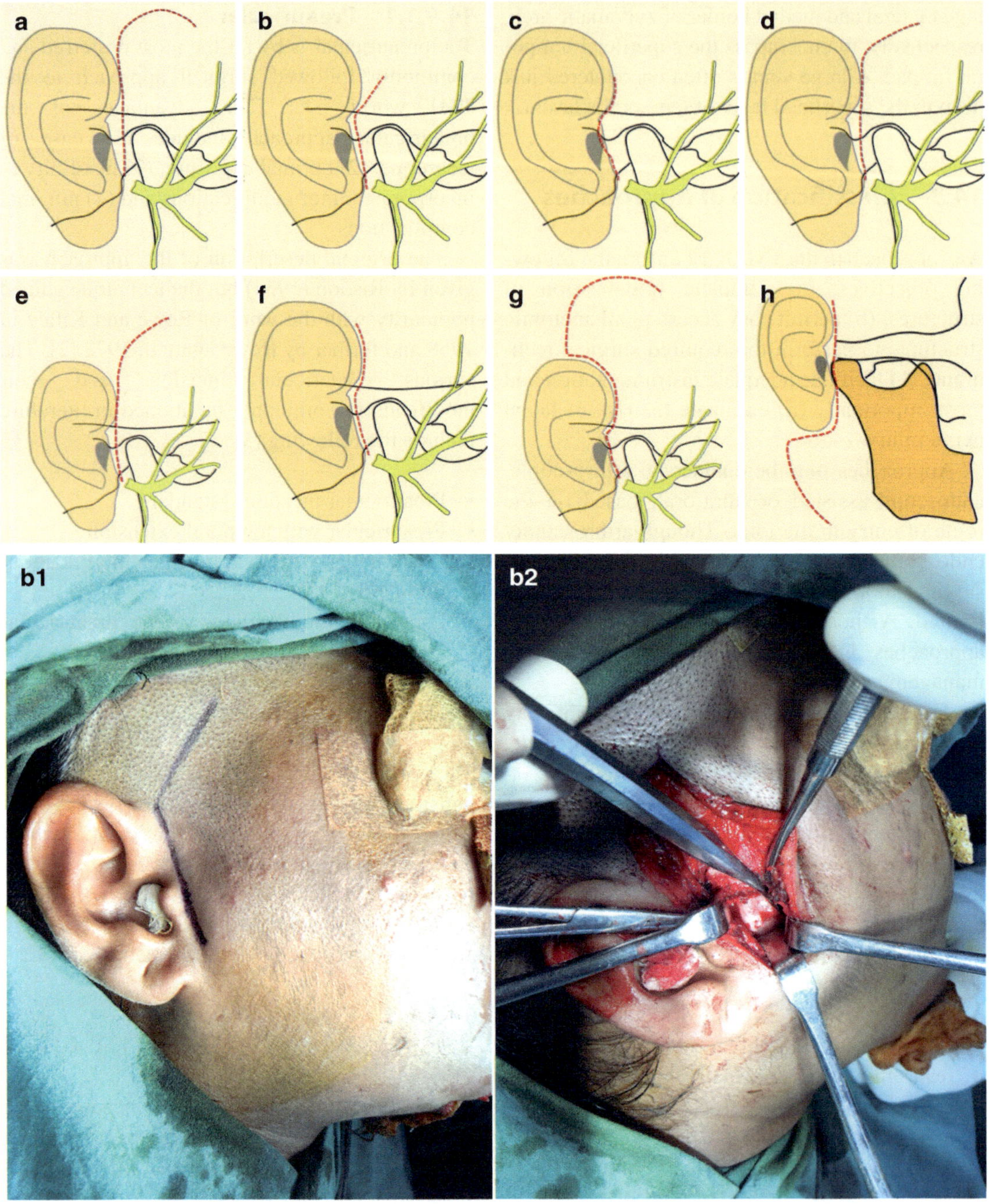

Fig. 14.5 Preauricular incision and its variations (**a**–**h**). (**b**1) Preauricular incision as described by Thoma (1945); surgical marking. (**b**2) Preauricular incision as described by Thoma (1945); surgical exposure. (**e**1) Preauricular incision as described by Dingman. (**g**1) Preauricular incision with temporal extension as described by Al Kayat and Bramley (1979) [1]. (**h**1) Preauricular with lazy "S" modification; surgical marking. (**h**2) Preauricular with lazy "S" modification; surgical exposure

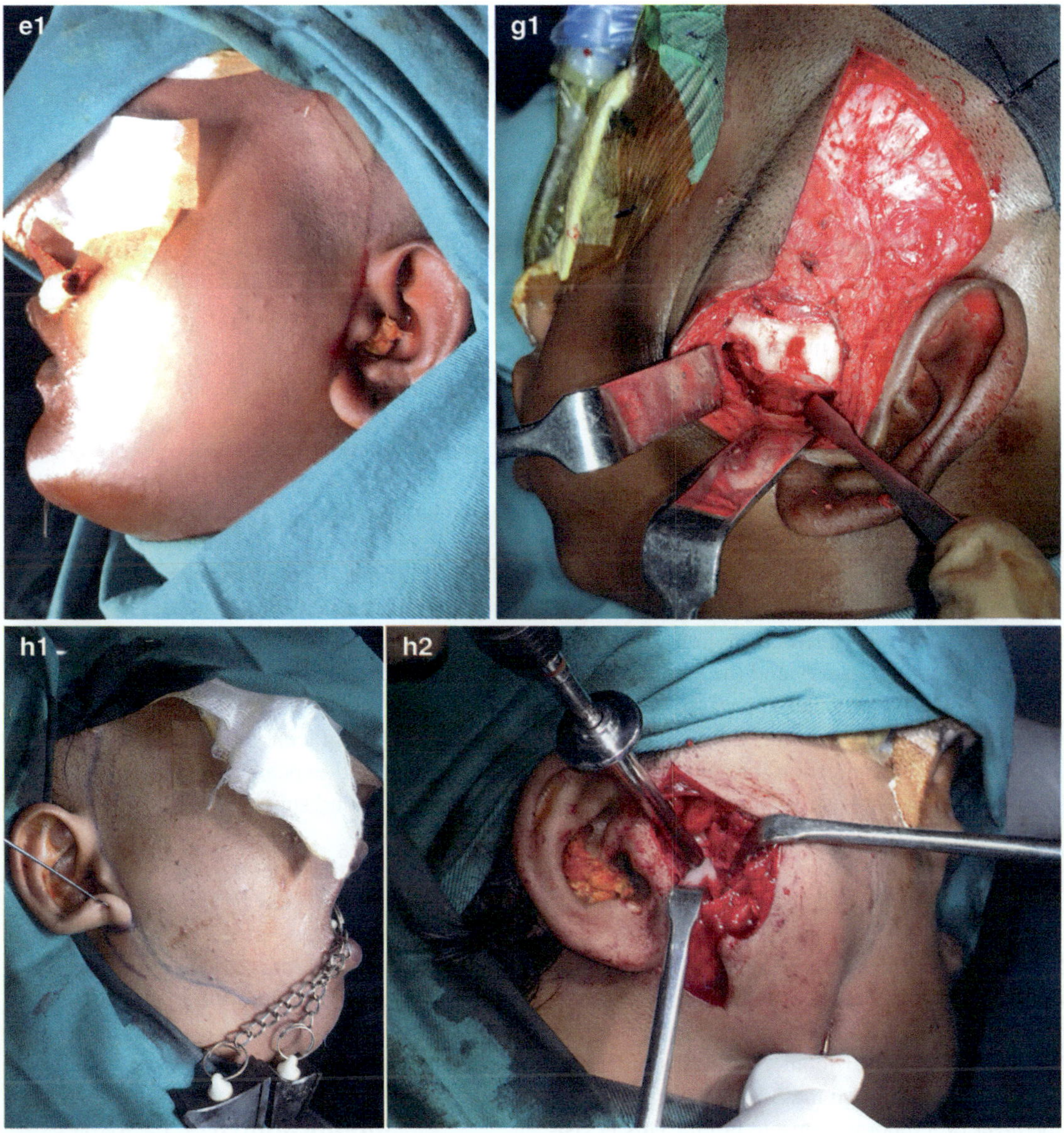

Fig. 14.5 (continued)

14.4.1.5 Preauricular—Dingman 1966 [6], 1974 (Fig. 14.5d, e, e1)

This involves a standard preauricular incision with a temporal and anterior extension. The dissection plane followed was subfascial.

14.4.1.6 Straight Line Preauricular Incision—Rowe and Killey 1968 (Fig. 14.5f)

This is a straight line incision that extends from the root of the helix superiorly to the attachment of the lobule on the face, inferiorly.

14.4.1.7 Preauricular with Temporal Extension—Al Kayat and Bramley 1979 [1] (Fig. 14.5g, g1)

This approach involves a 4–6 cm long skin incision placed in the pre-tragal region behind the superficial temporal artery and the auriculotemporal nerve. The preauricular approach may also be modified to include a small temporal extension depending on the indication for surgery. The temporal extension offers the advantages of (1) facilitating the "deep subfascial" approach for facial nerve preservation and (2) additional exposure over the zygomatic arch and (3) to enable the harvest of galea and the temporalis muscle when required. The incision is placed on the skin and taken down into the subcutaneous plane taking care not to extend the inferior limit beyond the attachment of the ear lobule. The incision is then carried deeper through the SMAS layer to expose the layer of temporalis muscle fascia. This is visible as a glistening white sheath that can be easily identified. The fascia is then incised sharply along a line which starts at the root of the zygomatic arch and extends anteriorly and superiorly at a 45-degree angle to the arch for a length of 4 cm. This ensures that the branches of the facial nerve lie superior to the temporalis fascial layer and thus significantly reduces incidence of facial nerve weakness following the surgery. Extension of this incision vertically below the level of the arch was described by Popowich [7]. The dissection of the joint and the arch of the zygoma in this plane provides a safe and an easy way to achieve optimal exposure in a safe and predictable manner. Identification of the joint is made by the visualization of the joint capsule, which can be incised in a sharp fashion to expose the joint proper.

Indications:

1. Surgery to the joint proper with exposure of both the condylar and the glenoid components
2. Exposure of the fractures of the condylar head and neck

Merits:

1. Good exposure of the entire joint
2. Additional exposure of the zygomatic arch and temporal regions
3. Predictable healing and satisfactory cosmesis
4. Flexibility for harvesting grafts and flaps like galea and temporalis muscle

Limitations:

1. Possibility for facial nerve damage
2. Compromised exposure for ORIF in the case of low neck and sub-condylar fractures

Exposure of the joint with this incision provides additional access to the zygomatic arch and temporal regions, which help in harvesting a temporalis fascia/muscle flap. This apporoach also helps in preserving the superficial temporal vessels.

14.4.1.8 Preauricular with Lazy "S" Modification (Fig. 14.5h, h1 and h2)

Aids in enhanced access to the joint along with the sub-condylar and the mandibular angle regions. This is a good approach for reconstructive surgery of the joint.

14.4.1.9 Endaural Approach (Fig. 14.6)

The endaural approach was originally described by Lempert for surgery of the middle ear. This was modified for use in TMJ surgery [8]. The commonly used modification is the Rongetti's limited length, intra-aural incision that extends along the depth of the external auditory meatus [9].

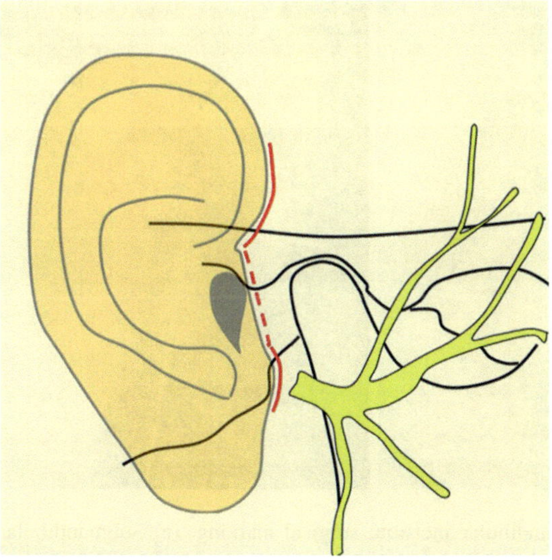

Fig. 14.6 Endaural approach (dotted line represents the endaural component of the incision)

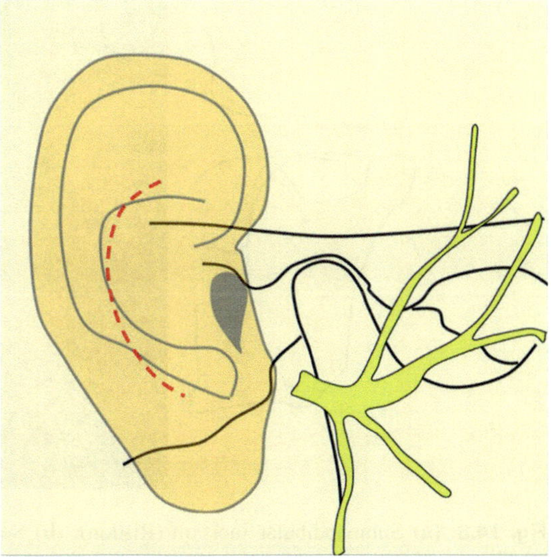

Fig. 14.7 Postauricular approach

Indications:

1. Open surgery to the TM joint
2. Surgery involving the condylar head and the superior aspect of the condylar neck.

Merits:

1. This approach provides cosmetic advantage over the traditional preauricular approach
2. Reduced iatrogenic damage to the superficial temporal artery and the auriculotemporal nerves

Limitations

1. Damage to the tragal cartilage may be a complication

14.4.1.10 Post-auricular Approach [10] (Fig. 14.7)

The first description of the post-auricular approach is credited to Bockenheimer in 1920 followed by Axhausen in the early 1930s. It utilizes the use of an incision posterior to the auricle followed by dissection in an anterior direction and division of the external auditory canal. The entire external ear is reflected anteriorly to expose the capsule of the TMJ. This is not a commonly used approach and has gradually taken its exit from mainstay TMJ surgery after reports of stenosis of the cartilaginous canal by Husted.

Common Indications

1. Exposure of TM joint proper
2. Exposure of the condylar head

Merits:

1. Inconspicuous scar behind the ear
2. Was preferred for use in patients with propensity to develop excessive scarring and keloids
3. Excellent exposure of the joint with good access to the retrodiscal tissue and posterior aspect of the condyle

Limitations:

1. Prone for stenosis of the cartilaginous auditory canal
2. Contra-indicated in patients with otitis media and infection of the TM joint

14.4.1.11 Sub-mandibular (Fig. 14.8a–c)

Risdon proposed the classical sub-mandibular approach which was placed between the man-

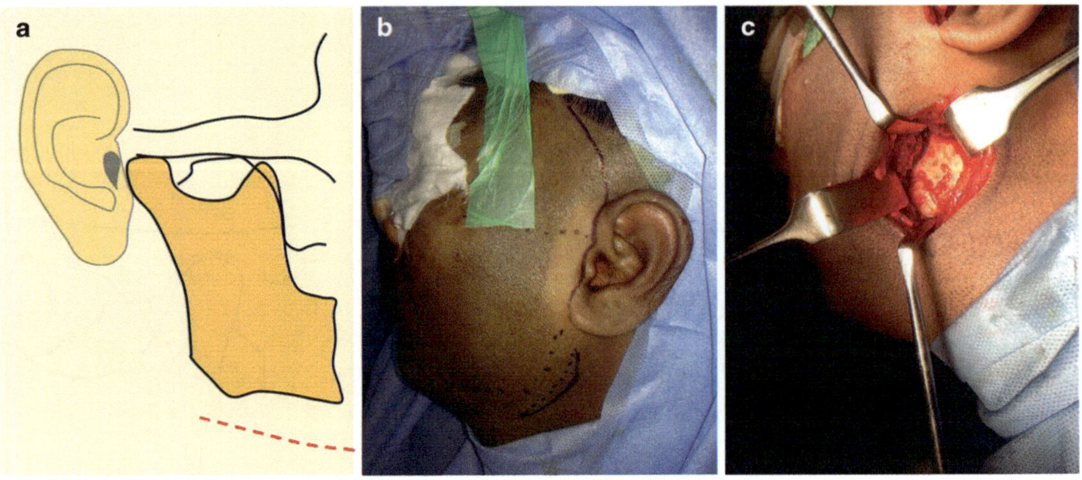

Fig. 14.8 (**a**) Submandibular incision (Risdon). (**b**) Submandibular incision; surgical marking. (**c**) Submandibular incision; surgical exposure

dibular and cervical branches of the facial nerve. This approach provided excellent exposure to the entire lateral aspect of the mandible. Though it did not offer the same degree of exposure of the TM joint as the techniques described above, it was a preferred method of accessing the sub-condylar region till the late 1980s. The Hayes Martin modification of the sub-mandibular approach for protection of the marginal mandibular nerve is the most commonly used surgical technique in current practice.

Indications:

1. Sub-condylar fractures
2. As an adjunct in reconstruction of the TM Joint using alloplastic prosthesis or autogenous grafts
3. Associated surgery of the mandibular angle and/or ramus

Merits:

1. Predictable approach used for more than a century for a wide exposure of the lateral mandible

Limitations:

1. Cannot be used for access of the TM joint proper
2. Limited access for high condylar fractures

14.4.1.12 Endoscopic Approach

Recent advances in the field of oral and maxillofacial surgery has increased the focus on minimally invasive approaches. This has led to popularization of endoscopic approaches to the TM joint both for diagnostic and therapeutic purposes. Arthroscopes are now being utilized to perform surgical procedures of the TMJ and for the ORIF of condylar fractures. While diagnostic arthroscopy involves the use of only one scope, surgical intervention to the joint may utilize a single or multiple scope approach using the "triangulation" concept. Triangulation involves the camera-cannula and the working cannula being triangulated in a way where the camera is used to visualize the working cannula. Basic instrumentation includes: (1) the arthroscope, (2) the working cannula which acts as the conduit for irrigation and instrumentation. Instrumentation includes forceps, rasps, sutures rotatory instruments.

Indications:

1. Diagnostic
2. Arthrocentesis, lavage and fibrolysis
3. Disc procedures and osseous recontouring within the joint
4. ORIF for condylar fractures may be performed with endoscopic assistance

Merits:

1. Minimally invasive technique
2. Less trauma with early recovery
3. Practically no incidence of neurological deficits

Limitations:

1. Steep learning curve
2. Technique and equipment—sensitive
3. Indications are specific
4. Back up to open surgery should always be an option. Hence the surgeon should also be trained for that

14.4.2 Exposure of Joint Space and Disc

The approaches to the TM joint that have been described earlier in the text are meant to access the macro-joint area. This involves the temporal region, the mandibular condyle and the associated soft tissues that maintain the integrity of the joint. However, indications for intra-capsular interventions necessitate exposure of the upper and lower joint compartments and the disc. The joint spaces and the disc are enclosed by the capsule laterally which is also called as the lateral ligament which need to be incised. This can be performed by the use of different incision designs (Fig. 14.9). Care is taken to plan the incision in a way that facilitates good re-approximation of the capsule after the surgery to the joint is completed.

14.4.3 Dissection Planes

14.4.3.1 Suprafascial, Subfascial and Deep Subfascial Dissections (Fig. 14.10)

After a pre-auricular skin incision, different planes of tissue dissection have been adopted by authors, with an attempt to negate facial nerve injury. Three possible planes of dissection are the following;

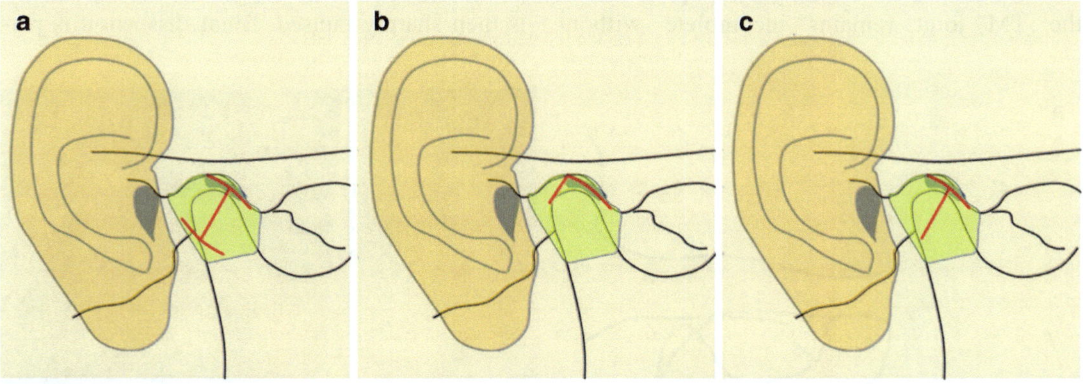

Fig. 14.9 Exposure of the joint space and the disc (**a**) "H" incision, (**b**) Inverted "L", (**c**) "T" incision

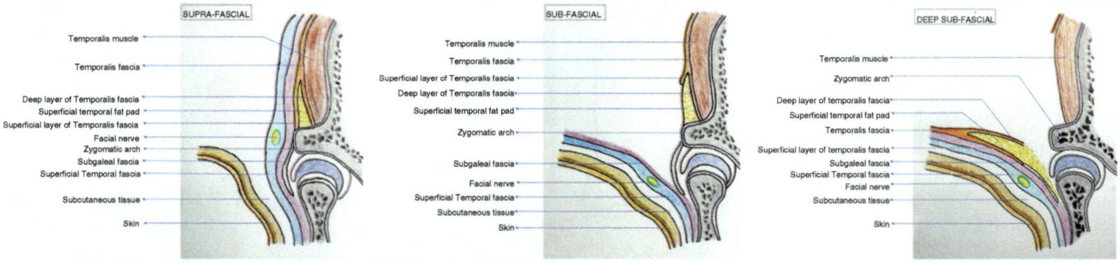

Fig. 14.10 Suprafascial, subfascial and deep subfascial dissections

- *Suprafascial*
- *Subfascial*
- *Deep subfascial*

Originally, the TMJ was approached by adopting a suprafascial plane which resulted in higher incidence for facial nerve injuries. Significant modification in technique came in with the publication of the subfascial approach of Al-Kayat and Bramley in 1979 which focused on the preservation of the integrity of the facial nerve in relation to the zygomatic arch. However, though the neurological deficits were reduced by this technique, it was still high enough to be bothersome. Politi in 2004 discussed the deep subfascial modification of the preauricular approach with the claim of no temporary or permanent neurological deficit to the facial nerve in his series of 21 patients.

14.5 Approaches for the Management of Condylar Fractures

A discussion involving surgical approaches to the TM joint remains incomplete without encompassing approaches to the fractured mandibular condyle. Surgical management of such condyles and subsequent derangement of the TMJ proper necessitate adequate exposure. These approaches to the mandibular condyle may be different from the approaches to the TM joint depending on the type of fracture and the degree of exposure needed for its reduction and fixation. A brief description of the contemporary approaches to the mandibular condyle is provided below.

14.5.1 Retromandibular Approach (Fig. 14.11a, b)

Described by Hinds and Girotti in 1967, this approach provides direct access to the neck of the mandibular condyle and the ramus of the mandible. A linear incision of 3 cm length is placed about 0.5 cm below the pinna and a centimeter behind the posterior border of the ramus. Dissection is carried out through the skin, subcutaneous tissues and scant platysma exposing the parotideomasseteric fascia (SMAS layer) which is then sharply incised. Blunt dissection is per-

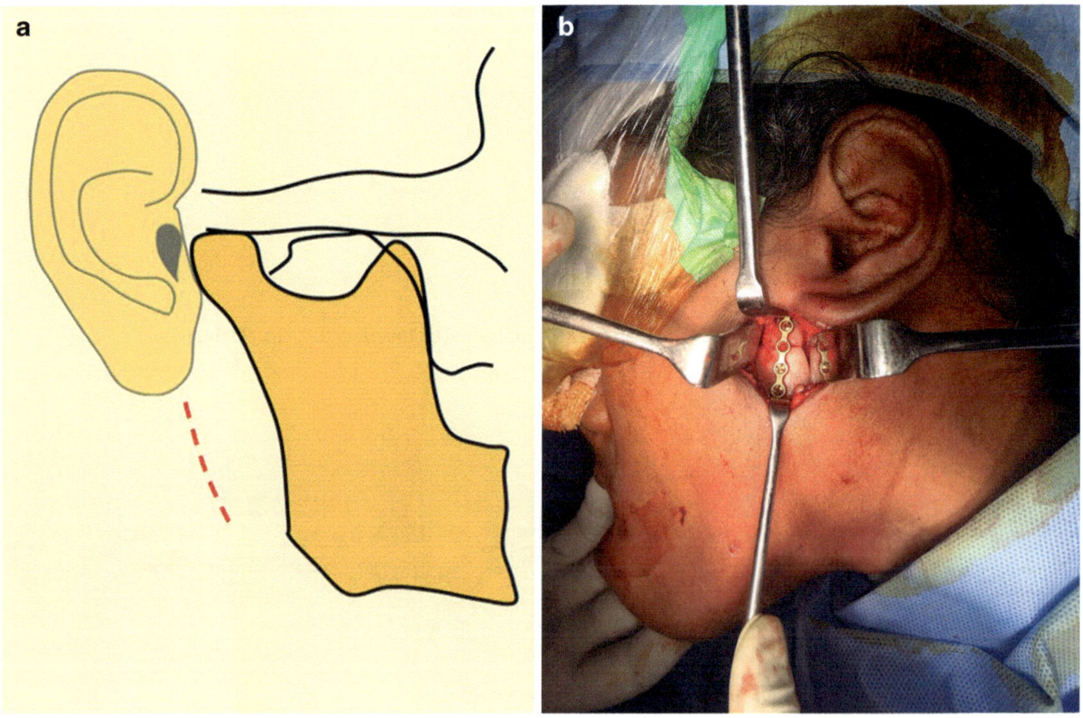

Fig. 14.11 (**a**) Retromandibular approach. (**b**) Retromandibular approach; surgical exposure

formed through the parotid substance. The area of dissection lies between the temporofacial and cervicofacial branches of the facial nerve and is performed parallel to the direction of the nerves to expose the masseter and the pterygomasseteric sling. The trans-masseteric dissection can be performed by two methods; it can either be divided sharp using a blade or cautery or can be cleaved bluntly along the direction of the muscle fibres to expose the bone beneath. Care should be taken to avoid injuring the retromandibular vein which lies immediately posterior. Subperiosteal dissection is continued superior and inferiorly to expose the sub-condylar region and part of the mandibular ramus. The transparotid dissection of the approach warrants careful and meticulous closure of the parotid capsule while suturing to avoid any salivary fistulas or sialoceles following surgery.

Indications:

1. Fractures involving condylar neck and subcondylar fractures
2. Fractures of the ramus of the mandible

Merits:

1. Direct approach
2. Good area of exposure
3. Favourable scar

Limitations:

1. Risk of injury to the buccal and marginal mandibular branches of facial nerve is high due to multiple cross-innervations.
2. Presence of vital structures such as facial nerve, parotid gland and duct, retromandibular vein exposing them to risk of iatrogenic injury.
3. Risk of salivary fistula/sialocele formation.
4. Not useful for high condylar fractures.
5. Though rare, risk of Frey's syndrome due to inadvertent injury and aberrant reinnervation of postganglionic parasympathetic nerve fibres to local sweat glands.

14.5.2 Periangular Approach (Fig. 14.12a–c)

The Periangular approach or high sub-mandibular approach described by Patel and Cronyn is a direct approach to posterior mandibular body and angle region. A 3–5 cm curvilinear incision is made 0.5–1 cm posterior-inferior to the angle of the mandible through skin and subcutaneous tissues exposing the platysma. Blunt dissection of the platysma is carried out creating a subplatysmal plane over the superficial layer of deep cervical fascia. The SMAS layer in the region including the masseteric fascia is divided to expose the pterygomasseteric sling. Sharp dissection of pterygomasseteric sling allows excellent exposure of lateral border of the mandible extending from the angle to the subcondylar region.

Indications:

1. Mandibular angle and posterior body fractures
2. Ramus fractures
3. Inferior distraction of mandible for reduction of condylar fractures.

Merits:

1. No reported incidence of facial nerve deficits
2. Does not necessitate ligation of facial artery and vein
3. Infero-superior dissection does not involve breach of the parotid capsule circumventing salivary gland complications such as sialoceles and salivary fistulas.
4. Sub-mandibular space is not violated and integrity of gland and lymphatics is maintained.
5. Excellent cosmesis as the scar is hidden behind the gonial angle prominence.
6. Technically simple and less time taking.

Limitations:

1. Limited access for high-level condyle fractures.

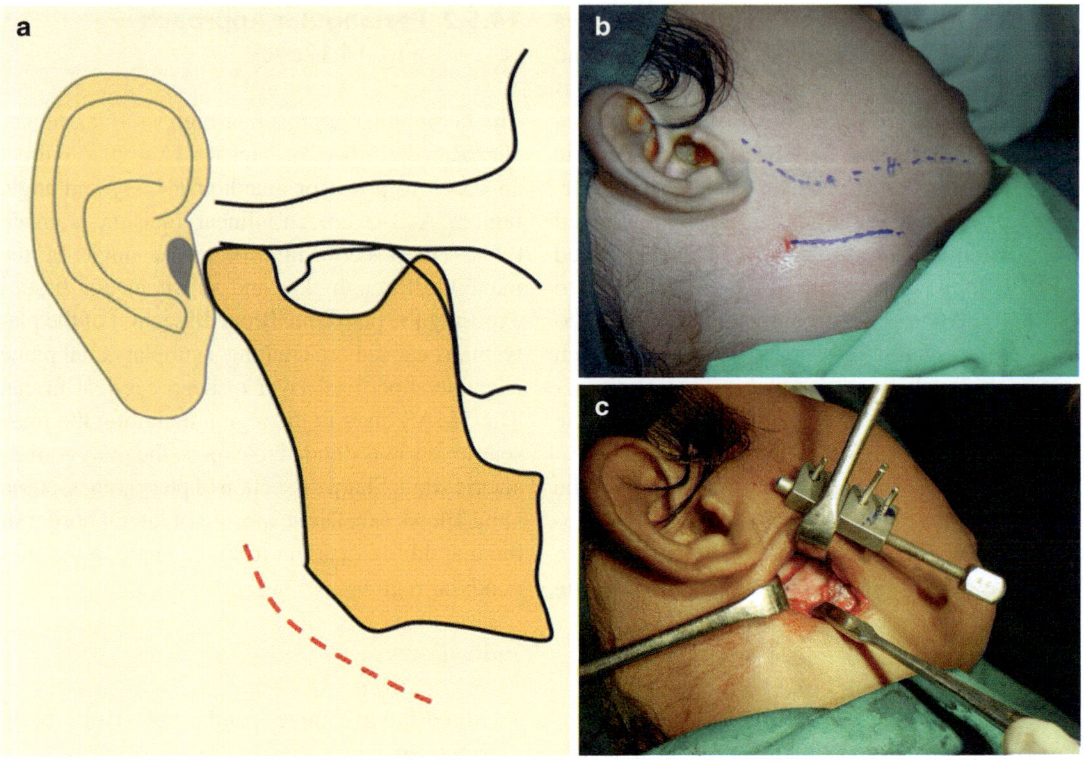

Fig. 14.12 (**a**) Periangular approach. (**b**) Periangular approach; surgical marking. (**c**) Periangular approach; surgical exposure

14.5.3 Rhytidectomy Approach [11] (Fig. 14.13)

Also known as the facelift approach, this provides a wide exposure of the mandibular condyle, ramus and angle of the mandible. This is similar to the trans-masseteric antero parotid approach but has a wider area of exposure. The skin incision is a long incision starting from the preauricular crease extending downwards and around the base of pinna over the posterior surface of the auricle and ends in an extension over the skin of the mastoid region. The pertinent anatomy of this particular approach requires careful dissection over the mastoid and post-auricular region wherein the great auricular nerve traverses in an antero-superior direction over the sternocleidomastoid muscle piercing the superficial layer of deep cervical fascia and lies beneath the subcutaneous plane. The initial incision is made through the skin, subcutaneous tissues and scant platysma, and a plane is created over the superficial musculoaponeurotic system through blunt dissection. The deeper dissection through the parotid capsule and gland can be performed similar to transparotid retromandibular or the trans-masseteric antero parotid approaches.

Indications:

1. Multiple fractures involving condyle, ramus and posterior body of the mandible.
2. Concomitant injuries requiring soft tissue resuspension.

Merits:

1. Wide surgical exposure
2. Direct access
3. Provision to accommodate soft tissue corrections for better cosmetic outcomes

4. Lengthy incision provides for better retraction
5. Favourable scar, as part of the scar is extended into the hairline and in post-auricular surface

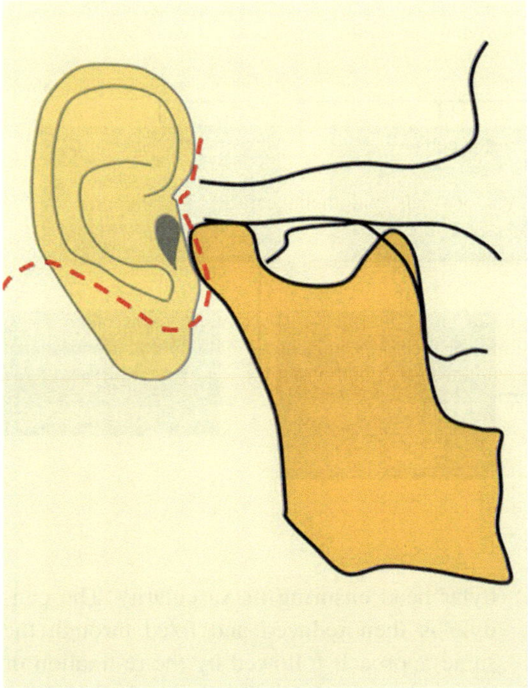

Fig. 14.13 Rhytidectomy approach

6. Accommodates for modifications in dissection into the deeper tissues.

Limitations:

1. Injury to great auricular nerve may result in paresthesia of skin over the angle and ear lobe.

14.5.4 Access Osteotomies (Fig. 14.14)

Medially displaced condyles, especially high-level fractures tend to be a challenge to retrieve, reduce and fix as the access to mobilize them and reduce them is very limited. The following text discusses two techniques of using access osteotomies for the retrieval, reduction and fixation of the displaced condylar head (osteotomy-osteosynthesis).

1. The use of vertical ramus osteotomies for accessing the medially displaced high condylar fractures started with the independent descriptions of Ellis et al. and Mikkonen et al., both in 1989. But these carried a significant disadvantage of compromised vascularity to the fractured condyles as both techniques advocated extra-corporeal fixation of the con-

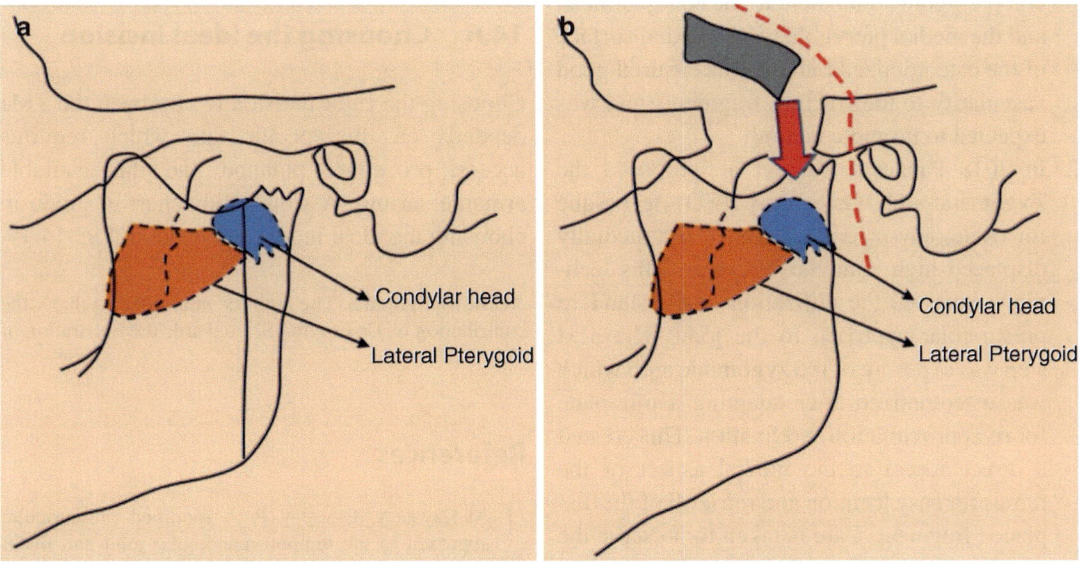

Fig. 14.14 Access osteotomies; (**a**) Vertical ramus osteotomy. (**b**) Zygomatic-arch Osteotomy

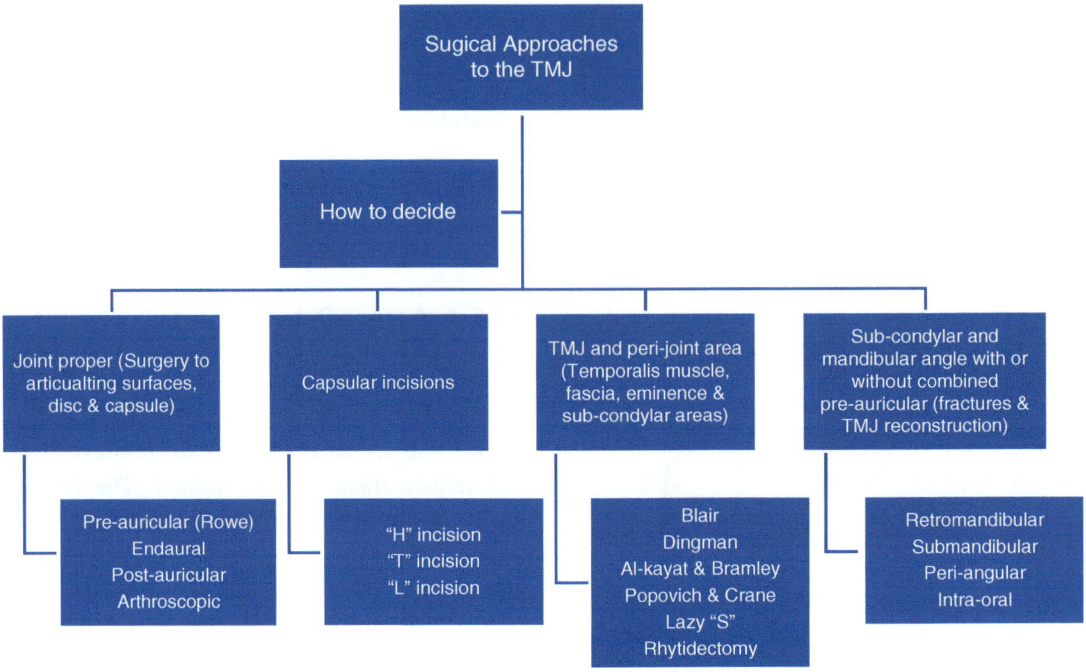

Fig. 14.15 Guide for choosing the ideal incision

dyle to the osteotomized ramus prior to anchoring the segments back to the distal fragment. These were overcome by the technique advocated by Sasaki et al. in 2002, which involved maintaining fragments internally with their muscular attachments; the lateral pterygoid attachment to the condylar head and the medial pterygoid to the medial surface of the osteotomized ramus. This ensured good vascularity to the fracture fragments and was expected to promote healing.

2. In 2018 Panneerselvam et al. proposed the Zygomatic-arch Osteotomy (ZO) technique for osteotomy-osteosynthesis of the medially displaced high condylar fractures. This technique involved the utilization of the standard preauricular approach to the joint. The next step was exposure of the zygomatic arch which was osteotomized after adapting a miniplate for re-approximation and fixation. This created a direct access to the medial aspect of the ramus for easy location and retrieval of the displaced fragment. Care is taken to preserve the attachment of the lateral pterygoid to the condylar head ensuring its vascularity. The condyle is then reduced and fixed through the same approach followed by the re-fixation of the osteotomized arch into its original position with the aid of the adapted miniplate.

14.6 Choosing the Ideal Incision

Choosing the right incision to approach the TMJ depends on the specific site which requires access, procedure planned and the available armamentarium. A simple flowchart to guide in choosing the ideal incision is given in Fig. 14.15.

Acknowledgments The authors would like to thank the contribution of Dr Logitha Sri, towards the illustration of Fig. 14.10.

References

1. Al-Kayat A, Bramley P. A modified pre-auricular approach to the temporomandibular joint and malar arch. Br J Oral Surg. 1979;17(2):91–103.

2. Rowe NL. Surgery of the temporomandibular joint. Proc R Soc Med. 1972;65(4):383–88.
3. Kreutziger KL. Surgery of the temporomandibular joint. I. Surgical anatomy and surgical incisions. Oral Surg Oral Med Oral Pathol. 1984;58(6):637–46.
4. Blair VP. Surgery and diseases of the mouth and jaws. 3rd ed. St Louis: The CV Mosby; 1917. p. 322–23.
5. Thoma KH. Oral surgery, vol. 1. St Louis: The CV Mosby; 1948. p. 634–43.
6. Dingman RO, Grabb WC. Intracapsular temporomandibular joint arthroplasty. Plast Reconstr Surg. 1966;38(3):179–85.
7. Popowich L, Crane RM Jr. Modified preauricular access to the temporomandibular apparatus. Experience with twenty-eight cases. Oral Surg Oral Med Oral Pathol. 1982;54(3):257–62.
8. Lempert J. Endaural, antauricular surgical approach to the temporal bone – principles involved in this new approach; summary report of 1,780 cases. Arch Otolaryngol. 1938;27(5):555–87.
9. Rongetti JR. Meniscectomy; a new approach to the temporomandibular joint. AMA Arch Otolaryngol. 1954;60(5):566–72.
10. Alexander RW, James RB. Postauricular approach for surgery of the temporomandibular articulation. J Oral Surg. 1975;33(5):346–50.
11. Block MS, Kent JN. Modified rhytidectomy approach for total temporomandibular joint reconstruction: a case report. J Oral Maxillofac Surg. 1989;47(2):187–90.

Internal Derangements of Temporomandibular Joint

15

Kishore Moturi

15.1 Introduction

Temporomandibular joint (TMJ) is one of the functionally complex joints in the human body. Intervening disc in the TMJ is an essential component for maintaining its normal function and should endure its dynamically anatomic position as well as shape for a balanced joint mechanics. Internal derangement (ID) of the TMJ is any interference with the smooth joint movement due to lost synchronization between the joint components. In the temporomandibular joint, the intervening disc lies between the condylar head and the articulating surface of the glenoid fossa in the temporal bone. In essence, condylar head articulates with the inferior surface of the fibrous disc and the cranial surface of the disc articulates with the glenoid fossa. The glenoid fossa in the temporal bone is a fixed bony landmark with disc and the condylar head of the mandible being dynamic in nature. The role of the disc is to maintain a functional pad between the superior temporal bone and the inferior head of the condyle during mandibular movements, effected by the movement at the temporomandibular joint bilaterally.

At rest and during initial pure joint rotation, when the mouth is closed or with slight opening, the disc rests between the condylar head and the bone of the glenoid fossa. Wider mouth opening is achieved by translation of the mandibular condyle in forward direction. At this dynamic state, the disc should accompany the head of the condyle and move anteriorly. Similarly, while closing the mouth, the disc should go back to its resting sandwich position smoothly. Disharmony in the dynamic functioning of the joint is referred to as internal derangement. It is synonymous with disc displacement/derangement (DD). Patients at onset or with initial progressive disharmonies may be symptom-free. When present, symptoms may range from pure joint sounds (click or a pop) to chronic pain with severely disturbed function. Muscle pain/tenderness, headache and disability including reduced jaw opening may add to a deterioration in quality of life for a patient with internal derangement of the temporomandibular joint [1].

Disc displacements (DD) are frequently divided into two broad classes:

1. DD with reduction (DDwR) (Fig. 15.1a, b)
2. DD without reduction (DDwoR) (Fig. 15.2a, b).

DDwR represents lost synchrony between the disc, condyle and the glenoid fossa, but the intervening disc manages to return to its functional position, on mandibular movements. Whereas, in cases with DDwoR, the disc does not return to its

K. Moturi (✉)
Department of Oral and Maxillofacial Surgery, Vishnu Dental College, Bhimavaram, Andhra Pradesh, India

D. Bhargava (ed.), *Temporomandibular Joint Disorders*,
https://doi.org/10.1007/978-981-16-2754-5_15

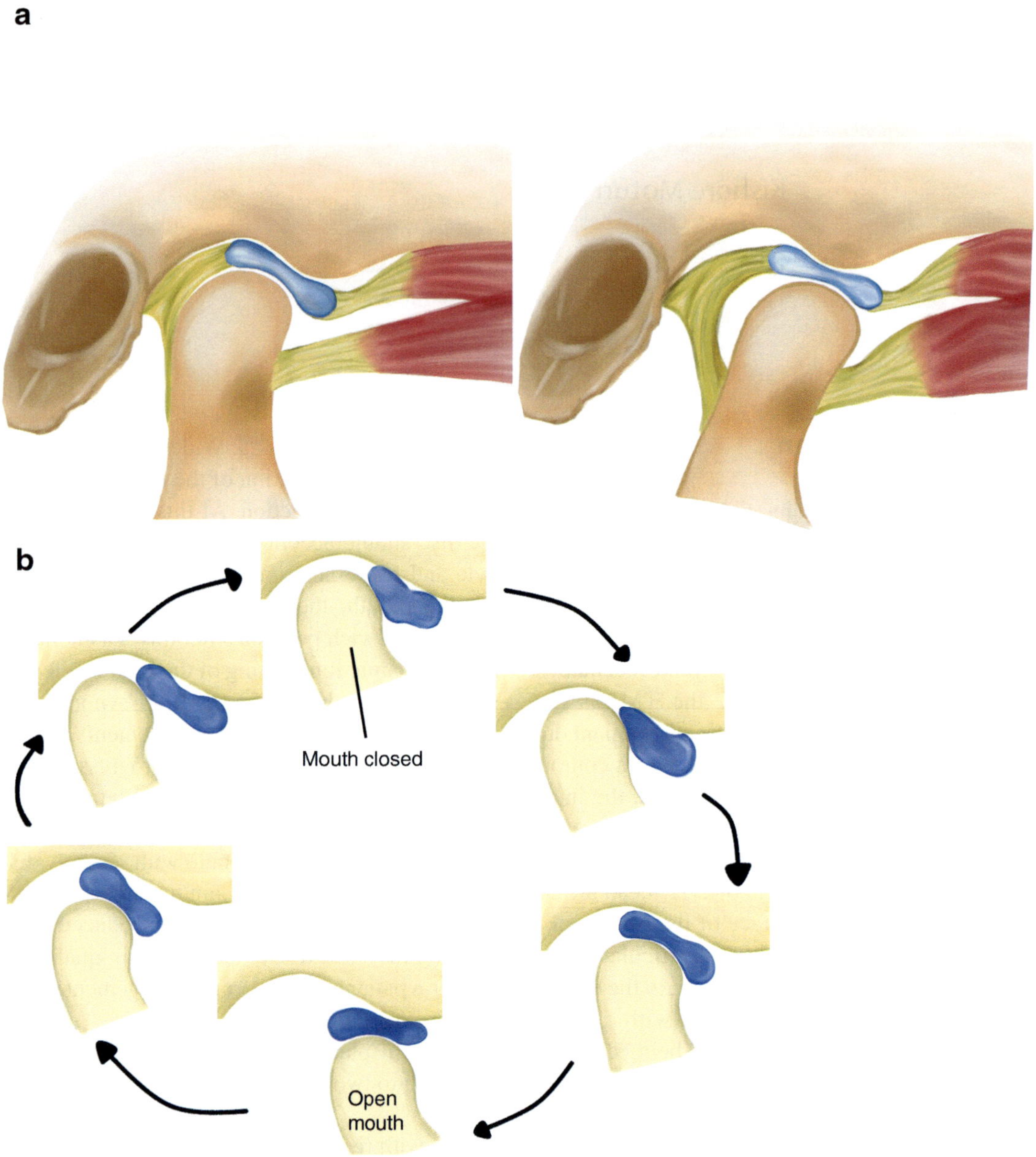

Fig. 15.1 (**a**) Relationship of the temporomandibular joint (TMJ) head to that of the discal tissue during closed and open mouth. (**b**) Anterior disc displacement with reduction

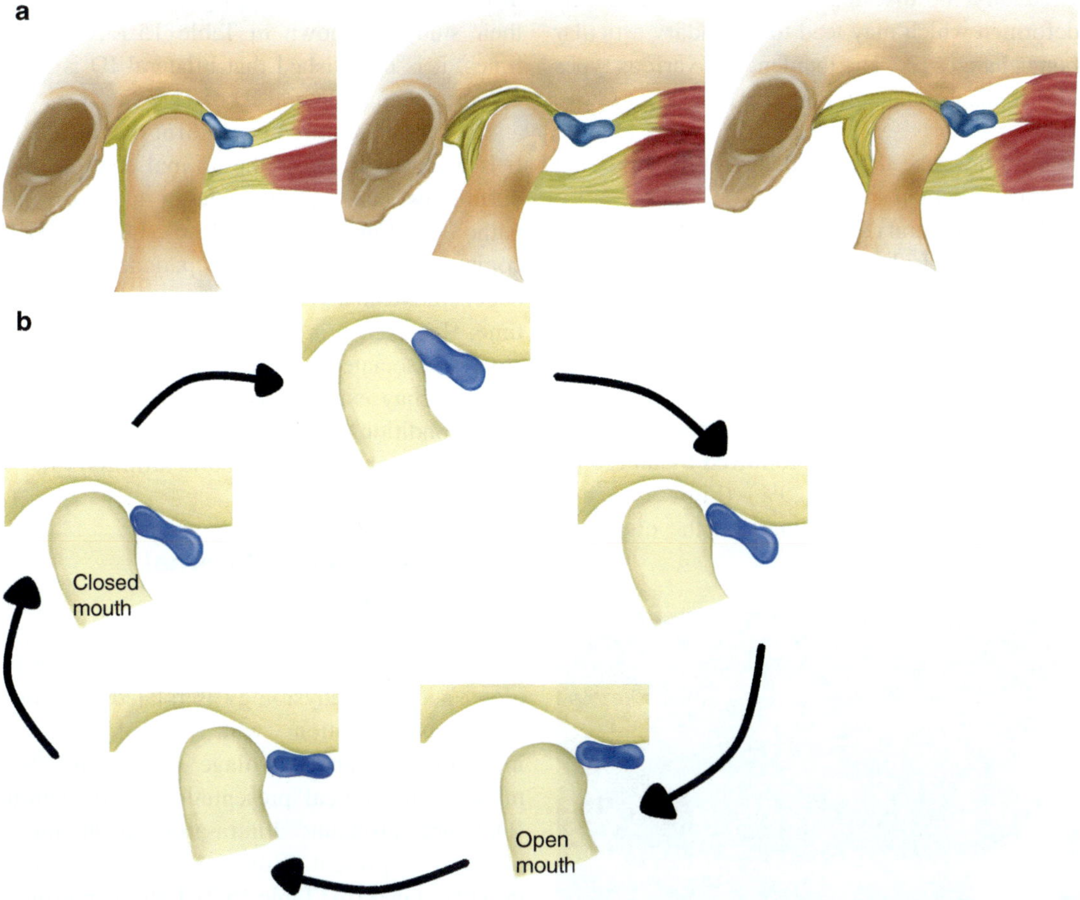

Fig. 15.2 (**a**) Disc displacement without reduction where the disc (blue) is seen to interfere with the condylar head. (**b**) Anterior disc displacement without reduction

functional or resting sandwich position between the condylar head and the glenoid fossa.

These derangements may further be divided into various sub-categories. The recently published Diagnostic Criteria for Temporomandibular Disorders (DC/TMD) has enumerated common intra-articular TMJ disorders such as DDwR, DDwR with intermittent locking, DDwoR with a limited opening, DDwoR without limited opening, degenerative joint disease (DJD) and sub-luxation.

15.1.1 Various Types of Disc Displacement

ID is usually a progressive disease process with the intervening disc displaced anterior, medial, lateral or posterior to its desired anatomic location in relation to the condylar head and the glenoid fossa at a resting closed mouth position. Initially, during the early course of this disharmony the intervening disc reduces to its functional position while opening the mouth.

Gradually the disc loses its elasticity and gets deformed which may lead to secondary articular bone changes [2]. The incidence of various types of disc displacement reported are:

1. Anterior disc displacement (80–90%), being most common
2. Medial/Lateral displacement (5%)
3. Posterior displacement (1%), least common
4. Stuck disc (4%)

Whyte et al. evaluated 288 displaced TMJ disc using magnetic resonance imaging (MRI) and concluded that anterior disc displacement (44%) is the most common type followed by anterolateral disc displacement (29%) (Figs. 15.3 and 15.4a, b). They also summarized the displaced disc position for bilateral, right and left TMJ in their study as shown in Table 15.1. In recent times, it is established that bilateral ID is more common than unilateral ID of TMJ [3, 4].

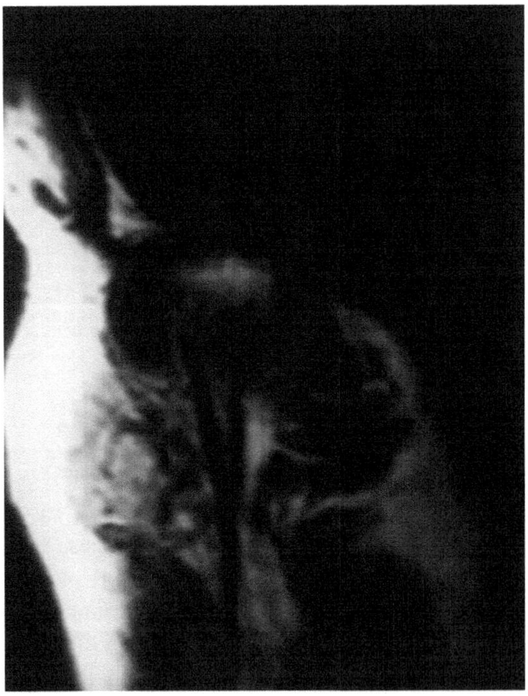

Fig. 15.3 Coronal T1-weighted magnetic resonance image (MRI) in closed-mouth position depicts lateral disc displacement, the disc crosses over the lines through the condylar poles. (Adapted with permission from Aoyama S, Kino K, Amagasa T, et al. Clinical and magnetic resonance imaging study of unilateral sideways disc displacements of the temporomandibular joint. J Med Dent Sci. 2002; 49(3):89–94)

Imaging is required to confirm the diagnosis. It is essential to know the normal disc position during rest and mouth opening to assess the pathology (Figs. 15.5 and 15.6). DD and DJD commonly co-exist. In some patients with DD, degenerative changes develop progressively with time. However, it is emphasized that DJD is not always associated with DD. Degenerative TMJ changes may exist solely or be associated with other conditions, such as systemic inflammatory joint disorders (e.g., rheumatoid arthritis) [5].

15.2 Aetiology of Internal Derangement

As the numerous emerging data suggest the aetiology and pathophysiology is related to a low-grade inflammation with the release of inflammatory and cartilage degrading biomarkers. In clinical presentations with painful ID, a more pronounced intra-articular inflammation may be present. Wilkes (1989) classified ID into five stages [6] (Table 15.2). Later Dimitroulis (2013) proposed the practical surgical classification for management of the TMJ disorders including ID [7] (Table 15.3). A new classification for juvenile anterior disc displacement has been proposed by Shen P et al. (2019) [8].

One of the common causes of ID is trauma which can be either micro- or macro-trauma [1]:

1. **Micro-trauma:** Excessive loading caused by para-functional habits, unstable occlusion, increased joint friction, hyper-mobility/subluxation of the joint cause prolonged repetitive atypical forces. If such force exceeds the physiologic limits, tissue degeneration is bound to occur.
2. **Macro-trauma:** Acute/Chronic trauma such as blow to the face, intubation induced trauma. There exists a balance between tissue breakdown and repair in synovial joints under normal physi-

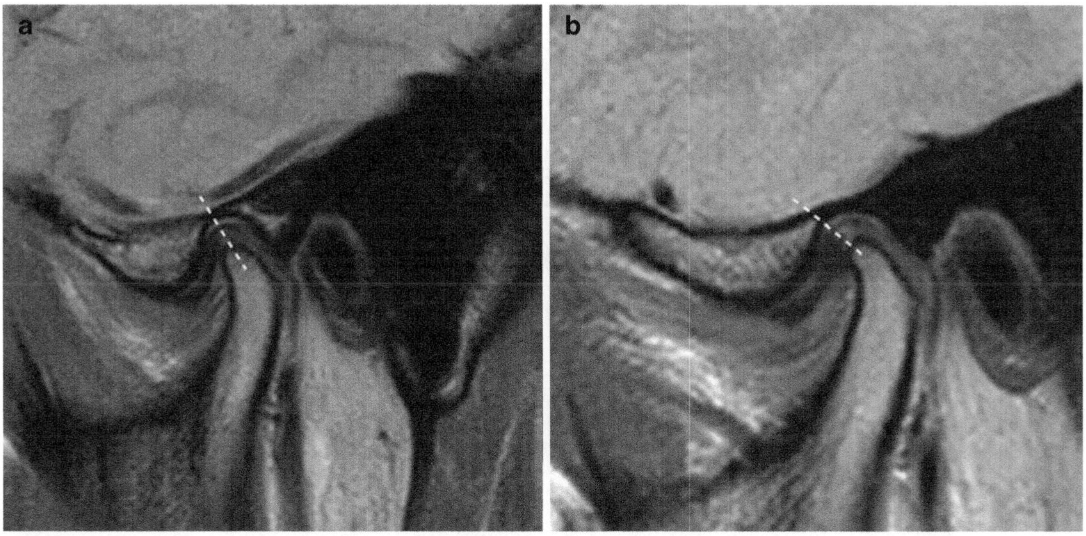

Fig. 15.4 (**a**, **b**) Same patient, right side (**a**) and left side (**b**). The disc can still be considered *non-dislocated* on the right side (**a**) since the border between the retrodiscal lamina and the posterior band lies at +15° (dotted line), even if the pars intermedia tends to slide anteriorly with respect to the condyle. The left disc instead (**b**) is dislocated. In fact, the border between the retrodiscal lamina and the posterior band lies at approximately +40° (dotted line), and the pars intermedia is not found between condyle and eminence any longer. [Reprinted/adapted by permission from Tanteri C., Robba T., Cimino R., Tanteri G. (2020) Joint Disorders. In: Robba T., Tanteri C., Tanteri G. (eds) MRI of the Temporomandibular Joint. Springer, Cham. https://doi.org/10.1007/978-3-030-25421-6_7]

Table 15.1 Summary of displaced disc in bilateral, right and left temporomandibular joint by Whyte AM et al.

Disc position/displacement	Bilateral (288 joints)	Right TMJ (143 joints)	Left TMJ (144 joints)
Normal	17%	20%	15%
Anterior	44%	40%	49%
Medial	1%	1%	1%
Lateral	3%	4%	2%
Antero-lateral	29%	30%	27%
Antero-medial	6%	5%	6%

ologic condition. If this balance is disrupted, it results in an increased tissue breakdown. It can contribute to the disc displacement due to stretching/tearing of the retro-discal tissue.

In the intra-articular compartment, an incessant process balances the free radical formation and neutralizing mechanisms. Local hypoxia occurs if there is increased mechanical loading in the joint. Increase in hypoxic cells in turn increases the free radical production leading to degradation of hyaluronic acid, which is an essential component of synovial fluid impairing the lubrication of the joint. This leads to indecorous friction between the joint components causing adhesions and DD [1] (Fig. 15.7).

15.3 Diagnosis of ID of TMJ

15.3.1 Clinical Examination

The common signs and symptoms include:

1. Pain/tenderness in the pre-auricular or TMJ region
2. Reduced mouth opening (Normal inter-incisal opening: 35–50 mm)

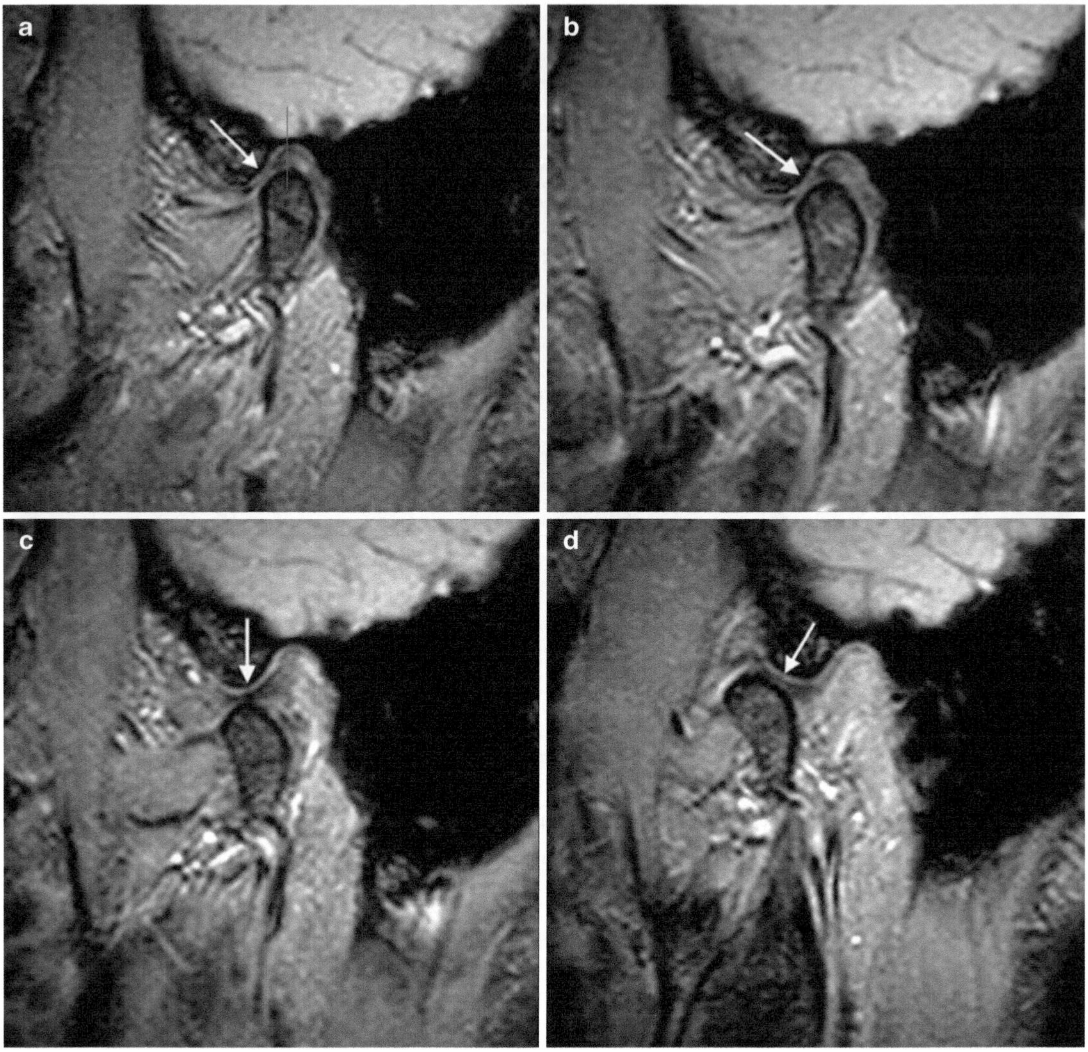

Fig. 15.5 Sequences of four images (**a–d**) have been selected from a kinematic-MR and show sequences from inter-cuspation (closed mouth) to maximum opening. During excursion, the pars intermedia of the disc (arrow) is constantly found between condyle and tubercle. Note that in normal conditions the disc will show mobility with respect to the condyle and the tubercle, thus resting between the two at all times, as shown in kinematic MRI images. At inter-cuspation (**a**), the pars intermedia is between the eminence and the condylar head (*arrow*), and the border between the retro-discal lamina and the posterior band lies at 12 o'clock (*blue line*) and the condyle-disc complex is cantered with respect to the fossa. Note the disc position, (**a**) at intercuspation (closed mouth); (**b**) on early opening of mouth – corresponding to rotation; (**c**) wider opening – corresponding to translation; (**d**) on maximum opening. [Reprinted/adapted by permission from Tanteri C., Robba T., Cimino R., Tanteri G. (2020) Joint Disorders. In: Robba T., Tanteri C., Tanteri G. (eds) MRI of the Temporomandibular Joint. Springer, Cham. https://doi.org/10.1007/978-3-030-25421-6_7]

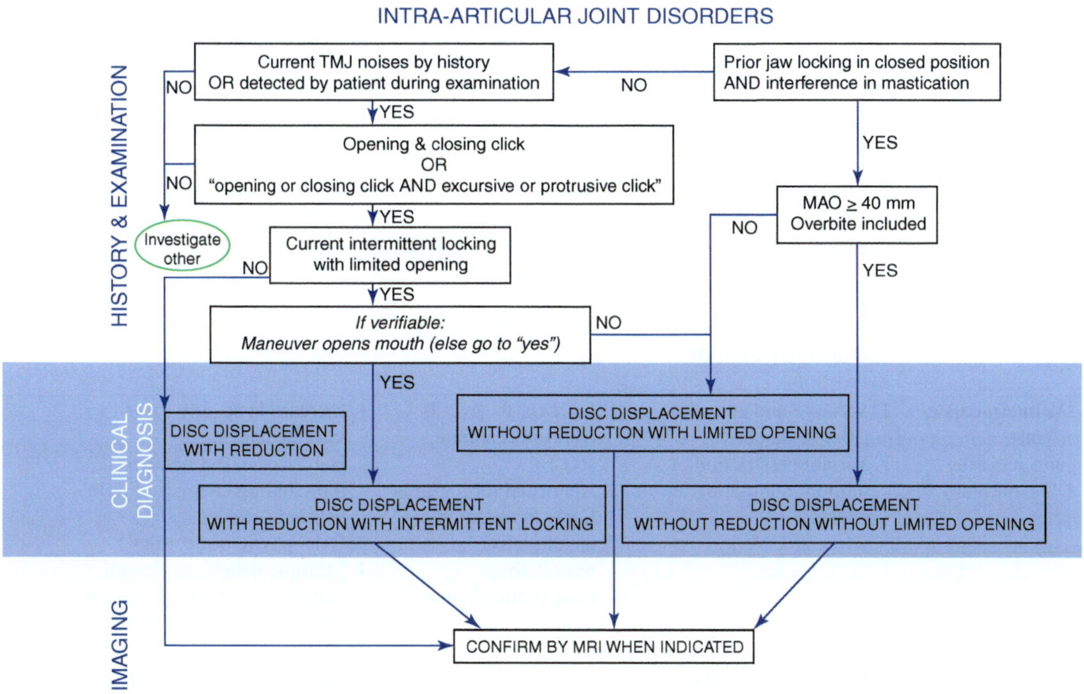

Fig. 15.6 Diagnostic flowchart based on history and clinical examination for disc displacements according to the TMD-diagnostic criteria. [Reprinted/adapted by permission from Tanteri C., Robba T., Cimino R., Tanteri G. (2020) Joint Disorders. In: Robba T., Tanteri C., Tanteri G. (eds) MRI of the Temporomandibular Joint. Springer, Cham. https://doi.org/10.1007/978-3-030-25421-6_7]

Table 15.2 Staging criteria for internal derangement of the temporomandibular joint by Wilkes CH (1989)

	Findings		
Stage	Clinical	Radiologic	Surgical
I. Early (early reducing DD)	1. No significant symptoms 2. Reciprocal clicking (early in opening movement, late in closing movement, and soft in intensity) 3. No pain or limitation of motion	1. Slight forward displacement 2. Good anatomical contour of disc 3. Normal tomograms	1. Normal anatomical form 2. Slight anterior displacement 3. Passive in-coordination (clicking) demonstrable
II. Early/intermediate (late reducing DD)	1. Few episodes of pain 2. Occasional joint tenderness and related temporal headaches 3. Initiation of major mechanical problems 4. Increase in intensity of clicking sounds 5. Joint sounds later in opening movement 6. Beginning of transient sub-luxation/joint catching and locking	1. Slight forward displacement 2. Slight thickening of posterior edge/beginning anatomical deformity of disc 3. Normal tomograms	1. Anterior displacement 2. Early anatomical deformity (slight to mild thickening of posterior edge) 3. Well-defined central articulating area

(continued)

Table 15.2 (continued)

Stage	Findings: Clinical	Radiologic	Surgical
III. Intermediate (Non-reducing DD—acute/ sub-acute)	1. Multiple pain episodes 2. Joint tenderness, temporal headaches 3. Major mechanical symptoms—transient catching, locking and sustained locking (closed locks) 4. Restriction of motion difficulty/pain with function	1. Anterior displacement with significant anatomical deformity 2. Prolapse of disc (moderate to marked thickening of posterior edge) 3. Normal tomograms	1. Marked anatomical deformity with displacement 2. Variable adhesions (anterior, lateral, and posterior recesses) 3. No hard-tissue changes
IV. Intermediate/ late (non-reducing DD—chronic)	1. Variable and episodic pain, headaches 2. Variable restriction of motion, undulating course	1. Increase in severity over intermediate stage 2. Abnormal tomograms 3. Early to moderate degenerative remodelling hard-tissue changes	1. Increase in severity over intermediate stage 2. Hard-tissue degenerative remodelling changes of both bearing surfaces 3. Osteophytic projections 4. Multiple adhesions (lateral, anterior, and posterior recesses) 5. No perforation of disc or attachment
V. Late (non-reducing DD with osteoarthritis)	1. It is characterized by crepitus on examination, scraping, grating, grinding symptoms 2. Variable and episodic pain 3. Chronic restriction of motion 4. Difficulty with function	1. Anterior displacement 2. Perforation with simultaneous filling of upper/lower compartments 3. Gross anatomical deformity of disc and hard tissues 4. Abnormal tomograms 5. Degenerative arthritic changes	1. Gross degenerative changes of disc and hard tissues 2. Perforation of posterior attachments 3. Erosions of bearing surfaces 4. Multiple adhesions equivalent to degenerative arthritis (sclerosis, flattening, anvil-shaped condyle, osteophytic projections, and subcortical cystic formation)

Table 15.3 TMJ surgical classification by Dimitroulis G (2013)

Category	TMJ condition	Management
1	Normal	Painful joint, joint shows normal smooth joint function Radiology confirms no joint pathology Surgical intervention is contra-indicated
2	Minor changes All components salvageable	Early stage ID of TMJ may result in closed lock. Arthrocentesis/arthroscopic lavage may be helpful in releasing the joint
3	Moderate changes Mostly salvageable	Non-reducing DD, recurrent TMJ dislocation where TMJ arthroscopy/ TMJ arthroplasty/disc repositioning may be appropriate
4	Severe changes Partly salvageable	Severely displaced/deformed discs resulting in a chronic pain and limited mouth opening Disc cannot be salvaged and require discectomy
5	Catastrophic changes Nothing is salvageable	End-stage joint disease such as severe osteoarthritis, ankylosis Best treated with total joint replacement

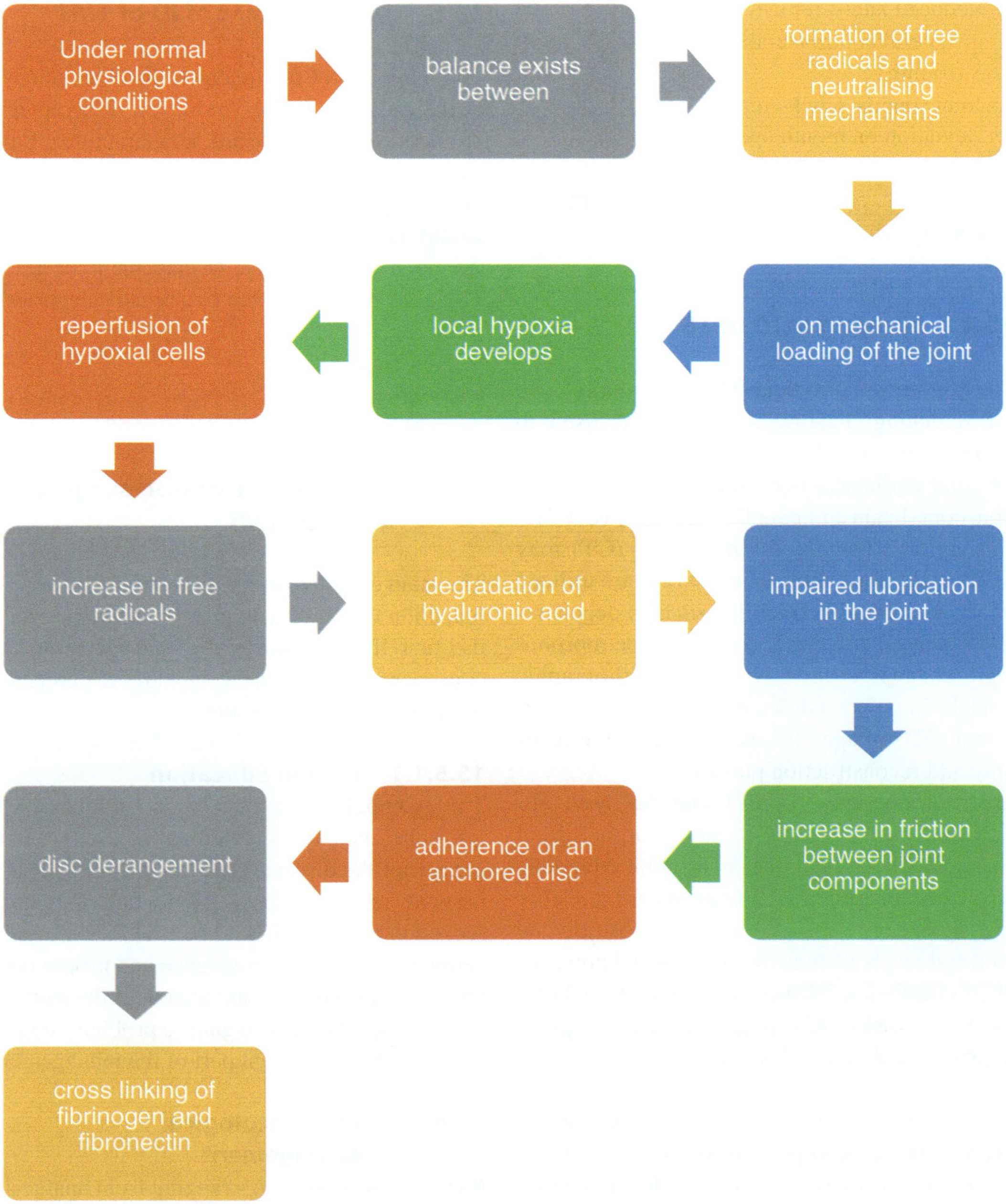

Fig. 15.7 Pathophysiology of internal derangement

3. Reduced latero-retrusive movements (Normal ipsilateral/contralateral movements of joint: 5–10 mm)
4. Joint sounds: Click/crepitation
5. Deviation on mouth opening
6. Locking
7. Presence of masticatory/cervical muscle tenderness

15.4 Imaging in ID of TMJ

The conventional radiographs are initially used for screening. Panoramic imaging is used to examine the condyle, glenoid fossa and the articular eminence. For a more detailed evaluation, cone-beam computed tomography (CBCT)/ conventional computed tomography (CT) may be advised. Bone study using X-rays are utilized to access joint abnormalities such as degenerative changes, osteoarthritis and other morphologic changes accurately. A stereolithographic model can be pre-fabricated using three-dimensional (3D) images for evaluation of the anatomy and reconstruction purposes.

Ultrasonography (USG) can be used for screening and to assess any morphological changes and the soft tissues of the joint. Magnetic resonance imaging (MRI) is a standard modality to visualize retro-discal tissue, disc position and morphology, bone marrow changes and presence of joint effusion. Newer advancement includes the use of MRI-CBCT image fusion technique to improve reliability and accuracy of disc position assessment. Real-time imaging using MRI allows to record data regarding the dynamics of entire articular components during jaw movement which is more consistent in diagnosing ID (Figs. 15.4 and 15.5).

If there is suspicion of systemic involvement (such as rheumatoid arthritis or juvenile idiopathic arthritis), appropriate tests such as human leukocyte antigen-B27, anti-nuclear factors and rheumatoid factors should be ordered [9].

15.5 Management of ID of TMJ

The main aim of the treatment involves removal of the causative factors, reduction of symptoms, promote healing of the articular structures. Early stages of ID can be managed by conservative or minimally invasive methods. Advanced stages would require surgical interventions including the open joint surgery. Management of ID of TMJ may be divided into two broad categories:

- Non-surgical
- Surgical

15.5.1 Conservative or Non-surgical Management

The main objective of the conservative therapy is reduction of joint loading and pain. It is usually the first line of therapeutic management. The conservative management includes a number of different treatment modalities.

15.5.1.1 Patient Education

The essential aspect of a treatment starts with informing the patient regarding the cause, pathogenesis of the disease. Diet modification, awareness of para-functional habits and the stress reduction protocols should be established by educating the patient. Re-assurance and proper communication from the clinician reduce the patient's anxiety regarding the diagnosed problem. It is the first and most important part of the management.

15.5.1.2 Pharmacological Management

It includes various drugs ranging from analgesics to immune suppressing agents such as corticosteroids. Ordinarily, management of TMDs require a combination of various group of drugs.

Analgesic drug Non-steroidal anti-inflammatory drugs (NSAIDs) are commonly used for the pain and/or inflammation reduction. In cases where NSAIDs are contraindicated, opioids may be utilized with the limitation to its anti-inflammatory property.

Muscle relaxants They reduce localized muscular spasms, which may be secondary to or leading to ID.

Chondro-protective drugs It aids in restoring the metabolic balance in articular cartilage.

Anti-anxiety and anti-depressants Anxiety, depression and stress are found to be associated with TMDs. Anti-anxiety and anti-depressants drugs resolve stress induced TMDs. They also act as an adjunct to improve sleep and reduce stress related para-functional habits. Benzodiazepines are potent group of drugs that can aid in reducing the muscle tonicity, when required.

Systemic corticosteroids Though rarely used for ID, may be utilized for its strong anti-inflammatory properties through leukotriene pathway suppression.

15.5.1.3 Thermotherapy

Thermal stimuli in the form of heat or cold application can be done in ID cases. Heat is frequently used in the form of hot compresses. Application of moist hot fomentation on the symptomatic area for 10–15 min not more than 30 min is beneficial. The primary goal is to increase blood supply through vasodilatation, leading to decreased pain and joint stiffness.

Cold compression reduces transmission of impulse by the nerve endings causing decreased perception of pain. It causes local vasoconstriction. The use of cold compress includes fomentation using an ice pack or cooling sprays such as ethyl chloride and fluoro-methane [9].

15.5.1.4 Physiotherapy

Physiotherapy is a common therapeutic method indicated in discopathy and hyper-mobility of TMJ. It helps in improving the strength of articular capsule, along with the improvement in the desired crusade of the masticatory/cervical muscles. The exercises should be performed at short intervals and multiple times daily than once a day for a longer period as it can cause overload of the joint and progression of pain. It should be performed to limit the pain and patient should not try to overcome pain by movement. It is essential to perform passive motion exercise for at least 2 months in the post-surgical period.

Manual therapy involves a group of supportive activities as an adjunct to the definitive treatment. It can enhance the outcome of the management for TMDs. They offer best outcomes when selected appropriately and combined with the customized need of a particular patient. The various techniques performed for the soft tissue or joint mobilization and muscle conditioning include deep massage, gentle distraction of the joint, passive or assisted muscle stretching, resistance exercise, postural training for aligning head, neck and shoulders.

1. **Isometric exercise:** Patient places the hand beneath the chin and starts exercising against palm resistance by slowly opening the mouth. It aids in strengthening of the active muscles and the articular capsule involved.
2. **Repositioning exercise:** It is indicated for alignment of dislocated disc and jaw mobilization.
3. **Massage of masticatory muscles:** It helps to improve blood flow enhancing muscles function and decreasing the pain. It contributes to movement co-ordination and stretching of spastic muscles. It can also be used for post-operative mouth opening.

15.5.1.5 Intraoral Appliance

Use of an intraoral orthodontic appliance finds application in management of many TMJ disorders. Specific malocclusions include the absence of posterior support, loss of vertical dimension of occlusion resulting in mandibular over closure and severe class II division II malocclusions benefit from an appliance therapy. Para-functional habits cause loss of occlusion from teeth wear. Using an intraoral appliance such as night guard in patients with known clenching/bruxism protects the dentition from wear, decreases the muscle hyperactivity to some degree and alters the joint loading, thereby improving the symptoms.

15.5.1.6 Occlusal Splints

It is a removable appliance with a thickness of 1.5–3 mm commonly made from acrylic resin. The splints can be fabricated for maxilla/mandible and can be partial/complete. It aids in reduction of the intra-articular pressure reducing overload and pain, balancing and deprograming occlusion, thus reducing the muscle spasm. The potential disadvantage of splint is, its long-term use can cause a malocclusion. Considerations for constructing an occlusal splint include

1. Symmetrical, bilateral articulating contacts of maxilla/mandible
2. Smooth edges
3. Proper retention
4. Should not irritate periodontal tissues. It should cover only the teeth
5. It should not cause functional obstacle by restricting tongue movement, phonation and deglutition.

Common types of occlusal splints that are put to use for treating various TMDs include: Stabilization splint, anterior repositioning splint and a soft or a resilient splint.

15.5.1.7 Diagnostic Blocks

Blocking the nerves supplying the TMJ with local anaesthetic solution (LA) can be an essential diagnostic aid to determine if this joint is the primary source of pain and if related areas of referred pain exist. Block can be accomplished through either intra- or extra-capsular injection.

Epinephrine containing aesthetic solutions should generally be avoided to prevent vasoconstriction in areas where circulation may already be compromised because of chronic muscle contraction or a spasm and presence of an on-going inflammatory process. An attempt to distinguish a local muscle soreness, muscle spasm and locating the trigger points can be made using local anaesthetics.

15.5.1.8 Ultrasound Therapy

It has the same concept of thermotherapy, but is found to be more effective as it acts on deeper tissues and not just the surface. Ultrasound not only increases the blood flow in deep tissues but also seems to separate collagen fibres, which improve the flexibility and extensibility of connective tissues, decrease joint stiffness, provide pain relief, improve mobility and reduce muscle spasm. Studies indicate that ultrasound therapy is effective in relieving myofascial pain caused by TMJ [10].

15.5.1.9 Trans-cutaneous Electrical Nerve Stimulation (TENS)

Electric stimulation devices for treatment of TMD are claimed to have two primary purposes of relieving pain and muscle hyperactivity or spasm. But studies have proved that TENS can be used only as an adjunct to other treatment modalities and not as the only treatment method [10, 11].

15.5.1.10 LASER (Light Amplification by Stimulated Emission of Radiation)

Low-level laser therapy (LLLT) may help in repair of tissues by its action as an analgesic and an anti-inflammatory. It claims to stimulate blood flow to tissues, increases lymphatic drainage and reduces muscle contraction. But the long-term effectiveness of LLLT in managing TMDs remains limited [12, 13].

15.5.1.11 Acupuncture

Acupuncture is a lesser known modality to relieve pain in TMJ disorder but there exist few reports pointing towards its effectiveness in selected cases [13, 14].

15.5.2 Surgical Treatment

Surgery to the TMJ plays an essential role in the management of patients who have late or advanced stage ID. Surgical intervention is generally indicated when non-surgical therapy is ineffective and is usually avoided for asymptomatic or minimally symptomatic cases. ID of TMJ is not considered

Table 15.4 Surgical management for ID of the TMJ

Surgical procedure	Techniques
Closed/minimally invasive technique	
Arthrocentesis	Single puncture Double puncture
Arthroscopy	Diagnostic followed by therapeutic Discopexy
Open technique	
Disc plication	Partial Complete
Discopexy	Temporal supported Mitek anchor
Lysis of adhesions in superior and inferior joint spaces without disc repositioning	Can be undertaken in conjunction with eminoplasty
Meniscectomy (discectomy) without replacement	Platelet-rich plasma injection, may be utilized simultaneously to prevent dead space formation
Meniscectomy with replacement	*Autogenous material* (a) Auricular cartilage (b) Temporalis muscle/fascia (c) Dermal graft *Alloplastic material* (a) PTFE interpositional implants (b) Silicone pull out implants
Condylotomy	Conventional Intra-oral condylotomy Closed condylotomy (Kostecka's technique)

as a condition of TMJ disc alone but of the entire joint and associated structures. Patients categorized to the initial stages of Wilkes classification can be managed effectively with conservative to minimally invasive modalities. Advanced and non-salvageable stages may require open joint surgeries. The various techniques include minimally invasive to open surgical procedures which are discussed as under (Table 15.4).

15.5.2.1 Arthrocentesis

Arthrocentesis is a least invasive and an effective procedure performed for the ID of TMJ consisting of joint lavage and administration of medications into the joint [15]. It is usually an office-based procedure under local anaesthesia (LA) occasionally assisted with conscious sedation. This technique involves the insertion of two adequate-gauge needles into the superior joint space of the TMJ in a double puncture technique. Through the first or an inflow needle, 100–300 ml of Ringer's lactate solution is injected into the superior joint space. The second needle acts as an outflow portal allowing lavage of the joint cavity.

Steroids, sodium hyaluronate or platelet rich plasma (PRP) may be injected at the end of the lavage to alleviate intra-capsular inflammation and improve joint function. The patient is placed on a soft diet and physiotherapy for a few days after the procedure with regular follow-up. The main goal of arthrocentesis is lysis of the adhesions and lavage of the joint, to flush the inflammatory mediators and reduce the intra-articular oxidative stress. Various techniques have been described to execute arthrocentesis which may depend on the number of joint access points, single puncture technique or double puncture technique (Refer Chap. 19).

15.5.2.2 Arthroscopy

Arthroscopy is another treatment modality employed in the management of ID of TMJ. It involves the use of endoscope introduced into the joint cavity which allows the intra-articular examination or treatment. Usually a diameter of 1.9–2.7 mm endoscope is used to perform TMJ arthroscopy. It is as effective and sometimes superior to arthrocentesis to remove articular adhesions, improve function and reduces pain in ID. It can be diagnostic or therapeutic (Refer Chaps. 20 and 21).

15.5.2.3 Diagnostic Arthroscopy

It aids in visualization of various areas in the joint space subsequently allowing lysis of the adhesions and lavage of the joint. Diagnosis of the stage of the ID, changes in the synovium caused by the inflammation can be identified and recorded followed by administration of medicaments into the joint space. Patients with DDwoR may present with pronounced fibrous adhesions and enhanced inflammatory changes. Lysis and lavage under arthroscopic view is effective in such patients provided ID (DDwoR) is of shorter duration.

15.5.2.4 Surgical Arthroscopy

It involves performing a surgical intervention in and around the joint under arthroscopic view.

Along with the endoscope, surgical instruments such as needles and knifes for releasing, hooks, probes, scissors, forceps or shavers are introduced into the joint through a separate surgical working port. It may be employed to remove adhesions, repair the disc, disc recapitulation/plication, synovectomy, discectomy and eminectomy. Specimens also can be obtained for histopathologic examination under arthroscopic view [9, 15].

15.5.2.5 Open Surgical Methods

The various open surgical methods for ID of TMJ are listed in Table 15.4. They are aimed to effectively reduce pain and increase the range of motion in the post-operative period. For an open arthroplasty procedure, the joint is exposed after layered dissection through a pre-auricular incision (Refer Chap. 14). Following adequate manipulation of the mandible, the lateral pole of the condyle can be palpated with capsular depression evident between the glenoid fossa and the lateral pole. A small incision is placed in the lateral capsule after administration of LA to enter the superior joint space which is confirmed by the presence of the synovial fluid. Depressing the posterior mandible increases the joint space at this stage. Further incising results in the visualization of the superior aspect of entire disc along with the anterior and posterior recess.

A freer elevator should be used to break adhesions by sweeping across gently. Care should be taken to note the position and function of the disc along its medial-lateral dimension during mouth opening and closing movements. If both the disc and condyle function properly, the joint space is irrigated thoroughly followed by closure. If there are presence of adhesions/deformities in the inferior joint space, they should be removed/contoured followed by copious irrigation while the condyle is retracted inferiorly and anteriorly [16, 17].

15.5.2.6 Disc Plication

It may be a partial or a complete plication procedure. In partial disc plication, a small wedge-shaped (pie shaped) tissue is removed followed by repositioning the disc in a posterior and lateral plane. Contrary to this, a full wedge of retro-discal tissue is removed and disc repositioning is done by suturing the salvaged retro-discal tissue to the posterior ligament for complete plication. Repair is usually performed using 4-0 resorbable suture. If there is still an obstruction in the mandibular movement, the surgeon may opt to undertake an eminoplasty [17].

15.5.2.7 Discopexy

After entering the superior and inferior joint space, lysis of adhesions is performed followed by freeing the displaced disc. A small hole is made in the postero-anterior direction in the lateral condylar pole. A 3-0 non-resorbable suture is placed through the hole and the disc at the junction of anterior and intermediate bands. The success of this procedure depends on the degree of deformity and extent of degenerative changes. The same procedure can be performed by using Mitek anchors. It can secure the disc in a more physiologic position. It involves a metal insert into the condylar head with a suture attached to it (Refer Chap. 18) [17, 18].

15.5.2.8 Discectomy (Meniscectomy) Without Replacement

It is performed when the disc is irreparable and is considered as the main treatment modality after failure of non-surgical and arthroscopic interventions and even in the presence of disc perforations. The central avascular part of the disc and perforated area are removed. It is difficult to remove the medial part of the discal tissue. To control haemorrhage, thrombin-soaked sponges or LA containing epinephrine may be used. A Wilkes retractor can be used to push the condyle in an antero-inferior direction providing maximum access to the medial part of the disc. Care should be taken not to extend the incision through the medial capsular wall to prevent damage to the middle meningeal artery.

A temporary silicone implant placement may be considered to prevent any adhesion between condyle and the glenoid fossa. It also aids in formation of fibrous tissue lining. The implant is usually removed after 6–12 weeks. Although, may be retained for several months post-operatively without any adverse reactions unless if any.

Another feasible option instead of an alloplastic material is to inject autogenous platelet rich plasma (PRP) or use platelet rich fibrin into the joint space. It prevents the formation of dead space and promotes healing as it contains various growth factors and has a wound healing potential [17, 19].

15.5.2.9 Discectomy with Replacement

There are several autogenous and alloplastic materials available to replace the disc after meniscectomy. Although, many patients do not require any tissue replacement and perform well in the long term. Several investigators have tried various replacement materials to reconstruct the disc after surgery. The commonly used materials include autogenous grafts like dermal graft, auricular cartilage graft and temporalis muscle or fascia.

Dermal Graft

A full thickness graft involving both the epidermis and dermis can be harvested from the thigh or abdomen using a 15# bard parker blade. The harvested graft should be larger than the defect as it can contract during harvesting and handling before replacing. It should be harvested from non-hair bearing areas. It may also be harvested using a dermatome [17, 20].

Auricular Cartilage Graft

A posterior approach may be used to harvest an auricular cartilage that will leave a minimal scar. While using the anterior approach, incision should be placed between the anti-helix and outer helix. The rim of the anterior helix should not be violated during the graft harvest. The cartilage should be harvested in a curvilinear shape to match the glenoid fossa contour [17].

Temporalis Muscle/Fascia

The temporalis myofascial flap is a full thickness flap harvested using an preauricular or an endaural incision extending to the temporal region for 2–3 cm. The distal width of the inferiorly based flap should be wider than the actual dimensions of the joint space to compensate for the contraction. The dimensions of the flap are approximately 5–6 cm in length and 3 cm in width. The flap is rotated over the zygomatic arch laterally and lined into the glenoid fossa and secured with multiple 4-0 chromic/polyglactin 910 sutures [17].

15.5.2.10 Condylotomy

Condylotomy was described as a sub-condylar osteotomy mimicking a displaced sub-condylar fracture. This technique can be used in cases of ID instead of routine intra-capsular disc repositioning techniques. It was popularized by Hall and other investigators with several modifications. Following this procedure, patients should be kept under intermaxillary fixation (IMF) for 7 days followed by physiotherapy and inter-arch elastics [17, 21].

In 1928, the classic closed condylotomy was proposed by Kostecka, demonstrating a high vertical oblique osteotomy cut bilaterally on the condylar neck. Modifications of the technique were given by Ward, Smith and Sommer (1957), Banks and McKenzie (1975) who advocated a more vertical and less oblique condylotomy. A modified condylotomy technique was proposed by Upton and Sullivan (1991) by performing an osteotomy cut from the most anterior aspect of the sigmoid notch to angle of the mandible as it facilitates the overlapping of the condylar and distal segment. An intraoral sub-condylar condylotomy was performed by Shevel E (1991) [21–26].

Numerous authors have proposed newer technical modifications which involve use of the resorbable pins and newer suturing techniques for disc repositioning. These modifications are being investigated to improve the treatment outcome in such patients [27–33].

15.5.2.11 Orthognathic Surgery

With advancements in surgical procedures involving the jaws, interventions such as bilateral sagittal split osteotomy (BSSO) and the intraoral vertical ramus osteotomy (IVRO) to address the skeletal malocclusion in patients diagnosed with TMDs have been reported. The main goal should be to identify and correct the symptomatic TMDs along with the dento-facial deformity contributing to the cause (Fig. 15.8). Care should be taken to prevent and manage any intra-operative or post-operative complications and the risk of relapse. The patients diagnosed with class III skeletal malocclusion are least likely of all jaw relationships to have pre-operative TMDs. Literature suggests IVRO as the

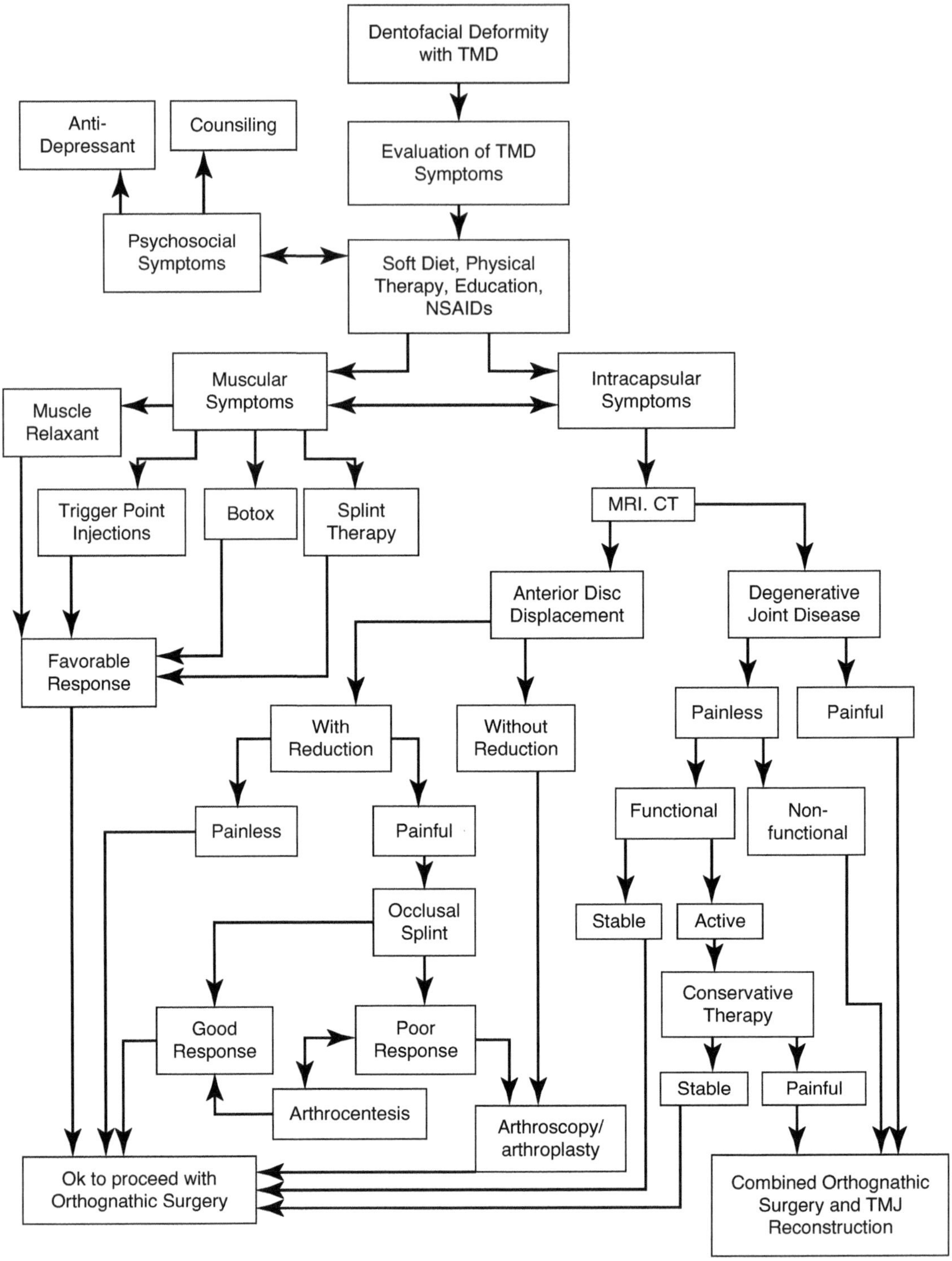

Fig. 15.8 Flow diagram and treatment algorithm for patients with a dento-facial deformity and TMD symptoms. (Reprinted from Orthognathic Surgery, Vol 26/Issue 4, John C. Nale, Orthognathic Surgery and the Temporomandibular Joint Patient, Pg.554., Copyright (2014), with permission from Elsevier)

technique of choice in TMD patients with a Class II skeletal malocclusion causing an anterior and inferior displacement of the condyle which increases the joint space and disc reduction in joints with disc displacement with reduction or recent progression to a disc displacement without reduction. Occasionally, patient may present with both skeletal-facial deformity and end-stage TMJ disease where orthognathic surgery along with an alloplastic total joint reconstruction (TJR) for TMJ may be considered (Refer Chap. 22).

The role of orthognathic surgery in the treatment of TMD has been debated for years due to the difficulty to establish a cause-and-effect relationship between orthognathic surgery and improvement in signs and symptoms owing to the multi-factorial nature of TMDs [34].

15.6 Conclusion

Post-operative follow-up and care is an essential aspect in managing patients diagnosed with ID of TMJ. Patient counselling, diet modification, pharmacological and minimally invasive management protocols usually provide relief to majority of the patients. In cases where surgery is required, early aggressive physiotherapy and rehabilitation of the joint improves the outcome.

15.7 Definitions

1. Internal derangement is a localized mechanical fault interfering with the smooth action of a joint—Hey and Davies, 1814
2. Internal derangement is a disturbance in the healthy anatomic relationship between the disc and condyle which interferes with the smooth movement of the joint and causes momentary catching, clicking, popping, or locking—Laskin DM, 1994
3. Internal derangement is defined as any interference with smooth joint movement—de Leeuw R, 2008 [1]
4. Disc derangement (DD) is a malpositioning of the articular disc relative to the condyle and eminence
5. DD with reduction (DDwR) is a condition where the articular disc resumes its normal position on top of the condyle on mouth opening
6. DD without reduction (DDwoR) is a condition where the articular disc remains malpositioned on opening attempts, resulting in restricted mouth opening in acute cases
7. Disc adherence is a temporary sticking of the disc either to the fossa or to the condyle
8. Disc adhesion is a fibrotic connection between the disc and the condyle or the disc and the fossa
9. Subluxation (hyper-mobility) is an over extension of the disc–condyle complex on mouth opening, beyond the articular eminence
10. Joint dislocation is the dislocation of the entire disc–condyle complex beyond the eminence combined with the inability to return passively into the fossa
11. Discopexy is a disc tie-down procedure that anchors the disc to a condyle or fossa purchase point using a suture/pin/screw/anchor
12. Disc Plication is the surgical repositioning of disc by suturing it to retro-discal and/or lateral capsular tissue
13. Discoplasty is the repair of small perforation in the disc accompanied by degenerative changes by sutures in young patients
14. Discectomy/Meniscectomy is the removal of the discal tissue in the presence of extensive disc perforation or in ID patients with no improvement from conservative/minimally invasive methods.
15. Condyloplasty is the process of contouring the condylar surface when it is rough and uneven.
16. Condylar shaving is the removal of 3–5 mm bone from the superior surface of the condyle
17. Condylotomy is creating an osteotomy cut at the different levels of sub-condylar/ramus region to mimic a sub-condylar fracture
18. Condylectomy is the removal of condyle when the joint cannot be salvaged.

Acknowledgements 1. *V. Vidya Devi*, Consultant Medical Illustrator for the project, Senior Lecturer, Oral & Maxillofacial Surgery, Kamineni Institute of Dental Sciences. Sreepuram, Narketpally 508254 Nalgonda (dist), Telangana, India. 2. *Kalyani Muddapu*, for literature Search, Consultant Maxillofacial Surgery, Vishakapatnam, Andhra Pradesh, India.

References

1. de Leeuw R. Internal derangements of the temporomandibular joint. Oral Maxillofac Surg Clin North Am. 2008;20(2):159–68.
2. Aoyama S, Kino K, Amagasa T, et al. Clinical and magnetic resonance imaging study of unilateral sideways disc displacements of the temporomandibular joint. J Med Dent Sci. 2002;49(3):89–94.
3. Whyte AM, McNamara D, Rosenberg I, Whyte AW. Magnetic resonance imaging in the evaluation of temporomandibular joint disc displacement–a review of 144 cases. Int J Oral Maxillofac Surg. 2006;35(8):696–703.
4. Sanchez-Woodworth RE, et al. Bilateral internal derangements of the temporomandibular joint: evaluation by magnetic resonance imaging. Oral Surg Oral Med Oral Pathol. 1988;65:281–5.
5. Young AL. Internal derangements of the temporomandibular joint: a review of the anatomy, diagnosis, and management. J Indian Prosthodont Soc. 2015;15(1):2–7. https://doi.org/10.4103/0972-4052.156998.
6. Wilkes CH. Internal derangements of the temporomandibular joint. Pathological variations. Arch Otolaryngol Head Neck Surg. 1989;115(4):469–77.
7. Dimitroulis G. Management of temporomandibular joint disorders: a surgeon's perspective. Aust Dent J. 2018;63(1):79–90.
8. Shen P, Xie Q, Ma Z, Abdelrehem A, Zhang S, Yang C. Yang's classification of juvenile TMJ anterior disc displacement contributing to treatment protocols. Sci Rep. 2019;9(1):5644.
9. Tatli U, Machon V. Internal derangements of temporomandibular joint. Diagn Manag. 2017. https://doi.org/10.5772/intechopen.72585.
10. Rai S, Ranjan V, Misra D, Panjwani S. Management of myofascial pain by therapeutic ultrasound and transcutaneous electrical nerve stimulation: a comparative study. Eur J Dent. 2016;10(1):46–53. https://doi.org/10.4103/1305-7456.175680.
11. Shanavas M, Chatra L, Shenai P, et al. Transcutaneous electrical nerve stimulation therapy: an adjuvant pain controlling modality in TMD patients – a clinical study. Dent Res J (Isfahan). 2014;11(6):676–9.
12. Shukla D, Muthusekhar MR. Efficacy of low-level laser therapy in temporomandibular disorders: a systematic review. Natl J Maxillofac Surg. 2016;7(1):62–6. https://doi.org/10.4103/0975-5950.196127.
13. Madani A, Ahrari F, Fallahrastegar A, Daghestani N. A randomized clinical trial comparing the efficacy of low-level laser therapy (LLLT) and laser acupuncture therapy (LAT) in patients with temporomandibular disorders. Lasers Med Sci. 2019; https://doi.org/10.1007/s10103-019-02837-x.
14. Goldstein L, Gilbert S. Acupuncture: new approach for temporomandibular disorders. Practical Pain Management. 11(16).
15. González-García R, Rodríguez-Campo FJ. Arthroscopic lysis and lavage versus operative arthroscopy in the outcome of temporomandibular joint internal derangement: a comparative study based on Wilkes stages. J Oral Maxillofac Surg. 2011;69(10):2513–24.
16. Quinn P, et al. Atlas of temporomandibular joint surgery. 2nd ed. Wiley-Blackwell; 2015.
17. Laskin DM, et al. Temporomandibular disorders: an evidence-based approach to diagnosis and treatment. 1st ed. USA: Quintessence Publishing; 2006.
18. McCain JP, Hossameldin RH, Srouji S, Maher A. Arthroscopic discopexy is effective in managing temporomandibular joint internal derangement in patients with Wilkes stage II and III. J Oral Maxillofac Surg. 2015;73(3):391–401.
19. Miloro M, Henriksen B. Discectomy as the primary surgical option for internal derangement of the temporomandibular joint. J Oral Maxillofac Surg. 2010;68(4):782–9.
20. Dimitroulis G. The use of dermis grafts after discectomy for internal derangement of the temporomandibular joint. J Oral Maxillofac Surg. 2005;63(2):173–8.
21. Puricelli E, et al. Clinical – surgical treatment of temporomandibular joint disorder in a psoriatic arthritis patient. Head Face Med. 2013;9(11).
22. Kostecka KA. A contribution to the surgical management of open bite. J Orthodont. 1934;28:1082–92.
23. Banks P, Mackenzie I. Condylotomy. A clinical and experimental appraisal of a surgical technique. J Maxillofac Surg. 1975;3(3):170–81.
24. Tasanen A, Lamberg MA. Closed condylotomy in the treatment of recurrent dislocation of the mandibular condyle. Int J Oral Surg. 1978;7(1):1–6.
25. Upton LG, Sullivan SM. The treatment of temporomandibular joint internal derangements using a modified open condylotomy: a preliminary report. J Oral Maxillofac Surg. 1991;49(6):578–83.
26. Hall HD. Modification of the modified condylotomy. J Oral Maxillofac Surg. 1996;54(5):548–51.
27. Ogütcen-Toller M. Sound analysis of temporomandibular joint internal derangements with phonographic recordings. J Prosthet Dent. 2003;89(3):311–8.
28. Kirk WS Jr. Risk factors and initial surgical failures of TMJ arthrotomy and arthroplasty: a four to nine year evaluation of 303 surgical procedures. Cranio. 1998;16(3):154–61.
29. Zhang S, Yang C, Chen M, Liu X, Feng Z, Cai X, Wang L. Histologic study of adhesions in the upper joint compartment of the temporomandibular joint. J Oral Maxillofac Surg. 2009;67(6):1184–90.
30. Zhang SY, Liu XM, Yang C, Cai XY, Chen MJ, Haddad MS, Yun B, Chen ZZ. New arthroscopic

disc repositioning and suturing technique for treating internal derangement of the temporomandibular joint: Part II–Magnetic resonance imaging evaluation. J Oral Maxillofac Surg. 2010;68(8):1813–7.
31. Goizueta Adame CC, Muñoz-Guerra MF. The posterior double pass suture in repositioning of the temporomandibular disc during arthroscopic surgery: a report of 16 cases. J Craniomaxillofac Surg. 2012;40(1):86–91.
32. Yang C, Cai XY, Chen MJ, Zhang SY. New arthroscopic disc repositioning and suturing technique for treating an anteriorly displaced disc of the temporomandibular joint: Part I–Technique introduction. Int J Oral Maxillofac Surg. 2012;41(9):1058–63.
33. Goizueta-Adame CC, Pastor-Zuazaga D, Orts Bañón JE. Arthroscopic disc fixation to the condylar head. Use of resorbable pins for internal derangement of the temporomandibular joint (stage II-IV). Preliminary report of 34 joints. J Craniomaxillofac Surg. 2014;42(4):340–6.
34. Nale JC. Orthognathic surgery and the temporomandibular joint patient. Oral Maxillofac Surg Clin North Am. 2014;26(4):551–64. https://doi.org/10.1016/j.coms.2014.08.012.

16 Temporomandibular Joint Trauma

Darpan Bhargava, Yogesh Sharma, and Preeti Gurjar

16.1 Introduction

Condylar fractures and soft tissue injuries to the temporomandibular joint (TMJ) comprise 29% of all the mandibular fractures. These injuries are mostly overlooked and least diagnosed of all facial injuries. Fracture is the commonly documented result of trauma to TMJ apparatus. Other soft tissue injuries to joint apparatus should also be evaluated for appropriate diagnosis and to prevent resultant complications such as disturbed jaw function, internal derangement of joint, possibility of ankylosis and mandibular growth disturbance leading to hypoplasia [1].

Injury of TMJ apparatus includes

- Effusion (hemorrhagic or serous)
- Soft tissue injury of disc, capsule or ligaments
- Dislocation of condyle from the fossa
  - Without fracture
  - With fracture other than condyle
  - With associated condyle fracture
- Fracture
  - Non-displaced
  - Deviated
  - Displaced
  - Dislocated
  - Comminuted
  - Involving adjacent bony structures
  - Combinations of the above [2]

D. Bhargava (✉)
TMJ Consultancy Services, Bhopal, Madhya Pradesh, India

Oral and Maxillofacial Surgery, People's College of Dental Sciences and Research Centre, People's University, Bhopal, Madhya Pradesh, India
e-mail: drdarpanbhargava@gmail.com

Y. Sharma
Department of Dentistry, Netaji Subhash Chandra Bose Medical College, Jabalpur, Madhya Pradesh, India

P. Gurjar
Oral and Maxillofacial Surgery, TMJ Consultancy Services, Bhopal, Madhya Pradesh, India

16.2 Incidence of Condyle Fracture

Condylar fracture accounts for 29–35% (range based on percentage reported by various authors) of all mandibular fractures. Incidence of trauma varies as per various age groups described by Owusu and colleagues [3]. It comprises of about 74% in individuals aged between 13 and 18 years and 26% in children less than 12 years. Condylar fractures as documented are more common in males than females [4].

16.3 Aetiology

The most common causes of condylar fractures in children at different age groups are: bicycle associated fall (6–12 year), motor vehicle accidents (6–18 year), falls (1–12 year), child abuse

D. Bhargava (ed.), *Temporomandibular Joint Disorders*,
https://doi.org/10.1007/978-981-16-2754-5_16

(1–5 year), contact sports (12–18 year) [5]. In adults, motor vehicle accidents, assaults, falls and sporting accidents are major contributing factors. Falls in elderly group is a primary factor [6]. Other less frequent causes of injury to TMJ include oro-tracheal intubation, whiplash injury and childbirth [7].

16.4 Mechanism of Injury

Teeth provide cushioning effect to the TMJ when in occlusion and thus the impact of force applied to mandible is less in a closed dentate mouth as compared to open mouth. Type of condylar fracture depends on magnitude and direction of the force. When force is axially directed from chin, it results in unilateral or bilateral condylar fracture. As the condyles are positioned superiorly and posteriorly, due to the direction of the force transmitted, there is fracture of the condylar neck and thus, preventing the forces getting directed to the glenoid fossa. This mechanism prevents direct transmission of forces to the base of skull [8].

16.5 Pathophysiology

Anatomy of mandibular condyle at various growth stages determines the pattern of fracture and response to trauma. In children less than 5 years of age condylar fractures often are intra-capsular than extra-capsular as the condylar neck is short, broad and highly vascular, comprising more of cancellous bone and thin cortical bone. Intra-capsular fractures consequential to chin impact due to fall, disperses force on the condyle, resulting in a crush type of injury to condylar head. In 5–12 years of age group, a condylar neck fracture is usually greenstick type or incomplete, as the anatomical configuration of the TMJ apparatus is more of adult type, with increased remodelling potential.

In adults, extra-capsular (condylar neck) fractures with medial or lateral displacement are more common, as it is the weakest point of the mandible. Likewise, in cases of intra-capsular fractures in adults vertical (sagittal split) is common and is most unnoticed variant of condyle fracture.

16.6 Classification of Condylar Fractures

16.6.1 Lindhal's Classification

Condylar fracture is basically classified based on anatomic location of the fracture and the relationship of fractured segment with mandible and the glenoid fossa. Lindhal L (1977) classified condylar fractures based on following factors [9] (Fig. 16.1)

1. ***Anatomic location of fracture*** *(Fig. 16.1a)*
   - (a) *Fracture of condylar head*: These are intra-capsular fractures which are further divided into Vertical (antero-posterior sagittal split), Compression ('mushroom' type expansion) and Comminuted.
   - (b) *Fracture of condylar neck:* Extra-capsular type inferior to attachment of joint capsule.
   - (c) *Sub-condylar fracture:* Extends antero-posteriorly from deepest part of sigmoid notch till point of maximum concavity on ramus of mandible. It may be further described as high or low sub-condylar fractures.
2. ***Relationship of fractured condyle to mandible***
   - (a) Undisplaced (Fig. 16.1b)
   - (b) Deviated (Fig. 16.1c)
   - (c) Displaced with medial or lateral overlap (Figs. 16.1d and 16.1e)
   - (d) Displaced with anterior or posterior overlap (Fig. 16.1f)
   - (e) No contact between the fracture segments (Fig. 16.1g)
3. ***Relationship of condylar head to glenoid fossa***
   - (a) Non-displaced (Fig. 16.1h)
   - (b) Displacement: Condylar head within the fossa, with alteration in joint space (Fig. 16.1i).
   - (c) Dislocation: Mostly antero-medial dislocation of fractured condylar head out of the fossa (Fig. 16.1j).

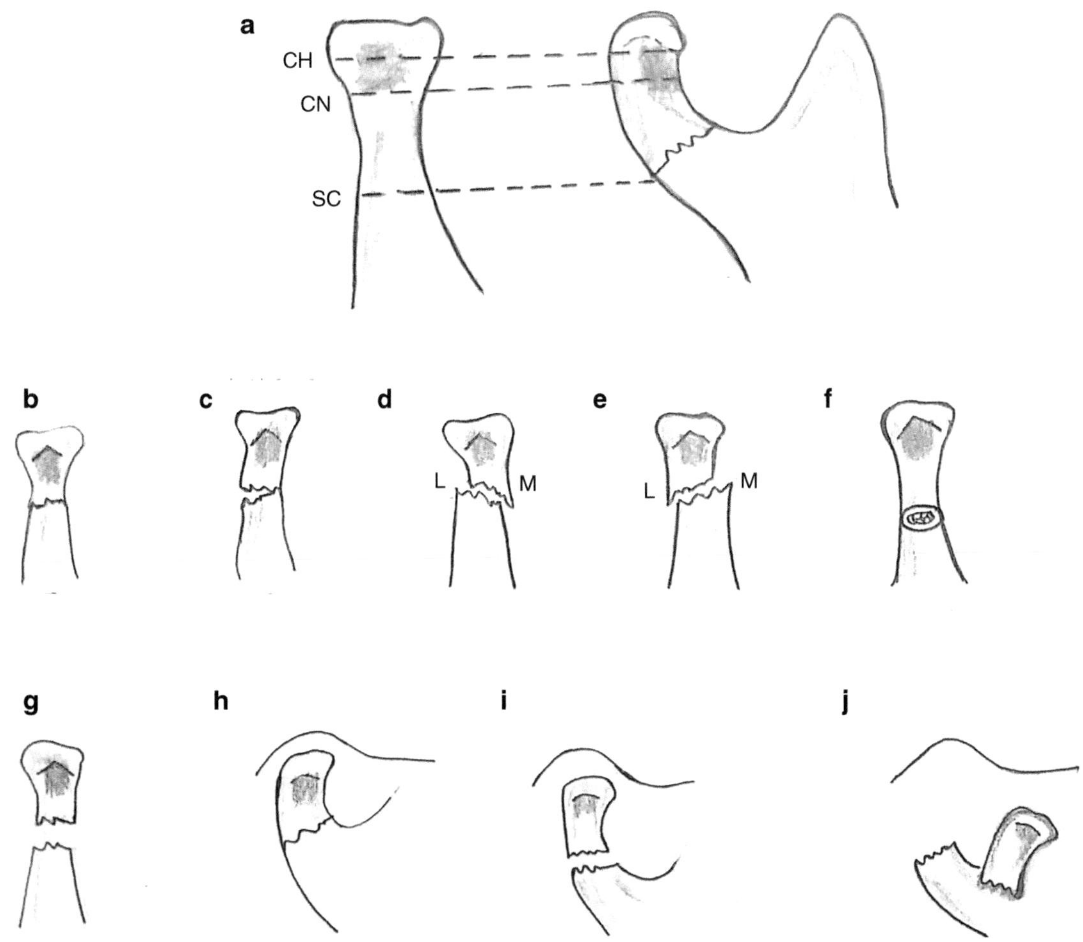

Fig. 16.1 Lindhal's classification of condylar fracture based on anatomic fracture location, relationship of the fracture condyle to mandible and the glenoid fossa. (*CH*: Condylar Head; *CN*: Neck of the condyle; *SC*: Sub-condylar; *L*: Lateral; *M*: Medial)

Displacement of the condylar head and shortening of ramus are considered to be two useful determinants for condylar fracture. Other classification systems with clinical significance which are based on anatomic location and propose an algorithm for treatment of condylar fractures are as under.

16.6.2 Classification proposed by Strasbourg Osteosynthesis Research Group (Loukota et al., 2005) (Fig. 16.2)

This system categorizes condylar fractures on anatomic position and clinical significance. It includes:

- *Dicapitular fracture*—fracture line starting from the condylar head, which may extend outside the capsule.

Condylar neck and base fractures are differentiated with the relationship of fracture segment with an imaginary line (line A) drawn from the inferiormost point of sigmoid notch perpendicular to the tangent of the ramus.

- *Fracture of condylar neck*—More than half of fracture is superior to line A.
- *Fracture of condylar base*—More than half of the fracture is inferior to line A.
- *Displacement*—It refers to fracture line status which may be mild (<10 degrees), moderate

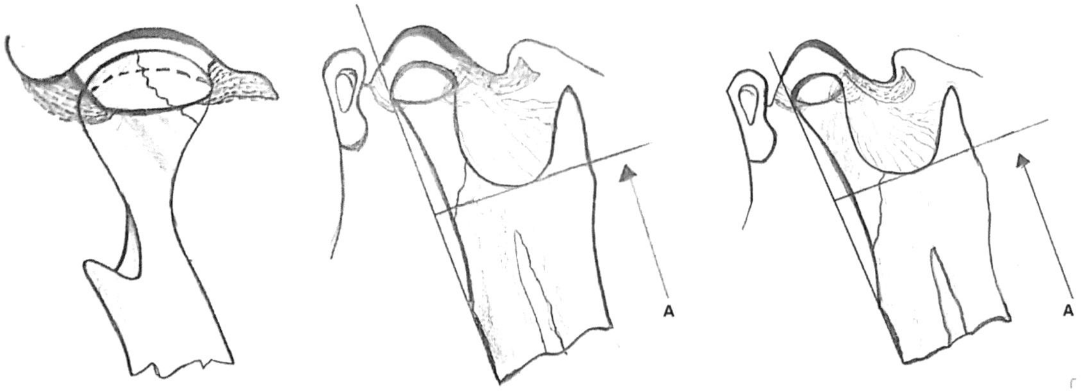

Fig. 16.2 Classification proposed by Loukota et al., 2005 and adopted by Strasbourg Osteosynthesis Research Group (SORG) for mandibular condyle fractures

(10–45 degrees) or severe (≥45 degrees). Condylar fractures with displacement ≥10 degrees and ramus height shortening with ≥2 mm are indicated for open reduction and internal fixation.

16.6.3 Classification for Management of Sub-condylar Fractures

This system includes pattern of sub-condylar fractures and corresponding treatment guidelines:

- *Class 1*: Minimally displaced fracture indicative of closed reduction (shortening of ramus height <2 mm; degree of fracture displacement <10 degrees).
- *Class 2*: Moderately displaced indicated for ORIF (shortening of ramus height 2–15 mm; degree of fracture displacement 10–45 degrees). [ORIF: Open reduction and internal fixation].
- *Class 3*: Severely displaced indicated for ORIF (shortening of ramus height >15 mm; degree of fracture displacement >45 degrees) [8].

16.7 Diagnosis of TMJ Injuries

Diagnosis of various hard and soft tissue injuries to TMJ can be elicited based on clinical features and appropriate radiological examination (Table 16.1).

Table 16.1 Clinical features of condylar fracture

• Evidence of trauma (laceration abrasion contusion over chin or haematoma over pre-auricular region)
• Facial asymmetry (foreshortening of ramus due to overlap of fracture segments)
• Pain and swelling in pre-auricular region
• Bleeding from external auditory canal (fracture of anterior tympanic plate)
• Trismus (due to muscle spasm, hemarthrosis or pain)
• Restricted mouth opening with deviation towards fractured side on mouth opening
• Malocclusion
– Fractured side: premature molars contact
– Non-fractured side: posterior open bite
– Bilateral condylar fracture with displacement: anterior open bite and gagging of posterior teeth.

16.7.1 Imaging of TMJ Injuries

Radiological examination helps in definitive diagnosis of the condylar fractures. Orthopantomogram (OPG), mandibular lateral oblique view and reverse Towne's view are considered as baseline investigation for condylar fractures. Advanced imaging techniques such as computed tomography (CT) and magnetic resonance imaging (MRI) are reserved for detailed evaluation of complex injuries including displaced or dislocated condylar fractures, intracranial penetration with related soft tissue injury to the temporomandibular joint and adjacent tissues (Figs. 16.3, 16.4, 16.5, and 16.6).

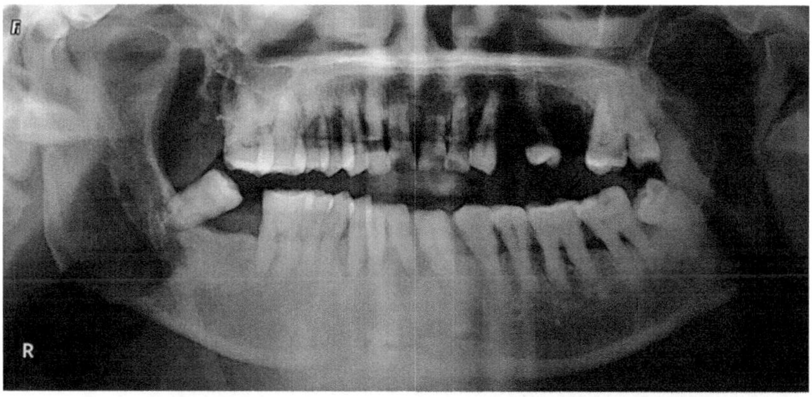

Fig. 16.3 Panoramic radiograph depicting left sub-condylar fracture with displacement of the condyle from the glenoid fossa

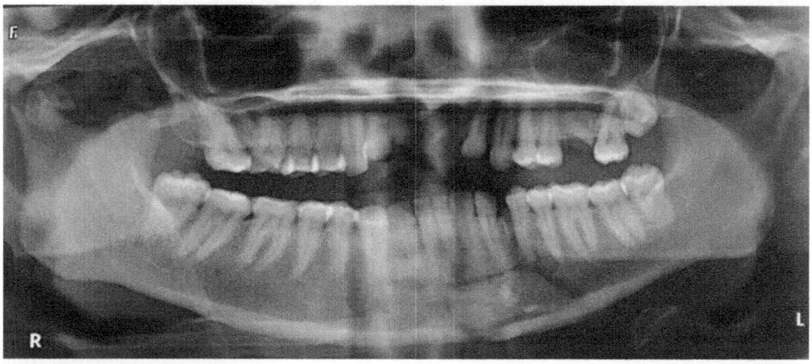

Fig. 16.4 Note the right-side fracture of the condylar head suggestive of high-condylar fracture and fracture of the coronoid process as an indirect trauma due to blow on the left parasymphysis and body of the mandible

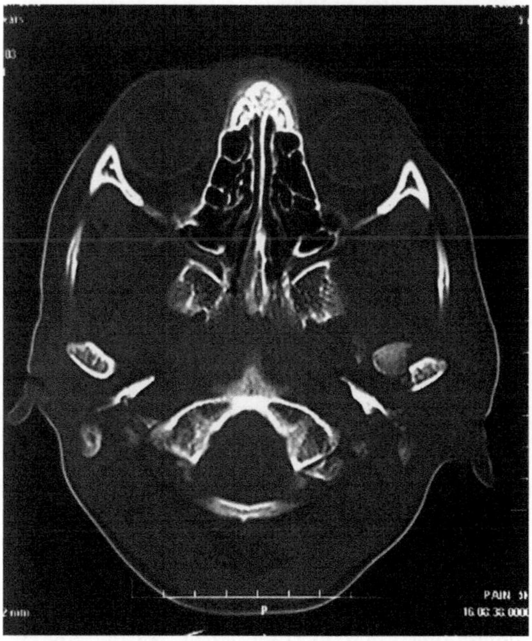

Fig. 16.5 Computed tomographic (CT) scan of a patient with a sagittal fracture of the mandibular condyle

16.8 Treatment of Condylar Fractures

The primary goal of treatment for condylar fractures is restoration of pre-operative masticatory function, occlusion and facial symmetry. Unlike fractures of other bones in the body, precise approximation of fracture segments may not be obligatory in case where reduction cannot be achieved, evaluating the risk-benefit ratio. Owing to remarkable remodelling and reconstructive properties of the condyle, opting conservative treatment in cases with minimally displaced and dislocated condyle, a perfectly functional and morphologically reconstituted condyle can be achieved. Treatment modalities for condylar fracture vary in different age groups and it follows either conservative or surgical approach based on the degree of displacement and facial asymmetry.

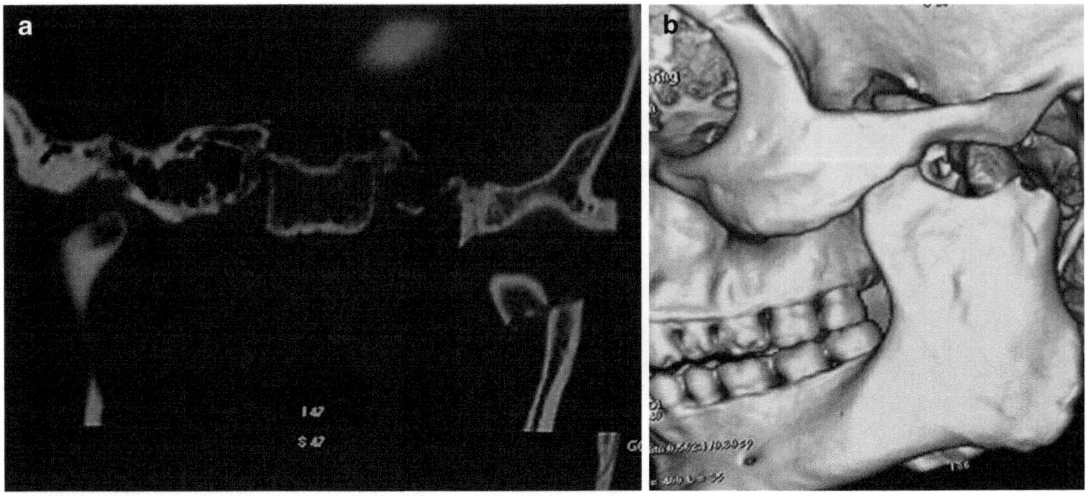

Fig. 16.6 Computed tomographic (CT) scan (**a**) coronal section, (**b**) 3D reconstructed image demonstrating an antero-medially displaced fractured mandibular condyle (pulled along the tangential force of the lateral pterygoid muscle)

16.8.1 Conservative Management

Observation, soft diet and analgesics are preferred treatment of choice in cases with minimal displacement of condyle and absence of any occlusal discrepancy. Cases with mild displacement, minimal inter-occlusal mal-relationship and deviated jaw on opening the mouth should be treated by immobilizing the mandible using splints, elastics and maxillo-mandibular fixation (MMF). There are several non-surgical protocols for the management of the condylar fractures which vary with the age of the patient (Table 16.2).

16.8.2 Surgical Management of Condyle Fractures

When indicated, open reduction and internal fixation (ORIF) aids in early restoration of form and function when compared to conservative methods. Meyer et al. have described the lines of osteosynthesis for the mandibular condyle with the zone of tension that lies along the anterior border of the condyle and the sigmoid notch and the zone of compression that lies along the posterior border of the ramus. Based on the Meyer's research, ideally two plate fixation along the lines of osteosynthesis will provide a stable fixation for the mandibular condyle (Fig. 16.7). As per the AO surgery reference recommendation for cases where there is limited bone available for plating, an alternative way of achieving the same stability

Table 16.2 Non-surgical management of condylar fractures

Age group	Management
0–2 years	Active jaw function and analgesics.
3–5 years	MMF using cap splints (with/without hooks; with/without occlusal coverage) or mini arch bars for 10–14 days followed by active physiotherapy. Myofunctional appliances to promote normal growth of the mandible.
6–12 years	MMF using arch bars or Ivy eyelets wiring for 2–3 weeks (14–21 days)* followed by active physiotherapy. (*This duration for MMF may be considered upto the age of 16 years, based on the operator preference and the extent of deviation or displacement of the fractured segment).
Adults	MMF for 4–6 weeks using Erich arch bars, Ivy eyelets or IMF screws and wires or elastics.
Geriatrics (edentulous patients)	MMF using 'gunning type splints' secured with per alveolar wires, fixed using piriform aperture or circum-palatal wires. Existing dentures may also be used for MMF.

MMF: Maxillo-mandibular fixation; IMF: Inter-maxillary fixation

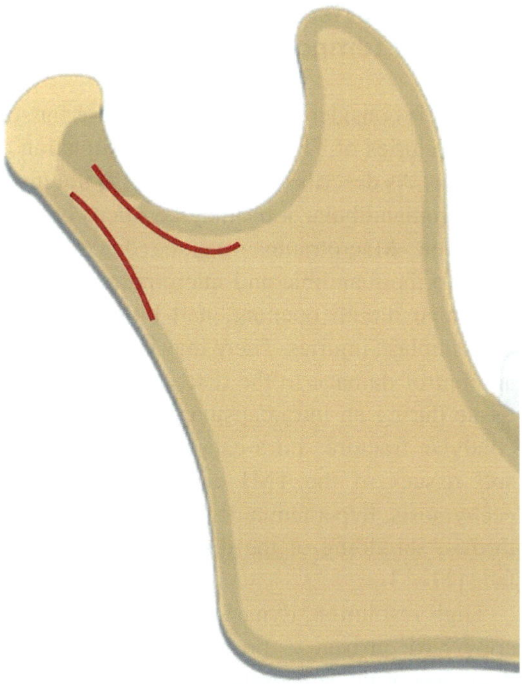

Fig. 16.7 The lines of osteosynthesis for the mandibular condyle (as described by Meyer et al. 2000)

is by using a single heavier plate for the mandibular condyle fixation. Fixation using wire osteosynthesis, intramedullary Kirschner(K)-wire or screw and external bone pins have been advocated by various authors in the past. Use of functional miniplates for fixation is the most preferred method of condylar fracture stabilization. Apart from miniplates, use of specialized geometric plates like Y plate, trapezoidal plate and delta plate (3D plates) have been proposed by various authors. Use of resorbable plating systems (poly-L-lactic acid and glycolic acid plates) have been documented for fracture fixation in growing mandible. Recommendations of the American Association of Oral and Maxillofacial Surgeons (AAOMS) Clinical Practice Guidelines for Oral and Maxillofacial Surgery (AAOMS ParCare, 2017) for the open reduction and internal fixation of the condylar fractures include the following cases: 1. Fracture dislocation of a mandibular condyle 2. Mechanical interference with mandibular function by the condyle or a foreign body 3. Condylar fractures with loss of anterior-posterior and vertical dimension that cannot be managed by closed reduction (eg, edentulous patient, multiple facial fractures) including internal fixation if indicated 4. Compound fracture 5. Displacement of a mandibular condyle into middle cranial fossa 6. Patient or surgeon preference for early or immediate mobilization or function [15]. Based on careful evaluation of cases, absolute and relative indications for open reduction and internal fixation were proposed by Zide and Kent [10], which are as follows:

Absolute Indications

1. Displacement of the condyle into middle cranial fossa
2. Impossibility of obtaining adequate occlusion by closed techniques
3. Lateral extra-capsular dislocation of the condyle
4. Foreign bodies within the capsule of the TMJ
5. Mechanical obstruction impeding the function of the TMJ
6. Open injury (penetrating, lacerating and avulsive) to the TMJ that requires immediate treatment

Relative Indications

1. Bilateral condylar fractures in an edentulous patient when splints are unavailable or impossible because of severe ridge atrophy
2. Unilateral or bilateral condylar fractures when splinting is not recommended because of concomitant medical conditions or when physiotherapy is not possible
3. Bilateral fractures associated with communited mid-facial fractures
4. Bilateral fractures associated with other gnathologic problems

16.9 Approaches for Open Reduction and Internal Fixation of Condyle

Based on the location of the fracture and the degree of displacement, selection of an appropriate surgical approach is made to access the fractured joint (Table 16.3) (Refer Chap. 14).

Table 16.3 Different surgical approaches to the temporomandibular joint for reduction and fixation of condylar fractures

Surgical approach	Indication
1. Pre-auricular approach	Intra-capsular or high condylar neck fracture
2. Sub-mandibular approach	Low sub-condylar fracture (good exposure for the level of neck and coronoid notch)
3. Retromandibular approach (Fig. 16.8)	Sub-condylar, angle and body fracture
4. Rhytidectomy (face-lift) approach	High-level condylar fractures
5. Post-auricular approach	Entire Joint
6. Intraoral approach (may be combined with endoscopic technique)	Low sub-condylar fracture, also all the extra-capsular fractures
7. Transparotid approach	Entire Joint

16.10 Soft Tissue Injuries of Temporomandibular Joint

Trauma is considered as a primary cause for soft tissue injuries of TMJ, leading to dysfunction of the joint. As described by Goldman [7] trauma to temporomandibular joint may be micro or macrotrauma. Macrotrauma may be due to direct blow to the mandible and microtrauma includes excessive mouth opening, nail biting, bruxism and whiplash injuries. There may be considerable amount of damage to the disc and adjacent soft tissue during an intra-capsular or extra-capsular condylar fracture. Intra-capsular trauma to the soft tissues of the TMJ can lead to synovial ecchymosis, hyperaemia of the capsule, haemarthrosis, shredding of the disc and articular surface [11–13].

High resolution, dynamic MRIs and arthroscopy have proven to be an accurate means in diagnosis of the soft tissue injuries such as effu-

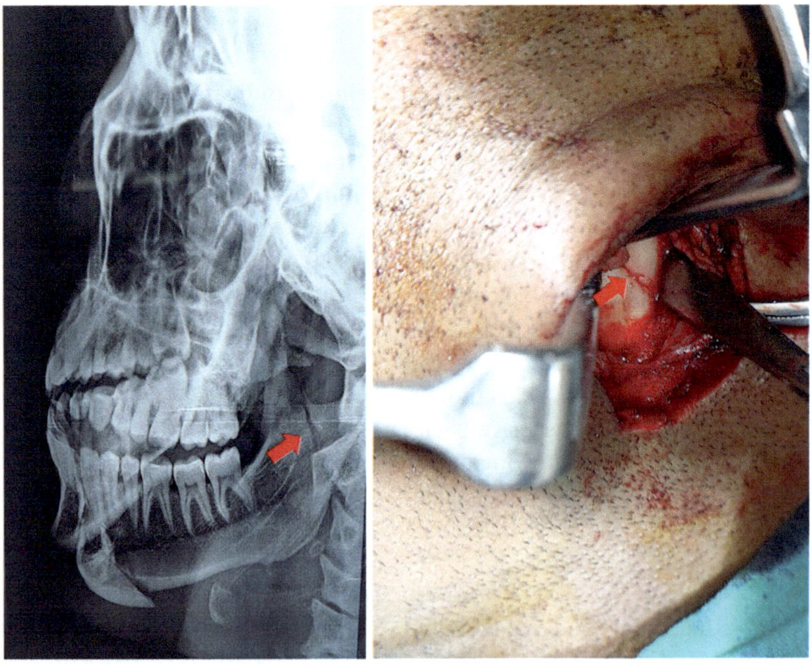

Fig. 16.8 Retromandibular approach for reduction and fixation of sub-condylar fracture (arrow)

sion of the joint, disc displacement and damage to the soft tissues surrounding the joint fossa.

Trauma induced soft tissue injuries to the temporomandibular joint can lead to internal derangement, osteoarthrosis and possibly fibrous ankylosis. Most often it is found that history of previous trauma to the temporomandibular joint is the precursor for internal derangement of the joint [14]. According to Merill et al. in their study on 1151 patients with internal derangement, 60% of the study population gave a history of mandibular trauma [11].

16.11 Conclusion

Following appropriate management protocols, patients with trauma to the temporomandibular joint should be evaluated periodically and followed up closely for any preceding joint derangements and for restoration of normal function.

References

1. Bradley PF. Condylar injuries. In: Rowe NL, Williams JL, editors. Maxillofacial injuries. Edinburgh: Churchill Livingstone; 1985.
2. Miloro, Michael, and Larry J. Peterson. Peterson's Principles of Oral and Maxillofacial Surgery. 6th Ed. Shelton, CT: People's Medical Pub. House-USA, 2012.
3. Owusu JA, Bellile E, Moyer JS, Sidman JD. Patterns of pediatric mandible fractures in the United States. JAMA Facial Plast Surg. 2016;18(1):37–41.
4. Sawazaki R, Lima Júnior SM, Asprino L, Moreira RW, de Moraes M. Incidence and patterns of mandibular condyle fractures. J Oral Maxillofac Surg. 2010;68(6):1252–9.
5. Myall RWT. Condylar injuries in children: what is different about them? In: Worthington P, Evans JR, editors. Controversies in oral and maxillofacial surgery. Philadelphia: WB Saunders; 1994. p. 191–200.
6. Marker P, Nielsen A, Bastian H. Fractures of the mandibular condyle. Part I: Patterns of distribution of types and causes of fractures in 348 patients. Br J Oral Maxillofac Surg. 2000;38:417–21.
7. Goldman J. Temporomandibular disorders: diagnosis and treatment. In: Kaplan AS, Assael LA, editors. Philadelphia: WB Saunders; 1991.
8. Fonseca, Raymond J., and Robert V. Walker. Oral and Maxillofacial Trauma. Philadelphia: Saunders, 1991.
9. Lindhal L. Condylar fractures of the mandible: classification and relation to age, occlusion, and concomitant injuries of the teeth and teeth-supporting structures, and fractures of the mandibular body. Int J Oral Surg. 1977;6:12.
10. Zide M, Kent J. Indications for open reduction of mandibular condyle fracture. J Oral Maxillofac Surg. 1983;41:89.
11. Goss AN, Bosanquet AG. The arthroscopic appearance of acute temporomandibular joint trauma. J Oral Maxillofac Surg. 1990;48:780–3.
12. Sullivan S, Banghart PR, Anderson O. Magnetic resonance imaging assessment of acute soft tissue injuries to the temporomandibular joint. J Oral Maxillofac Surg. 1995;53:763–6.
13. Sullivan SM, Banghart PR, Anderson Q. Magnetic resonance imaging assessment of acute soft tissue injuries to the temporomandibular joint. J Oral Maxillofac Surg. 1995;53(7):763–6; discussion 766–7. https://doi.org/10.1016/0278-2391(95)90326-7.
14. He D, Yang C, Chen M, Yang X, Li L. Effects of soft tissue injury to the temporomandibular joint: report of 8 cases. Br J Oral Maxillofac Surg. 2013;51(1):58–62.
15. Ochs M, Chung W, Powers D. Trauma Surgery. J Oral Maxillofac Surg. 2017;75(8S):e151-e194. https://doi.org/10.1016/j.joms.2017.04.023.

17 Temporomandibular Joint Ankylosis

Darpan Bhargava and Ankit Pandey

17.1 Introduction

Ankylosis otherwise colloquially referred to as a fused joint or a stiff joint. Temporomandibular Joint (TMJ) ankylosis or craniomandibular ankylosis is characterized by formation of a fibrous or bony mass, that replaces the normal joint architecture. The quality of life in such patients is greatly affected due to their deformed face and reduced jaw function affecting the speech, mastication and deglutition, thereby affecting the general health of the patient [1]. In growing patients, the early diagnosis and management of the condition is the only means to prevent progressive secondary deformity. The diagnosis of TMJ ankylosis is confirmed after the clinical and radiographic evaluation. The detailed description of this peculiar condition is outlined in this chapter including its aetiology, classification, clinical features, management and complications, that may arise.

TMJ ankylosis can result from a variety of aetiological factors affecting the joint and its surrounding structures. It can be classified by location (intra-/extra-articular), type of tissue involved (bony/fibrous/fibro-osseous) and extent of fusion (complete/incomplete).

D. Bhargava (✉)
TMJ Consultancy Services,
Bhopal, Madhya Pradesh, India

Oral and Maxillofacial Surgery, People's College of Dental Sciences and Research Centre,
People's University, Bhopal, Madhya Pradesh, India
e-mail: drdarpanbhargava@gmail.com

A. Pandey
Amrit Dental and TMJ Centre,
Bhopal, Madhya Pradesh, India

17.2 Aetiology

The common aetiology of TMJ ankylosis is trauma to the TMJ (haemarthosis), sequale to condylar fractures, injury during birth (forceps delivery was implicated in the past) and infection. There are several other aetiologies which may contribute to the development of this condition but are less common (Table 17.1) [2, 3].

Table 17.1 Aetiology of TMJ ankylosis

Aetiology	Condition
Trauma	Forceps delivery during birth Condylar fracture
Infection	Otitis media Osteomyelitis of mandible Actinomycosis Peri-articular abscess
Inflammation	Rheumatoid arthritis Ankylosing spondylitis Psoriatic arthritis Poliomyelitis
Systemic disease	Tuberculosis Gonorrhoea Scarlet fever
Miscellaneous	Congenital (Syndromes)

D. Bhargava (ed.), *Temporomandibular Joint Disorders*,
https://doi.org/10.1007/978-981-16-2754-5_17

17.3 Pathogenesis

There are numerous mechanisms hypothesized in literature to explain the predisposing factors leading to TMJ ankylosis. One such theory is the *interfragmentary strain theory* or *Perren's strain theory*. It states that the strain tolerance of bone, cartilage and fibrous tissue is associated with TMJ ankylosis. In a fractured condyle, the stress created in the area surrounding the joint space cause tissue deformation in varying degrees. Minimum strain or limited movement of the jaw will lead to endochondral ossification causing bone formation especially in areas of the lateral part of the joint [4].

The pathogenesis of bone formation following trauma is due to *haemarthrosis*. Intra-articular haematoma organizes, leading to bone formation from disrupted periosteum or metaplasia of the non-osseous connective tissues causing osseous ankylosis. Fractures of the paediatric condyle is more prone for development of ankylosis owing to the peculiar anatomy of the condyle, having a broad neck and highly vascularized head that has rich osteogenic potential when compared to an adult condyle. It is hypothesized that haemarthrosis, along with the disruption of the fibro-cartilage integrity allows the in-growth of fibrous connective tissue into the joint which later results in ossification. *Ferretti et al.* opined that the extra-articular haematoma may also contribute to the development of ankylosis owing to the fact that fusion occurs in the juxta-articular area [5–7].

Meng et al. proposed that a force similar to distraction osteogenesis (DO) by the lateral pterygoid muscle during the sagittal condylar fracture healing has a vital role in the development of TMJ ankylosis. Newly formed bone in DO responds to the direction of tensile strength obtained by the muscle force. The tensile strength from lateral pterygoid muscle is horizontal which contributes to the horizontal enlargement of the condyle. But the authors did not explain how the two joint surfaces fuse to each other [5].

Hall's hypothesis stated that genetic predisposition was responsible for TMJ ankylosis. However, this theory lacks sufficient support. *Bhatt et al.* postulated that hypercoagulability of blood could be a contributing factor in traumatic TMJ. All the above-mentioned theories do not completely explain the development of TMJ ankylosis with each one having its own flaws in elucidating the pathosis. There are various cellular and molecular mechanism involved in ankylosis formation which needs further research to establish the exact cause for ankylosis [5]. Hypothesis supporting *hypertrophic non-union* following TMJ trauma is proposed by Yan et al., which include two prerequisites for the development of the ankylosis: 1) TMJ trauma induces a suitable microenvironment for the bone healing of the two articular surfaces, namely creating the underlying condition of bony ankylosis; 2) the bone healing of the injured articular surfaces is inhibited by the interference due to the opening movement of the jaw. Considering the opening joint movement into account and the extended clinical course of bone formation, the narrow residual radiolucent zone in the bony ankylosis is clearly explained by this hypothesis. Yan et al. also suggested that the shear force was the cause of the radiolucent zone, and the increased compressive loading due to disc displacement could stimulate new bone formation around the joint following the joint trauma [5].

17.4 Classification of TMJ Ankylosis

There are various proposed classifications based on clinical presentation, type of tissue involved and the radiographic features. The salient ones are as under:

1. Based on anatomic site of fusion/union (Kazanjian's classification)
   Intra-articular/True ankylosis
   Extra-articular/False ankylosis
   Juxta-articular ankylosis
2. Based on the type of tissue
   Osseous ankylosis
   Fibrous ankylosis
   Fibro-osseous ankylosis
3. Based on the side involved
   Unilateral (Fig. 17.1)
   Bilateral (Fig. 17.2)

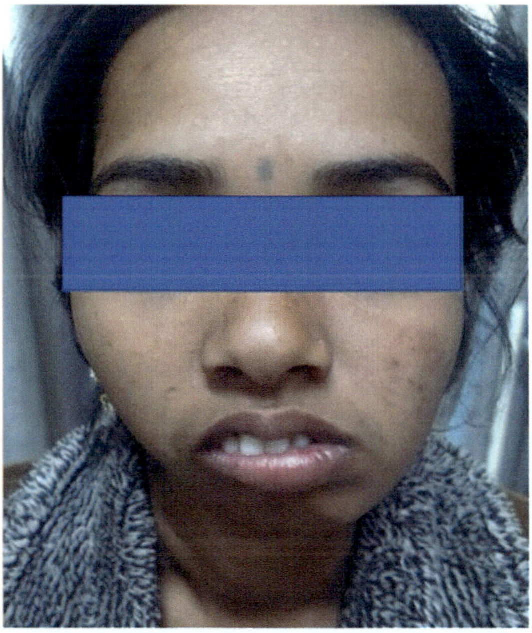

Fig. 17.1 Frontal profile of a patient depicting unilateral ankylosis of the left TMJ. Facial deformity can be appreciated with shortened facial height of the left lower half of the face and flattening of the right lower half of the face

4. Based on the extension of bone formation—Topazian's classification (Table 17.2) [8, 9]
5. Sawhney's classification—Based on radiographic and operative findings (Table 17.3) (Figs. 17.3a, b)
6. Turlington–Durr classification of heterotopic ossification in TMJ (Table 17.4) [10]
7. El-Hakim et al.'s radiographic classification (Table 17.5) [11]
8. Shanghai Ninth People's Hospital radiographic classification (Table 17.6) [12]

17.5 Clinical Features

Development of TMJ Ankylosis in early childhood leads to severe developmental deformities of the face whereas if it is of adult onset there is less or no facial deformity. The clinical features may vary based on the onset and the side involved (Table 17.7). All the patients generally present with poor oral hygiene leading to multiple carious teeth. The common presentation includes reduced or no mouth opening, retrognathia, micrognathia, elongated coronoid process which is evident on imaging (Figs. 17.4 and 17.5) and obstructive sleep apnoea (OSA). Usually, pain is never a presenting feature. The narrow airway leading to obstructive sleep apnoea in these patients is depicted in Fig. 17.6 [13–16]. A vital finding in these patients is the correlation of the age of occurrence and the degree of deformity. Younger patients with early onset of ankylosis during the growth phase will have more severe resultant secondary deformity as compared to an adult when the condition develops after growth completion.

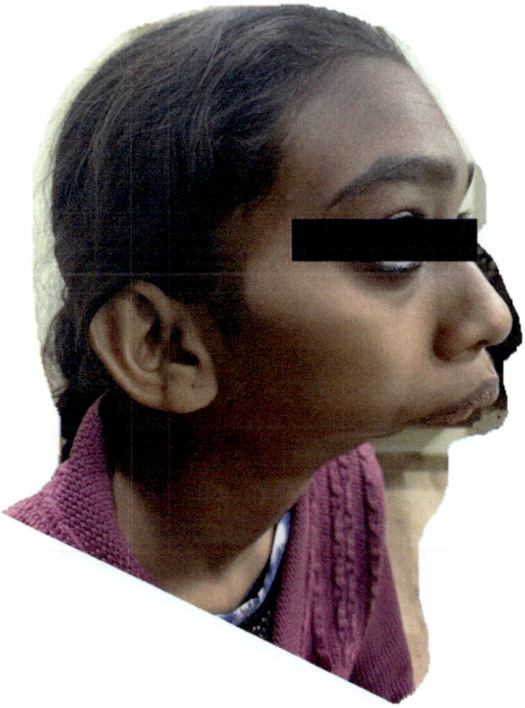

Fig. 17.2 Lateral profile of a patient having bilateral TMJ ankylosis. Severe facial deformity can be appreciated involving the mandible characterized by micrognathia and obtuse thyro-mental angle

Table 17.2 Topazian's classification of TMJ ankylosis (1966)

Stage	Extent of the ankylotic mass
I	Ankylotic bone limited to condylar process
II	Ankylotic bone extending to the sigmoid notch
III	Ankylotic bone extending to the coronoid process

Table 17.3 Sawhney's classification of TMJ Ankylosis based on the radiographic and operative findings (1986)

Type	Radiographic appearance
I	Extensive fibrous adhesions around the joint. Condylar head is present without much distortion
II	Bony fusion at the outer edge of the articular surface, but no fusion within the medial area of the joint. No involvement of sigmoid notch and coronoid process
III	Bony bridge between the mandible and the zygomatic arch. Medially atrophic dislocated fragment of former condyle head can be found Elongation of coronoid process
IV	Complete osseous block between ramus and skull base. Normal TMJ anatomy is completely disrupted

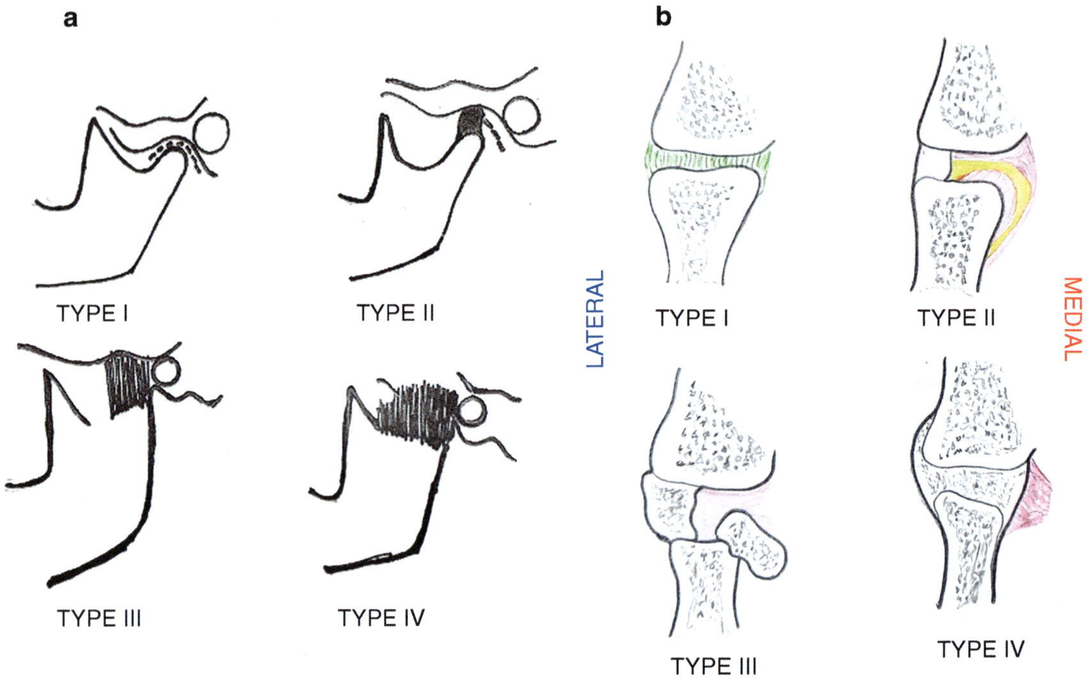

Fig. 17.3 Diagrammatic representation of Sawhney's classification of TMJ ankylosis, (**a**) lateral view, (**b**) coronal or anterio-posterior view

17.6 Growth Deformity

Facial asymmetry, retrognathia and OSA are usually present when onset or development of ankylosis occurs at an early age, as growth of the facial skeleton is affected in such individuals which can be explained by *Melvin Moss's Functional Matrix Theory*. The spacial anatomy of the hyoid bone and its associated musculature is also altered and is well demonstrated in Figs. 17.7 and 17.8. Rotation of the hyoid bone and the laryngeal inlet on the affected side in unilateral ankylosis may pose surgical and anaesthetic difficulties [17, 18]. Correlation between OSA and TMJ ankylosis is revealed in recent studies, resulting from the developmental deformity in mandible causing micrognathia, leading to narrowing of the pharyngeal space causing obstruction to air entry during sleep or when the patient is in supine position. This builds up to a complex syndrome of episodes of apnoea and hypopnoea resulting in marked reduction in oxygen saturation. This condition progresses to the systemic involvement of cardiovascular and respiratory systems. The correction of OSA simultaneous or prior to ankylosis release

Table 17.4 Turlington and Durr's classification (1993)

Grade	Feature
0	No bone islands visible
1	Islands of bone visible within the soft tissue around the joint
2	Peri-articular bone formation
3	Apparent bony ankylosis

Modified from classification of heterotopic ossification in hips
Grades 1, 2, 3 are subdivided into A—Asymptomatic, S—Symptomatic

Table 17.5 Ankylosed TMJ classified according to the relation of the ankylosed mass to the surrounding vital structures, especially at the base of the skull using axial and coronal CT image

Class I	Unilateral or bilateral fibrous ankylosis The condyle and glenoid fossa retain their original shape The maxillary artery is in normal anatomical relation to the ankylosed mass.
Class II	Unilateral or bilateral bony fusion between the condyle and the temporal bone The maxillary artery lies in normal anatomical relation to the ankylosed mass
Class III	The distance between maxillary artery and the medial pole of the mandibular condyle is less on the ankylosed than in the normal side or the maxillary artery runs within the ankylotic bony mass This is best seen on coronal CT
Class IV	The ankylosed mass appear fused to the base of the skull There is extensive bone formation, especially from the medial aspect of the condyle to the extent that the ankylosed bony mass is in close relationship to the vital structures at the base of the skull such as the pterygoid plates, the carotid and jugular foramina and foramen spinosum and no joint anatomy can be defined from the radiograph This is best visualized on axial CT.

and secondary deformity correction are important for the holistic management of these patients [19–21].

17.7 Investigations

The radiographic evaluation of the TMJ can distinguish between bony and fibrous ankylosis. The radiographic modalities used for evaluation are orthopantomogram (OPG) (Fig. 17.9), computed tomogram (CT) (Figs. 17.10 and 17.11) and cone beam computed tomogram (CBCT). Magnetic Resonance Imaging (MRI) can be used to accurately diagnose fibrous ankylosis or disc remnants between the bony ankylosis. The CT images reveal the fusion of bones in TMJ region involving the joint space, condylar head and the tempo-

Table 17.6 Shanghai Ninth People's hospital classification of TMJ ankylosis based on Coronal CT images

A1	Fibrous ankylosis without bony fusion of the joint
A2	Ankylosis with bony fusion on lateral side of the joint Residual condyle fragment is bigger than 0.5 of the medial condylar head
A3	Similar to A2 but the residual condylar fragment is smaller than 0.5 of the condylar head
A4	Ankylosis with complete bony fusion of the joint

Table 17.7 Clinical features differentiating between unilateral and bilateral ankylosis

Unilateral	Bilateral
Reduced or no mouth opening	Reduced or nil mouth opening
Facial asymmetry (fullness on affected side and flattening on unaffected side)	Retrognathia, micrognathia (bird face deformity), convex facial profile
Occlusal canting evident/ Ipsilateral maxillary growth may also get affected in growing patients which is restricted due to non growing mandibular opponent	No occlusal canting/ Bilateral posterior maxillary downward growth will be hindered in growing patients
Shortened ramus height on ipsilateral or affected side	Shortened ramus height bilaterally
Prominent ante-gonial notch on ipsilateral or affected side	Prominent ante-gonial notch on both the sides
Class II angles malocclusion with unilateral cross bite present at the affected side	Class II angles malocclusion may be present bilaterally Upper incisors may be protrusive with apparent anterior open bite
Deviation of the mandible to the affected side	Proclination of the lower anterior teeth
Elongated coronoid on the affected side or bilaterally (evident on imaging)	Elongated coronoids (evident on imaging)

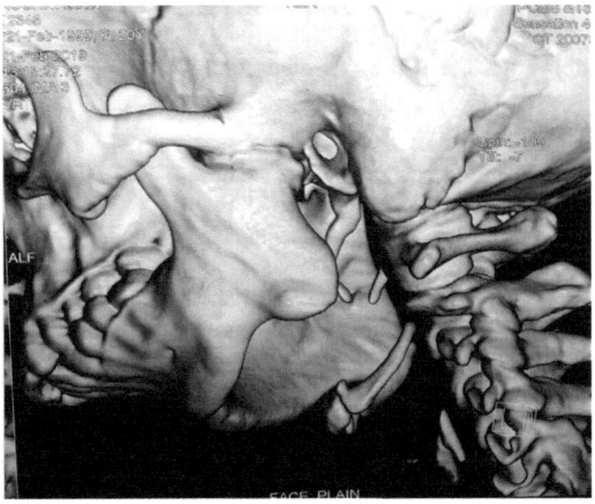

Fig. 17.4 A three-dimensional (3D) reconstructed image showing TMJ ankylosis with elongated coronoid process medial to the zygomatic arch

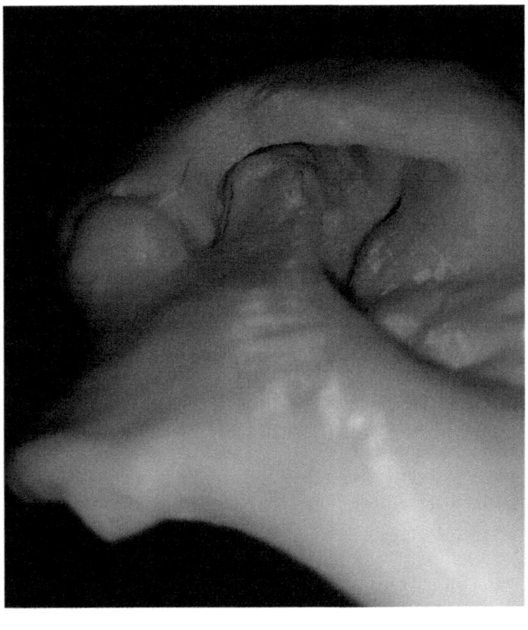

Fig. 17.5 Stereolithographic model reconstruction depicting the elongated coronoid process as seen from the inferior aspect of the mandible, medial to the zygomatic arch

ral bone. In extensive cases fusion of the coronoid process can be visualized with the zygomatic arch. A three-dimensional (3D) reconstruction CT enables fabrication of a stereolithographic model, which can be further utilized to analyse the extent of bony fusion and secondary deformity (Fig. 17.12). Such models also aid in pre surgical planning (Figs. 17.13 and 17.14) [22]. At instances, it may be wise to order an angiogram for assessment of the vasculature medial to or entrapped within the ankylotic mass.

In patients with OSA, polysomnography is considered the gold standard for diagnosis. The standard components of the polysomnogram include the electroencephalogram (EEG), electro-oculogram (EOG), electromyogram (EMG) and electrocardiogram (ECG, leadV2). Repeated episodes of pharyngeal airway obstruction are measured using apnoea-hypopnoea index (AHI) [20, 23].

17.8 Management of TMJ Ankylosis

The management of TMJ ankylosis differs with the age of the patient and the choice of reconstruction for the joint. In paediatric patients, there are growth deformities of facial bones and dental/occlusal derangements present which should be managed simultaneously involving a combination of surgical, orthodontic and psychological management. Contrary to this, in adults the TMJ ankylosis is usually caused by trauma which rarely causes significant facial asymmetry or occlusal alterations [24].

A variety of techniques for treating ankylosis have been described in the literature. No single method has proven to be completely efficacious. A treatment protocol for management of TMJ ankylosis was proposed by *Kaban, Perrott and Fisher*, in 1990 which is now universally accepted and practised (Table 17.8). In 2009, a modification of *Kaban's protocol* was proposed which included distraction osteogenesis (DO) in the surgical management of TMJ ankylosis (Table 17.9). DO has several advantages over costochondral grafts (CCG), as literature highlights that CCG may exhibit unpredictable growth which can further cause asymmetry or re-ankylosis [25, 26]. Most often, patients with TMJ ankylosis present with elongated coronoid process, which require coronoidectomy for eliminat-

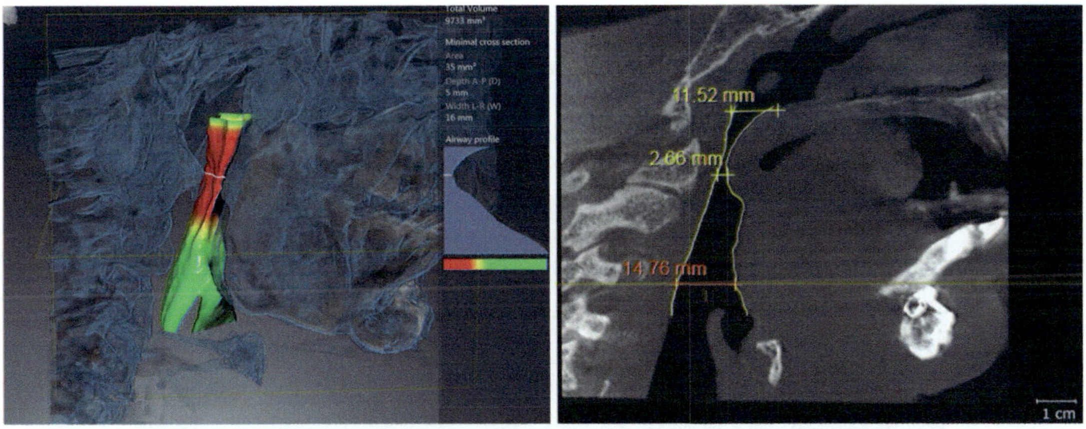

Fig. 17.6 Radiographic analysis of the airway passage depicting the narrow airway resulting in obstructive sleep apnoea in patients with temporomandibular joint ankylosis

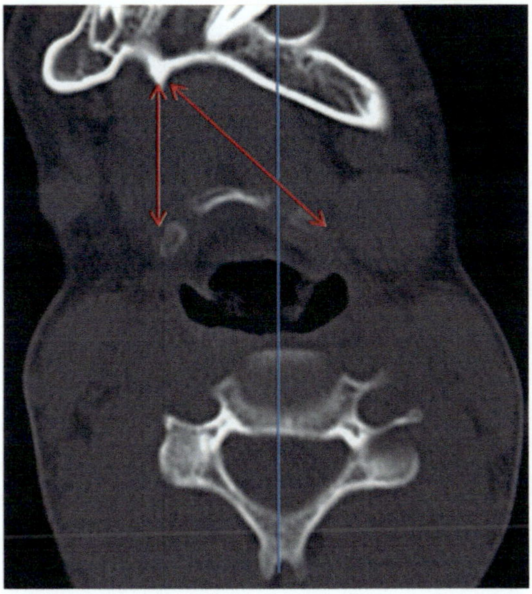

Fig. 17.7 Computed Tomography (CT) scan depicting the altered anatomy of the hyoid bone and its associated musculatures. Axial computed tomography section at the level of the hyoid in a 10-year-old patient with right temporomandibular joint ankylosis revealing shift of the hyoid complex and the laryngeal inlet to the ankylosed side. Note the shift of the genial tubercles to the ankylosed side with shortened suprahyoid musculature on the same side (*right red arrow*). Mid-sagittal plane is represented by a *blue line* (Adapted with permission from Computed tomography analysis of hyoid apparatus in temporomandibular joint ankylosis. J. Stomat. Occ. Med. (2012) 5:99–103. https://doi.org/10.1007/s12548-012-0046-7)

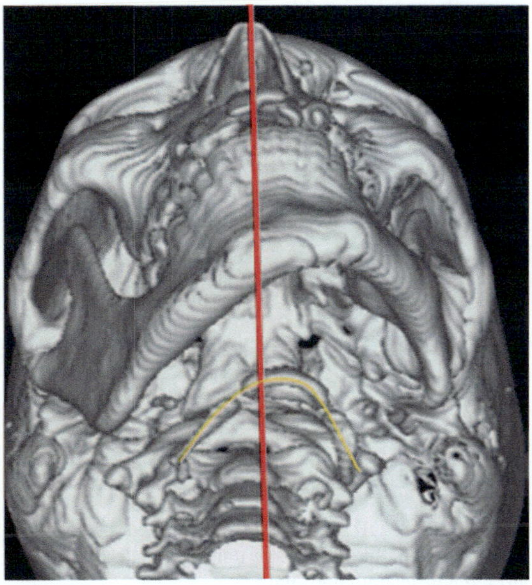

Fig. 17.8 A three-dimensional (3D) reconstructed computed tomography image of left temporomandibular joint ankylosis revealing a rotated hyoid complex to the left side (*Red line*: Mid sagittal plane; *Yellow curve*: rotated hyoid towards the side of ankylosis) (Reprinted with permission from **Springer Nature Customer Service Centre GmbH**, Computed tomography analysis of hyoid apparatus in temporomandibular joint ankylosis. J. Stomat. Occ. Med. (2012) 5:99–103. https://doi.org/10.1007/s12548-012-0046-7)

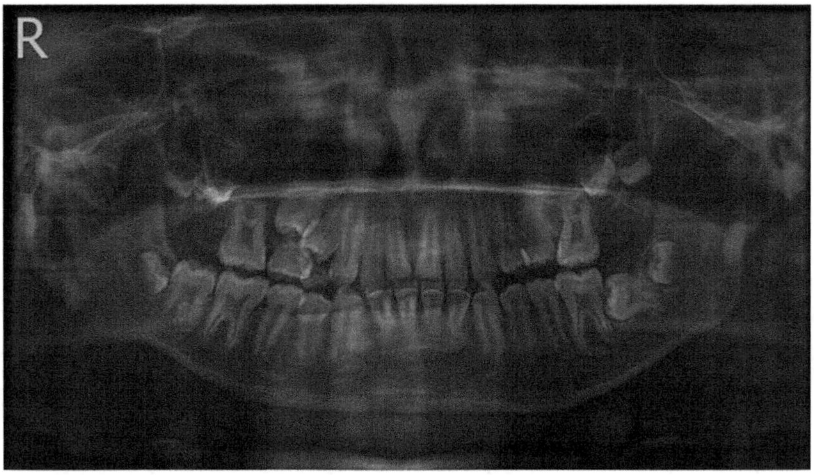

Fig. 17.9 Orthopantomogram (OPG) depicting bilateral radiopacity around the temporomandibular joint region suggestive of ankylosis with elongated coronoid process

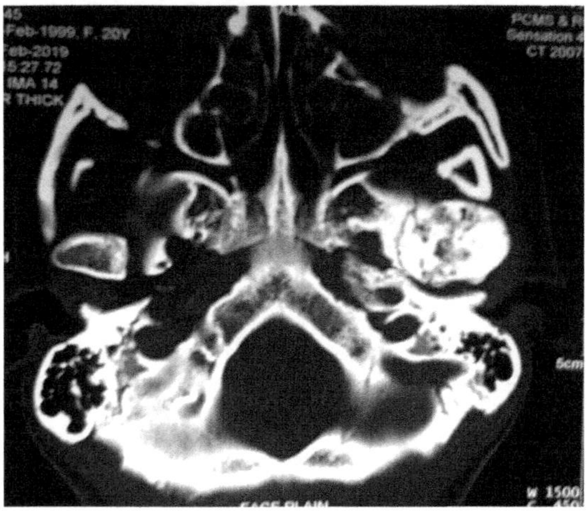

Fig. 17.10 Axial section of a computed tomography (CT) scan depicting extensive unilateral ankylosis of the left temporomandibular joint

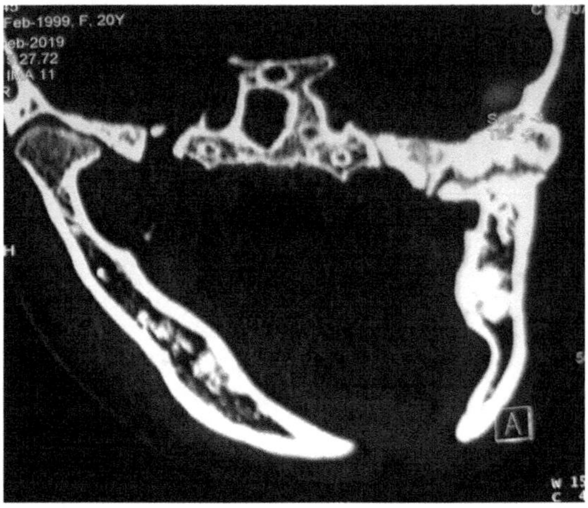

Fig. 17.11 Coronal section of a computed tomography (CT) scan depicting extensive ankylosis and rotation of the mandible with loss of radiographic mandibular morphology. Note the flattening and elongation on the normal side (Right) and shortning on the affected side (Left)

ing the mechanical hindrance with the zygomatic arch and this when done, has a 'drop down effect' to the mandible by eliminating the temporalis muscle pull.

There are several other techniques proposed for the management of TMJ ankylosis. *Esmarch operation* has been documented in literature where an osteotomy cut was placed at the angle region without involving the ankylotic mass or the ascending ramus of the mandible which aided in mandibular movements. It was later modified by Clarkson P et al. in 1949 [27]. *Salins PC* suggested that the ankylotic mass is non-neoplastic and the mass can be left in situ. He performed an osteotomy cut in the bone below the ankylotic mass resulting in the formation of pseudoarthrosis mimicking a sub-condylar fracture. He observed that this technique was effective in re-ankylosis cases with uneventful post-operative period considering it as an alternative to the conventional management [28]. *He et al.* proposed a new treatment protocol for managing TMJ ankylosis based on the proposed radiographic classification discussed earlier in this chapter [12]. The correction of the OSA is done either by DO or jaw advancement surgery (orthognathic surgery), or a combination of both [19, 20, 26]. For the correction of the secondry deformity including the facial

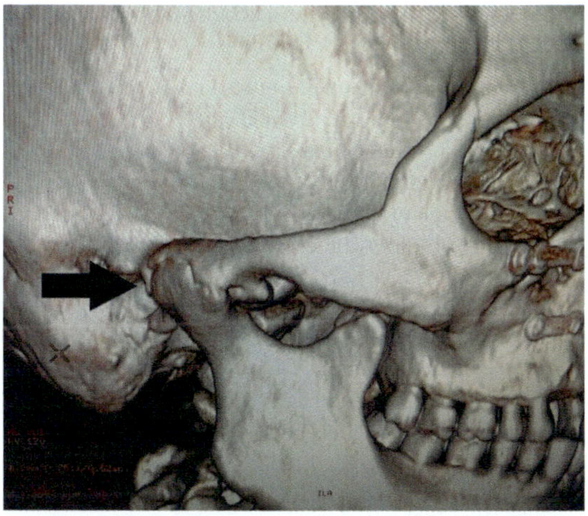

Fig. 17.12 A three-dimensional (3D) reconstructed image showing the lateral aspect of the skull demostrating ankylotic mass (*arrow*)

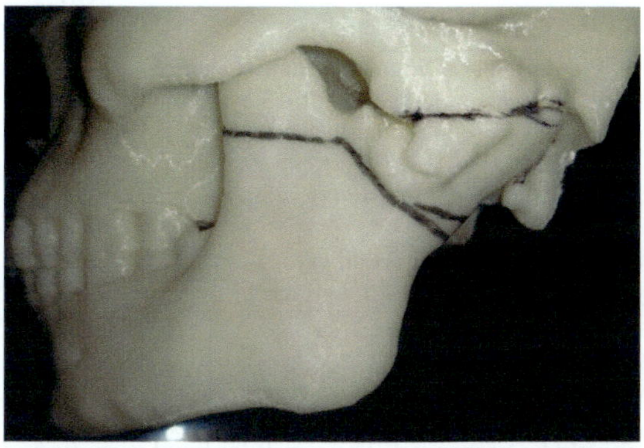

Fig. 17.13 Osteotomy cuts determined and marked on the lateral aspect pre-operatively on the stereolithographic model

asymmetry, micrograthia and occlusal cant, additional orthognathic procedures may have to be incorporated in the treatment plan.

17.9 Surgical Procedure

17.9.1 Anaesthesia

Anaesthetic management of the ankylosis patients is a challenge and demands training, expertise and additional instrumentation. The surgery should be performed under general anaesthesia (GA). Currently, the nasal fibre-optic intubation is the most acceptable method of administering inhalational anaesthesia (Refer

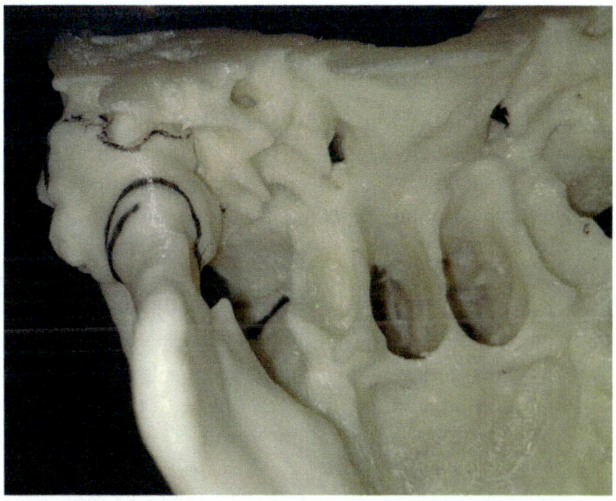

Fig. 17.14 Osteotomy cuts determined and marked in the medial and posterior aspect pre-operatively on the stereolithographic model

Chap. 27). Other intubation techniques may also be utilized that include GA via tracheostomy, retrograde intubation or blind intubation. Intubation and airway maintenance are vital aspects for a TMJ ankylosis surgery. A proper pre-anaesthetic evaluation must be done to prevent unexpected complications [16, 29]. The operating surgeon should discuss the surgical plan and possible complications that can occur in such patients with the team of anesthesiologists involved. Long-acting muscle relaxants should only be administered after securing the airway appropriately.

17.9.2 Brisement Forces

This technique may be advocated for cases with fibrous ankylosis for achieving adequate mouth opening. Forced mouth opening is done under GA (or adequate local anaesthesia) using manual force, jaw opening devices such as Heister/Fergusson's mouth gag, mouth props or a stack of wooden ice-cream sticks held together with a rubber band. This method helps in achieving adequate inter-incisal opening if the hindrance was caused due to haemarthrosis or fibrous ankylosis. The patient should be kept on active physiotherapy and should be followed up for at least 6 months post operatively [6, 30]. This method is inefficient for bony ankylosis release or in cases with long standing fibrous ankylosis, which would require more definitive management of the problem.

Table 17.8 Adaptation and modifications based on the protocol for management of TMJ ankylosis proposed by Kaban, Perrot and Fisher, 1990

1.	*Aggressive resection* of the ankylotic mass (Gap Arthroplasty)—Gap of at least 1–1.5 cm should be created between the cut bone ends (temporal and mandibular). Special attention should be directed to the medial aspect of the ankylosed bone mass (joint).
2.	*Ipsilateral Coronoidectomy*—Coronoidectomy on the side of ankylosis; this may be accompained with dissection and stripping of muscles: temporalis, when required, along with the fibers of masseter and medial pterygoid.
3.	*Contralateral coronoidectomy*—If the maximum inter-incisal opening is found less than 35 mm (with ipsilateral coronoidectomy), a contralateral coronoidectomy is performed via an intraoral approach.
4.	*Lining of TMJ* with temporalis fascia or cartilage—Temporalis fascia is interpositioned between the cut bone ends at the gap arthroplasty site. Alternatively, various authors have proposed the use of an intact disc, if identified, during the resection of ankylotic mass or cartilage from various sources (eg: auricular). Following resection of the ankylotic mass, coronoidectomy and lining of the joint, inter-maxillary fixation (IMF) is done for establishing the occlusion.
5.	Reconstruction of ramus is done with costochondral graft (CCG)
6.	Rigid fixation of the graft is assured
7.	Early mobilization and aggressive physiotherapy

Table 17.9 Modified Kaban's protocol for management of TMJ ankylosis in children (2009)

1.	Aggressive excision of fibrous and/or bony mass
2.	Coronoidectomy on affected side
3.	Coronoidectomy on opposite side if steps 1 and 2 do not result in MIO of >35 mm or to point of dislocation of opposite side
4.	Lining of joint with temporalis fascia or the native disc, if it can be salvaged
5.	Reconstruction of Ramus Condylar Unit with either Distraction osteogenesis (DO) or costochondral graft (CCG) and rigid fixation
6.	Early mobilization of Jaw; if DO is used to reconstruct the ramus condylar unit (RCU), mobilize on the day of surgery; if CCG used, early mobilization with minimal inter-maxillary fixation (not >10 days)
7.	Aggressive physiotherapy

Table 17.10 Approaches to TMJ for ankylosis management

- Pre-auricular (Dingman's/Blair's/Thomas/Popowich's modification of Alkayat-Bramley)
- Modified pre-auricular incision (Alkayat-Bramley Incision, 1980) [31]
- Sub-mandibular incision (Risdon's)
- Post-auricular
- Retro-mandibular (Hind's)
- Rhytidectomy/face-lift approach

17.9.3 Approaches to TMJ

There are several approaches stated in literature and are practised by various surgeons to access TMJ. They may vary according to the requirement and preference of the type of inter-positional grafts or choice of the modality adopted to reconstruct the joint. Various approaches used for surgical access to the TMJ region are enlisted in Table 17.10 (Refer Chap. 14).

17.9.4 Condylectomy

Condylectomy may be considered as an option in cases with fibrous joint ankylosis. After exposing the joint, the condylar head is identified. The vital structures on the medial aspect of the joint including internal maxillary artery, auriculotemporal nerve should be preserved. The condylar head is sectioned followed by contravention of the fibrous adhesions. The remaining condylar stump is smoothened which is followed by wound closure in layers. Unilateral condylectomy may cause deviation of the mandible towards the operated side on mouth opening. Anterior open bite may be seen in bilateral procedures. This further requires management of functional and occlusal discrepancy, where needed.

17.9.5 Gap Arthroplasty

After exposure of the ankylotic mass, resection of a segment of bone is performed to remove the ankylotic mass, creating a gap between the cranial (temporal) and caudal (mandibular) ends of the bone and is referred to as gap arthroplasty. For surgical bone removal, the superior and infe-

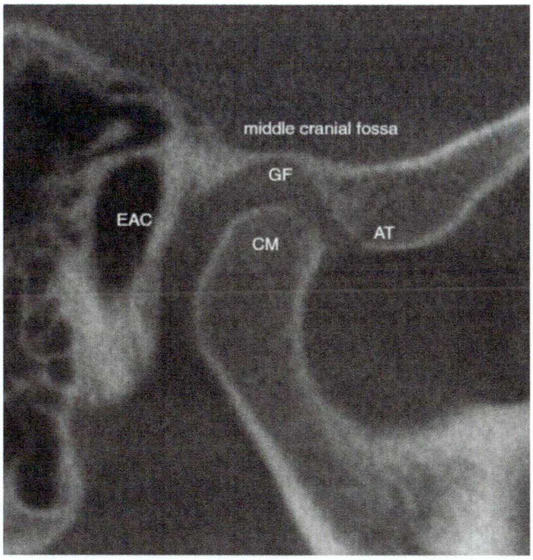

Fig. 17.15 Radiographic image shows the close proximity of the condylar head to the middle cranial fossa and external auditory canal. *CM* condylar mass, *GF* glenoid fossa, *AT* articular tubercle, *EAC* external auditory canal. (Reprinted/adapted by permission from T. von Arx, S. Lozanoff, Clinical Oral Anatomy, DOI 10.1007/978-3-319-41993-0_25)

rior limits are determined, usually by the identification of the coronoid process and the sigmoid notch, when not involved in ankylosis, are considered reliable indicators of the regional surgical anatomy by most surgeons. The limit of the superior bone cut should be planned with caution considering its proximity with the middle cranial fossa in this region (Fig. 17.15). Most reliably the superior cut can follow the inferior margin of the zygomatic arch, unless a modification is mandated based on the imaging study. Caution is essential for the prevention of any damage to the medial maxillary vessels, inferior alveolar neurovascular bundle and auditory canal posteriorly. Usually a segment of around 1–1.5 cm of bone is removed, en-block or piecemeal depending on the surgeon's preference. If motorized drill or a saw is utilized, it is wise to limit its use for the medial bone removal. Most surgeons prefer the cautious use of conventional "chisel and mallet" method for removing the bone on the medial aspect. It helps in releasing the ankylosed joint and re-instates the mobility of the mandible (Figs. 17.16 and 17.17). Babu L et al. proposed that aggressive gap arthroplasty may not be always essential but a minimal gap athroplasty of 5–8 mm with an appropriate inter-positional graft with complete resection of medio-lateral ankylotic mass would be sufficient to prevent re-ankylosis [32]. After sufficient mouth opening is achieved, the inter-positional graft or an alloplastic joint may be placed in order to prevent re-ankylosis and to reconstruct the joint.

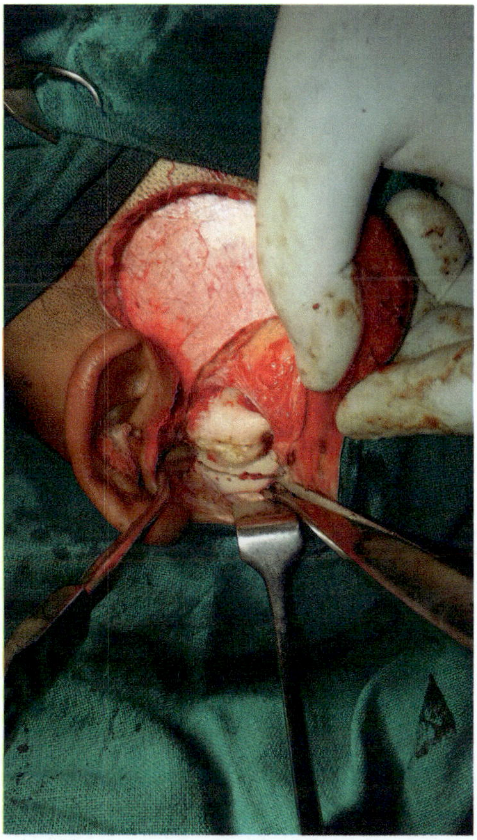

Fig. 17.16 Reference marking placed below the ankylotic mass for gap arthroplasty intra-operatively

17.9.6 Interpositional Grafts

Interpositional graft after a gap arthroplasty is considered to be an essential step to cover or separate the cut bone margins. The benefit of placing an inter-positional graft is to prevent the organization of haemotama and maintain mandibular function (Table 17.11) [33, 34]. In a

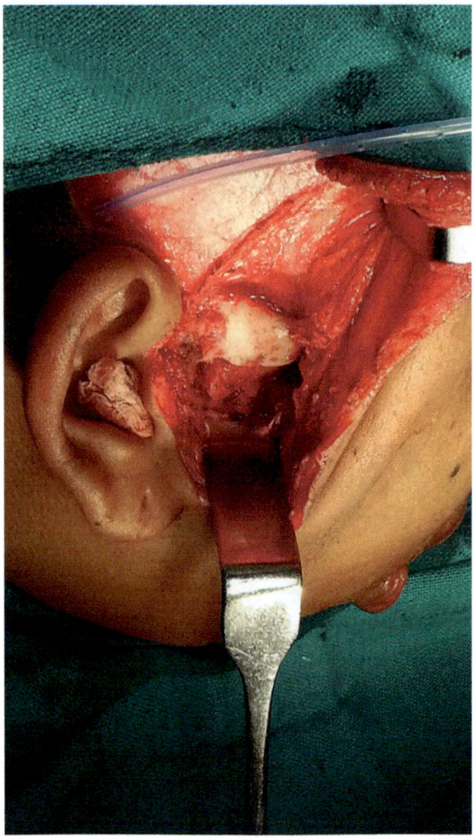

Fig. 17.17 Gap arthroplasty or gap created after resection of the ankylotic mass intra-operatively

technique proposed by Gunaseelan R, the ankylotic mass was recontoured and utilized to reconstruct the TMJ after ankylosis resection [35]. Zhu et al. reported the use of free grafting of autogenous coronoid process for condylar reconstruction in patients with temporomandibular joint ankylosis [36]. Use of autogenous coronoid process grafts pedicled on temporal muscle for reconstruction of the mandible condylar is also reported [37].

17.9.7 Reconstruction Using Autogenous Grafts and Alloplastic Prosthesis

TMJ can be reconstructed using CCG fixed to the remaining mandibular ramal bone on its lateral aspect. The evidence-based outcomes with the use of CCG are found to be unpredictable as there may

Table 17.11 Various interpositional graft materials documented in literature that were in use or are currently utilized for placement after gap arthroplasty

Autogenous	Alloplastic	Heterogenous
Temporalis muscle	Metallic 1. Tantalum plate 2. Gold 3. Stainless steel 4. Joint made from titanium	Chromatized sub-mucosa of pig bladder
Temporalis muscle and fascia		
Temporalis myofascial with dermal graft		
Dermal graft		
Buccal pad of fat		
Fascia lata		
Costachondral graft	Non-metallic 1. Silastic 2. Teflon 3. Acrylic 4. Proplast 5. Silicone 6. Ceramic implants	Lyophilized bovine cartilage
Auricular cartilage		
Sternoclavicular Joint		
Metatarsal		
Fibula graft		
Illiac crest graft		

be resorption or unwarranted growth in the graft, leading to an additional future problem requiring management. Alloplastic prosthesis has emerged as a novel standard modality that may be utilized to reconstruct the TMJ. Several prosthesis designs such as Techmedia/TMJ Concepts, Zimmer-Biomet, DARSN TM Joint prosthesis and may more have been widely studied and propose to reduce the donor site morbidity and are biocompatible, contributing to its gaining popularity over the recent years (Refer Chap. 22). They are available as stock or custom made prosthesis and can be advantageous in saving intra-operative time by reducing the need for an additional surgical site for graft harvest. However, alloplastic joints are not generally recommended for paediatric patients and autogenous reconstruction remains the preferred choice, considering the ongoing growth of the facial skeleton [38–40].

17.10 Post-operative Care

A preauricular pressure dressing is advised at most centres for a period of initial 12–24 h post surgery. If a vacuum suction drain is placed intra-operatively, requires emptying daily up to third post-operative day or when the collection is less than 25 ml. It is usually removed on the third to fourth day post-operatively (48–72 h) followed by application of a sterile dressing at the drain insertion site to cover the wound. Aggressive physiotherapy should be initiated at the earliest from the third post-operative day or when the patient can reasonably undertake such an exercise post-operatively. It should include an active hinge opening, lateral excursion and manual jaw stretching using fingers or mechanical devices. Soft, semi-solid diet may be adviced. The physiotherapy programme may include aids of mouth opening using a stack of wooden ice-cream sticks or wooden spatulas held together with a rubber band, acrylic cone and use of a mechanical mouth opener such as Heisters jaw stretcher for atleast 4–5 times daily for 15–20 min. The patient should be closely followed up for atleast 6 months post surgery.

17.11 Distraction Osteogenesis in TMJ Ankylosis

Anantanarayanan P et al. have used primary mandibular DO for managing nocturnal desaturation secondary to TMJ ankylosis [19]. Andrade NN et al. observed that these patients had a triad of TMJ ankylosis, micrognathia and OSA. The observations highlighted that patients developed bradycardia and respiratory distress during post-operative physiotherapy, when the ankylosis was released without addressing the micrognathia. To prevent this DO was performed as the first stage surgery and ankylosis release was undertaken at the later stage of the management at the time of distractor removal. Numerous studies have reported strong association of OSA with TMJ ankylosis [20, 21]. DO facilitates resolving the problem of OSA and is preferred at most centres (Fig. 17.18). The second stage of surgery may also be accompanied with orthognathic procedure(s) as per the requirement and surgeon's preference [41–44].

The treatment protocol followed at many craniofacial centres for the management of TMJ ankylosis has perceived a change since its association with OSA is established.

17.12 Complications

TMJ is surrounded by vital anatomical structures. Damage to these structures intra-operatively can lead to serious concern to patients post-operatively. The complications may be segregated into pre-operative, intra-operative and post-operative, for a better understanding and their prevention (Table 17.12) [45, 46] (Refer Chap. 25).

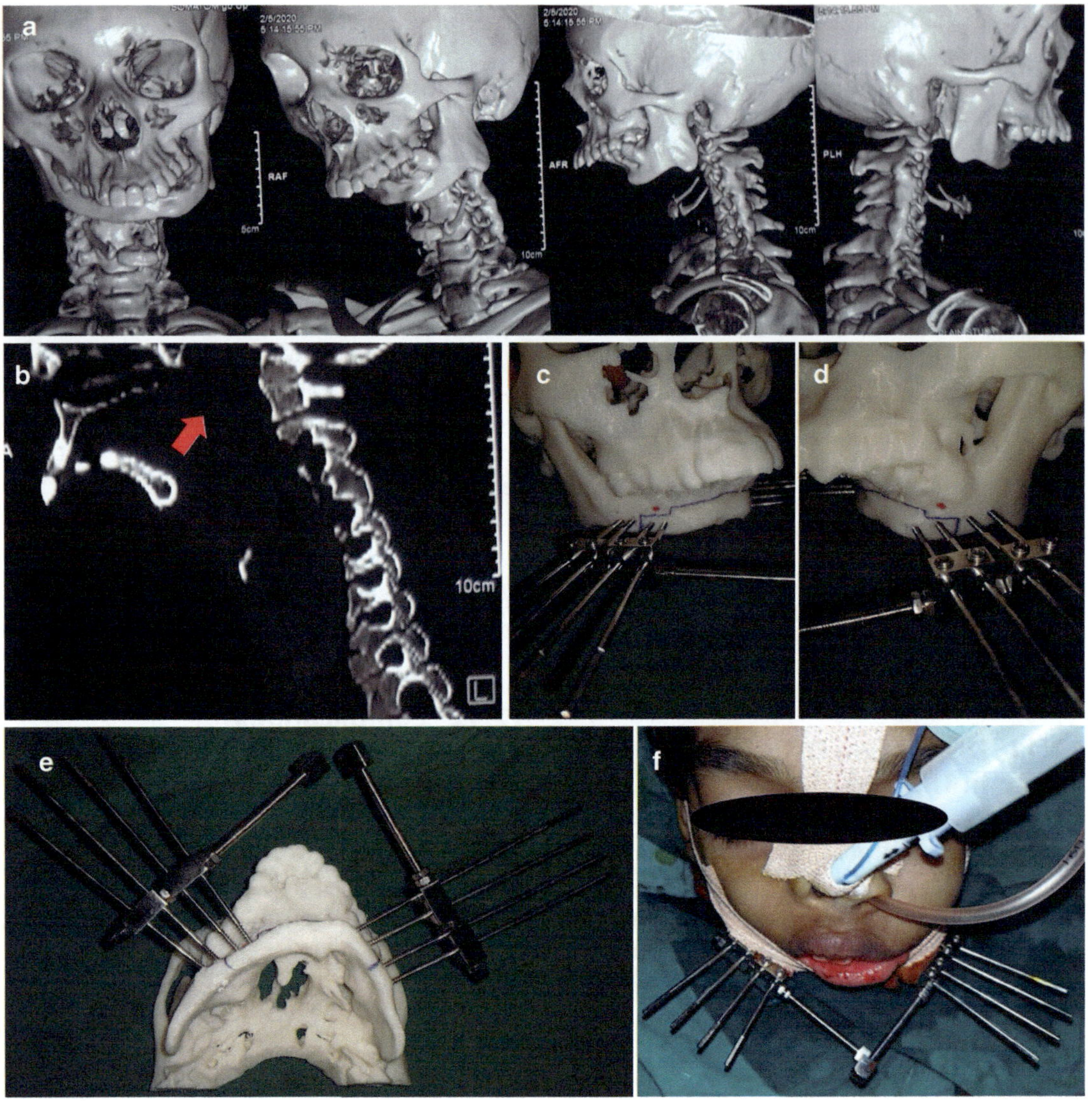

Fig. 17.18 Computer tomogram 3D reconstructed image of a patient with temporomandibular joint ankylosis and severe retrognathia with microgenia (**a**). Note the compromised airway (*arrow*), leading to OSA in these patients (**b**). Pre-ankylotic release extended genial distraction osteogenesis planning on the stereolithographic model, with bone cuts marked on the right (**c**) and on the left (**d**). Inferior view of the stereolithographic model highlighting the deformed mandibular anatomy and external pin distractor positioning (**e**). Final positioning of the distractors in the patient's mandible to correct retrognathia (**f**)

Table 17.12 Anticipated complications of the TMJ ankylosis surgery

Pre-operative	Intra-operative	Post-operative
During anaesthesia 1. Awake blind intubation requires patient co-operation 2. Micrognathia, retrognathia, altered larynx position poses difficulty for intubation	Haemorrhage caused by damage to internal maxillary artery, superficial temporal artery, transverse facial artery, inferior alveolar vessel, pterygoid plexus of veins.	Infection at the surgical site
	Damage to external auditory meatus	Open bite due to reduced vertical height
	Damage to zygomatic/temporal branch of facial nerve, auriculotemporal nerve	Recurrence/ re-ankylosis
	Aspiration of fluids, blood, foreign body as it is not possible to pack the throat prior to surgery	Hardware failure in alloplastic prosthesis
	Damage to glenoid fossa gaining entry to middle cranial fossa	Graft resorption or overgrowth
	Damage to parotid gland	Facial asymmetry
	Damage to teeth when using jaw stretcher	Facial nerve weakness/palsy
		Frey's syndrome

17.13 Conclusion

The essential goal of the surgery in temporomandibular joint ankylosis is to restore the mandibular form and function. The treatment plan and execution vary between an adult and a paediatric patient. A child should not be treated like a miniature adult owing to the difference in anatomy, physiology and the ongoing growth. Proper evaluation, surgical planning includes selection of a suitable modality for reconstruction after gap arthroplasty and executing the surgery with precision, evading the potential complications. Appropriate post-operative physiotherapy protocol and a long-term followup are the crucial factors in obtaining a successful outcome in such patients.

References

1. Sharma VK, Rattan V, Rai S, Malhi P. Quality of life assessment in temporomandibular joint ankylosis patients after interpositional arthroplasty: a prospective study. Int J Oral Maxillofac Surg. 2019;48(11):1448–55. https://doi.org/10.1016/j.ijom.2019.04.017.
2. Bello SA, Olokun BA, Olaitan AA, Ajike SO. Aetiology and presentation of ankylosis of the temporomandibular joint: report of 23 cases from Abuja, Nigeria. Br J Oral Maxillofac Surg. 2012;50(1):80–4.
3. Vasconcelos BC, Carvalho RW, Porto GG, Bessa-Nogueira RV, Nascimento MM. Surgical treatment of temporomandibular joint ankylosis: follow-up of 15 cases and literature review. Int J Oral Maxillofac Surg. 2011;40(10):1224.
4. Yan YB, Duan DH, Zhang Y, Gan YH. The development of traumatic temporomandibular joint bony ankylosis: a course similar to the hypertrophic non-union? Medical Hypotheses. 2012;78(2):273–6.
5. Yan YB, et al. Current concepts in the pathogenesis of traumatic temporomandibular joint ankylosis. Head Face Med. 2014;10:35.
6. Joshi UM, Patil SG, Shah K, Allurkar S. Brisement force in fibrous ankylosis: a technique revisited. Ind J Dent Res. 2016;27(6):661.
7. Laskin DM. Role of the meniscus in the etiology of post-traumatic temporomandibular joint ankylosis. Int J Oral Surg. 1978;7:340–5.
8. Topazian RG. Comparison of gap and interposition arthroplasty in the treatment of temporomandibular joint ankylosis. J Oral Surg (American Dental Association: 1965). 1966;24(5):405.
9. Yew CC, Ab Rahman S, Alam MK. Temporomandibular joint ankylosis in a child: an unusual case with delayed surgical intervention. BMC Pediat. 2015;15(1):169.

10. Durr ED, Turlington EG, Foote RL. Radiation treatment of heterotopic bone formation in the temporomandibular joint articulation. Int J Radiat Oncol Biol Phys. 1993;27(4):863–9.
11. El-Hakim IE, Metwalli SA. Imaging of temporomandibular joint ankylosis. A new radiographic classification. Dentomaxillofac Radiol. 2002;31:19–23.
12. He D, Yang C, Chen M, et al. Traumatic temporomandibular joint ankylosis: our classification and treatment experience. J Oral Maxillofac Surg. 2010;7:1600–7.
13. Behnia H, Tehranchi A, Younessian F. Comprehensive management of temporomandibular joint ankylosis—state of the art. A Textbook of Advanced Oral and Maxillofacial Surgery. 2015;2:2411.
14. Miloro M. Peterson's Principles of Oral and Maxillofacial Surgery. PMPH-USA; 2004. p. 1033–4.
15. Singh S, Kumar S, Pandey R, Passi D, Mehrotra D, Mohammad S. Dimensional differences in mandibular antegonial notches in temporomandibular joint ankylosis. J Oral Biol Craniofac Res. 2011;1(1):7–11.
16. Wahal R. Temporo-mandibular joint ankylosis – the difficult airway. J Oral Biol Craniofac Res. 2015;5:57–8.
17. Moss ML, Rankow RM. The role of the functional matrix in mandibular growth. Angle Orthodontist. 1968;38(2):95–103.
18. Deshpande A, Bhargava D, Kota S, Babu DG. Computed tomography analysis of hyoid apparatus in temporomandibular joint ankylosis. Int J Stomatol Occlusion Med. 2012;5(3):99–103.
19. Anatanarayanan P, Narayanan V, Manikandhan R, et al. Primary mandibular distraction for management of nocturnal desaturations secondary to TMJ ankylosis. Int J Pediatr Otorhinolaryngol. 2008;72:385–9.
20. Andrade NN, Kalra R, Shetye SP. New protocol to prevent TMJ reankylosis and potentially life threatening complications in triad patients. Int J Oral Maxillofac Surg. 2012;41(12):1495–500.
21. Shaeran TAT, Samsudin AR. Temporomandibular Joint Ankylosis Leading to Obstructive Sleep Apnea. J Craniofac Surg. 2019 Nov-Dec;30(8):e714-e717. https://doi.org/10.1097/SCS.0000000000005689.
22. Langdon J, Patel M, Ord R, Brennan P. Operative oral and maxillofacial surgery. 2nd ed. 2010. p. 567.
23. Akkoyunlu ME, Altın R, Kart L, et al. Investigation of obstructive sleep apnoea syndrome prevalence among long-distance drivers from Zonguldak, Turkey. Multidiscip Respir Med. 2013;8(1):10. https://doi.org/10.1186/2049-6958-8-10.
24. He D, Cai Y, et al. Analysis of temporomandibular joint ankylosis caused by condylar fracture in adults. J Oral Maxillofac Surg. 2013;12(15):763.e1–e9.
25. Kaban LB, Perrott DH, Fisher K. A protocol for management of temporomandibular joint ankylosis. J Oral Maxillofac Surg. 1990;48(11):1145–51.
26. Kaban LB, Bouchard C, Troulis MJ. A protocol for management of temporomandibular joint ankylosis in children. J Oral Maxillofac Surg. 2009;67(9):1966–78.
27. Clarkson P, Kenshole HH. Esmarch's operation for the relief of ankylosis and of pain in the temporomandibular joint; a modified operative technique. Br Dent J. 1949;87(10):257–64, illust
28. Salins PC. New perspectives in the management of temporomandibular joint ankylosis. Int J Oral Maxillofac Surg. 2000;29:337–40.
29. Mohan K, Mohana Rupa L, Gopala Krishna Murthy S, Greeshma PG, Bhavana U. Anaesthesia for TMJ ankylosis with the use of TIVA, followed by endotracheal intubation. J Clin Diag Res. 2012;6(10):1765.
30. Thakur R, Shigli AL, Thakur G, Ahuja R. Giving a second thought to brisement force–a case report. J Clin Pediat Dent. 2015;39(2):120–3.
31. Al-Kayat A, Bramley P. A modified pre-auricular approach to the temporomandibular joint and malar arch. Br J Oral Surg. 1979;17(2):91–103.
32. Babu L, Jain MK, Ramesh C, et al. Is aggressive gap arthroplasty essential in the management of temporomandibular joint ankylosis? – a prospective clinical study of 15 cases. Br J Oral Maxillofac Surg. 2013;51:473–8.
33. Tuncel U. Interpositional arthroplasty in the treatment of temporomandibular joint ankylosis: a review of literature. Surgery. 2011;1(103):2161–1076.
34. Rao JD, Dar N, Sharma A, Sheorain AK, Malhotra V, Arya V. Evaluation of the sternoclavicular graft for the reconstruction of temporomandibular joint after gap arthroplasty. Ann Maxillofac Surg. 2017;7(2):194.
35. Gunaseelan R. Condylar reconstruction in extensive ankylosis of temporomandibular joint in adults using resected segment as autograft: a new technique. Int J Oral Maxillofac Surg. 1997;26:405–7.
36. Zhu SS, Hu J, Li J, Luo E, Liang X, Feng G. Free grafting of autogenous coronoid process for condylar reconstruction in patients with temporomandibular joint ankylosis. Oral Surg Oral Med Oral Pathol Oral Radiol Endod. 2008;106(5):662–7.
37. Liu Y, Li J, Hu J, Zhu S, Luo E, Hsu Y. Autogenous coronoid process pedicled on temporal muscle grafts for reconstruction of the mandible condylar in patients with temporomandibular joint ankylosis. Oral Surg Oral Med Oral Pathol Oral Radiol Endod. 2010;109(2):203–10.
38. Wolford LM, Mercuri LG, Schneiderman ED, Movahed R, Allen W. Twenty-year follow-up study on a patient-fitted temporomandibular joint prosthesis: the Techmedia/TMJ concepts device. J Oral Maxillofac Surg. 2015;73:952–60.
39. Westermark A. Reconstruction of the temporomandibular joint. Up to 8 years follow-up of patients with Biomet total joint prostheses. Int J Oral Maxillofac Surg. 2010;39:951–5.
40. Bhargava D, Neelakandan RS, Sharma Y, Dalsingh V, Beena S, Gurjar P. Predictability and Feasibility of Total Alloplastic Temporomandibular Joint Reconstruction using DARSN TM Joint Prosthesis for patients in Indian subcontinent-A prospective clinical study. J Stomatol Oral Maxillofac Surg. 2020;121(1):2–8. https://doi.org/10.1016/j.jormas.2019.06.005.

41. Guruprasad Y, Hemavathy OR. Management of obstructive sleep apnea syndrome secondary to temporomandibular joint ankylosis by mandibular elongation using distraction osteogenesis. Contemp Clin Dent. 2012;3(1):69.
42. Gaur A, Singh G, Mishra M, Srivatsan KS, Sachdev V. Distraction osteogenesis for management of obstructive sleep apnea secondary to TMJ ankylosis. Nat J Maxillofac surg. 2013;4(1):104.
43. Tomonari H, Takada H, Hamada T, Kwon S, Sugiura T, Miyawaki S. Micrognathia with temporomandibular joint ankylosis and obstructive sleep apnea treated with mandibular distraction osteogenesis using skeletal anchorage: a case report. Head Face Med. 2017;13(1):20.
44. Li J, Zhu S, Wang T, Luo E, Xiao L, Hu J. Staged treatment of temporomandibular joint ankylosis with micrognathia using mandibular osteodistraction and advancement genioplasty. J Oral Maxillofac Surg. 2012;70(12):2884–92.
45. McKenzie WS, Louis PJ. Complications following temporomandibular joint replacement: a 10-year retrospective review. J Oral Maxillofac Surg. 2015;73(9):e21.
46. Jagannathan M, Munoli AV. Unfavourable results in temporomandibular joint ankylosis surgery. Indian J Plastic Surg. 2013;46(2):235.

Temporomandibular Joint Hypermobility Disorders

18

Darpan Bhargava and Beena Sivakumar

18.1 Introduction

Hypermobility of the temporomandibular joint (TMJ) is characterized by mandibular condyle having greater than normal range of motion (ROM) that can occur naturally in otherwise normal individual indicating a sign of joint instability. Several extrinsic or intrinsic predisposing factors are known to contribute to this condition (Table 18.1). Conservative methods of management should be initiated in such patients before considering the patients for surgery [1, 2].

While performing unstrained/normal mouth opening, the condylar head translates forward and stops in a position under the articular eminence. In hypermobility it translates anteriorly beyond the eminence (Fig. 18.1). Hypermobility disorders may be subdivided into subluxation and dislocation. Temporomandibular joint dislocation involves a non self-limiting displacement of the condyle, outside of its functional position within the glenoid fossa and posterior slope of the articular eminence [3]. Dislocation may be unilateral and/or bilateral (Table 18.2), acute or chronic. Chronic dislocation may further be divided into protracted or recurrent (Adekeye et al.) [3]. In subluxation, the joint is transiently displaced without complete loss of the articulating function and is self reducible by the patient at most instances.

Table 18.1 The various intrinsic and extrinsic factors for temporomandibular joint dislocation

Intrinsic factors (Related to joint structure or function)	Extrinsic factors (Systemic or other factors not related to joint architecture)
Laxity of ligaments, capsule and abnormality of skeletal structure	Previous injury to the mandible, occlusal disharmonies
Flattened eminence and/or shallow fossa	Ehlers-Danlos or other connective tissue diseases, neurodegenerative or neurodysfunctional diseases including epilepsy and Parkinson disease, Muscle dystrophies or dystonias (extra-pyramidal reactions)
Injury to the joint altering the joint anatomy and function	Anti-psychotic and neuroleptic drugs

D. Bhargava (✉)
TMJ Consultancy Services, Bhopal, Madhya Pradesh, India

Oral and Maxillofacial Surgery, People's College of Dental Sciences and Research Centre, People's University, Bhopal, Madhya Pradesh, India
e-mail: drdarpanbhargava@gmail.com

B. Sivakumar
Department of Oral and Maxillofacial Surgery, Meenakshi Ammal Dental College and Hospital, Chennai, Tamil Nadu, India

D. Bhargava (ed.), *Temporomandibular Joint Disorders*,
https://doi.org/10.1007/978-981-16-2754-5_18

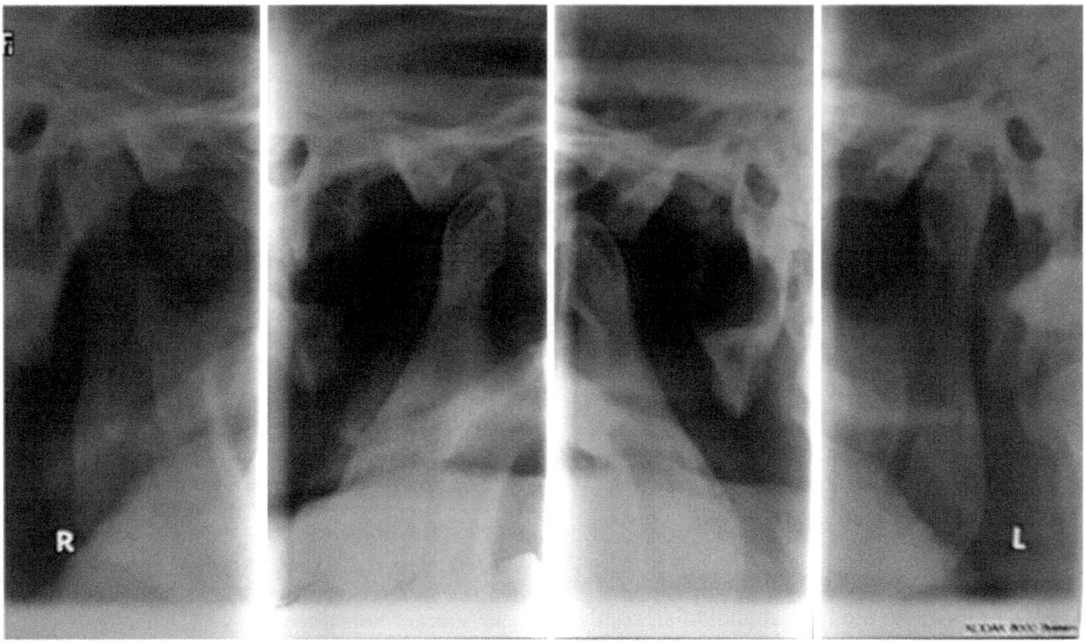

Fig. 18.1 TMJ tomogram depicting the position of condylar head during open and closed mouth position showing the condyle placed much anterior to the articular eminence during mouth opening. (Picture Courtesy: Dr. Darpan Bhargava, TMJ Consultancy Services, Bhopal, India)

Table 18.2 Clinical features of unilateral and bilateral temporomandibular joint dislocation

Unilateral acute dislocation	Bilateral acute dislocation
Difficulty in speech, mastication, deglutition Drooling of saliva Deviation of chin with lateral cross and open bite to the contralateral side Affected condylar movements may not be palpable. A depression may be noted in front of the tragus	Pain Inability to close mouth Contracted masticatory muscles Speech difficulty Excessive salivation and drooling Gagging of molar teeth with anterior open bite

In unilateral dislocation, deviation of the midline to the contralateral side with an ipsilateral open bite will be evident. Whereas bilateral dislocation is a more advanced hyper-translation where both the condyle locks out anterior to the eminence to a position where it cannot be self-reduced. Subluxation is the abnormal anterior excursion of condyle beyond the articular eminence where the patient can manipulate the joint back into normal position. It occurs when the condyle translates anterior to its normal range and the patient exhibits a temporary locking sensation that either abates spontaneously or can be reduced with manual self-manipulation. An incomplete recurrent, self-reducing, habitual dislocation is known as chronic subluxation (Table 18.3).

Table 18.3 Classification of temporomandibular joint hypermobility (Rowe and Killey)

Sub-luxation	**Dislocation** (non self-reducing)	
Reduces spontaniously or usually self-reduced by the patient	*Acute*	*Chronic*
	Isolated	
	Recurrent	

18.2 Clinical Examination

Clinical evaluation should include obtaining a history followed by examination of the patient. The common clinical features seen in dislocation include pre-auricular hollowing on maximal ROM, inability to close the mouth (open lock) caused by posterior disc displacement and reactive muscle spasm, difficulty in speech, drooling of saliva secondary to incompetent lips. The classic "click" in the terminal phases of mouth opening can be a sign of subluxation (a palpable preauricular feel of the condyle slipping at the eminence anterioly, on complete mouth opening). Chronic subluxation may become symptomatic, with pain as a presenting feature. Major cause of pain in subluxation is the compression of the intervening tissue between the condylar head and the height of the eminence along with the undue stretch in the retrodiscal area.

In acute dislocation, pain in the pre-auricular and temporal region may be present, but it is rarely a presenting feature in chronic recurrent dislocation. Emptiness in the joint space can be felt on palpation over the pre-auricular region. Predisposing factors for acute dislocation could be excessive mouth opening upon yawning, vomiting, laughing, prolonged dental procedures, facial trauma, epileptic attacks, and direct laryngoscopy [4, 5]. Acute dislocations are one time events, which when managed appropriately pose no long-term problems. Chronic dislocation include events of acute dislocations that are not self-reducing and require interceptive treatment to prevent its progession to chronic recurrent dislocations, which are non-self reducing and occur very frequently. Patients with Ehlers-Danlos or other connective tissue diseases, neurodegenerative or neurodysfunctional diseases including epilepsy and Parkinson's disease, muscle dystrophies or dystonias or patients on neuroleptic drugs may report with recurrent dislocation.

The optimal TMJ range of motion (ROM) is between 40 and 50 mm. Initial 20–25 mm of opening is achieved primarily through rotation which occurs in the lower half of the joint between the mandibular condyle and beneath the disc surface. The remaining 15–25 mm is achieved during forward gliding (anterior translation) motion that occurs between upper surface of the disc and the temporal bone (Fig. 18.2). Mostly in TMJ hypermobility ROM is beyond 50 mm following which the lock occurs. Various authors have classified the hypermobility based on the ROM, from 50 to 55 mm as mild hypermobility,

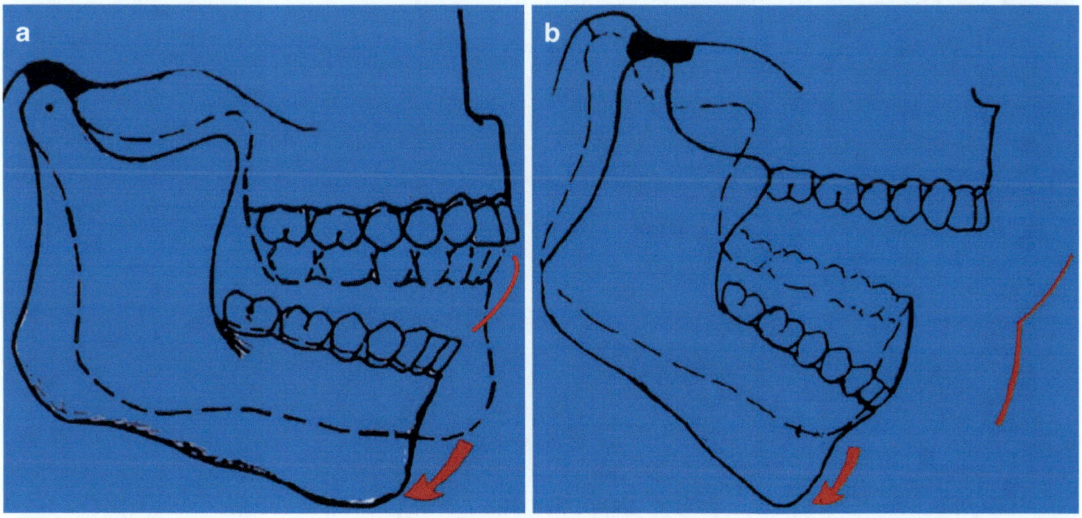

Fig. 18.2 (**a**) Mouth opening with hinge or rotational movement of the temporomandibular joint. (**b**) Mouth opening produced by a combination of rotation and translation movement of the temporomandibular joint. Note in the transition in the position of the disc and the mandibular condyle in relation to the articular eminence. (Adapted from Ozkan Y.K. (2018) Movements and Mechanics of Mandible Occlusion Concepts and Laws of Articulation. In: Ozkan Y. (eds) Complete Denture Prosthodontics. Springer, Cham. https://doi.org/10.1007/978-3-319-69032-2_8)

55–65 mm as moderate hypermobility, and > 65 mm as severe hypermobility disorder.

For establishing a diagnosis the instrumental movement analysis to assess the quantitative characteristics and analysis of performance of bilateral condyle may be used. It also records the condylar path length to determine hypermobility of the joint. It is performed using an electronic recording system, i.e. axiography for recording the mandibular movements based on ultrasonic measuring device [4]. Although, these equipments may not be universally available, and clinical assessment remains the best choice.

18.3 Pathogenesis of TMJ Hypermobility

The classic triad of chronic recurrent subluxation includes (1) Ligamentous and capsular flaccidity (2) Eminential erosion and flattening (Fig. 18.3) (3) trauma (macro or micro), myospasm, and aberrancy in masticatory movements. The dislocation is known to occur due to elevation of mandible caused by lack of muscular co-ordination. This is caused by lack of relaxation of the protractors (lateral pterygoid, digastric, mylohyoid, geniohyoid) with associated firing of the elevators (masseter, temporalis, medial pterygoid) causing myo-spastic contractions. It initiates a feedback loop that induces spastic contractions prohibiting self-reduction [3].

18.4 Radiographic Examination

TMJ hypermobility can be confirmed by the history of the patient and clinical examination. Radiographs such as open and closed mouth TMJ tomogram, computed tomography (CT) scan, dynamic magnetic resonance imaging (MRI, closed and open mouth with maximum ROM) can be obtained to evaluate the joint and periarticular tissues, and to aid in any surgical interventions that may be needed. Haghigah A et al. evaluated condylar distance in hypermobile TMJ with excessive mouth openings using CT. They

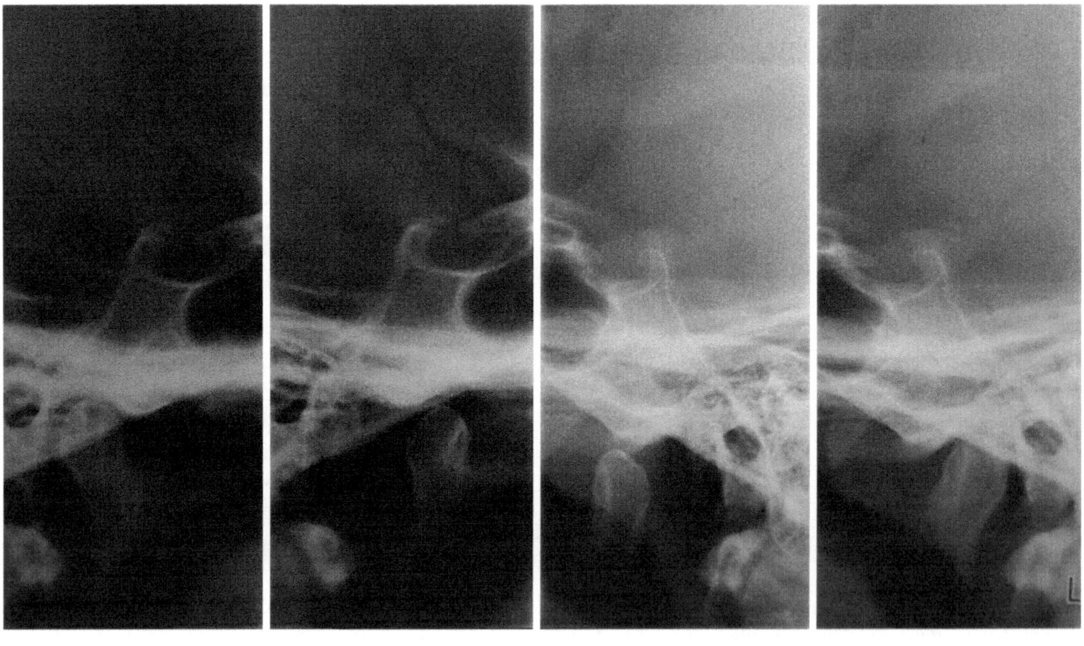

Fig. 18.3 TMJ tomogram depicting the position of condylar head during open and closed mouth position showing flattened articular eminence bilaterally allowing the condyle to slip anteriorly during mouth opening. (Picture Courtesy: Dr. Darpan Bhargava, TMJ Consultancy Services, Bhopal, India)

evaluated the position of the condyle from the articular eminence while MMO; and measured the distances from anterior, superior and posterior border of condyle and facing wall of glenoid fossa in closed mouth. The conclusion from the study indicate that the superior and posterior distances would be significantly higher in hypermobility patients when compared with healthy individuals [6–8].

18.5 Management of Hypermobility of TMJ

The management includes conservative, minimally invasive, and surgical methods depending upon the duration, severity and response to previous treatment methods. All the available treatment modalities fall in one of the following categories: 1) tightening of the capsule; 2) connecting the joint or mandible to adjecent fixed structure; 3) mechanical interferences for condylar translation; 4) elimination of interferences; 5) removal of lateral pterygoid pull preventing translation. Approaches to the condylar region have been discussed in detail elsewhere for open joint procedures (Refer Chap. 14). The history and various management methods for TMJ hypermobility are listed (Tables 18.4 and 18.5) [3, 9, 10].

Table 18.4 Management methods for TMJ hypermobility

Non-surgical/minimally invasive procedures
Intermaxillary fixation using elastics/Barton's bandage/Chin strap to limit oral opening
Administering Sclerosing agents/Proliferants in the joint space
Autologous blood injection (ABI)
Botulinum toxin injection
Surgical procedures
Capsule tightening procedures
- Arthroscopic capsulorrhaphy
- Open capsulorrhaphy
Surgical procedures that limits the condylar path
- Lindemann's procedure
- Mayor's procedure
- Dautrey's procedure
Placement of an obstacle using other materials
- L shaped plates, Steel pins
- Titanium screws
- Blocks of porous coralline hydroxyapatite
- Iliac/calvarial bone grafts
- Mitek bone anchors—Wolford
Creation of muscular balance
- Masticatory muscle myotomy
- Shortening of temporalis tendon

18.5.1 Conservative Method

Patient presenting with a locked jaw in open mouth position reports usually in a state of anxiety, specially when it is an acute dislocation experienced by the patient for the first time. Severe muscle spasm would be present surrounding the dislocated jaw. Initial management should aim at reducing the anxiety and limiting the muscle spasm by counselling, reassuring and with the use of pharmacotherapeutic agents that may include anxiolytic agents or sedative drugs (eg. Diazepam) before undertaking a reduction manoeuvre. The management of patients with chronic dislocation or chronic recurrent non-self reducing dislocation will have a better operator ease, as these patients are in a less anxious state from their previous experiences. Patients with symptomatic chronic subluxation may present with pain as the only presenting feature.

18.5.1.1 Conventional Intraoral Technique (Nélaton's Maneuver or the Hippocratic Technique)

Acute dislocation can be reduced under local anesthesia or general anesthesia or sometimes without the use of anesthesia using a bimanual intra-oral traction. Patient should be seated against a firm back and head rest and is instructed to remain calm which helps in relaxation of the elevator muscles of the mandible. The operator should stand in front of the patient grasping the mandible in the retro-molar region on both the sides firmly using the thumb intra-orally and the other fingers placed below the chin. Downward pressure should be exerted on the molars followed by a backward and an upward thrust below the lower border of the mandible extra-orally to push the mandible downward below

Table 18.5 History of treatment modalities for TMJ hypermobility

Year	Proposed by	Procedure
1945	Hudson	Plication of capsule to reduce the size of hollow viscus
1947	Schultz	Injection of sclerosing solution into joint to produce capsular fibrosis and restrict excessive condylar movements
1949	Bowman	Detachment of external pterygoid muscle from condyle along with a capsulorrhaphy
1951	Dingman	Meniscectomy to treat hypermobility
1961	Ward	Recommended condylotomy
1962	Litzow and Royer	Condylectomy should be reserved for long-standing dislocations
1964	Findlay	Inserted a stainless steel pin into the zygomatic process of temporal bone
1965	Georgiade	Ligation of condyle to zygomatic arch using mersilene (Dacron) strips
1968	Merril	Similar technique using Dacron strips in patient with Parkinson's disease
1968	Boudroux and Spire	Plication of capsule
1969	Thoma	Bone graft onlay to the articular eminence
1975	Sanders and Newman	Plication of capsule combined with a ligamentorraphy
1978	Howe and Kent	Attached a vitallium mesh to the zygoma
1978	Gould	Intra-oral scarification to effect a shortening of the temporalis tendon
1951	Myrhaug	Described the reduction in height of the articular eminence enabling the condyle to slip back into the fossa if sub-luxation occurs.
1957	Irby	
1972	Hale	
1975	Jacques Dautrey	Procedure describing an oblique cut through zygomatic arch posteriorly, arch is brought down and impacted under the articular eminence

the articular eminence and backward into the fossa (Fig. 18.4) [2, 3]. Combining the procedure with local anesthesia and/or sedation usually allows less painful reduction for the patient. Auriculotemporal nerve block through the preauricular approach helps in pain reduction due to dislocation and also aids for pain control during reduction. Young et al. (2009) have advocated the use of peripheral nerve blocks of the masseter and deep temporal nerve along with infiltration of the joint capsule for minimizing discomfort while reduction and also to, decreasing the muscle spasm.

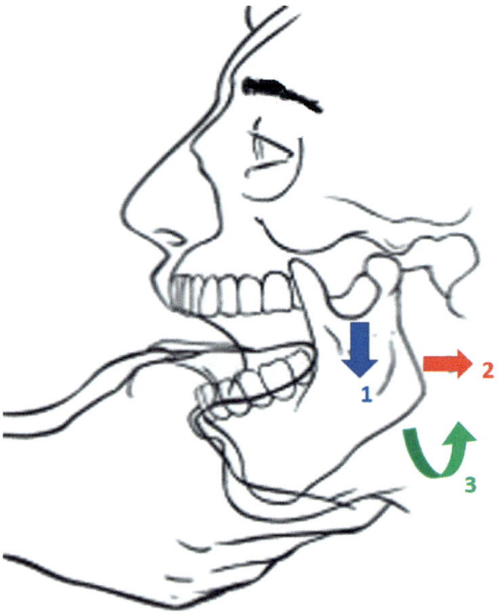

Fig. 18.4 Bimanual intra-oral traction manoeuvre for reduction of the dislocated mandible. Note the downward pressure (**1**) that should be exerted on the molars followed by a backward (**2**) and an upward thrust (**3**)

18.5.1.2 External Method (Ardehali et al.)

Ardehali et al. described an extraoral approach for condylar dislocation reduction where each joint is reduced separately. In this method, on one side, the thumb is placed just above the anteriorly displaced coronoid process, and the fingers are placed behind the mastoid process to provide a counteracting force. On the other side, the fingers hold the mandible angle and the thumb is placed over the malar eminence. To reduce the dislocated jaw, one side of the mandible angle is pulled anteriorly by the fingers, with the thumb over the malar eminence acting as a fulcrum. While the mandible angle is pulled anteriorly, steady pressure is applied on the coronoid process of the other side, with the fingers behind the mastoid process providing counteracting force. The mandible is rotated by this maneuver and the dislocated temporomandibular joint is usually reduced on one side. When one side of the dislocation is reduced, the other side will usually get reduced spontaneously [11].

18.5.1.3 Gag Reflex

Awang MN reported a technique of initiating a gag reflex to reduce acute dislocation using a mouth mirror to stimulate a gag by contacting the soft palate/pharynx. The impulse is carried to central nervous system causing stimulation of all the depressor and protruder muscles of the mandible along with reflex inhibition of elevator muscles causing mandible to relocate into the condylar fossa [12].

Following reduction, immobilization should be done to restrict the mouth opening using a Barton's bandage or inter-maxillary fixation (IMF) for 7 days. Diet modification should include liquid to semi-solid diet. Muscle relaxants should be prescribed. Long-standing cases, more than 15–30 days may not respond to the above-mentioned procedures. In such cases, reduction should be done under general anesthesia. For patients with persistant or protracted dislocations, who report late for the treatment, traction with wires at the angle under general anesthesia may be attempted. If manoeuvres described fail to achieve reduction, then surgical procedure should include osteotomising the mandible in the midline or paramidline region and reducing both the condyles individually, followed by fixation of the mandible. Alternatively, temporal myotomy via an intraoral anterior ramal incision is advocated (Laskin, 1972), which usually aids in repositioning of the condyles into the glenoid fossa.

18.5.2 Minimally Invasive Methods

18.5.2.1 Autologous Blood Injection

Autologous blood injection (ABI) was first described by Brachmann in 1964. The injected blood initiates an intra-capsular and peri-capsular inflammatory response caused by transferred platelets and blood constituents causing fibrosis and adhesions. Fibrosis and cicatricial maturation cause physiologic reduction in compliance to the peri-articular soft tissue causing a decreased ROM. Blood is injected following arthrocentesis procedure where the whole blood is drawn from the patient and deposited via the inflow needle into the superior joint space. The outflow needle is either removed or blocked during the blood injection. Some authors advocate the deposition of blood aditionally to the retrodiscal region and the pericapsular area apart from the superior joint space. The patient is advised to minimize mandibular function postoperatively. Based on clinical improvement, which should be assessed no earlier than 6-12 weeks post ABI, repeated injections may be administered. The advantages of ABI include reduced chance for allergic reactions and the technique is simple where the blood can be collected as a chair-side procedure. Autologous blood injections can be performed on an outpatient basis offering a safe and effective treatment [3, 13–16]. Autologous blood injections may be attempted for patients with chronic dislocation, symptomatic subluxation and recurrent acute dislocation with a suspected progression to chronic recurrent subluxation.

18.5.2.2 Sclerotherapy/Injection of a Sclerosing Agent

Injection of sclerosants produces an inflammatory response which causes fibrosis in the pericapsular region reducing the temporomandibular joint hypermobility. Several sclerosing agents are used in practice that include sodium tetradecyl sulfate, bleomycin, cyclophosphamide, tetracycline, iodine, alcohol, ethanolamine oleate and OK- 432 (Picibanil). Disadvantages of sclerotherapy include sensation of local irritation and the risk of allergic reaction to the sclerosant. There are documented reports on various sclerosing agents causing chondrocyte degeneration leading to the development of the degenerative joint disease [3, 17]. For this reason, repeated injections should be considered with caution.

While using the sclerosing agents, the control on the extent of fibrosis induced, is beyond clinical control. These injections are generally painful as they cause local irritation on injection, and thus requring the need for local anesthetic blocks before the injection.

18.5.2.3 Botulinum Toxin Injection

Botulinum toxin type A is known to cause a dose related weakness of skeletal muscle by inhibiting acetylcholine release at the neuromuscular junction. In TMJ dislocation it is used as a primary modality as a treatment or as an adjunct to other procedures. The target muscle is the lateral pterygoid as it is involved in spasm during dislocation.

Fu et al. assessed landmarks to approach lateral pterygoid belly percutaneously through the sigmoid notch inferior to the zygomatic arch. After aspiration, 25–50 units of Type A botulinum toxin should be injected directly into the muscle belly. It can also be injected trans-orally under electromyography (EMG) guidance. A single injection is usually effective.

However the disadvantage of botulinum injection includes hemorrhage on needle insertion. Rarely, toxin induced velopharyngeal insufficiency (VPI), dysphagia, and dysarthria is reported, which usually subside within 2–4 weeks [3, 18].

18.5.2.4 Prolotherapy

Prolotherapy for temporomandibular joint (Schultz, 1937), also known as proliferation treatment or regenerative injection therapy is infiltrating a non-pharmacologic agent around the peri-capsular tissue which initiates an inflammatory process causing local fibrous proliferation increasing the tissue robustness, thereby increasing joint stability and reducing laxity. Several agents have been used as proliferants for TMJ dysfunction since the 1930s such as dextrose, psyllium seed oil, glycerin, phenol and combinations. Commonly used proliferant is dextrose. 2 ml of 10–50% dextrose is injected in the superior joint space and the pericapsular area followed by diet modification and minimal jaw function for 2 weeks. Repeated injections may be required to achieve optimal therapeutic effects [3, 19]. *Refai et al. (2011)* conducted a prospective, randomized, double-blind, placebo-controlled clinical trial on twelve patients with painful subluxation or dislocation, where the study group received 4 injections of dextrose solution (2 mL of 10% dextrose and 1 mL of 2% mepivacaine) for each TMJ, each 6 weeks apart. Authors reported prolotherapy as a promising treatment for symptomatic TMJ hypermobility, as evidenced by the therapeutic benefits, simplicity, safety, patients' acceptance of the injection technique, and lack of any significant side effects. Injection of a proliferant is usually painful, mandating adequate use of local anaesthesia during prolotherapy. During the treatment with autologous blood, sclerosing agents or proliferants, use of anti-inflammatory medication, should be avoided including the non steroidal anti inflammatory drugs, as these management strategies utilize induction of an inflammatory response to induce fibrosis. The mainstay for pain management during the course of the treatment should be opioid class of analgesics, of which commonly used is tramadol. Dextrose, which is commonly used and is considered safe, is an osmotic proliferant which acts by dehydrating the cells at the injection site which utlimately leads to release of cellular fragments that act as chemoattractants and start the inflammatory cascade leading to deposition of collagen. Another proposed mechanism is by glycosylating tissues and making them appear foreign to the immune system thereby initiating an inflammatory response. Irrespective of the triger mechanism, the subsequent inflammatory reaction and the consequent wound healing cascade leads to the collagen formation by the fibroblasts in the due course [19].

18.5.3 Surgical Methods

Once the conservative and minimally invasive methods have failed to treat the patient symptomatically, surgery should be considered as an option. Approaches to the condylar region have been discussed in detail elsewhere (Refer Chap. 14). The various surgical procedures for management for hypermobility of TMJ are listed (Table 18.4).

18.5.3.1 Creation of Muscular Balance

Lateral Pterygoid Myotomy

Juxta-articular muscle alteration is a surgical method to correct the spastic muscle unit. The formation of resulting intra-muscular scar tissue facilitates hypomobility. Lateral pterygoid myotomy can be performed trans-orally or percutaneously using a pre-auricular incision. Under general anesthesia, after achieving maximal mouth opening, local anesthetic solution with a vasocontrictor should be infiltrated in the medial and lateral aspect of mandibular ramus. A vertical incision is placed extending from the coronoid process along the ascending ramus to the distal surface of the posterior most tooth. The soft tissues must be gently elevated from the medial aspect of the mandible to expose the lateral pterygoid. It is then detached from the anterior capsule of the condyle. Wound closure should be done followed by IMF for 7 days [3, 9].

Temporalis Scarification

Temporalis scarification creates a cicatricial restriction in dynamic muscular function, and reduce condylar translation. This technique was proposed by Gould JF [10, 20]. It is indicated for unacceptable late joint snapping on mouth opening associated with TMJ hypermobility and for recurrent dislocation. This procedure principally involves dissecting the tendinous fibres from the ascending ramus and suturing them to the surrounding periosteum and mucosa, this induces tightening of the tendon by scaring. The length of the tendon or the muscle may be surgically reduced depending on the amount of hypermobility.

18.5.3.2 Capsulorrhaphy

Arthroscopy is employed to identify the landmarks of the internal joint anatomy and facilitate posterior capsulorrhaphy using laser (Hol:YAG) or electro-thermal device. A cicatricial contracture is created with the removal of retrodiscal synovial tissue. The capsule is tightened and sutured to the desired position. External or open capsulorrhaphy procedure can be performed as an open joint surgical procedure [3]. MacFarlane (1977) has described capsular plication as a simple and effective method for recurrent dislocation of the temporomandibular joint (Fig. 18.5).

18.5.3.3 Open Surgical Methods

Eminectomy

Eminectomy, described by Myrhaug in 1951, reduces the vertical height of the articular eminence. The condyle slips posteriorly into the fossa without anatomic restriction in an episode of dislo-

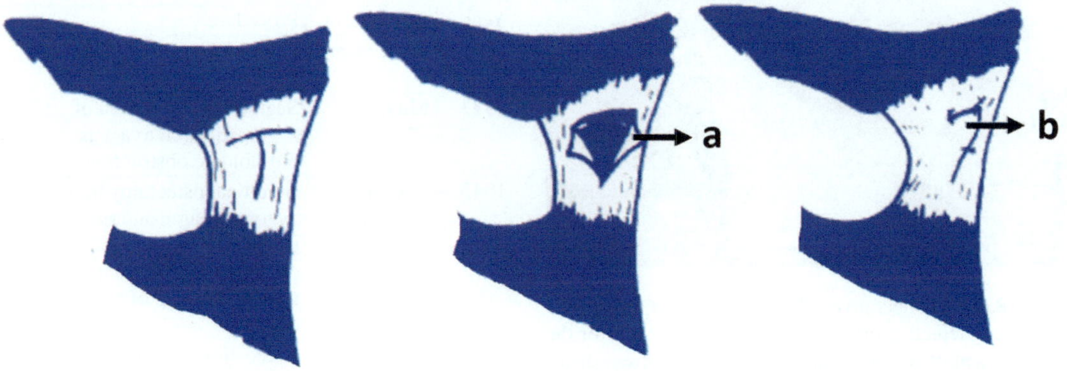

Fig. 18.5 MacFarlane's capsular plication procedure for recurrent dislocation. Note the 'T' shaped incision on the lateral capsule; (**a**) portion of capsule that is excised; (**b**) the flap is pulled and sutured. [Adapted from MacFarlane WI. Recurrent dislocation of the mandible: treatment of seven cases by a simple surgical method. Br J Oral Surg. 1977 Mar;14(3):227-9. https://doi.org/10.1016/0007-117x(77)90029-4.]

cation. A pre-auricular incision is placed, followed by layered dissection to expose the articular eminence. The articular eminence is reduced using a bone cutting bur or an osteotome in the medial aspect. The lateral tubercle may be removed or salvaged as a guide plane followed by layered wound closure. Post-operatively gentle physiotherapy with soft diet is advised to ensure functional mouth opening. Potential risks of this procedure include intra-cranial violation and damage to the surrounding neurovascular bundles [3, 10].

Dautrey's Procedure (Fig. 18.6)

There are few techniques documented in the literature wherein zygomatic arch is utilized to create a mechanical obstruction to the condylar translation (Table 18.6). Dautrey's procedure is done through a pre-auricular incision followed by layered dissection without violation of the TMJ capsule. An osteotomy cut is placed in the zygomatic arch anterior to the eminence. Slight pressure should be applied on the osteotomy site to create a greenstick fracture in the anterior region followed by mobilizing the fractured arch medially or laterally and inserting it under the articular eminence. It can be left passively or secured using a mini-plate followed by wound closure. Bone grafts can be placed as an interpositional material between the arch and articular eminence that can be secured using wires, screws, or mini-plates. Post-operatively soft diet with restriction of mandibular movements for 2 weeks followed by physiotherapy should be advocated [3, 9, 10].

Norman's procedure is an another documented technique where glenotemporal osteotomy is done along with the augmentation of the zygomatic root of the temporal bone by placing a bone graft from the iliac crest to prevent the forward movement of the condyle beyond the eminence. Modification to Norman's procedure for hypermobility of the temporomandibular joint is proposed by Sharma R (2021), where along with the conventional procedure, an inferiorly based pedicled flap from the temporal fascia was sutured to the antero-lateral aspect of the capsule. Authors proposed that an added modification of an additional intra-oral pterygoid disjunction should be executed in cases where hypermobility is associated with pain [21].

Neuro-sensory disturbances and risk of zygomatic arch fracture can be the possible complications. Fractured zygomatic arch may require stabilization.

Mechanical Obstruction with Mini-plate Placement

A 'L' shaped mini-plate can be secured with short arm fixed laterally to the eminence and long arm

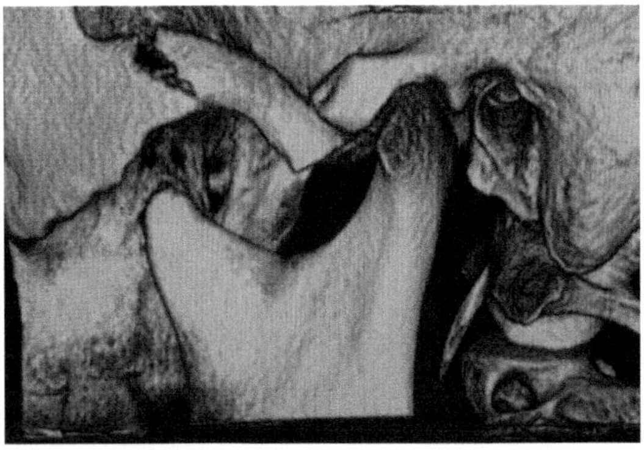

Fig. 18.6 Post-operative 3D reconstructed computed tomogram depicting osteotomized zygomatic arch for the management of temporomandibular joint recurrent dislocation using Dautrey's procedure. (Reproduced with permission from: Bhandari SK, et al. Management of temporomandibular joint recurrent dislocation using Dautrey's procedure: report and review. Int J Otorhinolaryngol Head Neck Surg 2019;5:1748–52)

Table 18.6 Glenotemporal osteotomy for TMJ hypermobility involving the zygomatic arch

Year	Proposal by	Procedure
1925	Lindemann	Utilized a bone chip from zygomatic arch
1933	Mayer	Segmental dislocation of zygomatic arch to act as physiologic obstruction
1943	LeClerc and Girard	A vertical osteotomy in the zygomatic arch anterior to the tubercle, inserting the osteotomized segment to impede the path of hypermobile condyle
1967	Gosserez and Dautrey	Greenstick fracture of zygomatic arch, with its displacement in downward and forward direction just in front of the articular eminence and locked under the eminence

can be contoured and fixed along the eminence inferiorly. The procedure should always be contained to the extra-capsular region and is relatively less morbid. There is a potential chance of plate fracture which requires a second surgery for hardware removal [3, 10].

Wolford's Procedure

Mitek anchor fixation for temporomandibular joint disorders work on the principle of using a bone anchor and artificial ligaments for disc stabilization.This procedure utilizes Mitek mini bone anchors which has osseointegration potential. Usually two Mitek anchors are utilized for the treatment of chronic mandibular dislocation. After exposing the zygomatic arch and lateral capsule, articular disc position is ensured. One anchor is placed in the lateral condylar pole and the second anchor is placed in the most posterior part of the zygomatic arch. The suture strings can be adjusted based on the desired mobility and tied. Eminectomy is not required with this procedure. The anchor sutures are tightened to a length that permits laxity for controlled translation of the mandible while preventing dislocation. The disadvantages are breakage of sutures or failure of the anchors [3, 5]. The use of Mitek anchor is also advocated for disc repositioning by Mehra and Wolford (2001) (Fig. 18.7). The modifications in the procedure for various clinical scenarios is summarized in the Table 18.7. Mitek anchors require specialized armamentarium which may not be universally available. An alternative to Mitek anchors, is the use of orthodontic mini-screw as advocated by Zachariah and Neelakandan (2015) (Fig. 18.8).

Tocaciu S et al. in their study proposed a new surgical treatment protocol for patients diagnosed with recurrent TMJ dislocation after retrospective observation of 14 patients over a period of 6 years. Successful long-term results were observed in the study population who underwent a combination of eminectomy and a disc plication (meniscopexy) procedure. The authors also emphasized that for the patients who are not eligible for surgery, may be treated using botulinum injections or sclerotherapy [22]. Very little literature evidence is available for dislocation of the TMJ in pediatric population as the treatment options can be limited in such age group. Ludovic S et al. proposed a management protocol for pediatric TMJ dislocation which can be useful for clinicians [23].

Stergiou GS et al. have described mini-plate eminoplasty for non-compliant patients and for patients with muscular disorders [24]. Krishnakumar Raja VB et al. have advocated inferior repositioning of the coronoid process to address subluxation or recurrent dislocation. This procedure is based on the principle of stretching of the muscle thereby increasing the neuromuscular activity and resistance training resulting in hypertrophy. They highlighted that there was an increase in mitochondrial content and the cross-sectional area of the muscle fibers. Ultrasonographic evaluation post-operatively revealed an increase in thickness and length of temporalis muscle which translated into better contraction [25].

The affected individual diagnosed with a hypermobility disorder must be screened for previous history of trauma, systemic disorders affecting the joint or connective tissue which can be a predisposing factor followed by devising a custom-made treatment plan, as no single modality of treatment is found to be effective in all the cases.

18.6 Goals of Treatment

Identification of the etiological factor causing the hypermobility, patient education, and reassurance followed by conservative to minimally invasive management are the important elements to achieve relief in such patients. If the non-surgical methods fail to provide relief, surgery should be considered as an option to improve the quality of life.

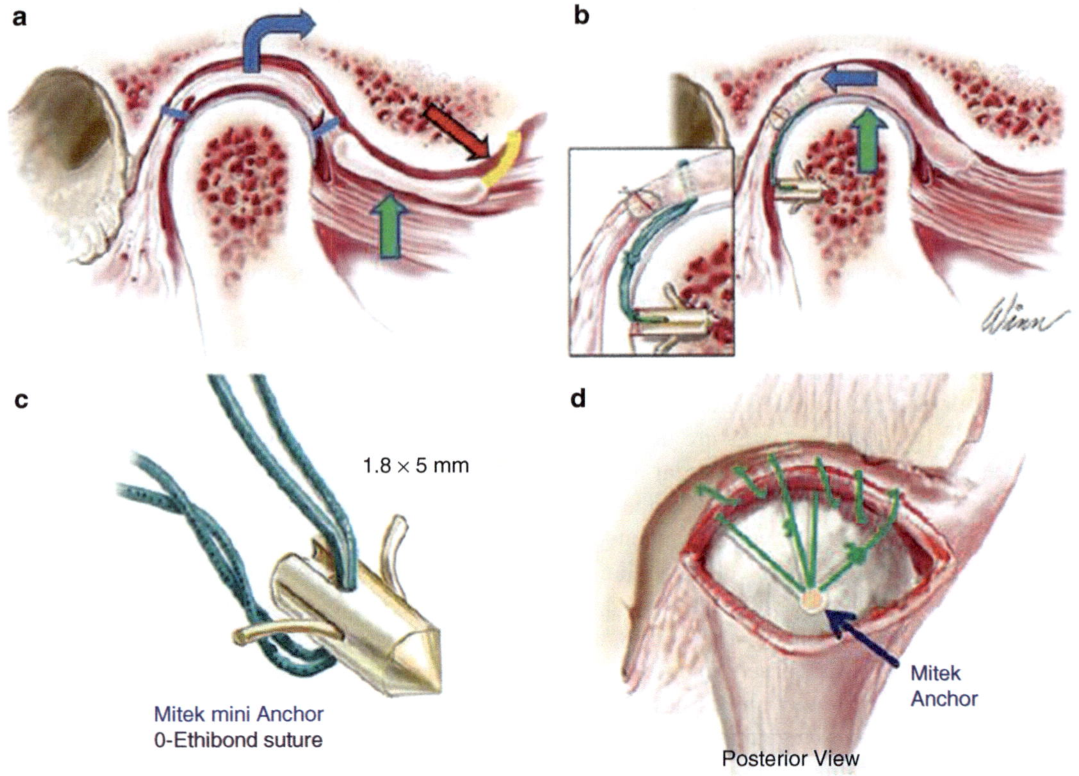

Fig. 18.7 (**a**) Sagittal view of the right TMJ. The TMJ articular disc is anteriorly displaced (green arrow). Bilaminar and synovial tissues cover the top of the condyle. This tissue is excised to eliminate excessive tissue when the disc is repositioned. The ligament that attaches from the anterior aspect of the disc to the anterior aspect of the articular eminence must be detached in order to mobilize the disc and reposition it passively over the condylar head (red arrow). (**b**) The disc has been mobilized and repositioned passively over the condyle. A hole is drilled into the posterior head of the condyle with the dedicated Mitek drill, and the Mitek anchor is inserted into the posterior head of the condyle into the medullary bone with the wings locking it in place against the cortical bone. The 0 Ethibond suture that was doubled and passed through the eyelet of the anchor provides two artificial ligaments to secure the disc in position. (**c**) The Mitek mini anchor is 1.8 mm in diameter and 5 mm in length. The body of the anchor is titanium alloy, and the wings are composed of nickel titanium with shape-memory technology to allow the wings to compress against the body of the device as it passes through the cortical bone of the condyle and then re-expand once into the medullary bone, locking the device in place against the cortical bone. (**d**) Posterior view of the anchor inserted into the condyle. The pilot hole is placed approximately 8 mm below the crown of the condylar head and just lateral to the midsagittal plane. The first suture (artificial ligament) is passed from beneath up through the posterior aspect of the posterior band of the disc toward the medial side. Two more throws are completed for a total of three throws. The second suture is passed in the same manner with three throws but positioned more laterally. The disc should be slightly overcorrected, and then the sutures are tied. Additional support sutures can be placed, for example, at the lateral pole area if additional support is required to stabilize the disc laterally. The 0 Ethibond suture can be passed through the lateral capsular tissue and up through the lateral aspect of the disc and secured to provide additional lateral support. (Reproduced with permission: Han, Michael et al. Surgery of the Temporomandibular Joint: Discectomy and Arthroplasty in, S. T. Connelly et al. (eds.), Contemporary Management of Temporomandibular Disorders, https://doi.org/10.1007/978-3-319-99909-8_6, Springer Nature Switzerland AG 2019)

Table 18.7 Wolford's procedure (modifications based on various clinical scenarios)

TMJ charateristics	Procedure
Chronic forward mandibular posture	Two artificial ligaments are tightened to retain the condyle seated in postero-superior aspect of the fossa, preventing forward translation
To prevent dislocation anterior to articular eminence	Artificial ligaments can be left loose to provide translation but limit forward movement by preventing condylar translation beyond the articular eminence
Dislocation of articular disc	Usage of third anchor to reposition the disc into a normal relation

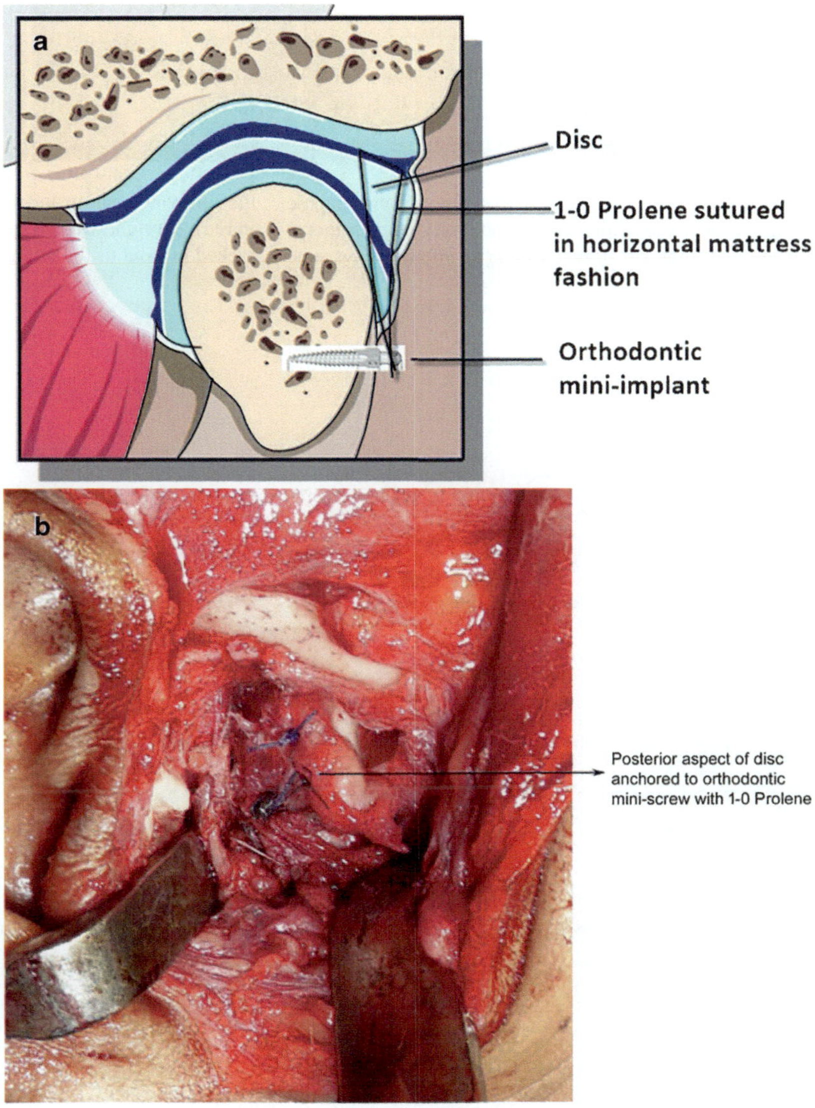

Fig. 18.8 Use of an orthodontic mini-screw for disc anchoring in cases with chronic meniscocondylar dislocation of the temporomandibular joint. Schematic diagram showing disc anchoring technique (**a**); Disc anchored to orthodontic miniscrew (**b**) [Adapted from Zachariah T, Neelakandan RS, Ahamed MI. Disc Anchoring with an Orthodontic Mini-Screw for Chronic Meniscocondylar Dislocation of TMJ. J Maxillofac Oral Surg. 2015;14(3):735–744. https://doi.org/10.1007/s12663-014-0729-2]

Appendix

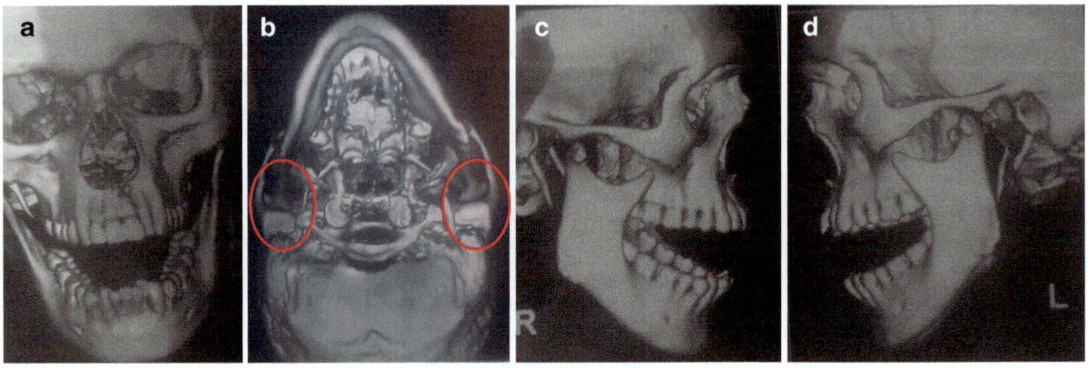

Atlas 18.1 3D reconstructed computed tomographic images of a patient with acute dislocation of the temporomandibular joint. (**a**) frontal view; (**b**) inferior view, note the condylar position and the empty glenoid fossa (marked in red); (**c**) right; (**d**) left, note the position of the condyle locked in front of the articular eminence

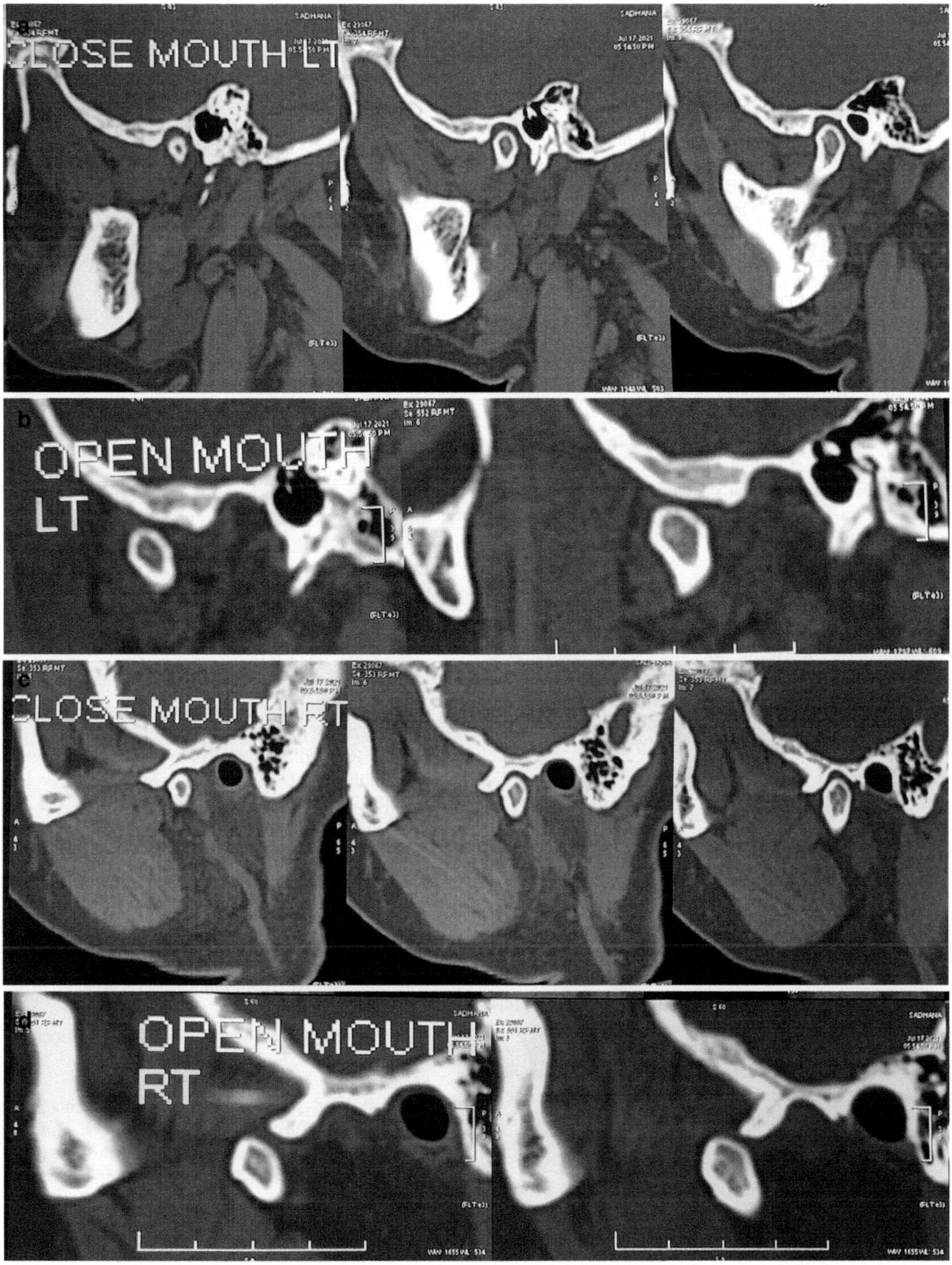

Atlas 18.2 Sagittal view of the computed tomographic images in a patient with chronic subluxation of the temporomandibular joint. (**a**) closed mouth view of the left joint; (**b**) open mouth view of the left joint, note the anterior translation of the condyle and its relation to the eminence; (**c**) closed mouth view of the right joint; (**d**) open mouth view of the right joint, note the anterior translation of the condyle and its relation to the eminence

References

1. Nosouhian S, Haghighat A, et al. Temporomandibular joint hypermobility manifestation based on clinical observations. J Int Oral Health. 2015;7(8):1–4.
2. Malik NA. Textbook of oral and maxillofacial surgery. 4th ed. New Delhi: Jaypee Publishers.
3. Liddell A, Perez DE. Temporomandibular joint dislocation. Oral Maxillofac Surg Clin N Am. 2015;27:125–36.
4. Badel T, Laškarin M, Zadravec D, Čimić S, Savić Pavičin I. Subluxation of temporomandibular joint – a clinical view. J Dent Probl Solut. 2018;5(2):029034.
5. Sharma NK, Singh AK, Pandey A, Verma V, Singh S. Temporomandibular joint dislocation. Natl J Maxillofac Surg. 2015;6(1):16–20. https://doi.org/10.4103/0975-5950.168212.
6. Haghigaht A, Davoudi A, Rybalov O, Hatami A. Condylar distances in hypermobile temporomandibular joints of patients with excessive mouth openings by using computed tomography. J Clin Exp Dent. 2014;6(5):e509–13. https://doi.org/10.4317/jced.51562.
7. Kalaykova S, Naeije M, Huddleston Slater JJR, Lobbezo F. Is condylar position a predictor for functional signs of TMJ hypermobility? J Oral Rehab. 2006;33:349–55.
8. Kalaykova S, Naeije M, Huddleston Slater JJR, Lobbezo F. Occupational differentiation in dentistry 3. Hypermobility of the temporomandibular joint and condylar position at maximal mouth opening. Ned Tijdschr Tandheelkd. 2006;113(10):391–6.
9. Martin WD, et al. Recurrent dislocation of the temporomandibular joint: a literature review and two case reports treated with eminectomy. J Craniomandibular Sleep Prac. 2014;32(2):110–7.
10. Lawlor MG. Recurrent dislocation of the mandible: treatment of ten cases by the Dautrey procedure. Br J Oral Surg. 1982;20:14–21.
11. Ardehali MM, et al. Temporomandibular Joint reduction technique: a new external method versus the traditional. Ann Plastic Surg. 2009;63(2):176–8.
12. Awang MN. A new approach to the reduction of acute dislocation of temporomandibular joint: a report of 3 cases. Br J Oral Maxillofac Surg. 1987;25:244–9.
13. Coser R, De Silveira H, Medeiros P, Ritto FG. Autologous blood injection for the treatment of recurrent mandibular dislocation. Int J Oral Maxillofac Surg. 2015; https://doi.org/10.1016/j.ijom.2015.05.004.
14. Hegab AF. Treatment of chronic recurrent dislocation of the temporomandibular joint with injection of autologous blood alone, intermaxillary fixation alone, or both together: a prospective randomized controlled clinical trial. Br J Oral Maxillofac Surg. 2013;51:813–7.
15. Varedi P, Bohluli P. Autologous blood injection for treatment of chronic recurrent TMJ dislocation: is it successful? Is it safe enough? A systematic review. Oral Maxillofac Surg. 2015; https://doi.org/10.1007/s10006-015-0500-y.
16. Oshiro N, Yoshida H, Uemura M, Suwa F, Morita S. Analysis of MRI findings in minimum invasive treatment for habitual temporomandibular joint dislocation by autologous blood injection around the temporomandibular joint capsule. J Cranio-Maxillofac Surg. 2014; https://doi.org/10.1016/j.jcms.2014.04.018.
17. Matthews NS. Dislocation of temporomandibular joint. A guide to diagnosis and management. Springer. In: Conservative management for TMJ dislocation. p. 67.
18. Ataran R, Bahramian A, Jamali Z, et al. The role of botulinum toxin A in treatment of temporomandibular joint disorders: a review. J Dent (Shiraz). 2017;18(3):157–64.
19. Majumdar SK, Krishna S, Chatterjee A, Chakraborty R, Ansari N. Single injection technique prolotherapy for hypermobility disorders of TMJ using 25% dextrose: a clinical study. J Maxillofac Oral Surg. 2017;16(2):226–30. https://doi.org/10.1007/s12663-016-0944-0.
20. Gould JF. Shortening of the temporalis tendon for hypermobility of the temporomandibular joint. J Oral Surg. 1978;36(10):781–3.
21. Sharma R. Modifications to Norman's procedure for hypermobility of TMJ. Med J Armed Forces Ind. 2012;68:231–5.
22. Tocaciu S, McCulloughb MJ, Dimitroulis G. Surgical management of recurrent dislocation of the temporomandibular joint: a new treatment protocol. Br J Oral Maxillofac Surg. 2018;56:936–40.
23. Ludovic S, O'hana D, Khonsari RH, Kaddour Brahim A. Bilateral dislocation of the Temporo-Mandibular Joint in children. J Oral Maxillofac Surg. 2018; https://doi.org/10.1016/j.joms.2018.04.004.
24. Stergiou GS, Obwegeser JA, Grätz KW, Zwahlen RA. Surgical treatment of anterior TMJ-dislocation with mini-plates: a case report (in German). Schweiz Monatsschr Zahnmed. 2007;117:523–6.
25. Krishnakumar Raja VB, Balasubramanian S, Sridharan G, Tarun S, Panneerselvam E. Inferior Repositioning of Coronoid Process for the Treatment of Temporomandibular Joint Subluxation/Dislocation. Ann Maxillofac Surg. 2019;9(2):397–9. https://doi.org/10.4103/ams.ams_137_19.

Arthrocentesis of the Temporomandibular Joint

19

Darpan Bhargava, M. Fatih Şentürk, Shaji Thomas, and Prateeksha Pawar

19.1 Introduction

Internal derangement (ID) of temporomandibular joint (TMJ) is defined as any abnormal anatomical or structural relationship between the articulating surfaces and the articular disc that interferes with the smooth functioning of the jaw joint. Disturbances in the joint movement in which the articular disc plays a central role are referred to as temporomandibular joint disc derangement [1]. For the better understanding of the disharmony in synchrony of the jaw joint movements, it is mandatory to understand the physiology behind the normal functioning of the temporomandibular joint while opening and closing the jaw (Figs. 19.1, 19.2, and 19.3).

D. Bhargava (✉)
TMJ Consultancy Services,
Bhopal, Madhya Pradesh, India

Oral and Maxillofacial Surgery, People's College of Dental Sciences and Research Centre,
People's University, Bhopal, Madhya Pradesh, India
e-mail: drdarpanbhargava@gmail.com

M. F. Şentürk
Oral and Maxillofacial Surgery, Ankara Yıldırım Beyazıt University Faculty of Dentistry,
Ankara, Turkey

S. Thomas
Department of Oral and Maxillofacial Surgery,
People's College of Dental Sciences and Research Centre, People's University,
Bhopal, Madhya Pradesh, India

P. Pawar
Oral and Maxillofacial Surgery, TMJ Consultancy Services, Bhopal, Madhya Pradesh, India

Internal derangement has been described to cause interferences with smooth movement of the joint through momentary "catching, clicking, popping, or locking". It may be with or/and without reduction of the displaced disc (Table 19.1) (Fig. 19.4) [2].

Derangement of the temporomandibular joint may have a progressive course, if not intercepted when indicated. Internal derangement usually advances from the preliminary stage, which is characterized by a clicking associated with normal maximal mouth opening (MMO) to the stage where clicking gradually ceases with occurrence of varying degrees of limitation in mouth opening (closed lock). The latter stage is commonly characterized by a non-reducible, (most frequently) anteriorly displaced disc which hinders the translating condyle [3, 4].

The treatment of choice for internal derangement still remains controversial, but on a progressive note, arthrocentesis; both needle and arthroscopic have been accepted as routine options for management in early stages. When the conservative methods fail to provide relief to the condition, surgical disc repositioning and repair are the possible options to re-establish the normal structural and functional relationship. Both TMJ needle arthrocentesis and arthroscopic lysis and lavage utilize high hydraulic pressure (within physiological limitations) in the

D. Bhargava (ed.), *Temporomandibular Joint Disorders*,
https://doi.org/10.1007/978-981-16-2754-5_19

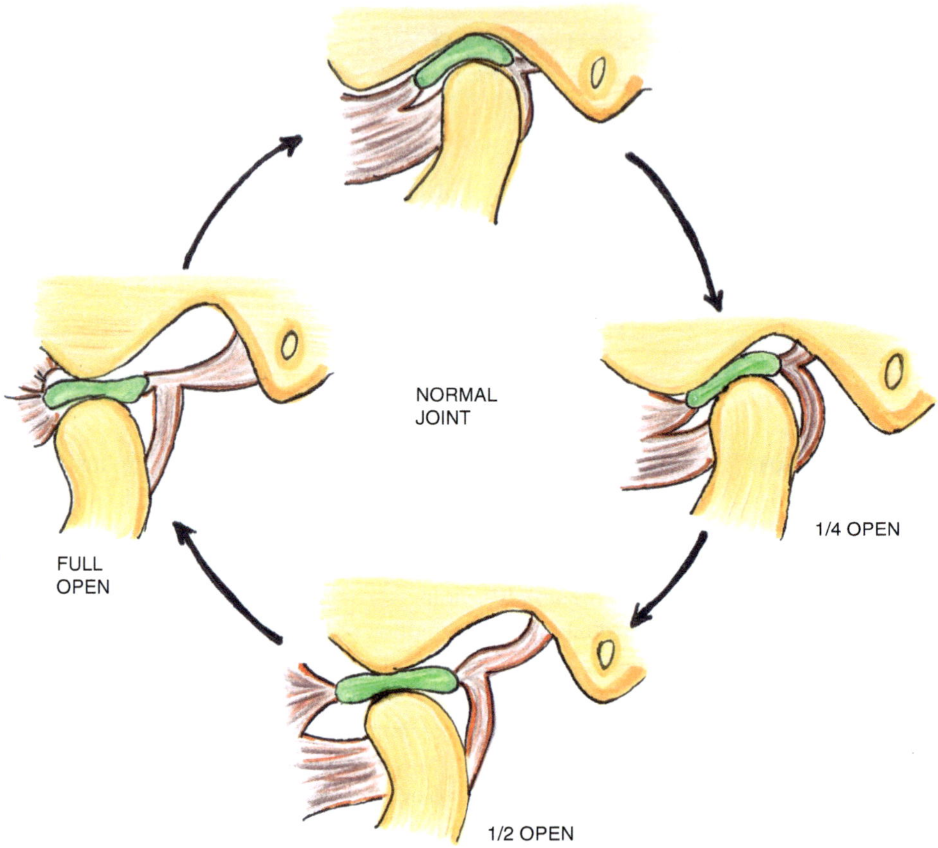

Fig. 19.1 Joint dynamics during function

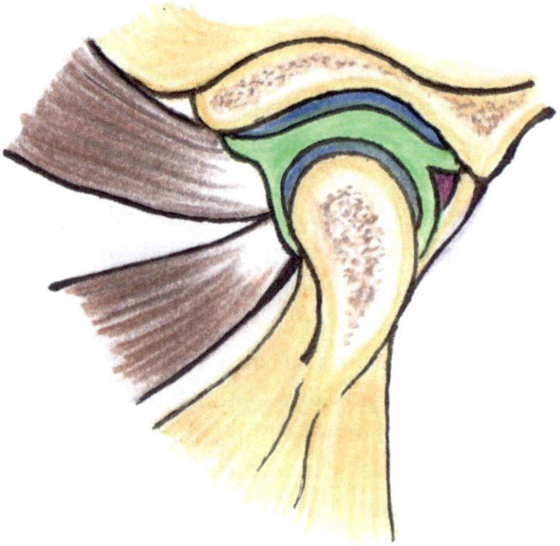

Fig. 19.2 Sagittal view of the joint architecture. Note the disc (green) dividing the joint into two distinct compartments (blue)

upper joint space to re-establish the internal anatomy and restore normal MMO in patients with symptomatic derangements and closed lock.

Several studies on temporomandibular joint disorders (TMDs) have suggested that minimally invasive TMJ surgeries should be considered as an early option in the management sequence for patients with ID, to avoid the progression of the disease to a more symptomatic and complex stages [5]. Arthrocentesis and arthroscopy are being widely practised in the field of orthopaedic surgery for various joints in the body. Over the last four decades it has gained much popularity in the field of Maxillofacial Surgery for the treatment for jaw joint disorders. Variety of techniques for performing arthroscopy and arthrocentesis of the TMJ have been proposed by

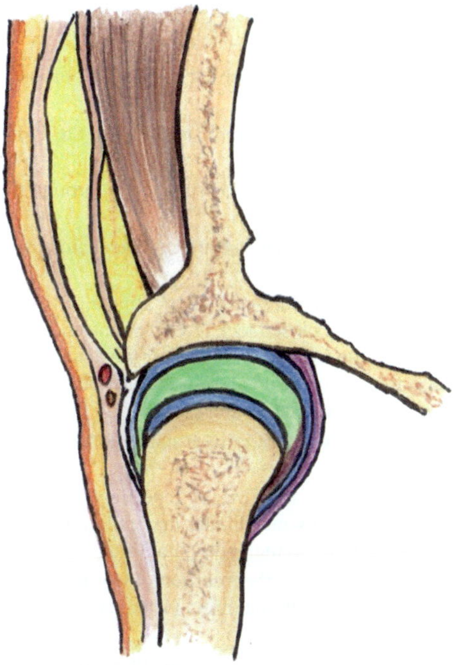

Fig. 19.3 Coronal anatomy of the joint architecture, note the disc (green) dividing the joint space into superior and inferior compartments (blue)

Table 19.1 Definition of internal derangement with/without reduction

Internal derangement with reduction	Internal derangement without reduction
A condition in which the articular disc of the TMJ is displaced (most often anteriorly) while the mouth is closed and the teeth are together in maximal occlusion. On opening, the condyle pushes against the posterior band of the disc until the condyle is able to slide or snap under the posterior band of the disc and the disc reduces to its position on the top of the condyle.	A condition in which the condyle is unable to slide or snap back underneath the disc. The displaced disc thus does not reduce to its position on top of the condyle during opening movement. In this condition, the posterior band of the disc shows significant plastic deformation as well as gradual flattening.

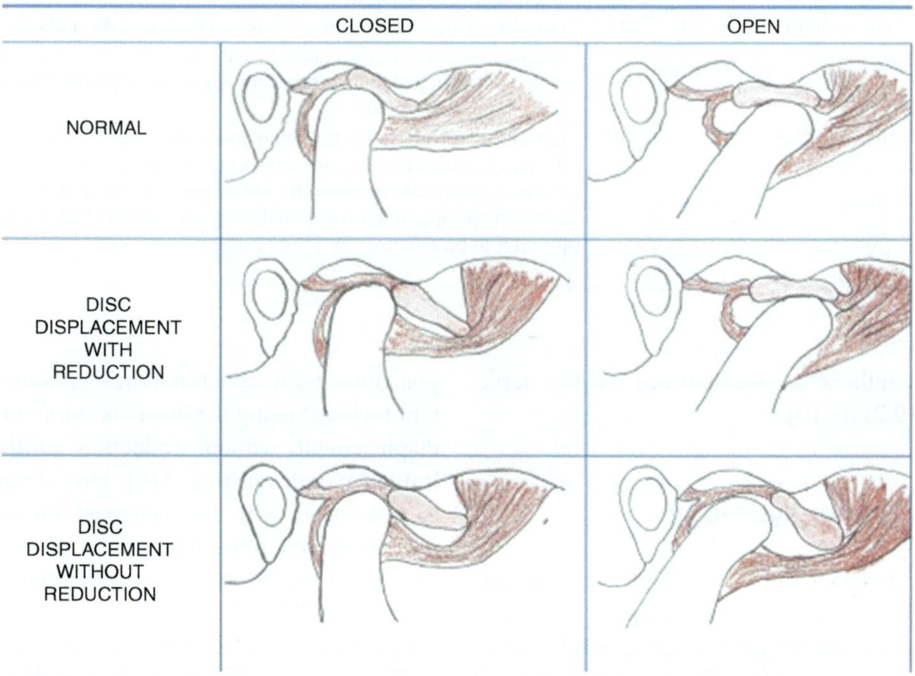

Fig. 19.4 Dynamics during normal joint function and in a deranged joint (Adapted from Bhargava D, et al. Temporomandibular joint arthrocentesis for internal derangement with disc displacement without reduction. *J Maxillofac Oral Surg*. 2015 Jun;14(2):454–9)

Table 19.2 History of development in arthroscopy and arthrocentesis for the temporomandibular joint

S. NO	Authors	Year	Study
1.	Onishi et al. [6]	1974	First reported the usage of the arthroscope for diagnostic purposes in TMJ.
2.	Murakami and Hoshino et al. [7]	1982	Explained the nomenclature for arthroscopic anatomy of the TMJ.
3.	McCain et al. [8]	1983	Favoured the development of routine TMJ arthroscopy through their cadaveric study with 67 joints.
4.	Holmlund and Hellsing et al. [9]	1985	Explained anatomic key points to make arthroscopy technique secure and standardized with a study on 54 cadavers.
5.	Sanders et al. [10]	1986	Outlined the advantages of arthroscopy for the treatment of temporomandibular joint acute closed lock (ACL) or chronic closed lock cases (CCL) and introduced the term lysis for the distension of the joint with an unsharpened trocar to abolish the suction effect of the disc to the fossa, and to breach the adherences.
6.	Murakami and Ono et al. [11]	1986	Described the arthroscopic removal of intra-articular adherences.
7.	Murakami et al. [12]	1987	First introduced arthrocentesis of the TMJ, by reporting the recapture of the anteriorly displaced disc by mandibular manipulation utilizing pumping and hydraulic pressure to the upper joint of the TMJ.
8.	Nitzan DW et al. [13]	1991	Introduced a modified method, with the insertion of two needles in the upper joint space for lavage without direct visualization of the joint.
9.	Dimitrilious G et al. [14]	1995	Evaluated the efficiency of arthrocentesis as a treatment for closed lock of the TMJ and advocated it to be a simple alternative to more invasive TMJ procedures.
10.	Alkan A et al. [15]	2007	Described temporomandibular joint lavage instrument with double needles in a single cannula as an alternative to classical arthrocentesis with two needles and found it to be simple to use with effective lysis and lavage with a single puncture.
11.	Dayisoylu EH et al. [16]	2013	Introduced ultrasound-guided lysis and lavage of the TMJ for the accurate insertion of the cannulas and concluded that the technique is more cost effective than arthroscopy, easy, and reproducible even by inexperienced surgeons
12.	Bhargava D et al. [17]	2019	Introduced a single-puncture, double-lumen, single-barrel needle for the temporomandibular joint arthrocentesis. They conducted a study to assist the needle insertion for single puncture arthrocentesis using ultrasonography in temporomandibular joint closed lock cases and found it to be effective for joint lavage.

various authors as summarized in the table. (Table 19.2) [6–17].

19.2 Pathophysiology

Internal derangement of the TMJ is a condition where the articular disc gets displaced from its original position relative to the condylar head. The displacement of the disc position can result in numerous presentations such as (1) disc displacement with reduction (with/without intermittent locking) being the most common, or (2) disc displacement without reduction (with/without limited mouth opening) [18]. Disc derangement is associated with an increased intra-articular friction which prevents smooth gliding of the joint resulting in progressive dilapidation of the joint tissues [1]. The pathophysiology of such a dilapidation process is summarized in Fig. 19.5.

Two major components responsible for free joint movement are:

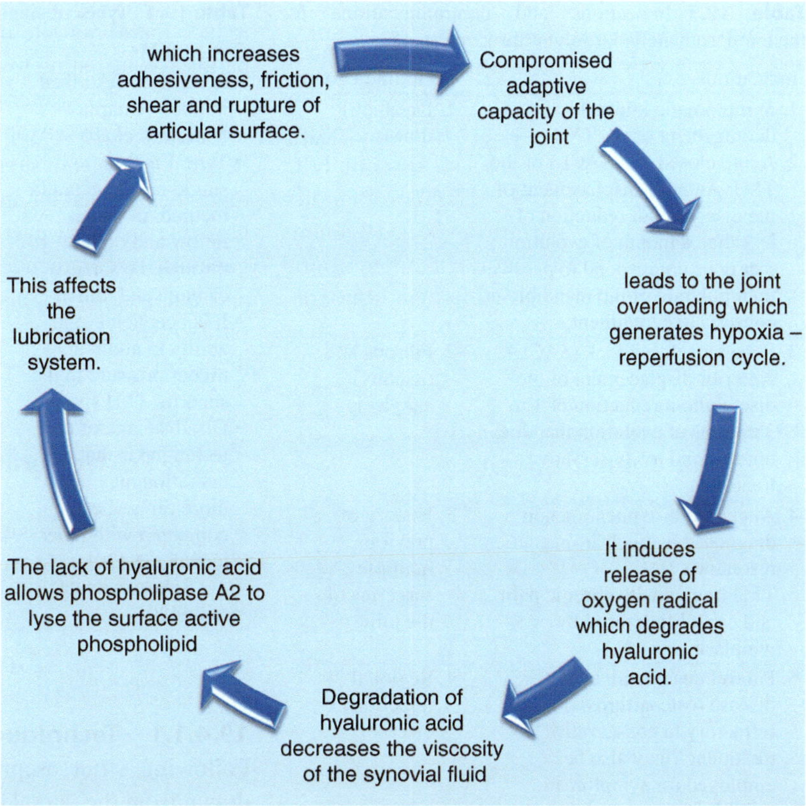

Fig. 19.5 Pathophysiology of degenerative progression in a TMJ disorder

1. Surface active phospholipid: is a major boundary lubricant protecting the articular surfaces.
2. Hyaluronic acid: is a high molecular weight mucopolysaccharide which forms a film that keeps the articular surfaces separated and prevents friction.

19.3 Arthrocentesis

Arthrocentesis is considered as the first line procedure and one of the least invasive intervention for internal derangements of the TMJ. It involves lysis and lavage of the joint space and is traditionally accomplished in a closed fashion, without viewing the joint. It involves active irrigation of the joint space together with joint manipulation. It aids in releasing adhesions, improves function, clears inflammatory mediators from the joint, and is also utilized for intra-articular administration of pharmacological agents. Like any other surgical procedure, arthrocentesis cannot be performed in all the patients diagnosed with TMDs and has definitive indications for a favourable outcome. The indications and contra-indications for arthrocentesis are summarized in Table 19.3 [5, 14].

19.4 Classification

Şentürk MF et al. have classified the TMJ arthrocentesis techniques, based on the number of punctures utilized to access the joint and accomplish the lavage [19].

(a) Single-puncture arthrocentesis (SPA)
(b) Double-puncture arthrocentesis (DPA).

SPA is further classified by the number of needles utilized (Table 19.4) [20–26].

Type 1: Single-needle cannula method (SPA Type 1)

Table 19.3 Indications and contraindications for the temporomandibular joint arthrocentesis [5]

Indications	Contraindications
1. Symptomatic internal derangement of the TMJ. 2. Acute closed lock (ACL) of the TMJ: Anterior displacement of the disc without reduction of less than a month of evolution that does not respond to passive manipulation of the mandible or conservative treatment.	1. Psychiatric illness.
3. Subacute closed lock (SACL): Anterior displacement of the disc without reduction of 1 to 3 months of evolution that does not respond to conservative treatment.	2. Fibrous and osseous ankylosis
4. Anchored disc phenomenon diagnosed by nuclear magnetic resonance. 5. TMJ trauma with chronic pain and capsulitis caused by whiplash.	3. History of previous multiple surgeries of the joint
6. Painful degenerative joint disease (osteoarthrosis) refractory to conservative treatment. (may also be employed for symptomatic relief in patients awaiting surgery)	4. Regional infectious disease
7. Patients who reject arthroscopy or who cannot be subjected to general anaesthesia.	5. Regional tumoural disease.

Type 2: Single-puncture method using a double/dual-needle cannula (SPA Type 2)

19.4.1 Double-Puncture Arthrocentesis (DPA)

This technique uses two needles inserted independently, that must be triangulated and located in the upper joint space for the lysis. Nitzan DW et al. described the traditional double-puncture arthrocentesis technique, which has remained the preferred method for most surgeons world over. This approach permits for large volume lavage of the joint as well as intra-articular aspiration and injection, where needed [13].

Table 19.4 Types of single puncture arthrocentesis

Type I SPA	Type II SPA
• It was first described in 2008 (Guarda-Nardini L et al.) • Type 1 is the single-needle cannula method, in which inflow and outflow go through the same cannula and lumen. • It is beneficial in its ability to attain a higher pressure in the superior TMJ space. • Disadvantage of this technique is that the operation may take more time when compared with other techniques [20]. E.g.: Single cannula needle [20]	• It was first described in 2007 (Alkan A et al.) • Type 2 is the double-needle, or dual-needle, cannula method, in which inflow and outflow go through the same cannula system but utilize different ports and lumens [15] E.g.: Double lumen single barrel needle [21, 22] Shepard cannula [23, 24] Concentric cannula [25] Intravenous catheter [26] Double-needle cannula [27]

19.4.1.1 Technique

Following strict aseptic precautions, a line is drawn from the lateral canthus to the most posterior and central point on the tragus, Holmlund-Hellsing line (HH line) (Fig. 19.6) followed by injection of a local anaesthetic (LA) solution to block the auriculotemporal nerve. The external auditory meatus (EAM) should be occluded using a cotton plug. In this technique, two 18-gauge (recommended) needles are used, one dedicated for the inflow of irrigant into the joint space and the second for the out flow of the irrigant and intra-articular debris [13].

The posterior point of entry (first needle) should be positioned along the cantho-tragal line, 10 mm from the middle of the tragus anteriorly and 2 mm below the cantho-tragal line (point A, Fig. 19.6). The anterior point of entry (second needle) is 20 mm anterior to the mid-tragal point on the cantho-tragal line and 10 mm below it (point B, Fig. 19.6). This marking specifies the location of TMJ eminence [13].

While the patient is asked to keep the mouth open, first the eighteen-gauge needle should be introduced directing upward, forward, and

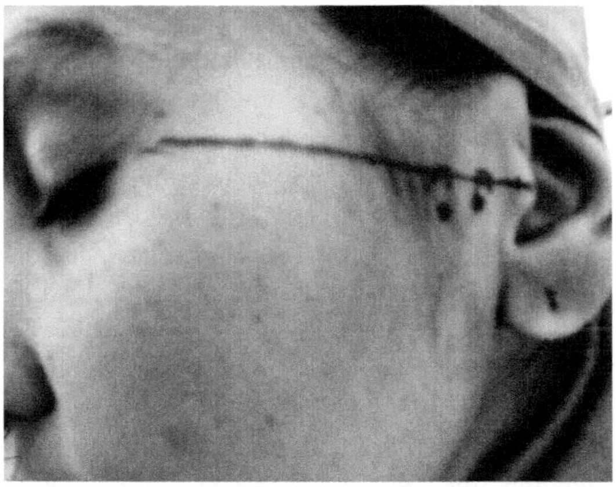

Fig. 19.6 Holmlund-Hellsing line (HH line) with points, A (10 mm in front of mid tragus; 2 mm below cantho-tragal line) and B (20 mm anterior to the mid-tragal point on the cantho-tragal line and 10 mm below it)

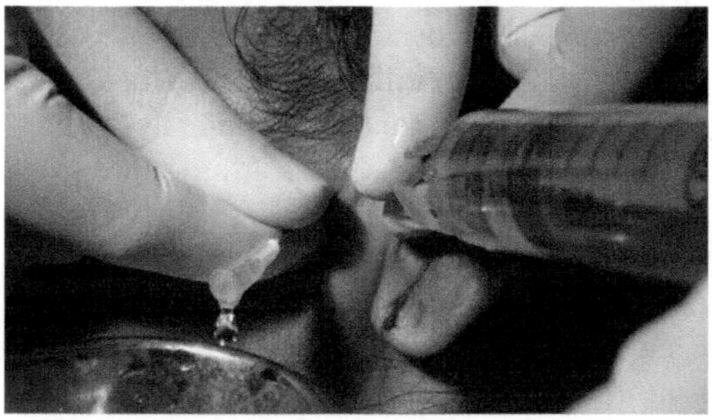

Fig. 19.7 Double needle arthrocentesis

inward to a depth of about 2 cm beyond the insertion point, where the tip of the needle comes into contact with the posterior wall of the articular eminence. This is followed by the injection of 2 to 3 ml of Ringer Lactate (RL) solution to expand the joint space and determine if the needle is inside the superior joint compartment. The second needle should be inserted using the landmark explained earlier. Commonly, 150–200 ml of RL solution is injected into the upper joint space over a period of 10–15 minutes via the first needle. The second needle is utilized for draining the solution (outflow), simultaneously, to establishe lavage of the joint cavity (Fig. 19.7) [13]. The role of the first and second needles as the inflow and outflow ports respectively, can be reversed to continue the lavage. On termination of the procedure, removal of the needles should be followed by a sterile pressure dressing for 24–48 hours post-operatively.

19.4.2 Single-Puncture Arthrocentesis (SPA)

Single-puncture arthrocentesis requires only one puncture to the upper joint compartment. It is considered to be safe, easy to perform with reduced procedural time, and is minimally invasive [19].

19.4.2.1 Technique

This procedure can be performed with two types of needles: (1) a concentric double needle that is available in different gauges, or (2) a single needle which has two adjoining lumens, one utilized for inflow and second as an outflow port.

The patient should be preferably seated at a 45-degree angle, with head turned to the unaffected side. Affected peri-auricular region must be prepared using an antiseptic/antimicrobial solution and strict aseptic measures should be followed for the joint access. Auriculotemporal nerve block should be administered just anterior to the junction of the tragus and the ear lobe with 1.8–2 ml of LA solution. The EAM on the affected side must be occluded with a cotton plug and marking for the needle should be placed using sterile marking ink. A line is drawn from the tragus to the outer canthus as described earlier. The needle should be inserted into the joint space 2 mm below and 10 mm anterior from the mid-tragus end of HH line (Point A) followed by lavage of the superior joint space with 150–200 ml of Ringer's Lactate solution (Fig.19.8).

19.5 Arthrocentesis with Irrigation Pump

Yura et al. described the effectiveness of arthrocentesis using an infusion accelerator under high pressure (maximum pressure, 40 KPa). The hypothesis claims that the high pressure elimi-

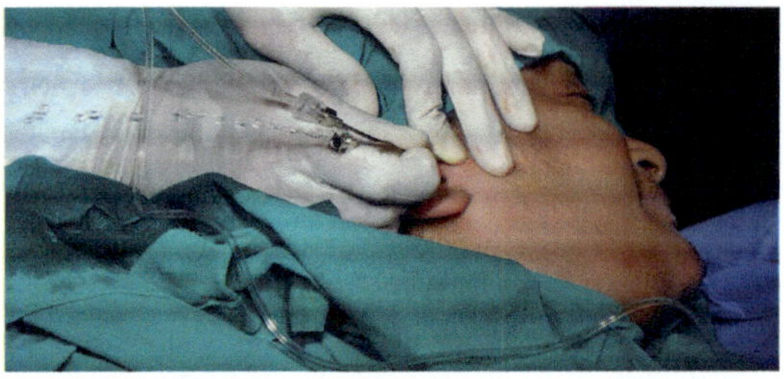

Fig. 19.8 Single needle arthrocentesis (using single-puncture technique, utilizing a double-lumen, single-barrel needle for patients with temporomandibular joint acute closed lock internal derangement as described by Bhargava D et al.)

nates adhesions, widens the joint spaces and concluded that arthrocentesis with sufficient pressure could be effective for closed lock cases with adhesions in the upper joint compartment. The possibility of complications with the use of mechanized high pressure in the intra-articular space and surrounding tissues should be kept in mind [27].

Alkan et al. described a modification in the arthrocentesis procedure which involves connecting an irrigation pump from a surgical/dental implant motor to the inflow needle, introducing automatic irrigation under high pressure. This modification delivers high hydraulic pressure in the intra-articular space [28].

19.6 Arthrocentesis with Intrarticular Injection

Following adequate irrigation, it is recommended that corticosteroids or sodium hyaluronate can be injected to reduce intra-capsular inflammation while improving function. They are also useful for reducing pain, and dysfunction associated with inflammatory process within the joints and reduce functional friction. Injecting the joint with sodium hyaluronate has shown a quicker and long-lasting analgesic effect as it is a viscous, high molecular weight polysaccharide which lubricates and allows subsequent protection of the joint cartilage.

According to Alpaslan et al. regardless of the improvement in the symptoms of TMDs as a result of intra-articular injections, the prognosis following their use is unpredictable since local side effects can influence outcomes. Side effects of the intra-articular injection of glucocorticoids include articular cartilage destruction, infection, and progression of already diagnosed degenerative joint disease [29]. Although many authors claim benefits of using post-surgical flushing of the joint with a single dose steroid (hydrocortisone sodium succinate) after the joint lavage with no obvious clinical adverse effects. The single dose steroid flush, gives the advantage of reducing the existing synovial inflammation along with reduction in post-surgical/arthrocentesis edema.

Kopp et al. found that TMJ arthrocentesis with intra-articular sodium hyaluronate and corticosteroid injections is known to reduce the clinical symptoms and dysfunction experienced by patients [30]. Girrardi GB et al. demonstrated that both betamethasone and sodium hyaluronate produce similar results after arthrocentesis and can safely be used [31].

A systematic review conducted by Davoudi A et al. on effects of various drugs used after arthrocentesis has concluded that there was no significant difference among the various steroids used by different operators and also when different class of drugs were used rendered no significant difference [32]. One sporadic study concluded that favourable outcomes were observed when lavage was performed using ozonized water followed by ozone injection into the TMJ as compared to the steroid study groups [33].

A bibliographic research on publications between 1991 and 2016 evaluating clinical outcomes such as mouth opening, intra-articular noises and pain emphasize that the commonly utilized pharmacological agents used for intra-articular injection include steroids, hyaluronic acid, morphine-based drugs, and platelet rich plasma. Majority of the available literature reports the superiority of protocols with intra-articular injections, irrespective of the agent used. However, no single pharmacological agent has shown any superiority over another in a randomised control trial setting [33, 34].

19.7 Summary and Conclusion

Nishimura M et al. evaluated the prognostic factors for effective arthrocentesis for internal derangement of the TMJ with a sample of 103 TMJs in 100 patients with internal derangement and assessed treatment outcomes in terms of the pre-operative and post-operative range of MMO and the degree of pain. They reported seventy-three cases (71%) as successful and 30 cases (29%) as ineffective one week after the procedure [38].

Monje-Gil F et al. reviewed clinical reports that were published regarding the critiques of TMJ arthrocentesis. 20 different articles with different designs fulfilling the selection guidelines were chosen and evaluated by the authors for the study. They reported a success rate of 83.5% in the review of 612 joints with acute closed lock (disc displacement without reduction or anchored disc phenomenon) from 586 patients. They concluded that arthrocentesis is a simple, non-invasive, inexpensive, and highly effective procedure apart from having a low morbidity rate [35]. Arthrocentesis may be utilized for acute disc-condyle conflicts, targeting an attempt to recapitulate the articular disc. One such condition described by Nitzan is temporomandibular joint "Open Lock". Open clock phenomenon is associated with the acute inability to close the mouth or painful closure on effort, usually in patients with internal derangement. In this condition the joint is locked in the open-mouth position, with the condyle of the affected joint located in front of the anterior band of the disc, thereby mechanically obstructing the posterior movement of the anteriorly displaced condyles into the articular fossa [39] (Fig. 19.9).

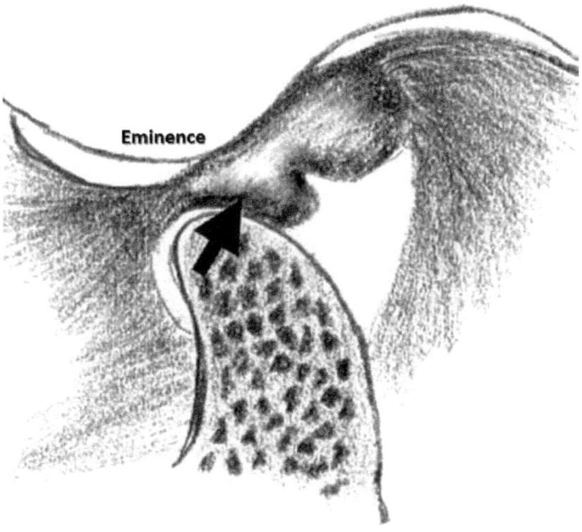

Fig. 19.9 Schematic representation of the temporomandibular joint. In open-lock, the condyle is trapped in front of the folded lagging disc (arrow) and cannot return to the fossa. Release of the disc after lavage of the upper compartment enables the reestablishment of simultaneous sliding of the disc together with the condyle. (Adapted with permission: Nitzan DW. Temporomandibular joint "open lock" versus condylar dislocation: signs and symptoms, imaging, treatment, and pathogenesis. J Oral Maxillofac Surg. 2002 May;60(5):506–11; discussion 512–3. https://doi.org/10.1053/joms.2002.31846)

19.8 Consideration for Arthrocentesis of TMJ

For patients who do not respond to the conservative management, arthrocentesis becomes the first line of intervention before subjecting the patient to a surgical open joint procedure. It is a simple and minimally invasive procedure with negligible risk of complications, while delivering significant benefits including improvement in MMO, clicking, pain, and jaw deviation on mouth opening.

Although the first line of treatment in every patient with internal derangement should be initiated with non-invasive methods aiming at control of para-functional habits, use of analgesics and anti-inflammatory drugs, altering the dietary habits and physiotherapy. Arthrocentesis should be considered if conservative methods fail to provide adequate relief to the patient [36–39].

References

1. Milaro M, Ghali GE, Larsen P, Waite PD. Peterson's principles of oral and maxillofacial surgery. 2nd ed. Hamilton, London: BC Decker Inc.; 2004.
2. Bhargava D, Jain M, Deshpande A, Singh A, Jaiswal J. Temporomandibular joint arthrocentesis for internal derangement with disc displacement without reduction. J Maxillofac Oral Surg. 2015;14 (2):454–9.

3. Ireland WE. The problems of "the clicking jaw". Proc R Sot Med. 1951;44:363.
4. Wilkes CH. Internal derangements of the temporomandibular joint: pathological variation. Arch Otolaryngol Head Neck Surg. 1989;115:469.
5. González-García R. The current role and the future of minimally invasive temporomandibular joint surgery. Oral Maxillofac Surg Clin N Am. 2015;27 (1):69–84. https://doi.org/10.1016/j.coms.2014.09.006.
6. Onishi M. Arthroscopy of the temporomandibular joint. Kokubyo Gakkai Zasshi. 1975;42:207–13.
7. Murakami K, Hoshino K. Regional anatomical nomenclature and arthroscopic terminology in human temporomandibular joints. Okajimas Folia Anat Jpn. 1982;58:745–60.
8. McCain J. Arthroscopy of the human temporomandibular joint. J Oral Maxillofac Surg. 1988;46:648–55.
9. Holmlund A, Hellsing G. Arthroscopy of the temporomandibular joint: an autopsy study. Int J Oral Maxillofac Surg. 1985;14:169–75.
10. Sanders B. Arthroscopic surgery of the temporomandibular joint: treatment of internal derangement with persistent closed lock. Oral Surg Oral Med Oral Pathol. 1986;62:361–72.
11. Murakami K, Ono T. TMJ arthroscopy by inferolateral approach. Int J Oral Maxillofac Surg. 1986;15:410–7.
12. Murakami K, Iizuka T, Matsuki M, et al. Recapturing the persistent anteriorly displaced disk by mandibular manipulation after pumping and hydraulic pressure to the upper joint cavity of the temporomandibular joint. Cranio. 1987;5:17–24.
13. Nitzan DW, Dolwick MF, Martinez GA. Temporomandibular joint arthrocentesis: a simplified treatment for severe, limited mouth opening. J Oral Maxillofac Surg. 1991;49:1163–7.
14. Dimitroulis G, Dolwick MF, Martinez A. Temporomandibular joint arthrocentesis and lavage for the treatment of closed lock: a follow-up study. Br J Oral Maxillofac Surg. 1995;33:23–7.
15. Alkan A, Baş B. The use of double- needle canula method for temporomandibular joint arthrocentesis: clinical report. Eur J Dent. 2007;1:179–82.
16. Dayisoylu EH, Cifci E, Uckan S. Ultrasound guided arthrocentesis of the temporomandibular joint. Br J Oral Maxillofac Surg. 2013;51:667–8.
17. Bhargava D, Thomas S, Pawar P, Jain M, Pathak P. (2019). Ultrasound-guided arthrocentesis using single-puncture, double-lumen, single-barrel needle for patients with temporomandibular joint acute closed lock internal derangement. Oral Maxillofac Surg. 2019;23 (2):159–65.
18. Young AL. Internal derangements of the temporomandibular joint: a review of the anatomy, diagnosis, and management. J Indian Prosthodont Soc. 2015;15 (1):2–7. https://doi.org/10.4103/0972-4052.156998.
19. Şentürk MF, Cambazoğlu M. A new classification for temporomandibular joint arthrocentesis techniques. Int J Oral Maxillofac Surg. 2015;44:417–8.
20. Guarda-Nardini L, Manfredini D, Ferronato G. Arthrocentesis of the temporomandibular joint: a proposal for a single-needle technique. Oral Surg Oral Med Oral Pathol Oral Radiol Endod. 2008;106:483–6.
21. Rehman KU, Hall T. Single needle arthrocentesis. Br J Oral Maxillofac Surg. 2009;47:403–4.
22. Bhargava D, Thomas S, Pawar P, Pathak P. Double lumen single barrel needle customization and fluid dynamics for single puncture temporomandibular joint arthrocentesis. Acta Scientific Orthopedics. 2018;1 (1):15–6.
23. Moran A, Kanatas AF, Worrall SF. Re: a new anatomical landmark to simplify temporomandibular joint arthrocentesis. Br J Oral Maxillofac Surg. 2010;48:486–8.
24. Talaat W, Ghoneim MM, Elsholkamy M. Single needle arthrocentesis (Shepard cannula) vs. double needle arthrocentesis for treating disc displacement without reduction. Cranio. 2016;34 (5):296–302.
25. Öreroğlu AR, Özkaya Ö, Öztürk MB, et al. Concentric needle cannula method for single- puncture arthrocentesis in temporomandibular joint disease. An inexpensive and feasible technique. J Oral Maxillofac Surg. 2011;69:2334–8.
26. Skármeta NP, Pesce MC, Espinoza-Mellado PA. A single puncture arthrocentesis technique, using a peripheral intravenous catheter. Int J Oral Maxillofac Surg. 2016;45:1123–5.
27. Yura S, Totsuka Y, Yoshikawa T, Inoue N. Can arthrocentesis release intracapsular adhesions? Arthroscopic findings before and after irrigation under sufficient hydraulic pressure. J Oral Maxillofac Surg. 2003;61:1253–6.
28. Alkan A, Kilic E. A new approach to arthrocentesis of the temporomandibular joint. Int J Oral Maxillofac Surg. 2009;38 (1):85–6.
29. Alpaslan GH, Alpaslan C. Efficacy of temporomandibular joint arthrocentesis with and without injection of sodium hyaluronate in treatment of internal derangements. J Oral Maxillofac Surg. 2001;59:613–8.
30. Kopp S, Wenneberg B, Haraldson T, et al. The short-term effect of intra-articular injections of sodium hyaluronate and corticosteroid on temporomandibular joint pain and dysfunction. J Oral Maxillofac Surg. 1985;43:429–35.
31. Giraddi GB, Siddaraju A, Kumar B, Singh C. Internal derangement of temporomandibular joint: an evaluation of effect of corticosteroid injection compared with injection of sodium hyaluronate after arthrocentesis. J Maxillofac Oral Surg. 2012;11 (3):258–63.
32. Davoudi A, Khaki H, Mohammadi I, et al. Is arthrocentesis of temporomandibular joint with corticosteroids beneficial? A systematic review. Med Oral Patol Oral Cir Bucal. 2018;23 (3):e367–75. https://doi.org/10.4317/medoral.21925. Published 2018 May 1.
33. Arafat SW, Chehata IM. Clinical and biochemical assessment of different injection materials following arthrocentesis for the treatment of internal derangement of the temporomandibular joint: a comparative study. Tanta Dent J. 2016;13:102–8.

34. Marty P, Louvrier A, Weber E, et al. Arthrocentesis of the temporomandibular joint and intra-articular injections: an update. Rev Stomatol Chir Maxillofac Chir Orale. 2016;117:266–72.
35. Monje-Gil F, Nitzan D, Gonzalez-Garcia R. Temporomandibular joint arthrocentesis. Review of the literature. Med Oral Patol Oral Cir Bucal. 2012 Jul 1;17 (4):575–81.
36. Emshoff R, Rudisch A. Temporomandibular joint internal derangement and osteoarthrosis: are effusion and bone marrow edema prognostic indicators for arthrocentesis and hydraulic distention? J Oral Maxillofac Surg. 2007 Jan;65 (1):66–73.
37. Kuruvilla VE, Prasad K. Arthrocentesis in TMJ internal derangement: a prospective study. J Maxillofac Oral Surg. 2012;11 (1):53–6. https://doi.org/10.1007/s12663-011-0288-8.
38. Nishimura M, Segami N, Kaneyama K, Suzuki T. Prognostic factors in arthrocentesis of the temporomandibular joint: evaluation of 100 patients with internal derangement. J Oral Maxillofac Surg. 2001;59:874–7.
39. Nitzan DW. Temporomandibular joint "open lock" versus condylar dislocation: signs and symptoms, imaging, treatment, and pathogenesis. J Oral Maxillofac Surg. 2002;60(5):506–11; discussion 512–3. https://doi.org/10.1053/joms.2002.31846.

20 Fundamentals of Temporomandibular Joint Arthroscopy

Ankit Pandey and Darpan Bhargava

20.1 Introduction

Temporomandibular Joint (TMJ) arthroscopy is one of the most advanced and a minimally invasive technique involving optical instrumentation and prescribed surgical armamentarium, used for the treatment of the TMJ disorders. It was introduced by Ohnishi in 1974 (Table 20.1). Arthroscopy emerged as a diagnostic tool, which now finds its application in the treatment of temporomandibular joint diseases. The advantage of this technique remains in direct visualization of all the anatomic regions inside the joint cavity for a definitive diagnosis, treatment, and predictable prognosis. Though, currently the equipment involved for a TMJ arthroscopy setup may be expensive and training regarding the same remains sparse, the future demands such minimally invasive and technologically sound advancement to diagnose and treat temporomandibular joint disorders [1].

Table 20.1 History of arthroscopy for TMJ

Pioneers involved in the evolution of TMJ arthroscopy	Development
Masatoshi Ohnishi 1974	Endoscopic access by Selfoc arthroscope with 1.7 mm diameter Published puncture technique as well as anatomic findings
Hilsabech and Laskin 1978	Proved arthroscopy as a safe technique in animal study for intra-articular adhesions
Williams and Laskin 1980	Diagnosis of pathologic conditions of TMJ in animal studies by arthroscopy
Ken-Ischiro Murakami and Kazumasa Hoshino 1982	Reported procedural terminology and arthroscopic anatomy with their study on 20 temporomandibular joints of 19 human cadavers
Joseph McCaine 1985	Acclaimed for his work on clinical arthroscopy for TMDs and introduced triangulation technique for the second puncture
J J Moses 1985	First hands-on course in cadavers for temporomandibular joint arthroscopy
Murakami and Hoshino 1985	Described histologic cellular characters of inner aspects of temporomandibular joint
Holmlund and Hellsing 1985	Concept of puncture sites correlating cantho-tragal line
Bruce sanders 1986	Executed arthroscopy clinically for TMDs
Holmlund et al. 1986	Endorsed the observations of Williams and Laskin

A. Pandey
Amrit Dental and TMJ Centre, Bhopal, Madhya Pradesh, India

D. Bhargava (✉)
TMJ Consultancy Services, Bhopal, Madhya Pradesh, India

Oral and Maxillofacial Surgery, People's College of Dental Sciences and Research Centre, People's University, Bhopal, Madhya Pradesh, India
e-mail: drdarpanbhargava@gmail.com

D. Bhargava (ed.), *Temporomandibular Joint Disorders*,
https://doi.org/10.1007/978-981-16-2754-5_20

Table 20.1 (continued)

Pioneers involved in the evolution of TMJ arthroscopy	Development
Murakami and Ono 1986	Research on improved surgical techniques for temporomandibular joint arthroscopy. Described arthroscopic suture for anterior disc displacement and chronic dislocation
Joseph McCain 1991	Described puncture technique and portals of entry for diagnostic and operative arthroscopy of the temporomandibular joint
Samer Srouji 2016	Described single cannula arthroscopy

20.2 Arthroscopic Anatomy of TMJ

Understanding the arthroscopic joint anatomy is the key to successful diagnosis and treatment. The various anatomic regions that need identification include: posterior pouch containing the recess, lateral pterygoid shadow, condylar disc, retro-discal tissue, and the anterior pouch including the junction of disc cartilage and lateral pterygoid muscle. The seven vital areas observed during arthroscopic examination are: medial synovial drape, pterygoid shadow, retrodiscal synovium, posterior slope of articular eminence and glenoid fossa, articular disc, intermediate zone, and anterior recess [2] (Fig. 20.1).

20.3 Armamentarium

Basic and advanced armamentarium utilized for TMJ arthroscopy is enlisted in Table 20.2 which is essential to execute level I (Diagnostic) to level III (Lysis, lavage, and discopexy) arthroscopic procedures (Fig. 20.2).

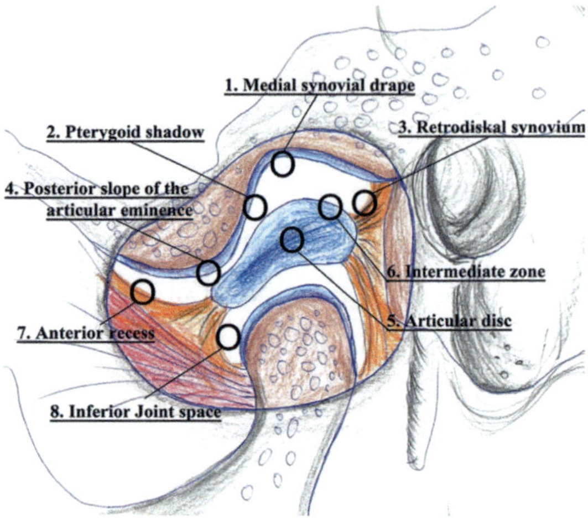

Fig. 20.1 During diagnostic temporomandibular joint arthroscopy, seven anatomic areas that need to be examined: (1) the medial synovial drape, (2) the pterygoid shadow, (3) the retrodiscal synovium and the posterior ligament, (4) the posterior slope of the articular eminence and glenoid fossa, (5) the articular disc, (6) the intermediate zone, and (7) the anterior recess. (8) The inferior joint space is not routinely explored. In cases of disc perforation, the inferior joint space can be examined by introducing the scope through the perforation [Reprinted/adapted by permission from S. T. Connelly et al. (eds.), Contemporary Management of Temporomandibular Disorders, https://doi.org/10.1007/978-3-319-99909-8_4]

Table 20.2 Armamentarium for TMJ arthroscopy

Instruments required from level I to III arthroscopy
TMJ arthroscope (preferably 30°) with sheath
Cannula with trocar and obturators (sharp and blunt)
Probes: Straight, hooked
Light source
Biopsy forceps: Serrated type, basket type
Scissors
Knife
High frequency ablation system/cautery long tip
Suction punch
Meniscus mender: Straight and curved needles with stylet and suture loop
Bone rasps
Curettes
Golden retriever
Motorized shavers and abraders
Laser Unit
Camera System
Needles (18G/16G)

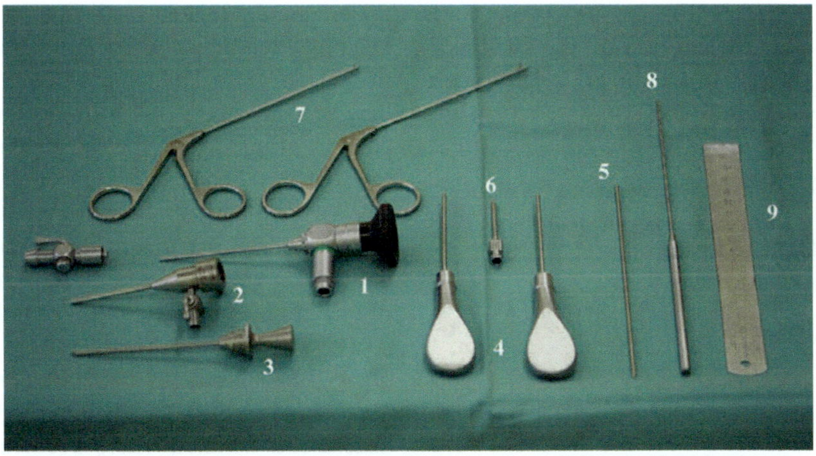

Fig. 20.2 The basic armamentarium for TMJ arthroscopy contains the (1) arthroscope, diameter 1.9 mm, length 6.5 cm; (2) high-flow arthroscope sheath; (3) trocar; (4) sharp and a blunt obturator; (5) changing rods for the sheath and (6) cannula; (7) biopsy forceps, single-action jaws; (8) hooked probe; and (9) ruler [Reprinted/adapted by permission from Seebauer C., Kaduk W., Sanroman J.F., Silva R.G. (2019) Surgery of the Temporomandibular Joint: Surgical Arthroscopy. In: Connelly S.T., Tartaglia G.M., Silva R.G. (eds) Contemporary Management of Temporomandibular Disorders. Springer, Cham. https://doi.org/10.1007/978-3-319-99909-8_4]

20.4 Patient and Surgeon Positioning

The patient should lie in supine position with head tilted laterally. The joint to be operated should lie parallel to the floor or the operating table. The face of the patient should be directed away and below the elbow level of the operating surgeon.

20.5 Surgeon's Position

When operating on the right temporomanibular joint region the surgeon should stand towards the right side of the patient. Left hand of the surgeon should be the working hand, i.e. the surgeon should hold and maipulate the scope with the left hand. While operating on the left side, the scope be should held and manipulated with the right hand standing on the left of the patient [2].

20.6 Arthroscopic Technique

There are various puncture techniques that can be employed for performing arthroscopy of the TMJ. They include single puncture, double puncture technique, triple puncture technique, and inferior joint space puncture technique for arthroscopic discopexy. Selection of the technique is based on individual patient's requirement, the working diagnosis, and the operator's preference [3]. The sequence of diagnostic arthroscopy has been summarized in Table 20.3.

Before initiating the procedure, the operating surgeon should always check all the connections properly and adjust the white balance (removing unrealistic colour casts) before performing the first puncture. Currently, the commonly practiced method for arthroscopy involves double puncture technique with placement of two cannulas in the superior joint space. One cannula is used for visualization with the scope while the other port is used for the outflow of the irrigation fluid and instrumentation.

Before proceeding for the procedure, it is important to identify and localize the landmarks for accurate entry into the superior joint space and insertion of the trocar appropriately. Once the prauricular region is palpated for the condylar head position by passively moving the mandible in open and closed mouth position, a line is drawn between the centre of the tragus and the lateral canthus of the eye on the same side (Holmlund-Hellsing line, HH). Insertion point for the first trocar is marked 1 cm from the centre of the tragus anteriorly and 2 mm downwards from the above point (Point A). This point denotes the area of maximum concavity of the glenoid fossa. The second puncture site is marked 2 cm from the tragus on the line anteriorly and 1 cm below the above marking (Point B) (Fig. 20.3). The local anaesthetic solution (LA, 2% Lignocaine) is injected, inserting from the junction of tragus and face, directing towards the condylar head. Once the bone is hit LA is injected into the superior

Table 20.3 Various steps involved during the procedure of TMJ arthroscopy

Sequence of diagnostic arthroscopy
Examination under anaesthesia
Identification of the anatomic landmarks (in the preauricular region)
Insufflation
Trocar and cannula insertion
Backwash
Confirmation of the scope entry
Outflow of the solution
Diagnostic sweep
Placement of medications

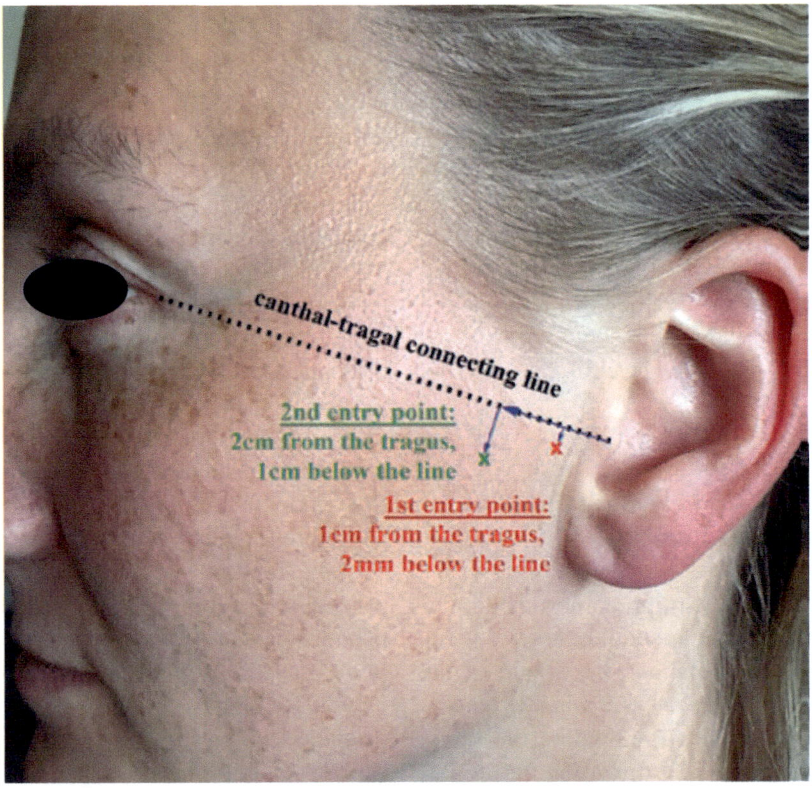

Fig. 20.3 On a line between the centre of the tragus and the lateral canthus, the insertion point for the first trocar is placed 1 cm from the tragus and 2 mm below the line. The second insertion point is placed 2 cm from the tragus and 1 cm below the line. [Reprinted/adapted by permission from Seebauer C., Kaduk W., Sanroman J.F., Silva R.G. (2019) Surgery of the Temporomandibular Joint: Surgical Arthroscopy. In: Connelly S.T., Tartaglia G.M., Silva R.G. (eds) Contemporary Management of Temporomandibular Disorders. Springer, Cham. https://doi.org/10.1007/978-3-319-99909-8_4]

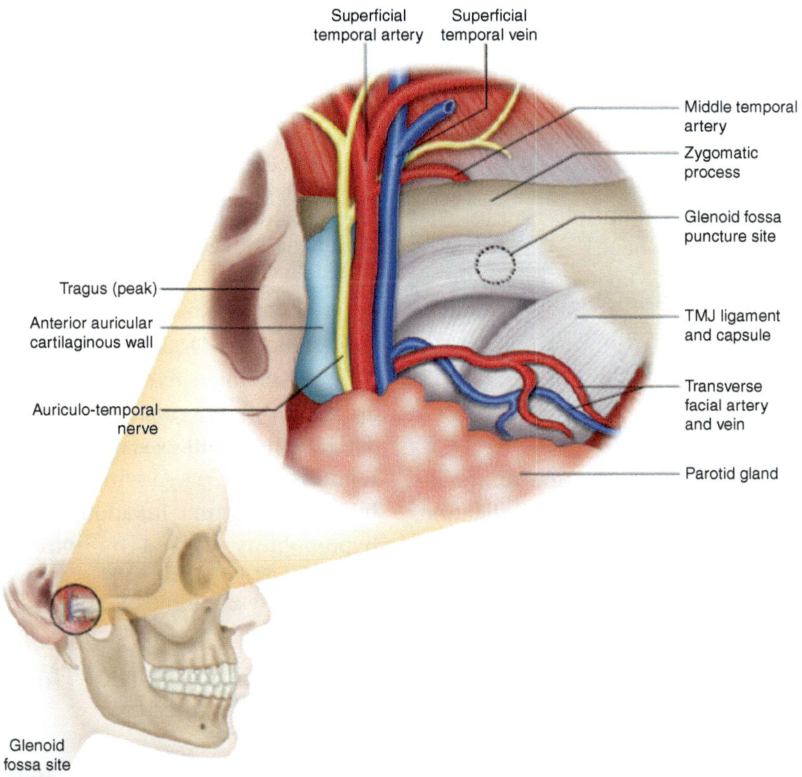

Fig. 20.4 Auriculotemporal nerve and temporal vessels running close the temporomandibular joint. Note the glenoid fossa puncture site. [Reprinted/adapted by permission from S. T. Connelly et al. (eds.), Contemporary Management of Temporomandibular Disorders, https://doi.org/10.1007/978-3-319-99915-9_4]

joint space, until plunging effect in the syringe is felt. Approximately 1.5 to 2 ml of LA may be required for insufflation [3]. The land mark for the first puncture is point A. The first insertion is done using a sharp trocar with sheath/sleeve by puncturing at point A without pulling the skin and palpating the concave part of the zygoma (Fig. 20.4). The zygoma is hit in the superio-inferior border with the trocar. The trocar is used to deglove the periosteum inferiorly until the superior joint space is punctured. The sharp trocar is retrieved and replaced with a blunt obturator after the initial skin penetration and the feel of loss of resistance of the capsular puncture before further advancing into the joint space, to prevent any intra-articular injury. The joint space can be accessed at an approximate distance of 25 mm from the skin puncture site, in an upward and inward direction below the initial bony contact of the trocar. Once the joint capsule is punctured and the trocar is replaced with the obturator before further advancing into the joint space, the outflow is checked. Once the outflow confirms the spatial location of the cannula in the joint space, the obturator is replaced with the arthroscope for visualization of the superior joint space (on the monitor/screen/output display). Solution (usually Ringer's lactate) for lysis and lavage is introduced into the joint and a second puncture is done for the solution outflow and inflammatory contents to drain out at Point B using a 18G needle or a working port cannula [3, 7].

During arthroscopy, "red-out" occurs if there is excess blood mixed with the irrigation fluid caused by insufficient flow to the joint. It indicates that the fluid inflow and outflow should be checked and adjusted to maintain the optimal flow of the irrigation fluid [4].

According to the requirements and the level of arthroscopic surgery further punctures may be required for the advanced intra-articular surgeries.

- **Level I:** Diagnostic arthroscopy
- **Level II:** Diagnostic sweep followed by lysis and lavage of the joint space
- **Level III:** Lysis and lavage followed by Discopexy [4]

20.7 Complications

TMJ arthroscopy is a relatively safe minimally invasive procedure but chances for complications does exist which may include instrument breakage, scar formation at the puncture site, VIIth cranial nerve trauma, parotid gland injury, arthrofibrosis, bleeding, and post-operative oedema. Fluid extravasation into the surrounding tissues during joint irrigation is also a possible complication, requring a continuous check for the fluid outflow during the procedure. Infection at the arthroscopy site or the joint per se may occur. The recurrence or relapse of joint derangement remains a possibility with patient turning symptomatic in the post-operative phase. Incorrect insertion of the trocar can cause perforation in to the ear canal or the medial synovial drape. Perforation of the glenoid fossa with subdural/epidural haematoma has been documented as a result of perforation into middle cranial fossa. Aborting the procedure is wise when one of the above complications are encountered, along with managing the complication appropriately. However, performing the procedure judiciously delivers the favourable results with this technique [2].

20.8 Indications and Contraindications

Meticulous patient selection is the key to successful treatment outcome. There are several indications and contra-indications that require consideration for arthroscopy of temporomandibular joint (Table 20.4). The American Association of Oral and Maxillofacial Surgeons have enumerated five main indications for TMJ arthroscopy: (1) internal derangement of the TMJ, mainly Wilkes stages 2–4, (2) degenerative joint disease, (3) synovitis, (4) painful hypermobility or recurrent luxation of the disc, and (5) hypomobility caused by intra-articular adherences [6, 7].

Table 20.4 Indications and contra-indications for TMJ arthroscopy

Indications	Contra-indications
Disc displacement/ deformity Intra-articular adhesions Osteoarthritis/ degenerative arthritis Post-traumatic changes Pseudo-tumours	Bony ankylosis Acute infection Tumours having risk of dissemination Systemic disorders and anatomic alterations to the joint architecture

20.9 Advantages of TMJ Arthroscopy

- Direct visualization of the joint space.
- Accurate diagnosis of the pathologic joint under direct vision.
- Biopsy and fluid collection can be performed.
- Minimally invasive procedure.

20.10 Limitations for TMJ Arthroscopy

- Availability of the equipment.
- Operator's proficiency and sufficient training is required. It is a technique sensitive procedure.
- Procedure should be aborted in cases of unfavourable puncture or when a complication is encountered.

20.11 Advanced Arthroscopy for TMJ

The advanced arthroscopy techniques are indicated when the joint disorder does not respond to medical management and minimally invasive procedures but require structural modifications in and surrounding the joint. There are several additional instruments which may be required for the advanced arthroscopic intervention listed in Table 20.2 [5] (Refer Chap. 21).

20.12 Other Additional Arthroscopic Treatment Modalities

There are several additional documented treatment modalities that may be combined with TMJ arthroscopy and the procedure can be performed for the management of joint dysfunction that includes use of water-jet treatment, lasers (CO_2, Nd:YAG and Holmium) and utilizing surgical navigation technique [4].

References

1. Peterson JL. Principles of oral and maxillofacial surgery, vol. 2. China: Pmph USA Ltd Series; 2004. p. 963–88.
2. Peterson JL. Operative oral and maxillofacial surgery, 2 ed. London: Hodder Arnold; 2011. p. 543–52.
3. McCain JP, Rua HLA, et al. Puncture techniques and portals of entry for diagnostic and operative arthroscopy of the temporomandibular joint. Arthroscopy. 1991;7(2):221–32.
4. Kaduk WMH. Arthroscopy of temporomandibular joint. Germany: Endo Press GmbH; 2006.
5. McCain JP, Hossameldin RH. Advanced arthroscopy of temporomandibular joint. Atlas Oral Maxillofac Surg Clin N Am. 2011;19:145–67.
6. Parameters of care for oral and maxillofacial surgery. A guide for practice, monitoring and evaluation (AAOMS Parameters of Care-92). American Association of Oral and Maxillofacial Surgeons. J Oral Maxillofac Surg. 1992;50(7 Suppl 2):i–xvi, 1–174.
7. Seebauer C, Kaduk W, Sanroman JF, Silva RG. Surgery of the Temporomandibular Joint: Surgical Arthroscopy. In: Connelly ST, Tartaglia GM, Silva RG. (eds) Contemporary Management of Temporomandibular Disorders. Springer, Cham. 2019. https://doi.org/10.1007/978-3-319-99909-8_4.

21 Temporomandibular Joint Arthroscopy Using Operative Single-Cannula Arthroscope

Samer Srouji and Daniel Oren

21.1 History and Goals

The first temporomandibular joint (TMJ) arthroscopy procedure was performed in 1974 by Masatoshi Ohnishi [1]. In 1982, Murakami and Hoshino developed the nomenclature of TMJ arthroscopic anatomy [2]. Modifications and new arthroscopy techniques have since been introduced by McCain [3, 4], Sanders [5], Holmlund and Hellsing [6], Nitzan and colleagues [7], Koslin [8] and others, with modified and alternative arthroscopy techniques to ensure safe and accurate diagnosis, effectively reduce pain and joint pathologies, and provide a joint environment that fosters functional restoration. TMJ arthroscopy is primarily performed using a single-puncture technique, appropriate for diagnostics and basic interventions only, or traditional double-puncture technique, which involves insertion of one cannula through which the arthroscope is introduced, and a second cannula, through which the surgery is performed [9]. While contemporary arthroscopy techniques aim to minimize invasiveness, advanced arthroscopy techniques are highly coordination-demanding and are associated with a steep learning curve, hindering their widespread adoption by maxillofacial surgeons. This chapter discusses in detail, the operative single-cannula arthroscopy (OSCA) technique, a single-track, advanced arthroscopy method appropriate for both diagnostic and interventional procedures [10].

21.2 Temporomandibular Joint (TMJ) Anatomy

The TMJ is a bilateral synovial articulation situated between the glenoid fossa and articular eminence of the temporal bone, the condylar head of the mandible, and the biconcave articular disk [11] (Fig. 21.1). The lower and superior compartments are separated by the articular disk. The anterior portion of the disk is penetrated by the superior head of the lateral pterygoid muscle, while its posterior end is connected to a highly vascularized and innervated retrodiscal tissue. The temporomandibular, stylomandibular, and sphenomandibular ligaments are associated with the TMJ, and define the range of mandibular movement.

S. Srouji (✉)
Oral and Maxillofacial Surgery, Oral Medicine and Dentistry Institute, Galilee Medical Center, Nahariya, Israel

Galilee College of Dental Sciences, Galilee Medical Center, Nahariya, Israel

The Azrieli Faculty of Medicine, Bar-Ilan University, Zefat, Israel

Bone Regeneration Lab, Galilee Medical Center, Nahariya, Israel

D. Oren
Oral and Maxillofacial Surgery, Oral Medicine and Dentistry Institute, Galilee Medical Center, Nahariya, Israel

The Azrieli Faculty of Medicine, Bar-Ilan University, Zefat, Israel

D. Bhargava (ed.), *Temporomandibular Joint Disorders*,
https://doi.org/10.1007/978-981-16-2754-5_21

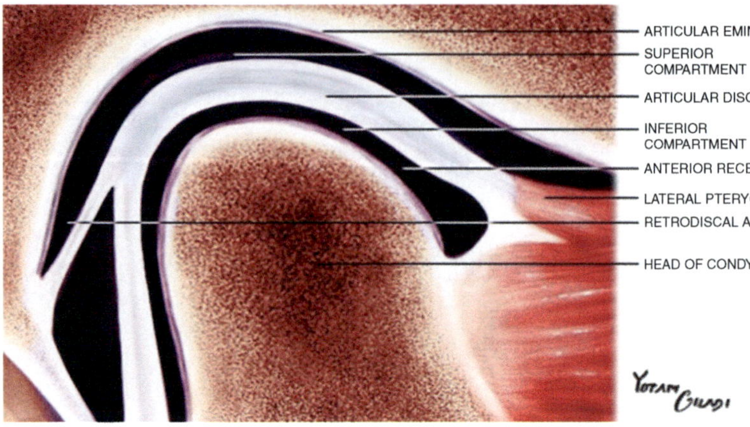

Fig. 21.1 A lateral view of the temporomandibular joint

The auriculotemporal nerve is a branch of the mandibular nerve (V_1) that runs parallel to the superficial temporal artery and vein. It passes between the neck of the mandible and the sphenomandibular ligament in proximity to the fossa puncture site. The most important blood vessels in this region are the superficial temporal artery and vein (Fig. 21.2).

21.3 Temporomandibular Joint Disorders

21.3.1 Diagnosis

Initial assessment of temporomandibular joint disorders (TMD) should include a detailed history and clinical examination and imaging of the region using conventional radiography or/and a panoramic X ray to observe the bony elements of the TMJ, or using computed tomography (CT), for evaluation of the bony elements of the TMJ and limited information of the surrounding soft tissues. Magnetic resonance imaging (MRI) provides information necessary to assess the shape, position, mobility, and structural integrity of the disk, as well as the status of the soft tissue. Maximal inter-incisal opening (MIO) should be measured (Fig. 21.3a), and joint noises should be assessed. The Mahan test assesses the presence of joint inflammation, reflected by contralateral pain on biting on the two wooden spatulas placed between the posterior teeth (Fig. 21.3b). Patients are asked to rate the pain using the 10-point Visual Analog Scale (VAS), to describe any changes in diet and use of non-steroidal anti-inflammatory drugs (NSAIDs) or any other over-the-counter medication. The Wilkes classification system (I-V) is the most widely accepted classification and terminology used to define internal derangement (ID) disorders and its severity (Table 21.1) [12].

21.3.2 Treatment Options

TMD is generally first conservatively addressed, which includes recommendation of changes in habits, NSAIDs administration, nocturnal use of a stabilization (flat-plane) device, for at least 3 months and physical therapy [3]. Diagnostic arthroscopy is recommended in patients suffering from persistent pain and presenting with hypo- or hypermobility, degenerative joint diseases, subluxation, or dislocation (Fig. 21.4).

21.4 Indications for Arthroscopy

The main indications for arthroscopy as set forth by the American Association of Oral and Maxillofacial Surgeons (AAOMS) include [11, 13–15]: degenerative joint disease (osteoarthritis), synovitis, internal derangement of TMJ (mainly Wilkes II-IV), hypermobility, hypomobility, inflammatory arthropathies, and

Fig. 21.2 Anatomy of the temporomandibular joint region

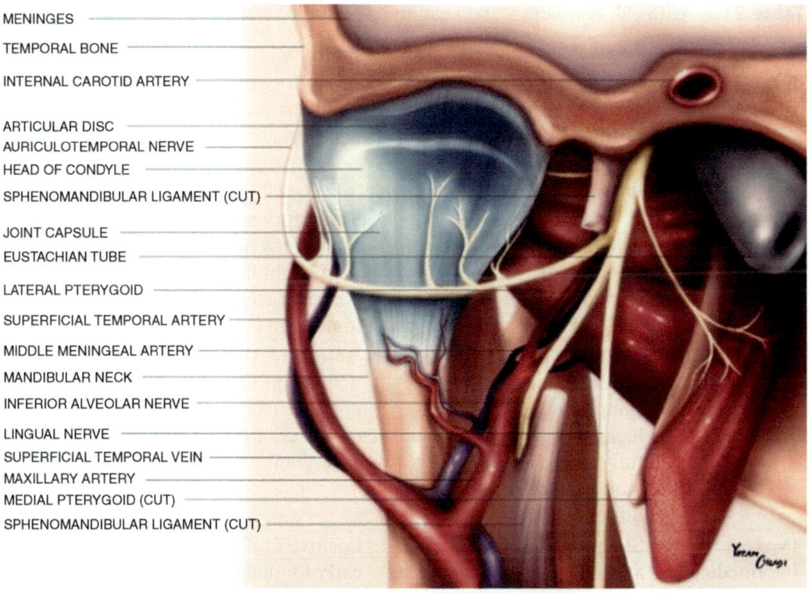

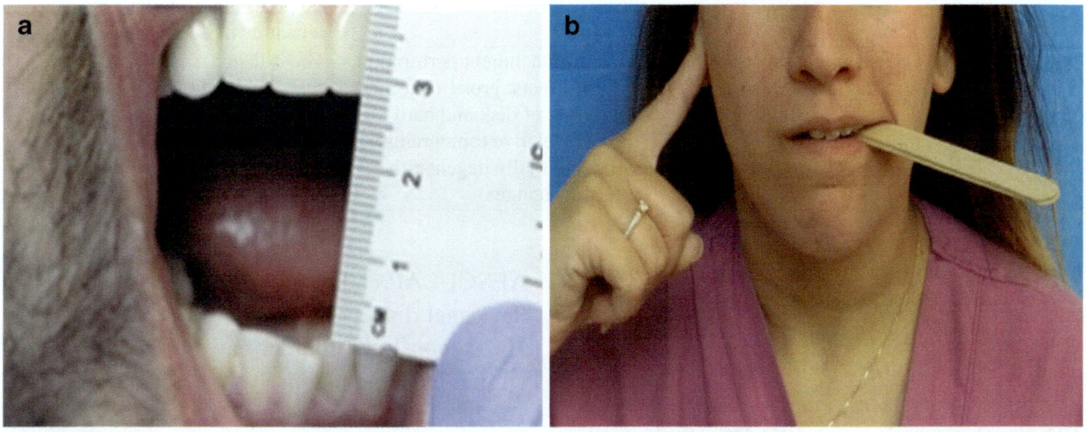

Fig. 21.3 (a) A patient with limited maximal inter-incisal opening. (b) Mahan test to assess contralateral pain upon biting, suggestive of joint inflammation

articular symptoms secondary to orthognathic surgery.

21.5 Contraindications

Arthroscopy is contraindicated in cases of severe fibrous or osseous ankyloses and tumor or metastasis in the TMJ. Risk of contamination of the join space is increased in cases of skin infection at the puncture site. In addition, the procedure should not be performed in patients with any medical conditions for which general anesthesia or surgery is contraindicated.

21.6 Surgical Tools

21.6.1 The Arthroscope

Arthroscopic systems should provide an angle of view of ≥30°, and a close-to-zero focal distance. Image resolution is optimal at a color temperature of 5000 K, which closely simulates natural day-

Table 21.1 Clinical, radiologic, and anatomical/pathological signs for Wilkes classification of TMJ ID

Stage	Clinical	Radiologic	Anatomic/Pathologic
I. Early stage	No significant mechanical symptoms other than early opening, reciprocal clicking; no pain or limitation of motion	Slight forward displacement; good anatomic contour of the disk; negative tomograms	Excellent anatomic form; slight anterior displacement; passive incoordination demonstrable
II. Early/intermediate stage	One or more episodes of pain; beginning major mechanical problems, loud clicking, transient catching, and locking	Slight forward displacement; early signs of disk deformity with slight thickening of posterior edge; negative tomograms	Anterior disk displacement; early anatomic disk deformity; good central articulating area
III. Intermediate stage	Multiple episodes of pain; major mechanical symptoms including locking (intermittent or fully closed), restricted motion, and functional difficulty	Anterior disk displacement with significant disk deformity/prolapse (increased thickening of posterior edge); negative tomograms	Marked anatomic disk deformity with anterior displacement; no hard tissue changes
IV. Intermediate/late stage	Slight increase in severity as compared to intermediate stage	Positive tomograms showing early to moderate degenerative changes—Flattening of eminence; deformed condylar head; sclerosis	Hard tissue degenerative remodeling of both bearing surfaces; multiple adhesions in anterior and posterior recesses; no perforation of disk or attachments
V. Late stage	Crepitus; scraping, grating, grinding; episodic or continuous pain; chronic motion restriction; functional difficulty	Disk or attachment perforation; filling defects; gross anatomic deformity of disk and hard tissues; positive tomograms with essentially degenerative arthritic changes	Gross degenerative changes of disk and hard tissues; perforation of posterior attachment; multiple adhesions; flattening of condyle and eminence; subcortical cystic formation

light. Color response, brightness, and "white balance" capacities of each system should be assessed. In the OSCA technique, the developers used a Polydiagnost (Hallbergmoos, Germany) interdisciplinary semirigid, 0.9 mm diameter, 181 mm-long endoscope (PD-DS-1083), with a standard light connection (ACMI/Storz/Wolf), which provides 10,000 pixel resolution, a 120° viewing angle, and a focal distance of 1–15 mm (Fig. 21.5a). The endoscope is connected in tandem to a 3-way female Luer lock connection handle and optic shifter as shown in Fig. 21.6.

The optic fiber is passed through the middle connection of a 3-way female Luer lock connection handle, while the other two connections are used for irrigation and instrumentation (Fig. 21.5b). The length of the optic fiber is then adjusted with a 26 mm optic shifter (Fig. 21.5c).

A multitude of recording and visualization instruments can be used. The authors use an AESCULAP endoscopy cart with a 26″ full HD flat panel display, full HD 3-chip Camera, AXel 300 xenon light source, and an Eddy Full HD Digital Documentation System (Fig. 21.7).

21.6.2 Cannulas

The authors use a unique a set of 1.6 mm, 2 mm, and 2.4 mm diameter cannulas (Fig. 21.8). The 2 mm cannula limits the diameter of introduced instruments and laser fiber to <1 mm, while the 2.4 mm cannula can accommodate a wider instrument. A sharp trocar (Fig. 21.9a) is introduced into the superior joint space and removed after penetrating the joint. Soft tissue is then separated using a blunt obturator (Fig. 21.9b). To monitor the depth of penetration, the cannula should be marked 25 mm from the working end, using an appropriate elastic rubber (Fig. 21.10).

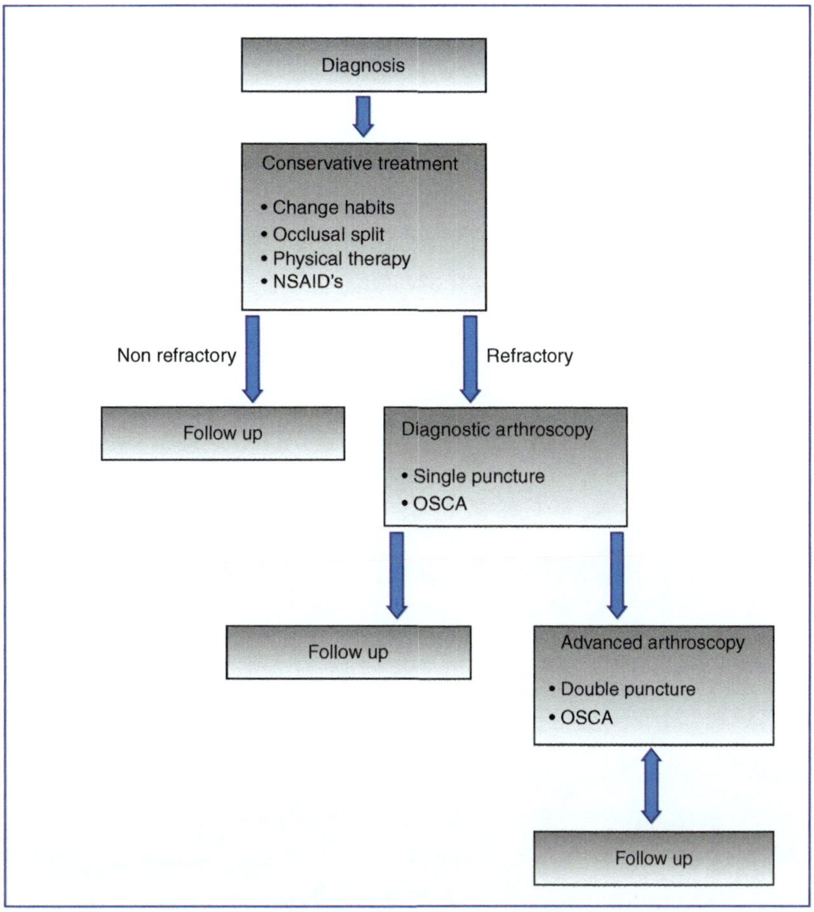

Fig. 21.4 Algorithm for TMD management

21.6.3 Probes

The probe is used for manual palpation, severing of adhesions, and to temporarily immobilize or to mobilize tissue. The probe must be of a diameter <1 mm and can be straight or hooked probe. The hooked probe is preferred for palpation in cases of chondromalacia, to elevate the anterior aspect of the disk after performing anterior releasing procedures and to complete disk dissection from the capsule and the pterygoid muscle.

21.6.4 Graspers and Biopsy Forceps

Graspers and biopsy forceps are used during biopsy collection and for debridement (Fig. 21.11).

21.6.5 Spinal Needles

Spinal needles used should be long (≥150 mm) and with a diameter of <1 mm. These are deployed to inject medications into the joint space or adjacent structures (Fig. 21.12).

21.6.6 Laser

Lasers can be deployed for synovectomy, retrodiscal scarification, tissue dissection, and debridement [9], each requiring different settings (Table 21.2). The authors recommend use of the air-cooling Holmium:YAG laser, and use the LISA LASER PRODUCTS Sphinx jr. Holmium:YAG laser (Fig. 21.13), which provides an optical power of 30 W at the fiber tip,

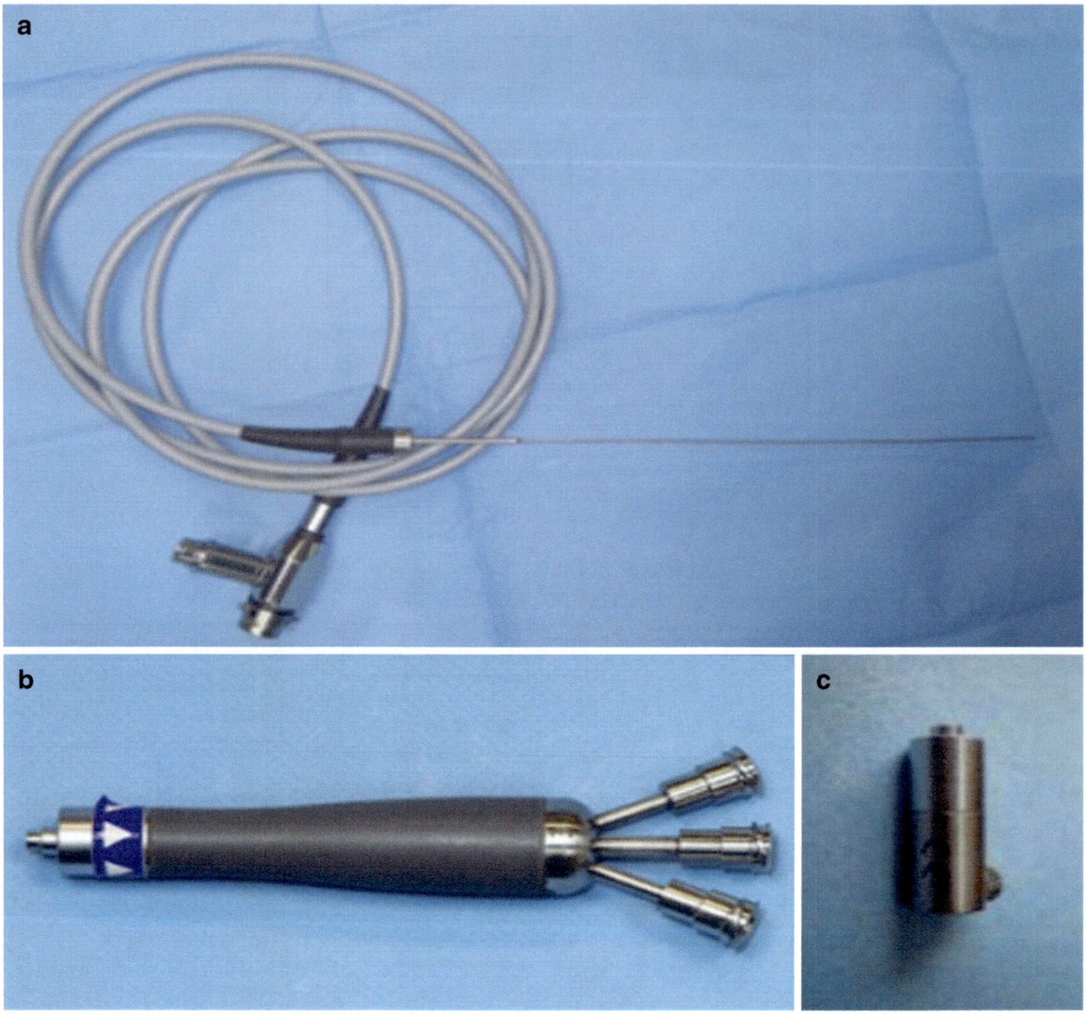

Fig. 21.5 (**a**) Polydiagnost interdisciplinary semirigid endoscope. (**b**) 3-way female Luer lock connection handle. **c**. Optic shifter

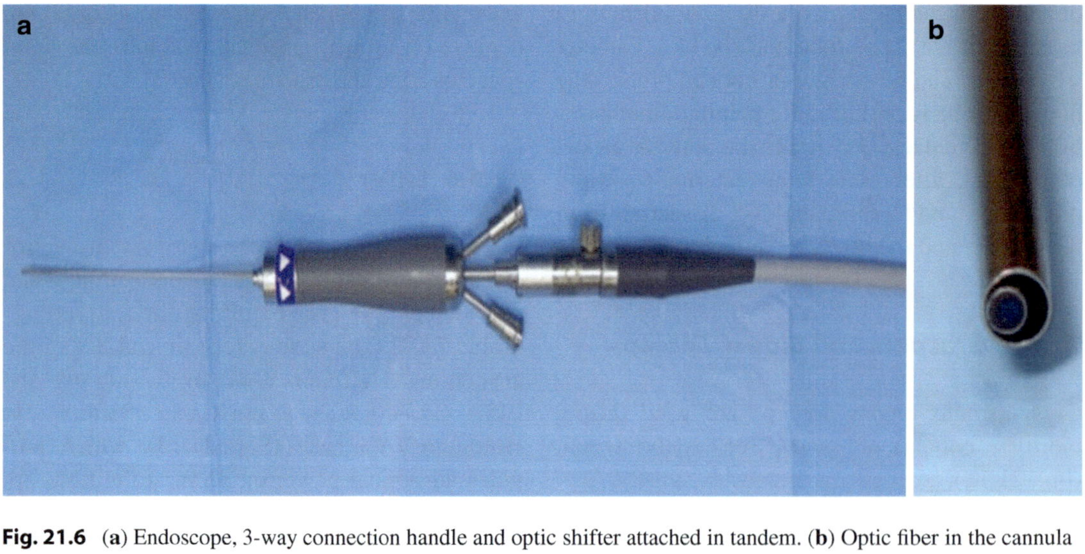

Fig. 21.6 (**a**) Endoscope, 3-way connection handle and optic shifter attached in tandem. (**b**) Optic fiber in the cannula

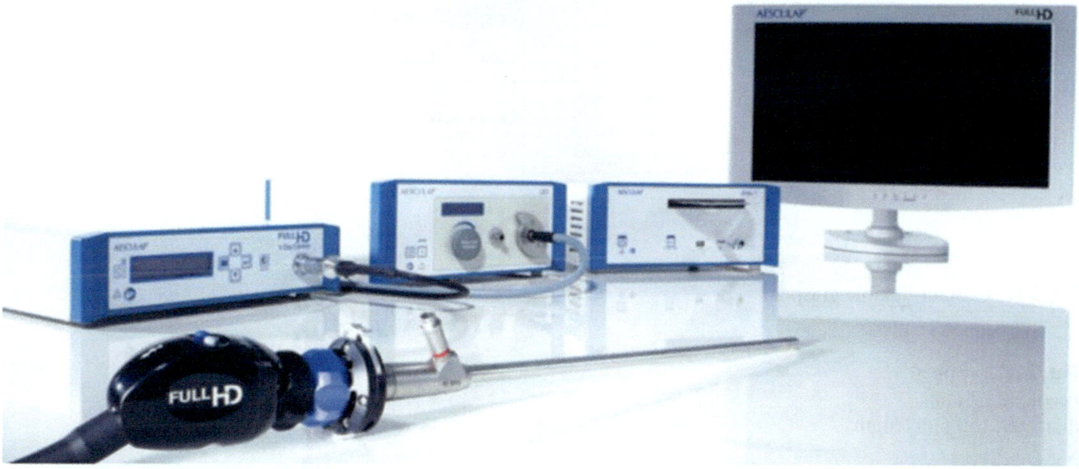

Fig. 21.7 AESCULAP endoscopy system

Fig. 21.8 1.6 mm, 2 mm, or 2.4 mm cannulas

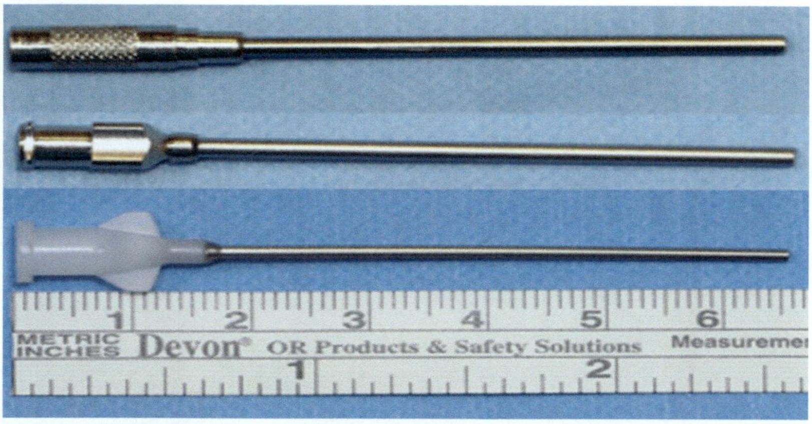

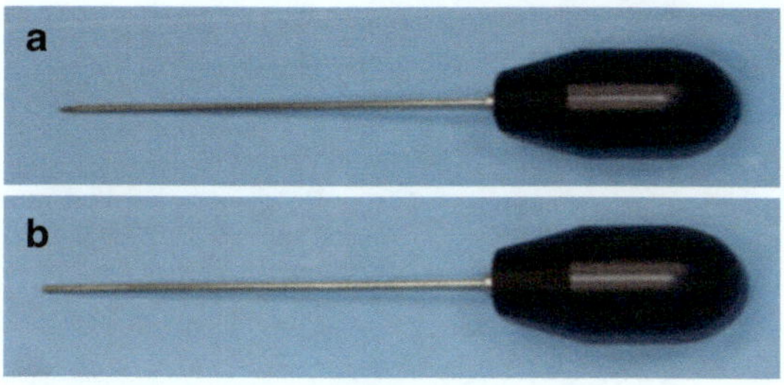

Fig. 21.9 (**a**) Sharp trocar. (**b**) Blunt obturator

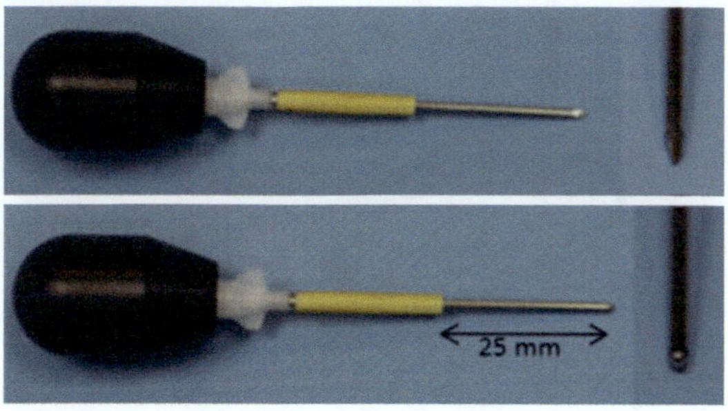

Fig. 21.10 Sharp trocar and blunt obturator inserted into a 1.6 mm cannula bearing a mark 25 mm from the working end

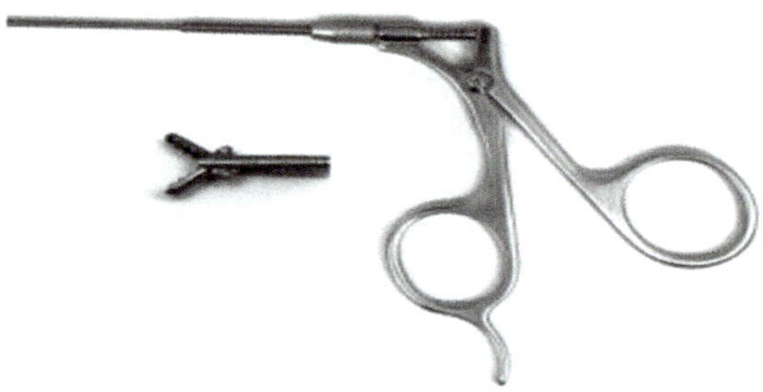

Fig. 21.11 Semi-flexible grasper

Table 21.2 Recommended Holmium:YAG laser settings for specific surgical activities

Laser setting for cutting	10 Hz	9 W	0.09 J
Laser setting for ablation	8 Hz	4 W	0.5 J
Laser setting for contracture	5 Hz	2 W	0.4 J

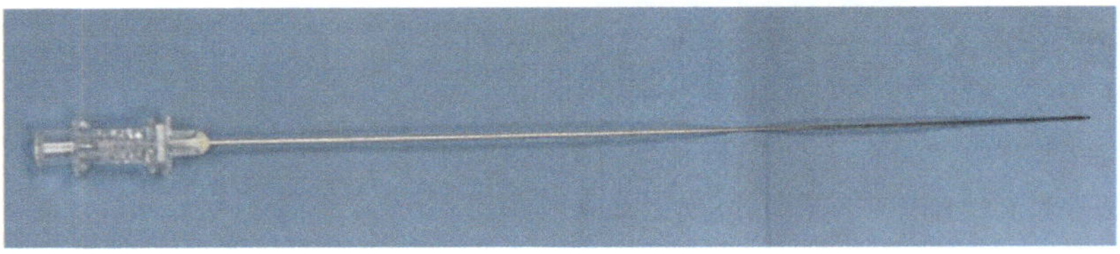

Fig. 21.12 Spinal needle: 0.72 mm diameter, 150 mm length

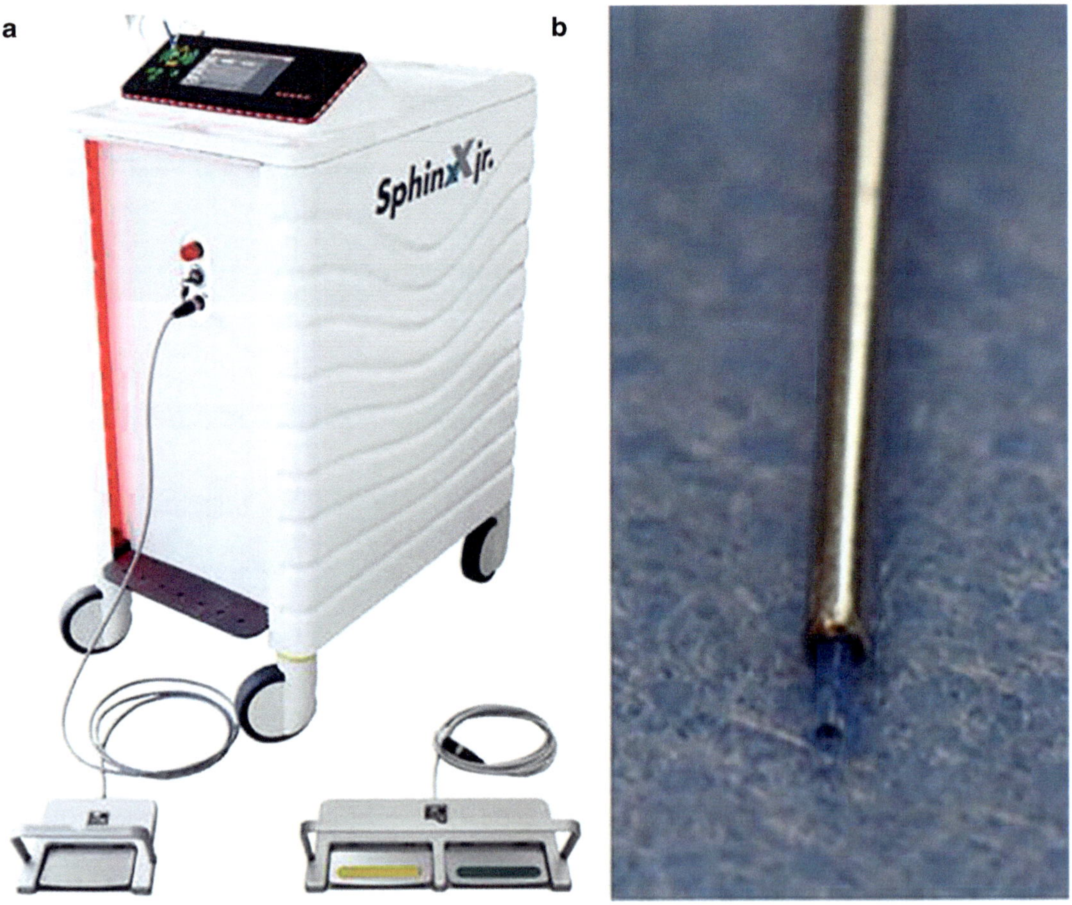

Fig. 21.13 (**a**) LISA LASER PRODUCTS Sphinx Jr. Holmium:YAG laser. (**b**) The laser fiber emerging from a metal protector

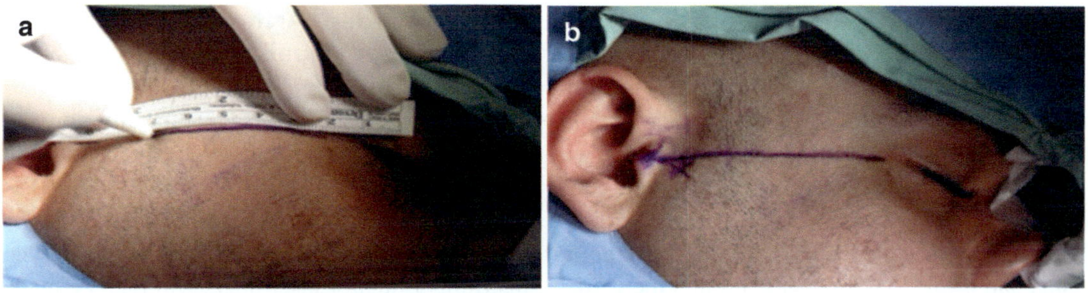

Fig. 21.14 (**a**) Marking the tragocanthal line. (**b**) The marked tragocanthal line and penetration point of the cannula, 10 mm anterior to the midtragus and 5 mm caudal to the tragocanthal line

0.3–5 J pulse energy, 100–650 μs pulse duration, and 1–25 Hz frequency. Its wavelength is strongly absorbed by water, and depth of penetration is limited to 0.3–0.5 mm, rendering it most appropriate for targeting most biologic tissues and safe for intraarticular use. For the OSCA technique, a 230 μm fiber laser is used, which is sufficiently small to safely access the TMJ.

21.7 OSCA Technique

OSCA can be performed under either sedation and local anesthesia or general anesthesia. Preoperative antibiotics and glucocorticosteroids are generally intravenously administered to prevent skin contamination and minimize edema, respectively. The patient is then placed in a supine position and an airway is established using nasotracheal intubation. The surgical site is prepared using an appropriate antiseptic solution, e.g., chlorhexidine gluconate (Unisept) or povidone iodine, isolating the surgical field and identifying anatomical landmarks to avoid complications. A tragocanthal line is established, and the cannula penetration point is planned 10 mm anterior to the midtragus and 5 mm caudal to the tragocanthal line (Fig. 21.14a, b).

Then, using a 22G needle, 2 ml bupivacaine is injected into the superior joint capsule, to expand the structures. When using a 3-mL syringe, backpressure can be felt when the joint space is penetrated (Fig. 21.15).

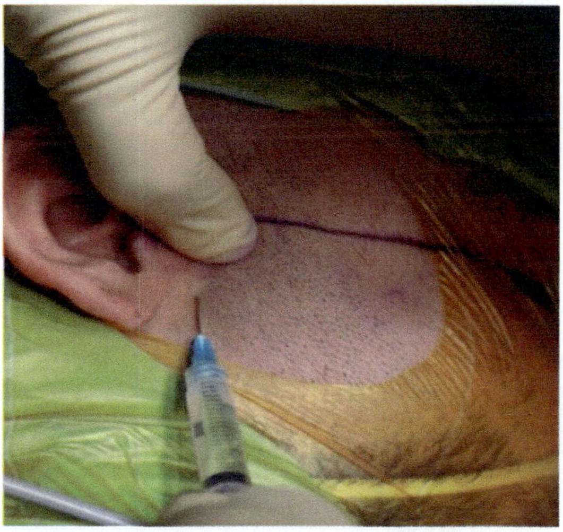

Fig. 21.15 Injection of bupivacaine into the superior joint capsule, using a 22G needle

Injection of epinephrine directly into the joint space can impair visualization of the synovial vasculature, which is critical for assessing inflammation. Therefore, vasoconstrictors should only be delivered after an initial evaluation. Using a standard inferiolateral technique, a sharp trocar is inserted to introduce a cannula to a depth of 25 mm, into the superior joint space [16] (Fig. 21.16).

The sharp trocar is removed and a blunt obturator is then deployed, using a sweeping motion, to separate the soft tissues within the TMJ (Fig. 21.17). The arthroscope is then inserted through the middle connection of the three-way female Luer lock, while the other two connections serve as the irrigation and working canals.

21.7.1 One-Track Arthrocentesis

One-track arthrocentesis enables initial location of the TMJ, in addition to its visualization while performing irrigation and arthrocentesis. Two female Luer lock connector pipe lines are connected to the other two ports. “One-track arthrocentesis” is performed through the irrigation canal and lavage outflow exits through the working canal (Fig. 21.18). The TMJ is irrigated with Ringer’s lactate solution or standard normal saline, introduced via a 50 mL syringe with a pumping motion, or continuously infused via a bag placed in a pressure cuff (Fig. 21.19). Fluid extravasation must be avoided.

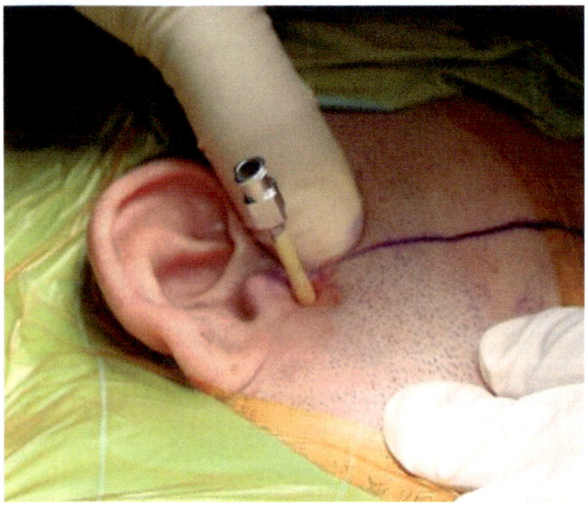

Fig. 21.16 A cannula is introduced into the superior joint space, to a depth of 25 mm

21.7.2 Standard Arthrocentesis under Visualization

An 18G needle is inserted 5 mm anterior and 5 mm caudal to the puncture point (Fig. 21.20), to serve as an outflow port. The outflow canal is then used as the operating canal of the OSCA system. Decisions regarding the most appropriate instruments and/or laser fibers will then be made based on the pathological findings within the superior space of the TMJ.

The medial synovial drape, pterygoid shadow, retrodiscal synovium, posterior slope of the articular eminence, articular disk, intermediate zone, and anterior recess of the TMJ are then visualized and assessed (Fig. 21.21):

1. The **medial synovial drape** has a gray-white, translucent, tense lining, with distinct superior to inferior striae (Fig. 21.22). Its appearance is one of the key indicators of TMJ synovitis (Fig. 21.23), with increased capillary proliferation and hyperemia of the medial synovial drape suggesting acute inflammatory state, whereas a fibrotic or whitish appearance indicating chronic synovitis.
2. The **Pterygoid shadow** is situated anterior to the medial synovial drape. In pathologic states, marked erythema and hypervascularization may be observed. In addition, the shadow may thin to the extent of perforation, followed by herniation of the pterygoid muscle directly into the anteromedial aspect of the superior joint space (Fig. 21.24).

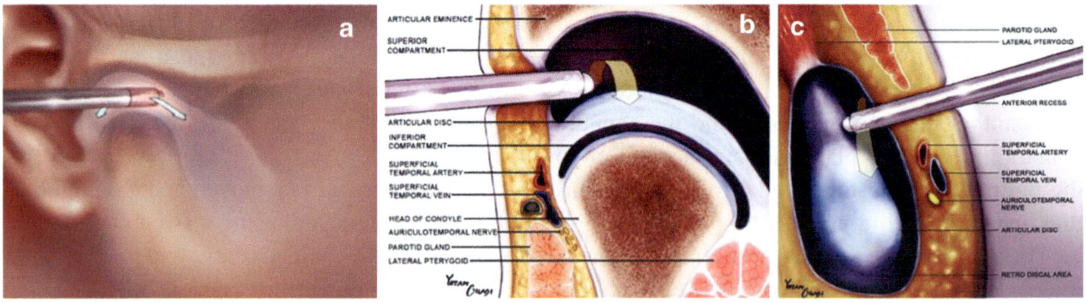

Fig. 21.17 (**a**) Sweeping motion of the obturator used to separate soft tissue. b-c. Introduction of the obturator and cannula into the upper compartment of the TMJ [coronary (**b**) and horizontal (**c**) views]

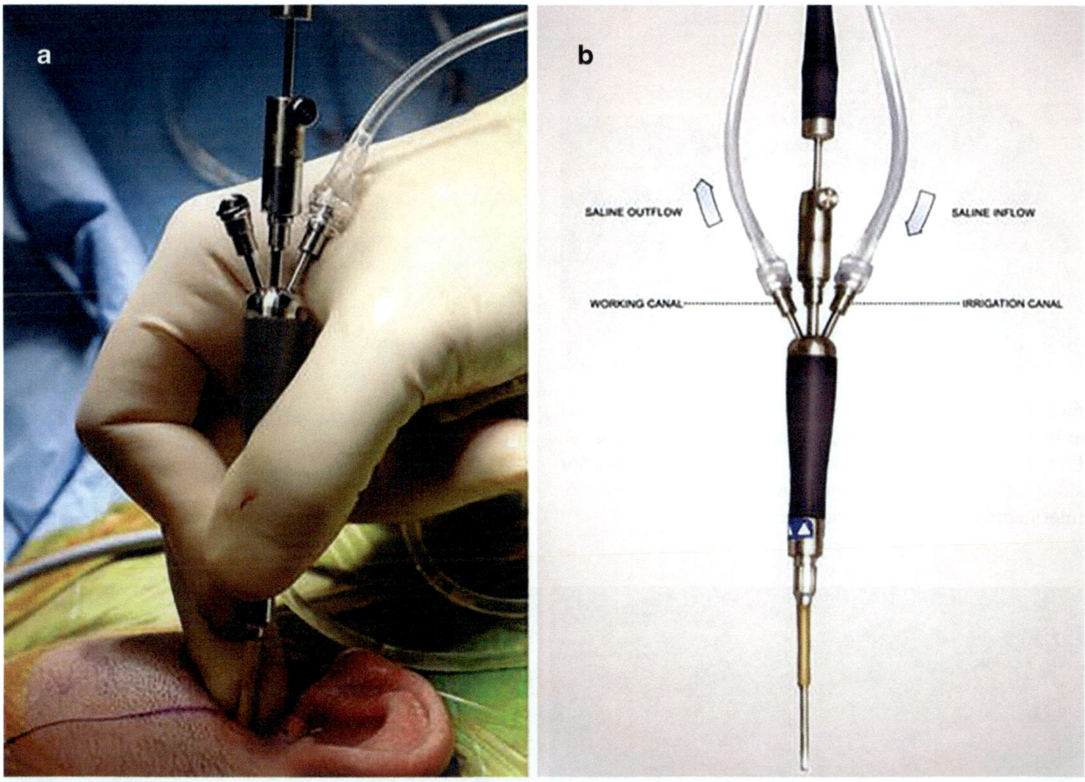

Fig. 21.18 One-track arthrocentesis. (**a**) The arthroscope is introduced into the TMJ through the middle connection of the three-way female Luer lock; the irrigation line is also seen. (**b**) Illustration of the arthroscope, showing inflow through the irrigation canal and outflow through the working canal

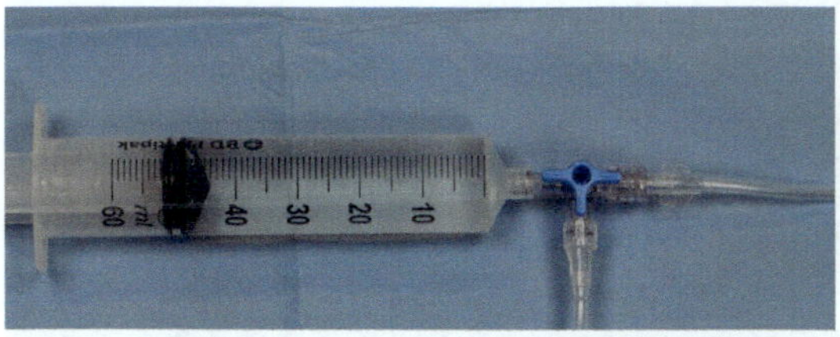

Fig. 21.19 Intermittent TMJ irrigation is achieved using a 50 mL syringe

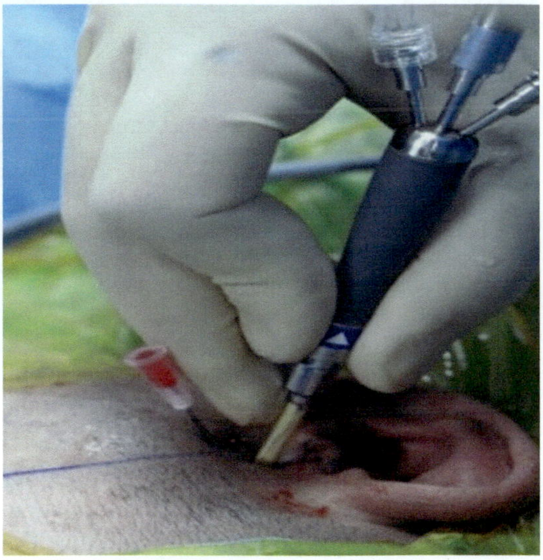

Fig. 21.20 Standard arthrocentesis under diagnostic visualization

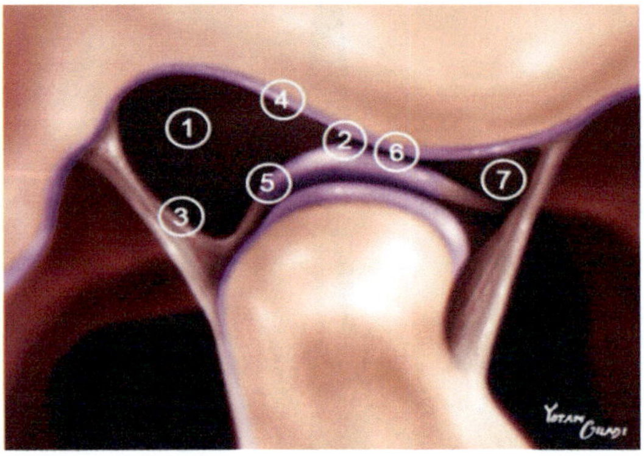

Fig. 21.21 The seven points of interest of the TMJ arthroscopic examination. 1. Medial synovial drape. 2. Pterygoid shadow. 3. Retrodiscal synovium. 4. Posterior slope of the articular eminence. 5. Articular disk. 6. Intermediate zone. 7. Anterior recess

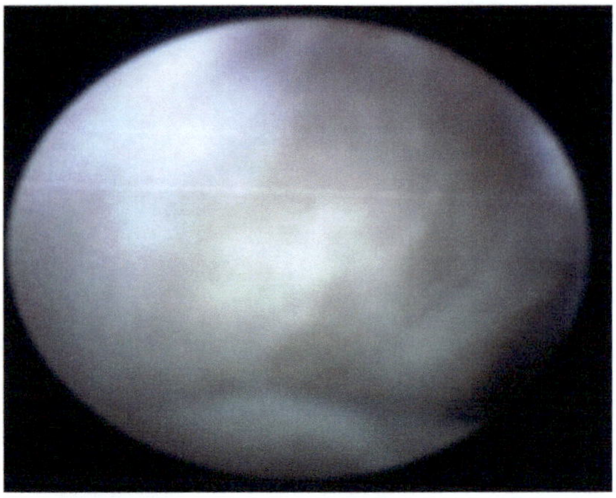

Fig. 21.22 Medial synovial drape

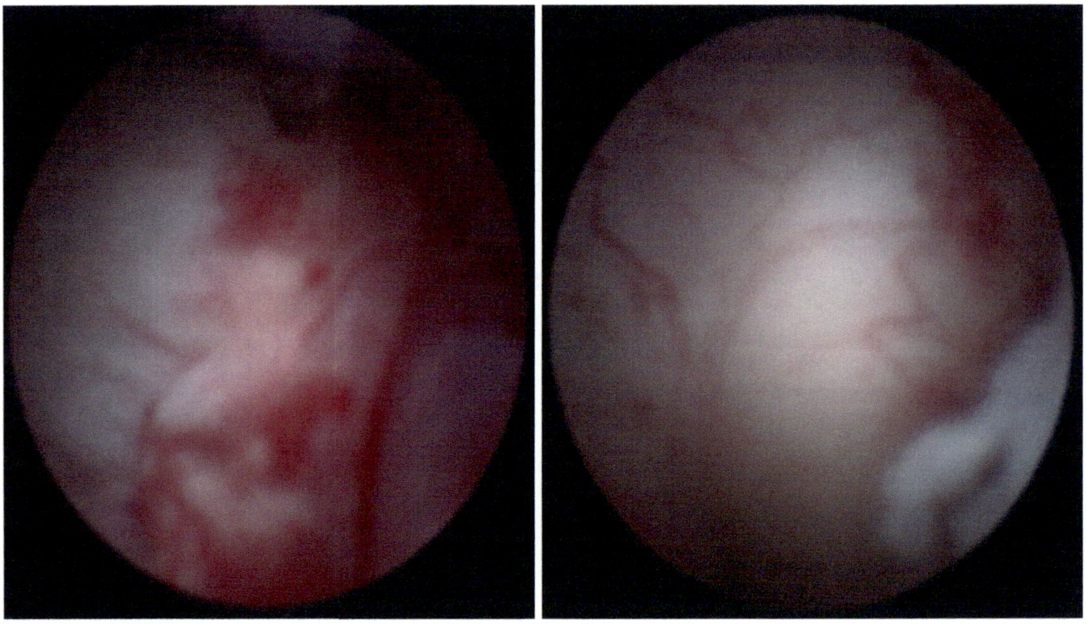

Fig. 21.23 TMJ synovitis with capillary proliferation

3. The **retrodiscal synovium**. The synovial membrane covers the posterior insertion of the disk and is related superiorly to the temporal fossa. When the mouth is open, the posterior insertion takes on a crest-like conformation, called the oblique protuberance (zone 1). The retrodiscal tissue is situated posterosuperiorly, attached to the posterior glenoid process (zone 2). Its lateral recess can be lateral to the oblique protuberance (zone 3), and confers a hyperemic or petechial appearance to the synovium in pathological states. Chronic synovitis is characterized by synovial hyperplasia, with increased tissue fold proliferation (Fig. 21.25).
4. The **posterior slope of the articular eminence** bears characteristically thick, white,

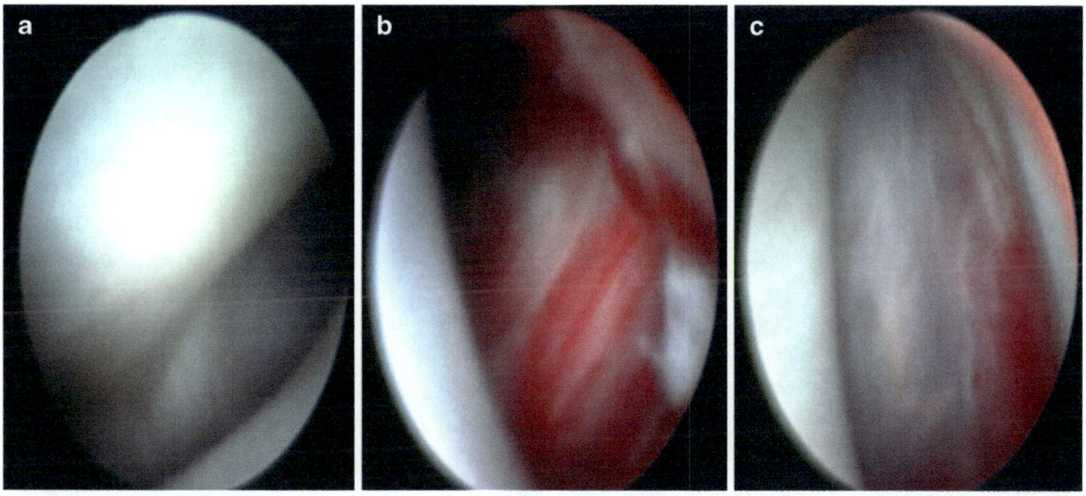

Fig. 21.24 (**a**) Normal appearance of the Pterygoid shadow. (**b**, **c**) Erythema in the Pterygoid shadow region

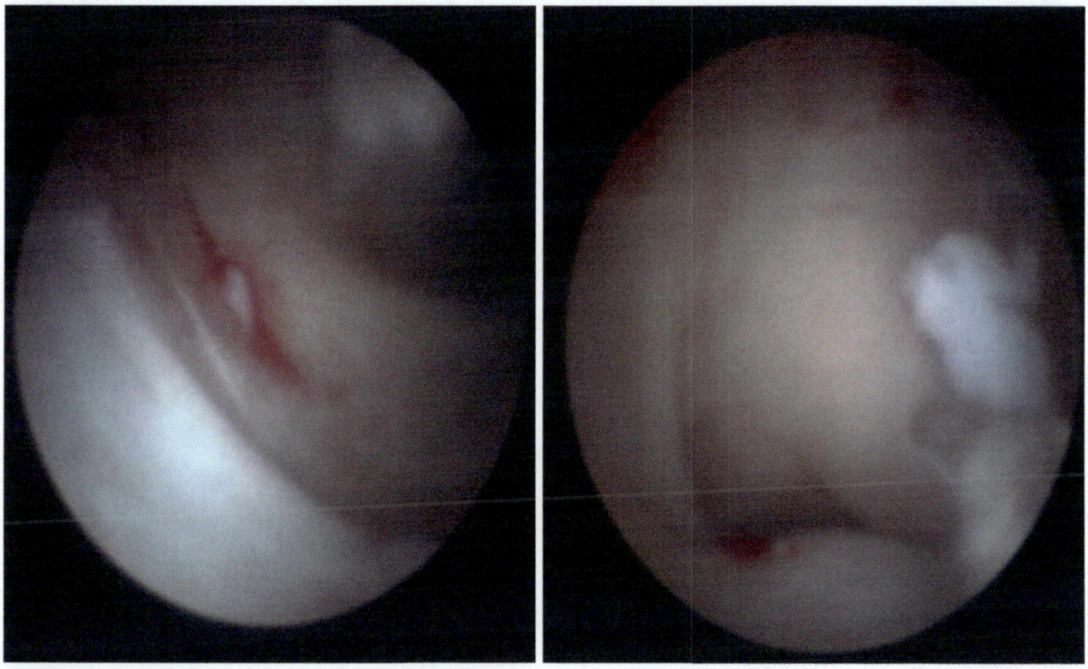

Fig. 21.25 Retrodiscal area

and highly reflective fibrocartilage, with interspersed anteroposterior striae. In pathological states, various stages of chondromalacia are often detectable, which may deteriorate to crater formation and exposure of the subchondral bone. In inflammatory states, synovial tissue creeping is often observed in the glenoid fossa and in the posterior slope of the eminence (Fig. 21.26).

5. The **articular disk** has a milky, highly reflective appearance, with no striae. In pathologic states, synovium creeping onto the surface of

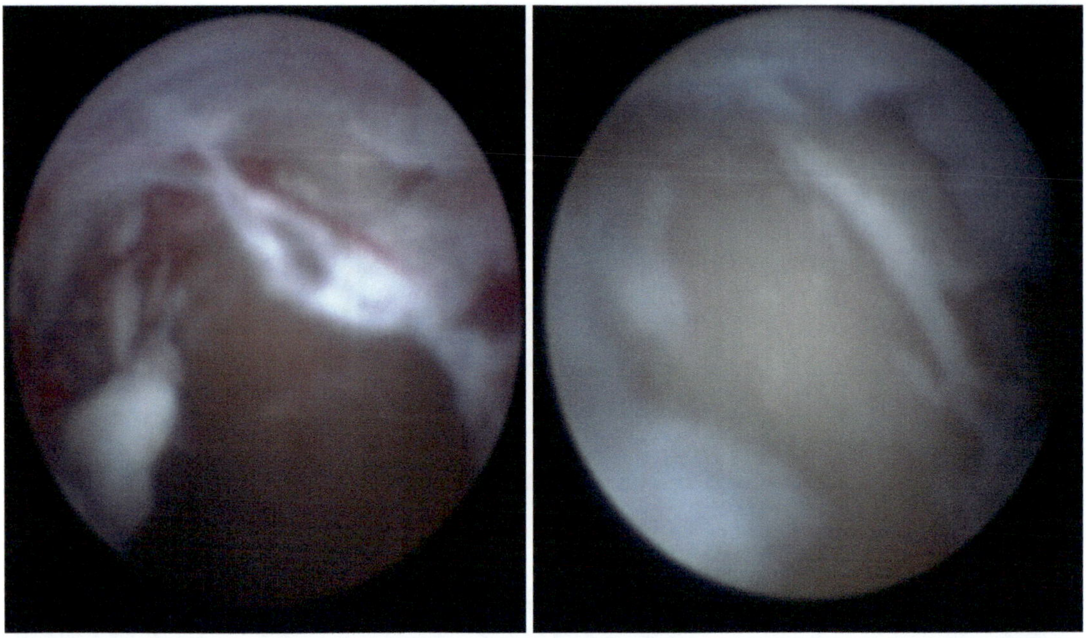

Fig. 21.26 Various stages of chondromalacia

the disk is observed, with fragmentation of the surface generally an indication of imminent or existing disk perforation. In cases of disk perforation, the scope can be introduced through the perforation to examine the inferior joint space (Fig. 21.27).

6. The **intermediate zone** has a white-on-white appearance, and the concavity of the disk can be seen.
7. The **anterior recess** is examined at the most extreme medioanterior corner of the crease and the pterygoid shadow. The union between the lateral synovial capsule and the anterior disk-synovial crease can be observed at the anterolateral site. In pathological states, the increased anterior synovial pouch vascularity and signs of synovial inflammation may be observed, occasionally with synovial redundancy and synovial plicae (Fig. 21.28).

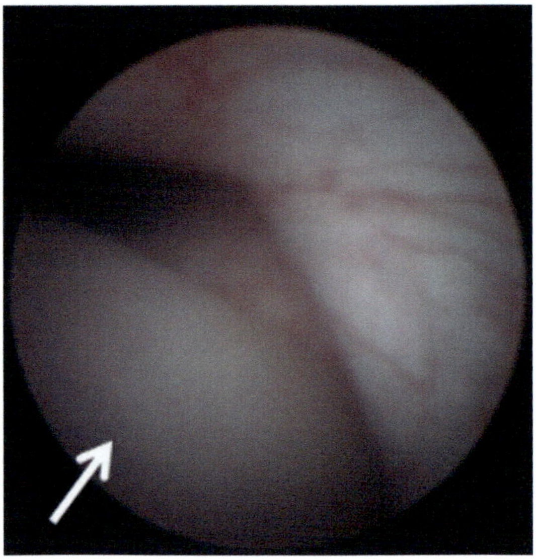

Fig. 21.27 Normal appearance of the articular disk (arrow)

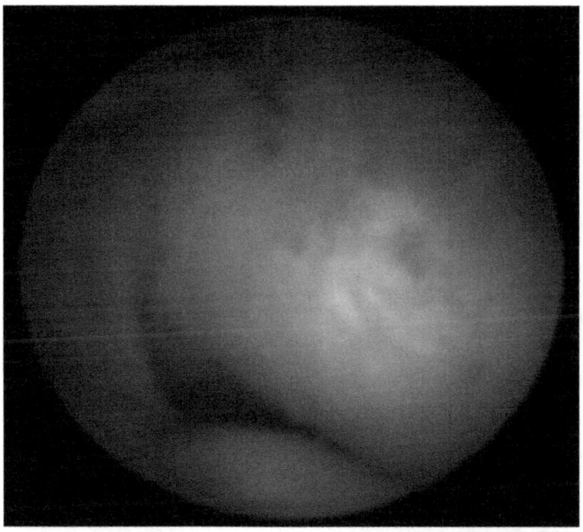

Fig. 21.28 Normal appearance of the anterior recess

21.7.3 Visually-Guided OSCA

A variety of hand or mechanical instruments can be used during OSCA; pathological findings or indication will dictate instrument suitability (Fig. 21.29). The Ho:YAG laser is both precise and safe and can be deployed for a broad range of interventions addressing internal pathologies and derangements of the joint (Figs. 21.30 and 21.31). Its cutting capacities can be applied to severe adhesions and execute anterior release with discopexy. It can also be used to ablate dilated vessels of the synovial tissue. Contraction of the retrodiscal synovial tissue to achieve posterior disk repositioning can be induced using its contracture mode.

21.7.4 Surgical Interventions Using the OSCA Technique

21.7.4.1 Release of Anterior and Posterior Recess Adhesions

Volume and architecture of the joint can be restored by sequential, anterior-to-posterior lysis of adhesions in the superior joint space, while avoiding repeated motion of instrumentation and subsequent risk of unnecessary articular surface scuffing. The probe of the Ho:YAG laser, set on cutting mode, is placed in the most medial aspect of the joint and then swept laterally along the disk-synovial junction with an inferoanterior maneuver. The lysis is completed by sweeping medially-to-laterally along the articular eminence, using a superoanterior maneuver. The two maneuvers are repeated until adequate recess volume is restored. Anterior recess lysis is often followed by posterior recess lysis. A marked increase in the range of movement (ROM) of the condyle is immediately achieved.

21.7.4.2 Synovectomy

Ho:YAG-assisted OSCA can also be used for effective reduction of redundant synovium, most commonly observed in the posterior pouch, especially after disk reduction procedures, and occasionally, in the anterior recess. Positive response is manifested by a color change from bright red to light brown or off-white (Fig. 21.32).

21.7.4.3 Anterior Release

Conditions such as chronic disk dislocation, fibrosis, adhesive bands, or pseudowall formation can obliterate the disk-synovial crease. A blunt probe is used for the lysis procedure. If the anteroposterior disk dimension appears adequate and relatively normal, disk shape is ascertained, and the release procedure is initiated in the medial half of the disk-synovial crease. Using Ho:YAG laser in cutting mode, the synovial capsule is incised just anterior and parallel to the anterior margin of the disk, after which the muscle fibers penetrating into the disk and capsule can be observed. Dissection should be performed to a depth of up to 5 mm or until the anterior band is fully mobile, without tethering. Myotomy at the most anteromedial corner must be executed with caution, with attempts made to identify the 1–2-mm-diameter artery that generally runs sub-adjacently to the anteromedial synovial drape-disk junction. The vessel is arthroscopically observed as a white tubular structure. If inadvertently incised, intraarticular hemorrhage will occur, with no effective means of cauterization or ligation. In cases of bleeding, all instruments must be removed and continuous lateral pressure applied on the joint for 8–10 full minutes, while the condyle is maintained in a forward and contralateral position. Once controlled, the OSCA technique is repeated and the joint is lavaged and clots are suctioned.

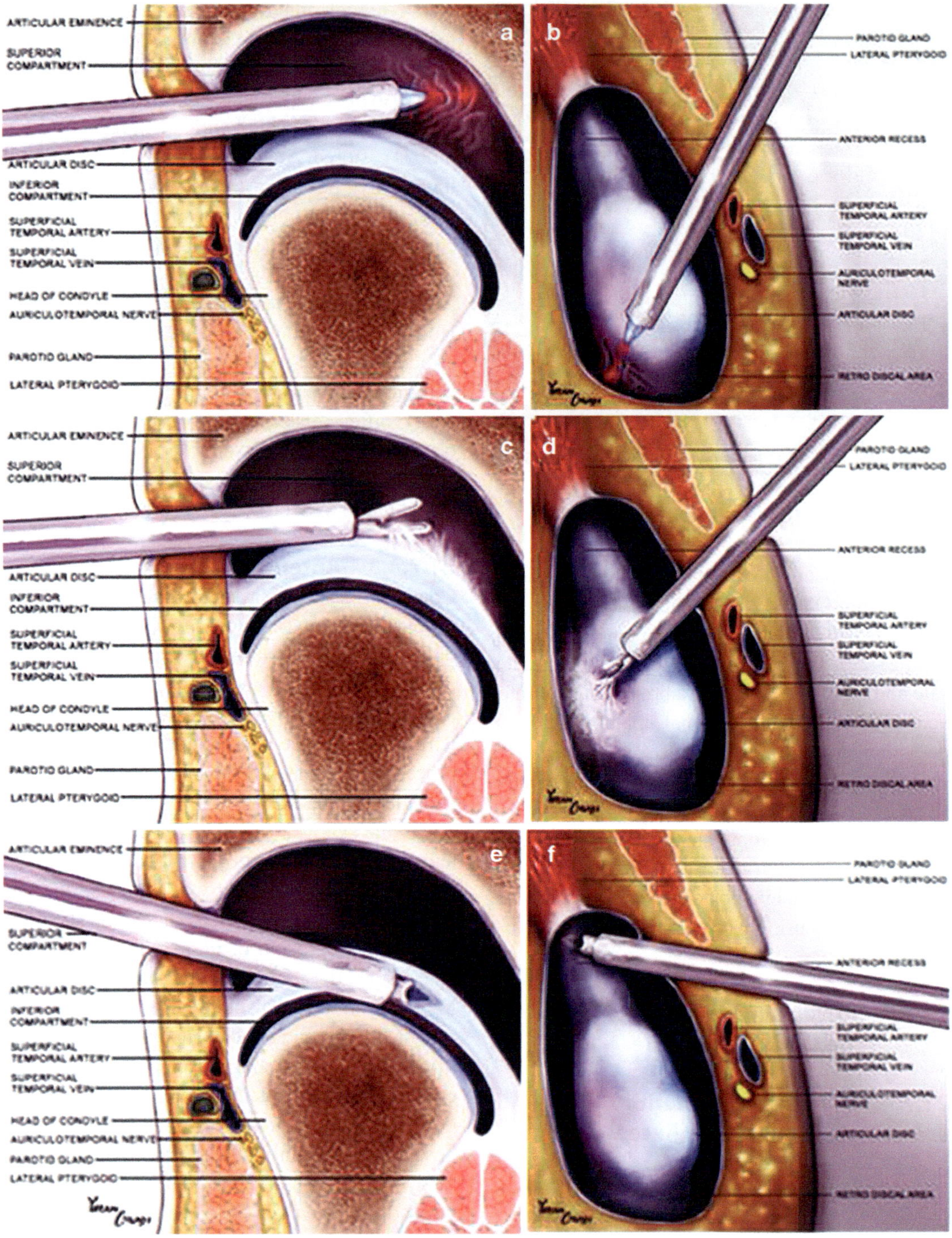

Fig. 21.29 Illustrations of instruments introduced into the TMJ during various visually-guided OSCA procedures. (**a**, **b**) Ho:YAG laser to elicit contraction of the retrodiscal synovial tissue. (**c**, **d**) Grasper for biopsy or chondromalacia removal. (**e**, **f**) Spinal needle for injection of drugs into the lateral pterygoid muscle

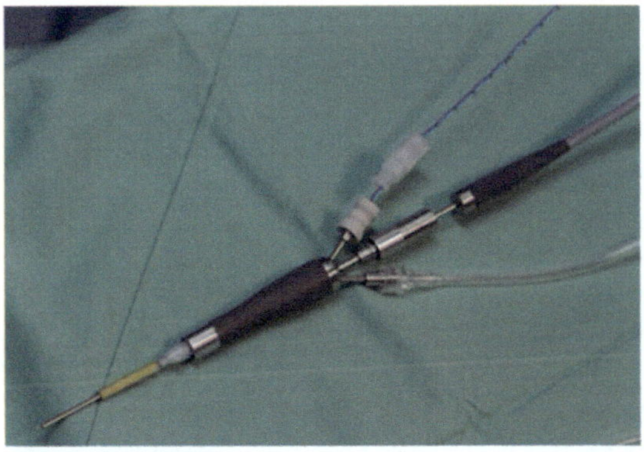

Fig. 21.30 Ho:YAG laser fiber and the arthroscope, setup in tandem

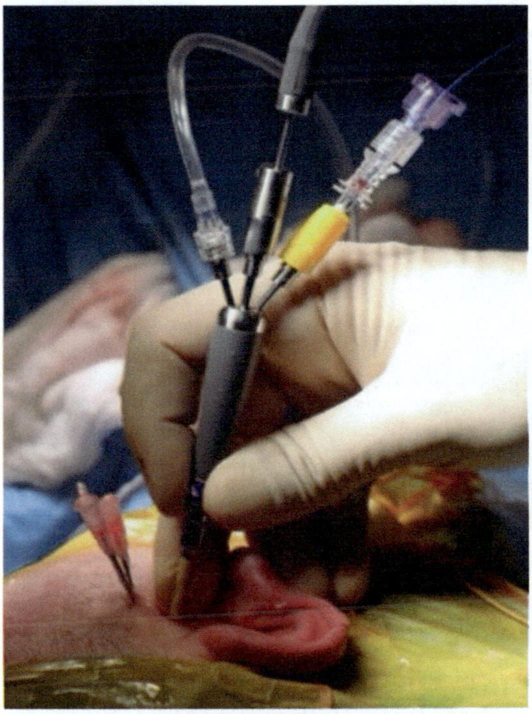

Fig. 21.31 Visually-guided OSCA. Intraoperative setup of the Ho:YAG laser fiber

21.7.4.4 Posterior Scarification/Contracture

Once disk reduction is achieved, excessive redundant synovium will be noted in the retrodiscal flexure. Even with minor disk repositioning and less evidence of redundancy, when discopexy is not performed, posterior scarification/contracture is executed. The retrodiscal tissue typically, "reefs," or bunches up, requiring bulk reduction using a Ho:YAG laser, to avoid tissue fibrosis which can ultimately displace the disk upon postoperative settling. Retrodiscal ablation should be executed until a normal-shaped retrodiscal flexure is obtained and the inflamed synovium and excess tissue bulk are ablated. Thereafter, deep-laser contracture of the oblique protuberance is performed, followed by examination of the anterior and posterior pouches (Fig. 21.33).

21.8 Advantages and Disadvantages of OSCA

The OSCA technique enables advanced visually-guided arthroscopy through a single cannula, associated with pain relief and mouth opening improvements similar to those reported for traditional techniques (Fig. 21.34a, b) [10]. The procedure is simpler, requires less expertise and coordination, is associated with a shorter learning curve, and is more cost-effective than the armamentarium used for the traditional double-puncture arthroscopy technique (Fig. 21.34c) [10]. In addition, its single-puncture nature reduces facial scarring, with possible impacts on limiting the incidence of facial nerve injury. Moreover, during OSCA, medications can be injected to a specific tissue region under visual guidance. Although image quality of conventional TMJ arthroscopes has been found satisfactory, with adequate observation of all anatomical and pathological structures, the relatively higher focal distance in OSCA procedures may result in relatively lower image quality (Table 21.3).

21.9 Intraarticular Drug Delivery Via OSCA

Before the advent of arthroscopy, intraarticular medications were blindly injected into the TMJ. The OSCA technique enables visually-guided injection of medications, into specific anatomic articular sites.

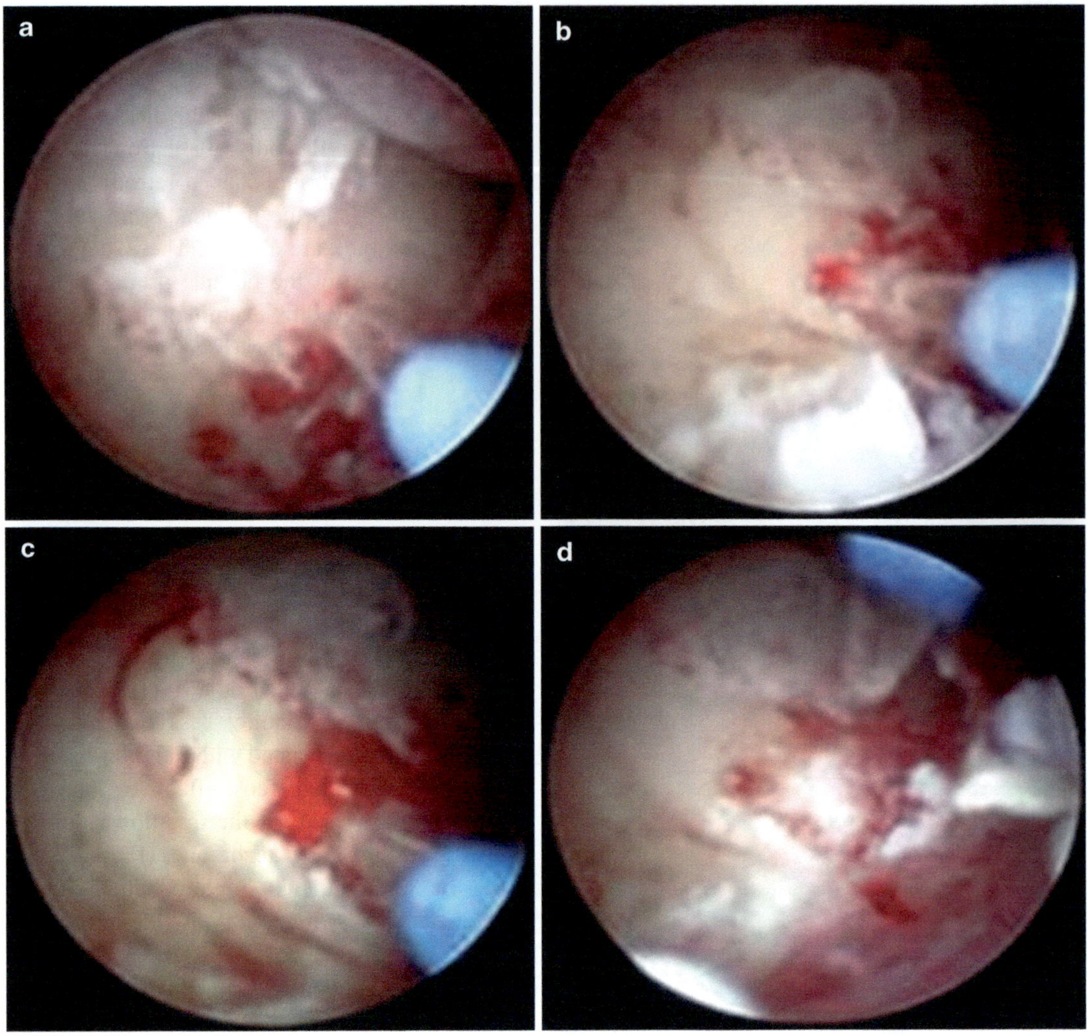

Fig. 21.32 (**a–d**) Intraoperative treatment of adhesions, fibrillations, and synovitis treated using Ho:YAG-assisted OSCA

21.9.1 Steroids

The authors' experience and research support the claimed benefit of steroid (e.g., methylprednisolone acetate (depo-medrol by Pfizer Inc.)) injection in reducing muscular irritation and spasm, consequently decreasing joint pain during function. The drugs can be introduced intraarticularly using a 3 mL syringe with a 25G spinal needle directly to specific TMJ structures, under visual guidance (Figs. 21.35 and 21.36).

21.9.2 Botulinum Toxin A

Botulinum toxin type A (Botox) has a well-documented therapeutic effect on functional disorders and provides symptomatic relief in cases of

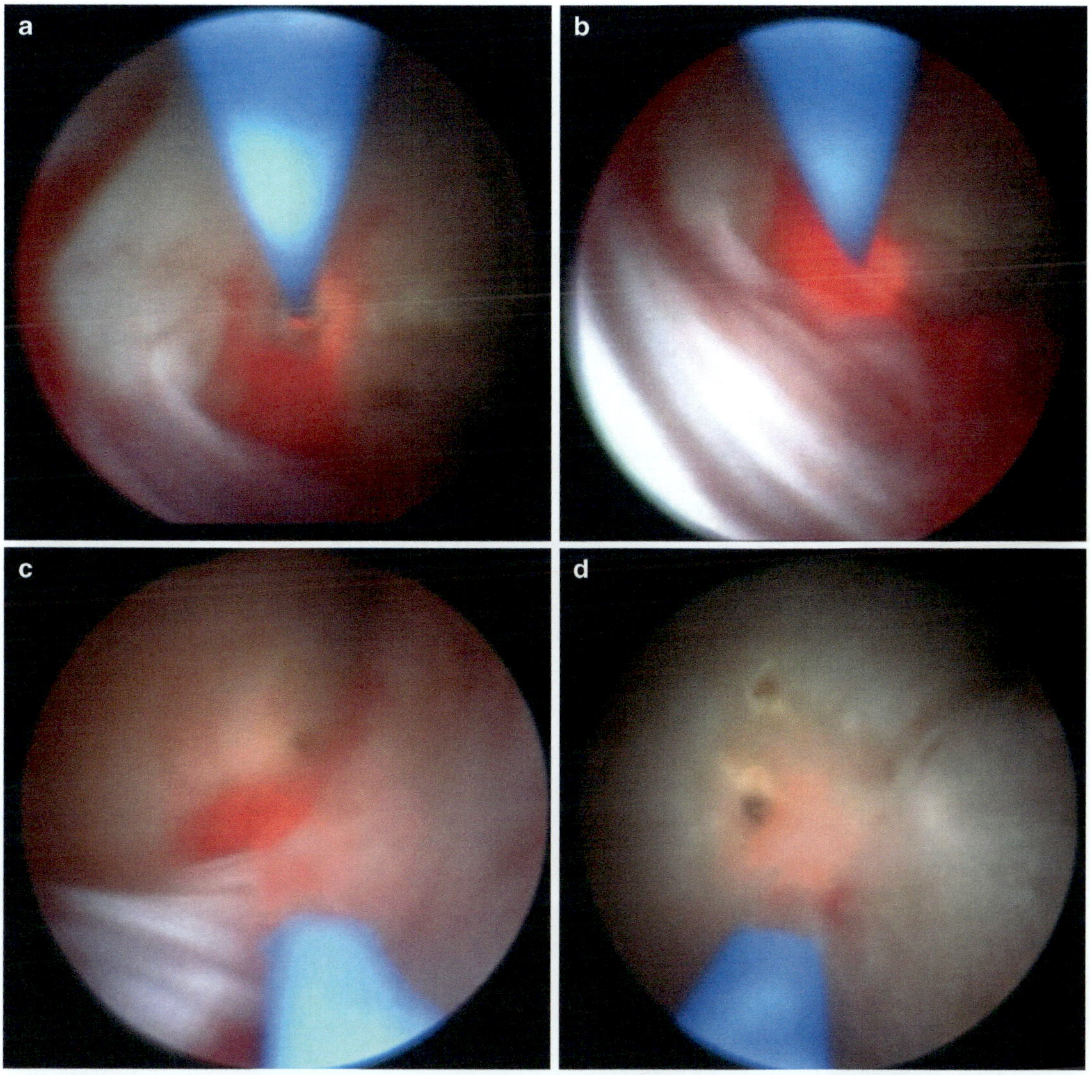

Fig. 21.33 (**a–d**) Contracture of retrodiscal synovium using Ho:YAG-assisted OSCA

dystonia. Recent reports by von Lindern, Israel, Mendes, and others have shown promising outcomes upon local injection of Botox in patients suffering from chronic facial pain secondary to hyperactive masticatory muscles. Research assessing the efficacy of direct injection of Botox into the superior head of the lateral pterygoid at the pterygoid shadow is still ongoing.

21.9.3 Hyaluronic Acid

Hyaluronic acid, a glycosaminoglycan polysaccharide produced by the articular chondrocytes and synoviocytes, and is a component of many extracellular tissues, including the synovial fluid and cartilage. Hyaluronate injection into the TMJ stimulates endogenous synthesis of hyaluronic

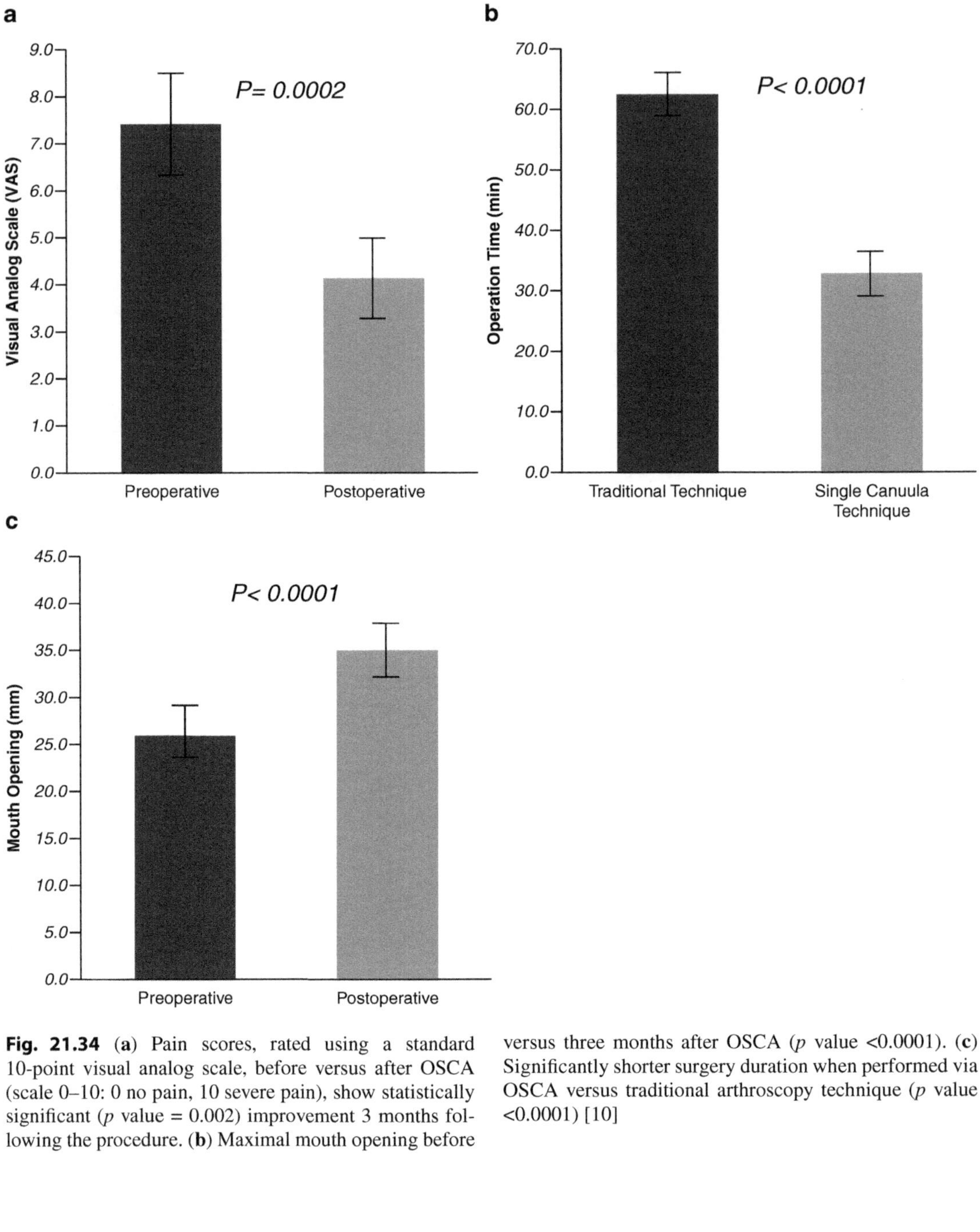

Fig. 21.34 (**a**) Pain scores, rated using a standard 10-point visual analog scale, before versus after OSCA (scale 0–10: 0 no pain, 10 severe pain), show statistically significant (p value = 0.002) improvement 3 months following the procedure. (**b**) Maximal mouth opening before versus three months after OSCA (p value <0.0001). (**c**) Significantly shorter surgery duration when performed via OSCA versus traditional arthroscopy technique (p value <0.0001) [10]

Table 21.3 Comparison of OSCA to single- and double-puncture arthroscopy techniques

Parameter	Single puncture	Double puncture	OSCA
Main indication	Diagnosis and basic interventions	Advanced arthroscopy	Advanced arthroscopy
Proficiency required	Low	High	Low
Duration of operation	Short	Long	Short
Number of punctures	1	2	1
Number of working cannulas	1	2	1
Risk for facial nerve injury	Low	High	Low
Risk for facial scar	Low	High	Low
Effectiveness in pain relief	Low	High	High
Effectiveness in mouth opening improvement	Low	High	High

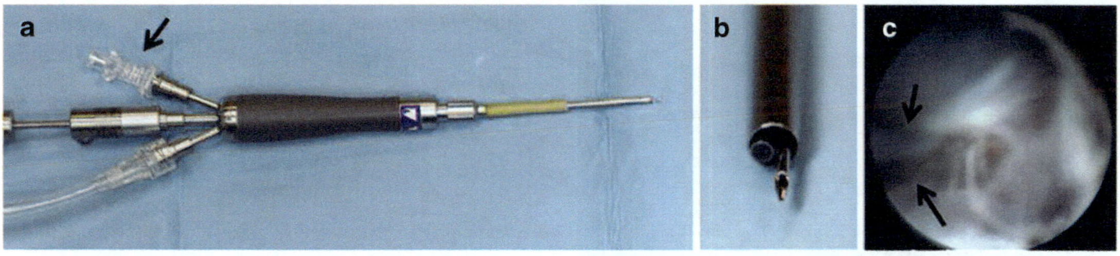

Fig. 21.35 Visually-guided drug injection. (**a**) Spinal needle (150 mm length, 0.72 mm diameter) with an arthroscope. (**b**) Optic fiber and needle passing through the cannula. (**c**) Injection of Depo-Medrol (white solution) into the joint space using a spinal needle (arrows)

acid, which can improve intraarticular lubrication, facilitating navigation and minimizing risk of iatrogenic intraarticular injury.

21.9.4 Platelet Concentrates (PC)

Autologous platelet concentrates (PCs) contain a highly concentrated cocktail of platelet-derived growth factors and endogenous fibrin scaffold components, which promote regenerative and other biological processes [17], including healing and chondrogenesis during cartilage repair [18]. Recent reports on the effective and safe use of platelet-rich plasma (PRP), a subtype of PC, in treating early-stage knee osteoarthritis (OA) are available for review [19, 20]. Furthermore, a number of randomized clinical studies have demonstrated the superiority of PC injection as compared to hyaluronic acid (HA) in symptomatic alleviation of mild to moderate knee OA [21, 22].

21.10 Patient Management After OSCA

21.10.1 Anti-Inflammatory and Pain Management

Tapered doses of intravenous/oral steroids should be administered over the 18–24-hour in the postoperative period and NSAIDs should be prescribed for up to 5–7 days.

21.10.2 Antibiotics

Patients should be switched from intravenous to oral antibiotics, e.g., cephalexin or amoxicillin

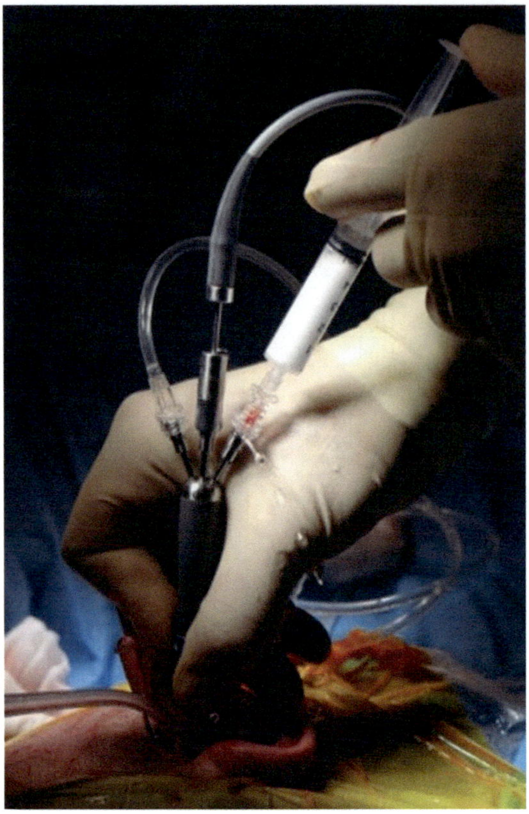

Fig. 21.36 Visually-guided intraoperative injection of Depo-Medrol

and clavulanic acid, for up to 7 days, unless there are signs of intolerance or hypersensitivity.

21.10.3 Diet

Patients can be gradually transferred from a fully liquid diet to a strictly soft diet and then to a normal diet.

21.11 Complications of Traditional Arthroscopy Versus OSCA

Owing to its minimally invasive nature, arthroscopy is generally associated with low complication rate, which is particularly low following OSCA techniques, due to its reduced invasiveness. Complications include fibrocartilage scuffing, damage to the VII cranial nerve, auriculotemporal nerve (branch of the mandibular nerve-V3), or vestibulocochlear nerve (VIII cranial nerve), tympanic membrane perforation and subsequent conductive hearing loss, damage to the superficial temporal artery and vein may lead to hamartosis. Other reported complications include glenoid fossa perforation and iatrogenic instrument failure.

Disclaimer Content of the chapter has original research of the authors. Portions of the text and figures of the chapter are reprinted/adapted with permission from Springer Nature; Originally published by the authors, Srouji S. McCain J. (2018) Modern Temporomandibular Joint Arthroscopy: Operative Single-Cannula Arthroscopy. In: Nahlieli O. (eds) Minimally Invasive Oral and Maxillofacial Surgery. Springer, Berlin, Heidelberg.

References

1. Onishi M. Arthroscopy of the temporomandibular joint. Kokubyo Gakkai Zasshi. 1975;42:207–13.
2. Murakami K, Hoshino K. Regional anatomical nomenclature and arthroscopic terminology in human temporomandibular joints. Okajimas Folia Anat Jpn. 1982;58:745–60.
3. McCain J. Arthroscopy of the human temporomandibular joint. J Oral Maxillofac Surg. 1988;46:648–55.
4. McCain JP. Principles and practice of temporomandibular joint arthroscopy. St. Louis: Mosby; 1996.
5. Sanders B. Arthroscopic surgery of the temporomandibular joint: treatment of internal derangement with persistent closed lock. Oral Surg Oral Med Oral Pathol. 1986;62:361–72.
6. Holmlund A, Hellsing G. Arthroscopy of the temporomandibular joint: an autopsy study. Int J Oral Maxillofac Surg. 1985;14:169–75.
7. Nitzan DW, Dolwick MF, Martinez GA. Temporomandibular joint arthrocentesis: a simplified treatment for severe, limited mouth opening. J Oral Maxillofac Surg. 1991;49:1163–7.
8. Koslin MG, Martin JA. TMJ arthroscopic surgery. Clinical results in 79 cases. J Ala Dent Assoc. 1990 Winter;74(1):26–31.
9. McCain JP, Hossameldin RH. Advanced arthroscopy of the temporomandibular joint. Atlas Oral Maxillofac Surg Clin North Am. 2011;19:145–67.
10. Srouji S, Oren D, Zoabi A, Ronen O, Zraik H. Temporomandibular joint arthroscopy technique using a single working cannula. Int J Oral Maxillofac Surg. 2016;45:1490–4.
11. Gonza'lez-Garcı'a R, Gil-Dı'ez Usandizaga JL, Rodrı´-guez-Campo FJ. Arthroscopic anatomy and lysis and lavage of the temporomandibular

joint. Atlas Oral Maxillofac Surg Clin North Am 2011;19:131–144.
12. Wilkes CH. Internal derangements of the temporomandibular joint: pathological variations. Arch Otolaryngol Head Neck Surg. 1989;115:469–77.
13. Barkin S, Weinberg S. Internal derangements of the temporomandibular joint: the role of arthroscopic surgery and arthrocentesis. J Can Dent Assoc. 2000;66:199–203.
14. American Association of Oral and Maxillofacial Surgeons. Position paper on TMJ arthroscopy 1988. In: Thomas M, Bronstein S, editors. Arthroscopy of the temporomandibular joint. Philadelphia, PA: WB Saunders; 1991. p. 347–50.
15. Israel H. Arthroscopy of the temporomandibular joint. In: Indresano T, Marciani R, et al., editors. Peterson L. JB Lippincott: Principles of oral and maxillofacial surgery. Philadelphia; 1992. p. 2015–40.
16. Murakami K, Ono T. Temporomandibular joint arthroscopy by inferolateral approach. J Oral Maxillofac Surg. 1986;15:410.
17. Ferna'ndez Sanroma'n J, Ferna'ndez Sanroma'n M, Costas Lo'pez A, Arenaz Bua J, Lo'pez A. Does injection of plasma rich in growth factors after temporomandibular joint arthroscopy improve outcomes in patients with Wilkes stage IV internal derangement? A randomized prospective clinical study. Int J Oral Maxillofac Surg. 2016;45:828–35.
18. Everts PAM, Knape JTA, Weibrich G, et al. Platelet-rich plasma and platelet gel: A review. J Extra Corpor Technol. 2006;38:174.
19. Chang KV, Hung CY, Aliwarga F, Wang TG, Han DS, Chen WS. Comparative effectiveness of platelet-rich plasma injections for treating knee joint cartilage degenerative pathology: a systematic review and meta-analysis. Arch Phys Med Rehabil. 2014;95:562–75.
20. Khoshbin A, Leroux T, Wasserstein D, Marks P, Theodoropoulos J, Ogilvie-Harris D, et al. The efficacy of platelet-rich plasma in the treatment of symptomatic knee osteoarthritis: a systematic review with quantitative synthesis. Arthroscopy. 2013;29:2037–48.
21. Sa'nchez M, Fiz N, Azofra J, Usabiaga J, Aduriz Recalled E, Garcia Gutierrez A, et al. A randomized clinical trial evaluating plasma rich in growth factors (PRGF-Endoret) versus hyaluronic acid in the short-term treatment of symptomatic knee osteoarthritis. Arthroscopy. 2012;28:1070–8.
22. Vaquerizo V, Plasencia M.A´, Arribas I, Sei-jas R, Padilla S, Orive G, et al. Comparison of intra-articular injections of plasma rich in growth factors (PRGF-Endoret) versus Durolane hyaluronic acid in the treatment of patients with symptomatic osteoarthritis: a randomized controlled trial. Arthroscopy 2013;29:1635–1643.

22 Alloplastic Total Joint Reconstruction for the Temporomandibular Joint

Darpan Bhargava, R. S. Neelakandan, and Beena Sivakumar

22.1 Introduction

Total joint replacement and reconstruction is a common practice in the field of orthopedic surgery for hip and knee joints, but it persisted to remain less popular for the craniomandibular joint till the 1980s due to the "Kent-Vitek mishap" in the 1970s. With recent advancements in the biomaterial science and better understanding of the regional surgical anatomy, alloplastic total joint reconstruction (TJR) for the temporomandibular joint (TMJ) has become popular and a feasible option in treating patients with end stage temporomandibular joint disease (ESJD), having history of previous surgeries resulting in joint deformities leading to considerable disability, for congenital deformities affecting the joint and for the craniomandibular ankylosis.

A thorough clinical and radiographic work-up followed by formulation of a rigorous treatment plan including the decision on the choice of prosthesis based on the patient's requirement is an essential aspect of the pre-surgical work-up. Several advances in alloplastic prosthesis design, bio-materials, and the surgical approaches have enhanced the overall quality of life (QoL) for the patients with restoration of function as well as esthetics rehabilitated with alloplastic prosthesis. However, there remain several factors that demand consideration while placing the alloplastic TMJ prosthesis as the outcome greatly depends on multi-factorial facets.

22.2 Alloplastic Prosthesis for Joint Replacement

The first successful alloplastic TJR device was designed by Sir John Charnley in the 1960s leading a way for various advancements in the prosthesis design and bio-compatible material science aimed at providing a better QoL for the patients post-surgically [1]. TMJ TJR has been an option since the nineteenth century but it remained less popular due to the intricate anatomy of the small joint in connotation with the complex maxillofacial skeleton and lack of understanding of the bio-

D. Bhargava (✉)
TMJ Consultancy Services, Bhopal, Madhya Pradesh, India

Oral and Maxillofacial Surgery, People's College of Dental Sciences and Research Centre, People's University, Bhopal, Madhya Pradesh, India
e-mail: drdarpanbhargava@gmail.com

R. S. Neelakandan
Meenakshi Academy of Higher Education and Research (Meenakshi University), Chennai, Tamil Nadu, India

Department of Oral and Maxillofacial Surgery, Meenakshi Ammal Dental College and Hospital, Chennai, Tamil Nadu, India

B. Sivakumar
Department of Oral and Maxillofacial Surgery, Meenakshi Ammal Dental College and Hospital, Chennai, Tamil Nadu, India

D. Bhargava (ed.), *Temporomandibular Joint Disorders*,
https://doi.org/10.1007/978-981-16-2754-5_22

compatible alloplastic materials that may be used for these prosthetic devices. Joint replacement systems containing Proplast-Teflon (Vitek Kent, Houston, Texas) was a setback to this growing science in the 1970s as these devices had to be withdrawn from the market due to foreign body giant cell reaction resulting in enormous failure rates.

Alloplastic TMJ reconstruction restores the form and function of the joint. With the increasing evidence of success of alloplastic prosthesis, various artificial prosthesis designs are being investigated and some of them are in use. Pain and dysfunction associated with TMDs has a significant psychosocial impact among the patients with a strong female predilection, which when progresses to a non-salvageable stage, is given a consideration for TJRs [2]. Several challenges tangled with alloplastic prosthesis include financial factors, achieving harmony in function between the alloplastic joint, osseous structure, and muscles controlling the movement, along with the masticatory function.

22.3 Factors for Assessment

There are various subjective and objective parameters utilized by several authors to assess the performance of various available alloplastic prosthesis, to name a few include, maximum inter-incisal opening (MIO), jaw function (JF), and diet intake (DI). Wolford LM et al. assessed objective evaluation for incisal opening, lateral excursions, and occlusal stability, whereas the subjective parameters assessed were pain and jaw function. In another study by the same author, apart from the conventional parameter assessment, evaluation of the patients' post-operative overall quality of life was highlighted [3]. Ferreira et al. evaluated various factors leading to joint failure. The clinical parameters assessed by them included severity of pain and mandibular function. The symptom severity was evaluated using Symptom Severity Index and the mandibular function using modified mandibular function impairment questionnaire [mMFIQ]. They concluded that facial pain was a significant factor correlated to perforation and breakdown of the alloplastic temporomandibular interpositional implants, and was the most likely reason for implant removal [4]. Leandro et al. additionally assessed speech apart from the above-mentioned clinical parameters [5]. Bhargava D et al. assessed nutritional status of the patients using mid-upper arm circumference along with the overall QoL post-surgically as compared to the patients' pre-surgical status as one of the study parameters [6].

22.4 Patient Selection for TMJ TJR

TMJ TJR surgery is an intricate science in itself considering the complexity in anatomy of TMJ and its proximity to various vital structures in the maxillofacial region. Any voids at the initial stage of the patient selection, surgical planning, or execution may pose a risk to the patient in terms of device failure, sub optimal function, or even to the extent of damage to the vital anatomical structures, if the surgery is not accurately undertaken. It is critical that an alloplastic TJR should be considered only when the joint and the surrounding structures cannot be salvaged. A range of conservative and minimally invasive surgical modalities must be considered prior to the total joint replacement surgery. In an adult patient, a successful alloplastic TJR may offer numerous advantages including occlusal stability, as autogenous grafts can exhibit variable resorption rates, lack of donor site morbidity leading to reduced surgical duration, and early mobilization with significant dietary improvement [7].

The indications for TJR include a wide range of disorders such as joint ankylosis, inflammatory, and neoplastic disease process involving the condyle, trauma, and congenital disorders affecting the condylar development (Table 22.1). Various authorities have proposed the criteria for indications of TMJ TJR. These include, the National Institute for Health and Care Excellence (NICE), British Association of Oral and Maxillofacial Surgeons, the Japanese Regulatory Society apart from various individual authors that contribute to a reliable database for reference [8–10]. These guidelines may offer expediency in augmenting surgeon's decision on appropriate patient selection for TMJ TJR. Absolute contraindications for alloplastic prosthesis include local infection and systemically compromised patients including patients with poor glycemic control. A patient who is grouped under the American Society of Anesthesiologists (ASA) category III having a severe disease process is considered as a relative contra-indication to TJR (Table 22.2) [11].

Table 22.1 Indications for alloplastic TMJ total joint replacement (TJR)

S. NO.	Indications
1	Severe degenerative joint disease—*Osteoarthritis*
2	Inflammatory joint disease—*Rheumatoid or psoriatic arthritis, ankylosing spondylitis*
3	Ankylosis—*Post-traumatic, re-ankylosis*
4	Irreparable condylar fracture/damage
5	Avascular necrosis (AVN)/osteochondritis dissecans (OCD) of the TMJ
6	Neoplastic ablation leading to post-surgical condylar loss
7	Failed reconstruction with autogenous grafts
8	Congenital disorders—*Hemifacial microsomia, Treacher Collins syndrome*
9	Multiple operated TMJ with inadequate results
10	Severe functional limitations and ongoing symptoms despite previous alloplastic implant

Table 22.2 Contra-indications for total prosthetic replacement

S. NO.	Contra-indications
1	Ongoing local infective process—Intra-capsular and peri-capsular infection
2	Severe immune compromise/uncontrolled systemic disease
3	Severe ASA III disease process

22.5 Radiographic Evaluation

Every patient planned for alloplastic TMJ prosthesis must be subjected to a computed tomography (CT) scan for the evaluation of an accurate bone anatomy in detail. The CT data usually in DICOM along with its three-dimensional (3D) reconstruction is a useful aid for the construction of stereolithographic models (Fig. 22.1). A custom made prosthesis can be constructed using computer aided replication and designing of the patient's mandible and cranial components (Fig. 22.2). This reduces intra-operative time as aligning the prosthesis or modifying the bone for a right fit is not necessary. Evaluation of the vascular anatomy in the infra-temporal fossa may require a Magnetic Resonance (MR) Angiography study [11]. A cone beam computed tomography (CBCT) can also be used for assessing the bone morphology. Other conventional two-dimensional (2D) radiographic imaging modalities are also useful in demonstrating the bony deformity but do not allow accurate evaluation of disease extent, therefore are limited for screening.

22.6 Components of Alloplastic Prosthesis

Alloplastic TMJ prosthesis usually consists of a fossa component and the ramus-condyle component. These components are stabilized using anchor screws against the bone. Various materials

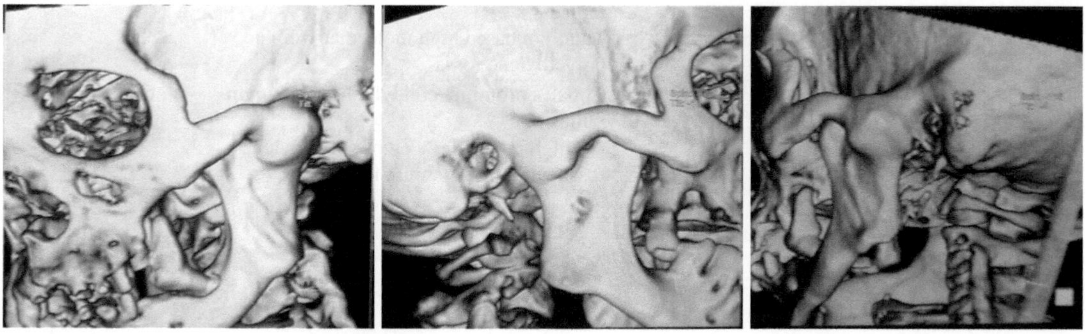

Fig. 22.1 Three-dimensional (3D) reconstructed CT image depicting the ankylosed mandibular condyle to the temporal fossa

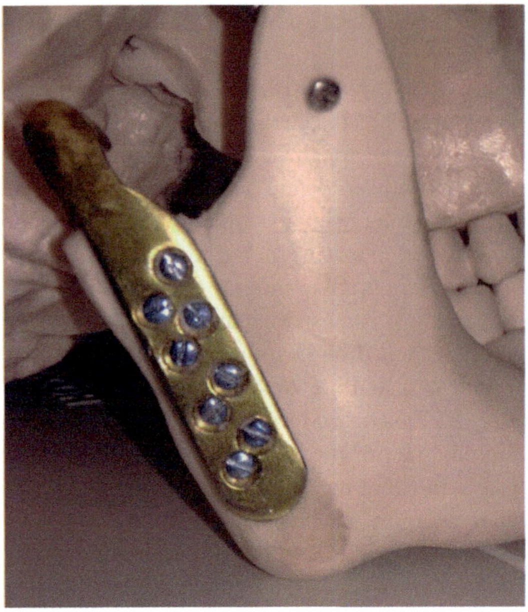

Fig. 22.2 Stereolithographic skull model showing one of the initial prototype of an alloplastic DARSN TMJ prosthesis, ramal component fixed using titanium screws

have been tested and tried to obtain a bio-compatible and biomechanically stable prosthesis. Recent studies favor the use of titanium (Ti) and high molecular weight polyethylene as they exhibit reasonable biomechanical properties and are bio-acceptable [7] (Tables 22.3 and 22.4) (Figs. 22.2, 22.3, 22.4, and 22.5). To enhance the wear properties of the articular surface of the joint head, few designs do incorporate chrome-cobalt alloy.

22.7 Alloplastic Prosthesis Design for TMJ TJR

The selection of an alloplastic prosthesis is multifactorial and depends on various parameters including the trust with post marketing surveillance reports, prosthesis cost, age and systemic condition of the patient, and surgeon's proficiency with the particular joint system to accurately place the alloplastic prosthesis. The currently available

Table 22.3 Evolution of alloplastic prosthesis for joint reconstruction

Year	Prosthesis	Description	Type
1963	Christensen (Type I)	Cobalt-chromium alloy fossa Ramus component with acrylic condylar cap	Stock/custom
1977	Christensen (Type II)	Cobalt-chromium alloy fossa Ramus component with cobalt-chromium condylar cap *Metal-on-metal prosthesis*	Stock/custom
1970s	Kent-Vitek (KV I) prosthesis Kent-Vitek (KV II) prosthesis (Fig. 22.3)	Fitting surface had a proplast laminant—Foreign body reaction to proplast causing destructive osteolysis. Manufacturing stopped due to associated litigation with the predecessor.	Stock
1989	Techmedia Now, TMJ concepts (Ventura, CA, USA) (Fig. 22.4)	Cobalt-chromium condylar head/titanium ramus Titanium based high molecular weight polyethylene fossa	Custom
2000	Lorenz Now, Zimmer Biomet (Fig. 22.5)	Cobalt-chromium condylar head/titanium ramus All high molecular weight polyethylene fossa without a titanium mesh	Stock/custom

Table 22.4 Bio-materials used in ramus and fossa component of various alloplastic prosthesis

Year	Alloplastic prosthesis/Surgeon	Ramus component	Fossa component
1963	Christensen Type I	Acrylic	Co-Cr
1965	Christensen Type II	Co-Cr with PMMA condyle	Co-Cr
1974	Kiehn	Co-Cr	Co-Cr with PMMA cement
1976	Morgan	Co-Cr with acrylic condyle	Co-Cr
1977	Momma	Co-Cr	Co-Cr
1977	Kummoona	Co-Cr with PMMA cement	Co-Cr
1983	Vitek Kent Type I	Teflon	Proplast +UHMWPE
1983	Sonnenburg and Fethke	Ti + palladium	Polyethylene with PMMA cement
1983	Sonnenburg and Sonnenburg	Ti + palladium	Polyethylene with PMMA cement
1986	Vitek Kent Type II	Proplast	Proplast+UHMWPE
1989	Techmedia/TMJ concepts	Ti + co-Cr-Mo condyle	Ti mesh back UHMWPE
1992	Butow	Nitride coated Ti	Nitride coated Ti
1993	Hoffman and Pappas	Ti + nitride coated condyle	Ti + UHMWPE
1993	Biomet micro-fixation	Co-Cr head	UHMWPE
1996	Nexus CMF	Co-Cr	Co-Cr
1999	Groningen TMJ	Ti + zirconia condyle	Ti and zirconia
2000	Lorenz/Zimmer Biomet	Co-Cr head/ Ti ramus	UHMWPE
2017	Melbourne prosthetic TMJ	Ti 64	High density polyethylene
2018	DARSN TM Joint prosthesis	Grade V Ti	UHMWPE
2019	Chinese TMJ prosthesis	Co-Cr	UHMWPE

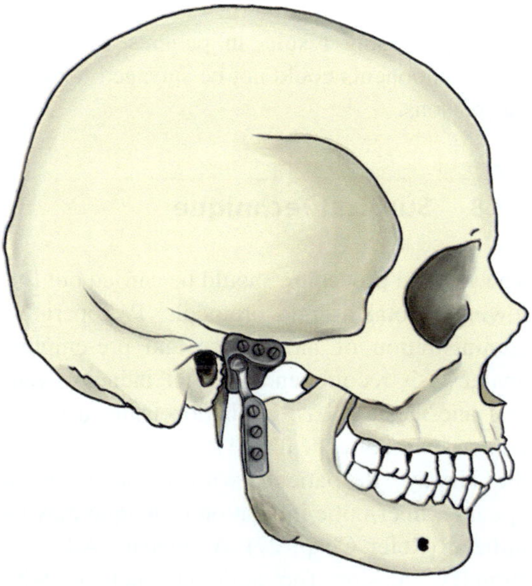

Fig. 22.3 Illustration depicting Type II Kent–Vitak alloplastic prosthesis

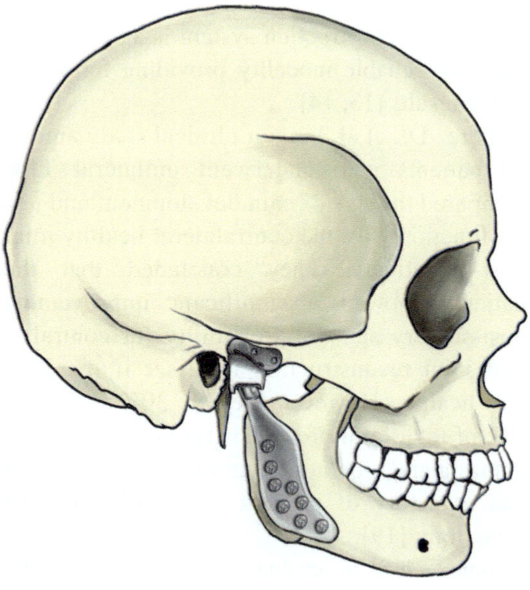

Fig. 22.4 Illustration depicting TMJ concepts alloplastic prosthesis

prosthesis can be either stock or a custom made. No single system can be endorsed superior to another in all aspects including the cost, biomechanical properties, bio-compatibility, ease of availability, and use [12–18].

Mercuri LG et al. assessed the safety and effectiveness of custom made alloplastic TMJ (Techmedia/TMJ concepts) device among patients who underwent TJR with a follow-up of 14 years. They observed significant improvement

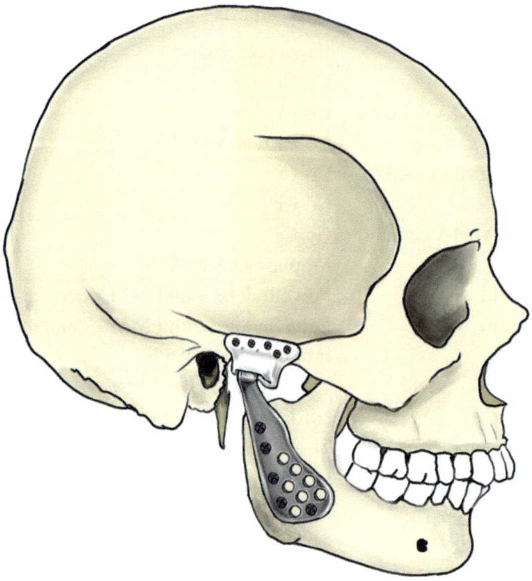

Fig. 22.5 Illustration depicting Biomet alloplastic prosthesis

in various subjective and objective parameters post-operatively concluding that patient fitted total TMJ reconstruction system is a safe, effective, and reliable modality providing long-term stable results [13, 14].

Perez DE et al. in their clinical study among 70 patients who underwent unilateral TJR, compared the risk of pain development and jaw dysfunction with the contralateral healthy joint post-operatively. They concluded that the patients showed a significant improvement post-surgery and the probability for contralateral joint reconstruction is lesser if the joint was healthy. However, there is 30% increased risk of total joint prosthesis replacement of the contralateral side at a later stage, if the patient had a history of previous surgeries with the same joint [19].

Sanovich et al. evaluated the total alloplastic temporomandibular joint reconstruction using Biomet stock prosthesis with their conclusions being consistent with literature of TJR being effective and safe [15]. Westermark observed that patients among his study population gained significant weight post-operatively after TMJ replacement which could be attributed to the improvement in diet intake (DI) factor [16]. The diet intake was further evaluated by Bhargava D et al. in patients who underwent TMJ TJR and found satisfactory improvement in the nutritional status of the patients post-operatively [6]. Jones conducted a preliminary study where he compared the use of the TMJ Concepts and Biomet Lorenz total joint replacement systems for the reconstruction of TMJ and observed that the results of his study were consistent with the individual studies on various joint systems performed by Mercuri LG et al., Wolford LM et al., and Quinn et al. reporting overall improved patient outcomes. Region specific data by Bhargava D et al. (DARSN TMJoint prosthesis; study population included patients of the Indian subcontinent) and Machon V et al. (Biomet TJR System; Czech and Slovakian population) found that TJR was an effective method in their preliminary studies [13–15, 20].

Similarly, other alloplastic devices such as Groningen prosthesis [21, 22], DARSN TM Joint prosthesis, [6, 20, 23, 24], Melbourne prosthetic TMJ [25], and Chinese prosthesis [26] used by various investigators for their study population found promising results in patients where the joint components could not be salvaged for various reasons.

22.8 Surgical Technique

The surgical procedure should be carried out following pivotal aseptic protocols. Pre-operative administration of anti-biotics and pre-emptive analgesia is recommended. After inducing general anesthesia (GA), intubation using a north-pole naso-endotracheal tube is preferred to secure the airway. In patients with reduced mouth opening, fiber-optic intubation technique may be utilized (Refer Chap. 27). A standard Alkayat–Bramley incision (pre-auricular incision with temporal extension) and Hind's incision should be placed after administering local anesthesia (LA) with epinephrine followed by careful layered dissection to expose the region of interest. Care must be taken to preserve retromandibular vessels and facial artery, facial and auriculotemporal nerve during the dissection (Refer Chap. 14 for approaches to TMJ).

The joint (ankylotic mass/deformed joint or region in case of an absent joint) should be exposed from above and below before the condylectomy (or gap arthroplasty) is carried out. The dissection should not extend too medial and caution should be summoned to save the injury to the maxillary, meningeal, masseteric vessels, and mandibular neurovascular bundle that lie in the vicinity. The disc and capsular tissue should be removed after the condylectomy to allow sufficient space for the prosthesis (Fig. 22.6). The fossa component is adapted at the predetermined position on the zygomatic arch keeping it parallel to the Frankfort horizontal plane and is fixed using 3 to 5 titanium screws. The length of the screws may be predetermined using CT data and confirmed on the model surgery. The check of the fossa fit should be examined and adjusted if there is any rocking movement observed followed by stabilization. Inter-maxillary fixation (IMF) should be placed to achieve a satisfactory occlusion once the fossa component is stable. Copious irrigation using saline should be done intra-operatively to prevent thermal injury to the bone/soft tissues while using rotary instruments and to remove any debris.

The Hind's incision should be utilized to check the fit of the condylar component. Necessity to trim the lateral border of mandible near the gonial angle and the region around antilingula should be determined in the steriolithographic model during pre-operative planning. The ramal component is secured in position along the posterior border of the ramus using 2.5 mm (predetermined length) bi-cortical titanium screws preserving the inferior alveolar nerve anteriorly. The orientation of the fossa component is confirmed in relation to the alloplastic condyle with lateral ramal plate and is then secured using screws. The relationship

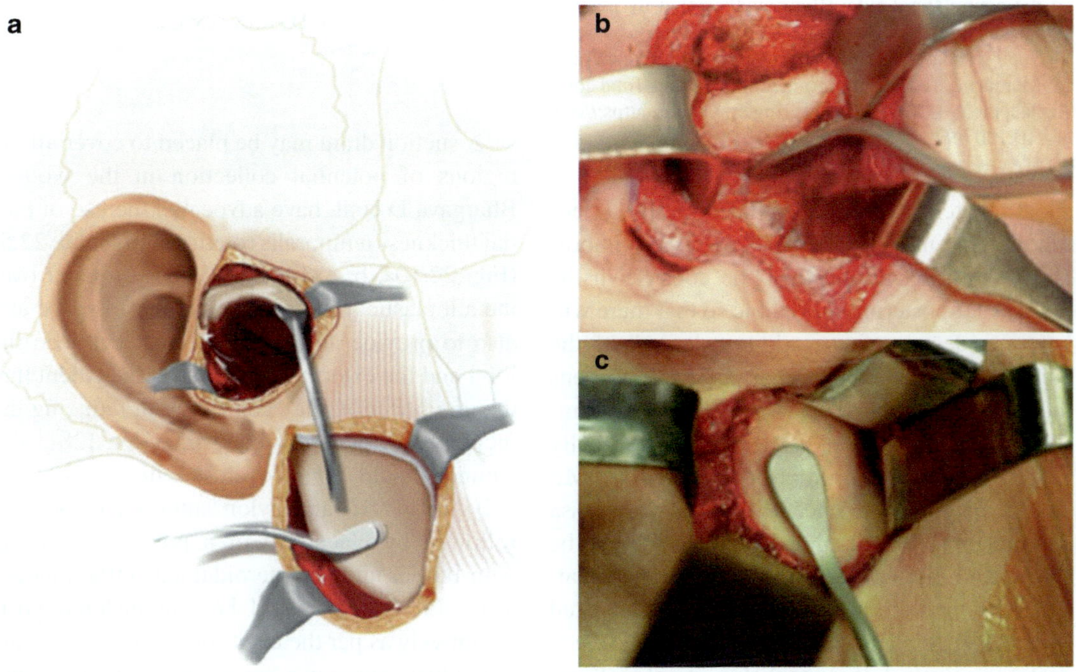

Fig. 22.6 (**a**) Diagram showing the use of the diamond rasp to perform the eminoplasty and, if necessary, remove a small amount of bone along the lateral aspect of the ramus to ensure a stable seating of the mandibular component and proper prosthesis orientation. (**b**) Intraoperative image showing the use of the diamond rasp for the eminoplasty. Bone is carefully removed to ensure tripod stability of the prosthesis and correct orientation. (**c**) Intraoperative image showing the diamond rasp removing a small amount of bone along the lateral aspect of the mandible. [Reprinted/adapted by permission from Quinn P., Granquist E.J. (2016) Stock Prostheses for Total Reconstruction of the Temporomandibular Joint. In: Mercuri L. (eds) Temporomandibular Joint Total Joint Replacement – TMJ TJR. Springer, Cham. https://doi.org/10.1007/978-3-319-21389-7_4]

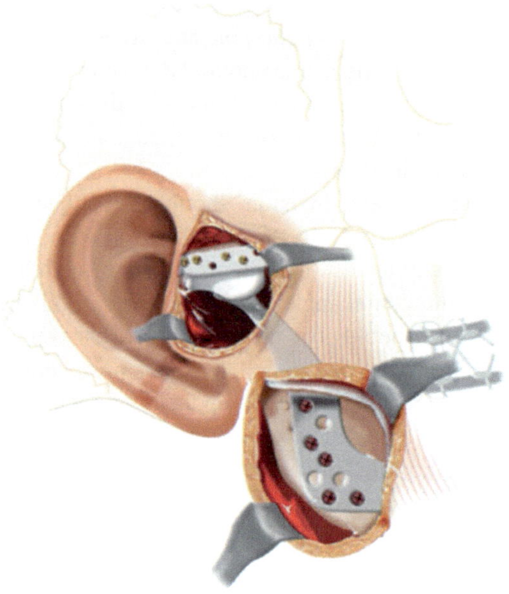

Fig. 22.7 Demonstration of pseudo-translation of the prosthesis. This occurs when a unilateral prosthesis is placed and the patient has a functioning lateral pterygoid on the contralateral side. [Reprinted/adapted by permission from Quinn P., Granquist E.J. (2016) Stock Prostheses for Total Reconstruction of the Temporomandibular Joint. In: Mercuri L. (eds) Temporomandibular Joint Total Joint Replacement – TMJ TJR. Springer, Cham. https://doi.org/10.1007/978-3-319-21389-7_4]

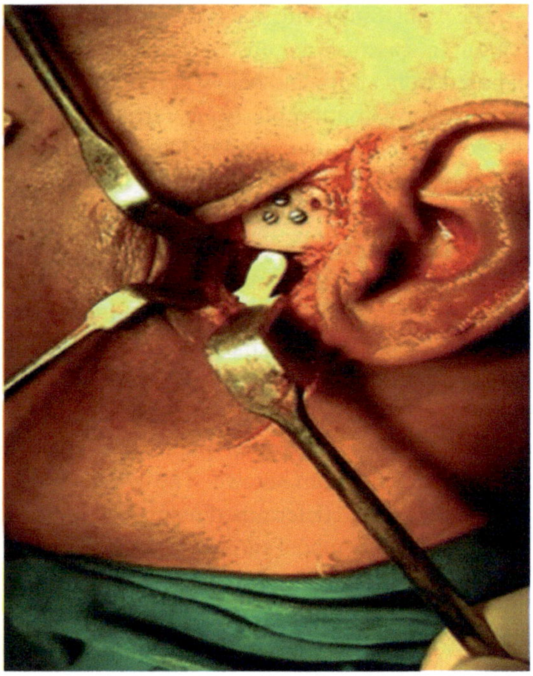

Fig. 22.8 Intra-operative image showing the fossa and ramal component of DARSN TMJ prosthesis secured using titanium screws

should match with the fit obtained on the stereolithographic model. It remains extremely important to position the head of the condyle in the fossa as far posterior as possible so that there will be some degree of "pseudo-translation" of the condylar head in the fossa as the patient opens the mouth to the expected range (32–35 mm) (Figs. 22.7 and 22.8). The prosthesis usually moves in the supero-inferior plane. The IMF should be removed once the ramal and fossa components are secured and occlusion should be re-checked. If the occlusion is found to be unsatisfactory, then the prosthesis should be adjusted (Fig. 22.9). IMF may be placed for one week post-operatively to re-establish vertical stability if dislocation of the prosthesis is observed.

A suction drain may be placed to cover all the regions of potential collection in the wound. Bhargava D et al. have advocated the use of partial thickness temporalis rotation flap (Table 22.5) (Fig. 22.10a, b, c) [27] that can be rotated over the alloplastic joint to reduce the dead space and also to provide an additional layer between the joint and the external skin layer. It is evident that this modification may contribute in reducing the incidence of peri-prosthetic infection [28]. The wound should then be closed in layers using polyglactin 910 and nylon sutures for the skin followed by placement of a pressure dressing. Anti-biotics and non-steroidal anti-inflammatory drugs (NSAIDs) should be administered post-operatively as per the institution's protocol or the individual surgeon's preference. Drains and sutures should be removed any day between third

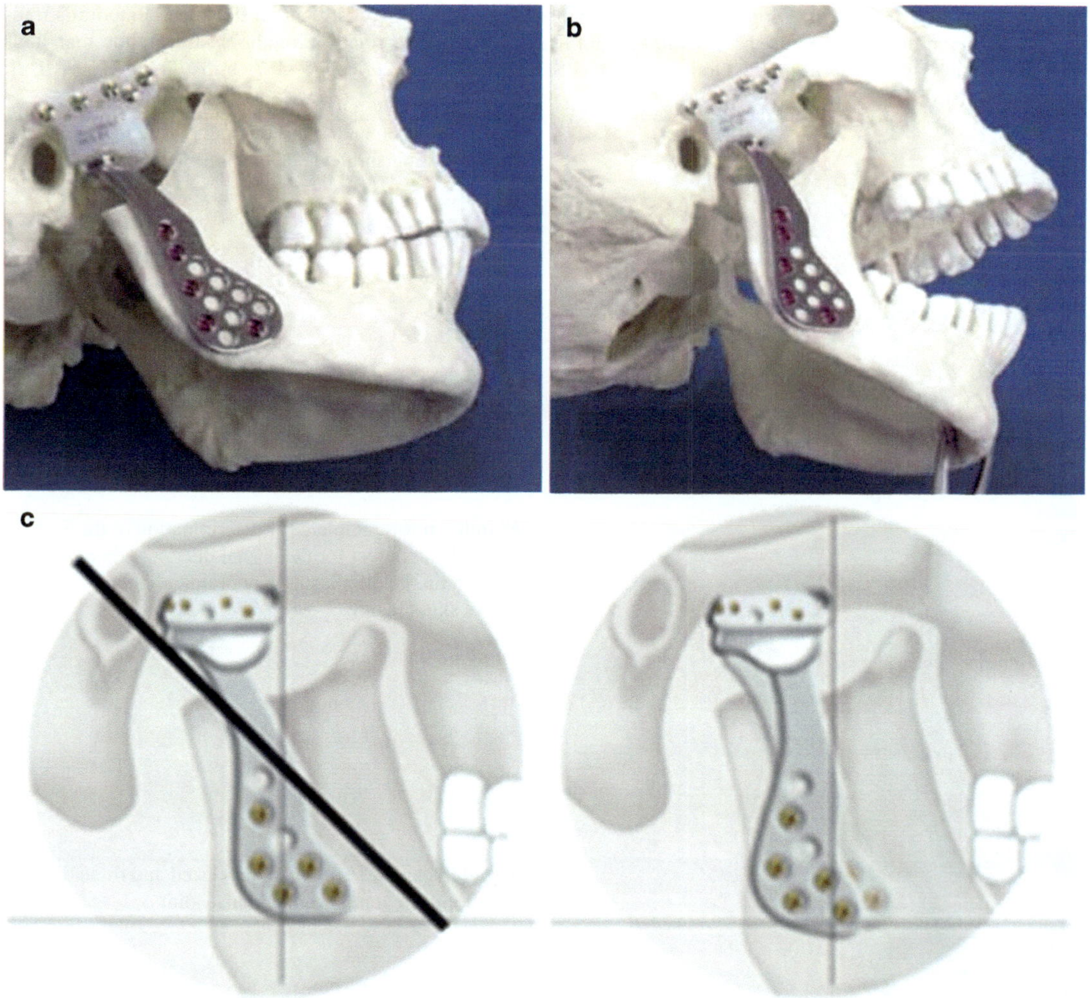

Fig. 22.9 *The left diagram* shows correct posterior position of the prosthesis while the *right diagram* shows incorrect positioning [Reprinted/adapted by permission from Quinn P., Granquist E.J. (2016) Stock Prostheses for Total Reconstruction of the Temporomandibular Joint. In: Mercuri L. (eds) Temporomandibular Joint Total Joint Replacement – TMJ TJR. Springer, Cham. https://doi.org/10.1007/978-3-319-21389-7_4]

to fourth and seventh to tenth post-operative days, respectively. Passive physiotherapy should be started from first post-operative day and continued up to six months. Post-operative evaluation of the device function may be assessed by periodical recording of the MIO, JF, DI, QoL, and nutritional status to measure the outcome. Post-operative radiographs may be ordered to evaluate the prosthesis adaptation and for the medical record data (Figs. 22.11 and 22.12).

However, prior to TJR, patients should be made aware about the possibility of device failure and its probable causes, as each patient's biological response remains different. Patients should also be counseled about the fact that the revision surgery poses more risk and difficulty.

Table 22.5 Surgical steps for alloplastic temporomandibular joint coverage with partial thickness temporalis rotation (Procedure proposed by Bhargava D et al. Partial thickness temporalis rotation for alloplastic temporomandibular joint - how I do it. J Stomatol Oral Maxillofac Surg. 2019 Sep;120(4):355–357. https://doi.org/10.1016/j.jormas.2019.01.001.)

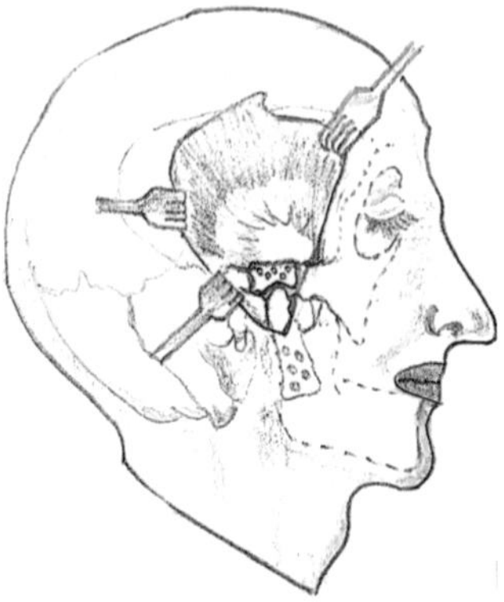	Total Temporomandibular joint alloplastic replacement demonstrating surgical site exposed with artificial joint in situ.
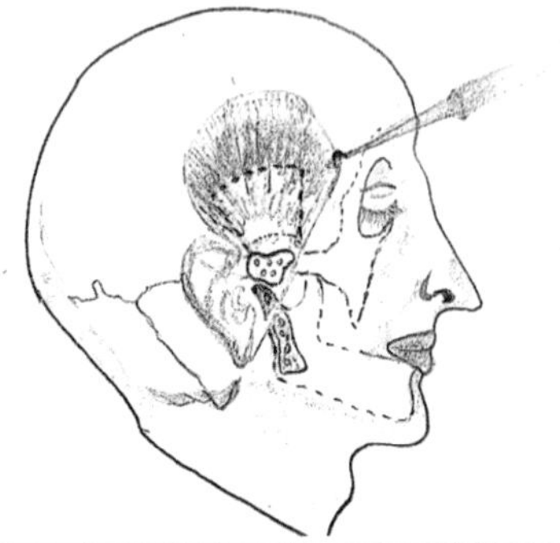	Aluminum foil template for determination of the surgical site defect for the partial thickness temporalis rotation on the alloplastic temporomandibular joint before skin closure.
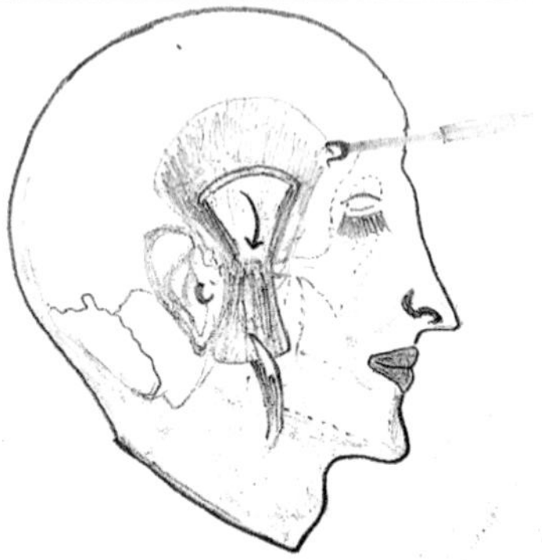	Partial thickness temporalis, harvested and rotated on the alloplastic temporomandibular joint
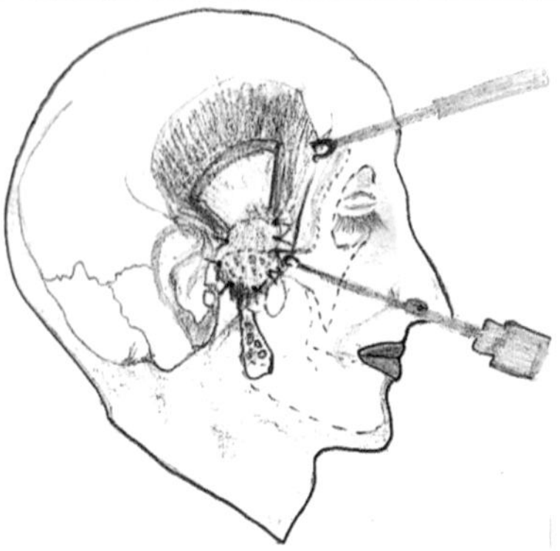	Rotated partial thickness temporalis secured with absorbable sutures around the lateral aspect of the alloplastic temporomandibular joint before subcutaneous and skin closure

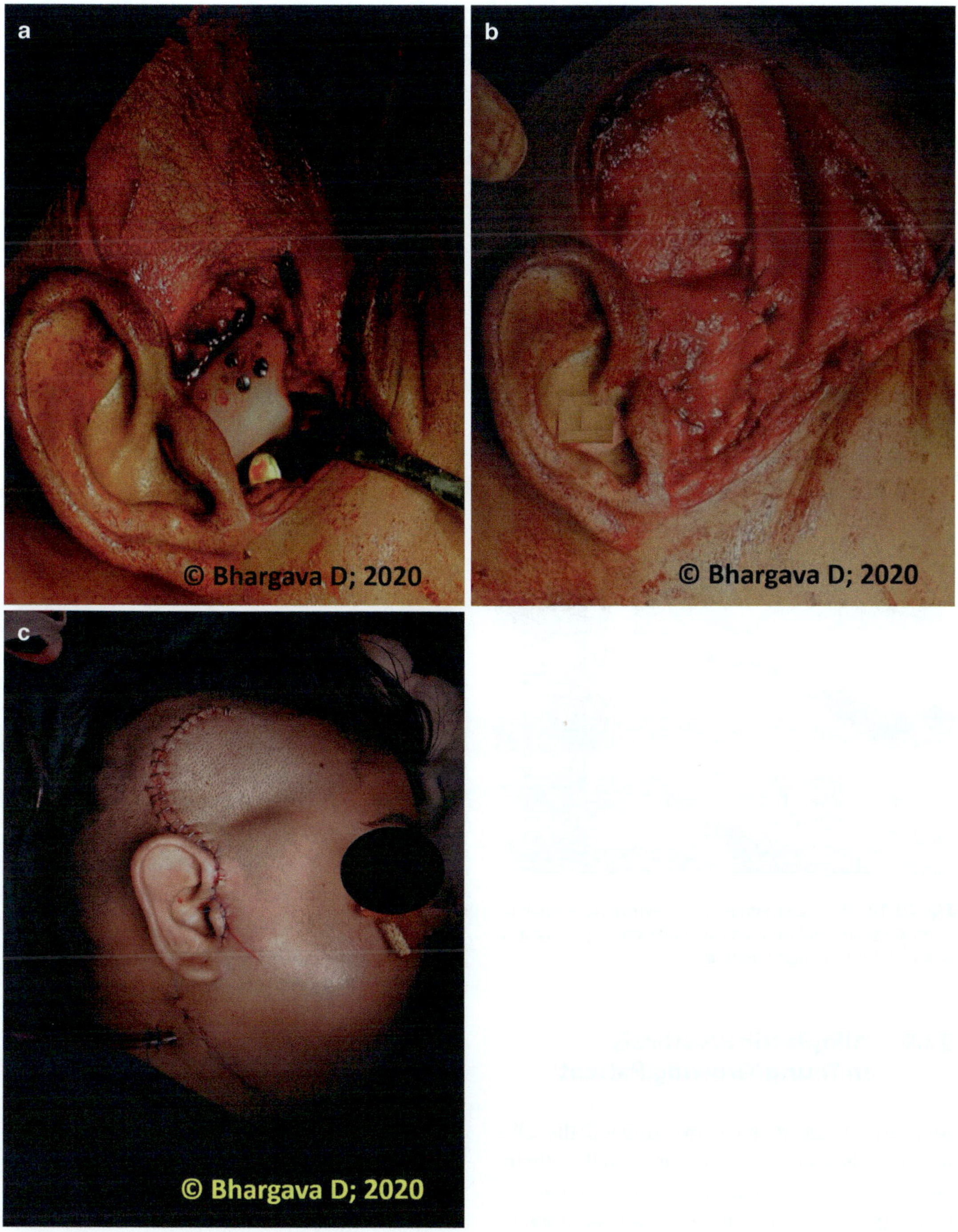

Fig. 22.10 (**a**) alloplastic joint placement through the pre-auricular incision. Note the condylar head component and the ultrahigh molecular weight polyethylene fossa. (**b**) Partial thickness temporalis muscle flap used to cover the alloplastic joint and is secured in position with absorbable sutures before preauricular skin closure. (**c**) Note the temporal hollowing and zygomatic bulge caused due to the partial thickness temporalis muscle flap rotation, in author's experience the preauricular zygomatic bulge reduces with time in the post-operative 8–12 months for most of the patients. The temporal hollowing is hidden inside the hairline in the immediate post-operative period. With residual functional muscle hypertrophy, temporal hollowing gets shallower with time

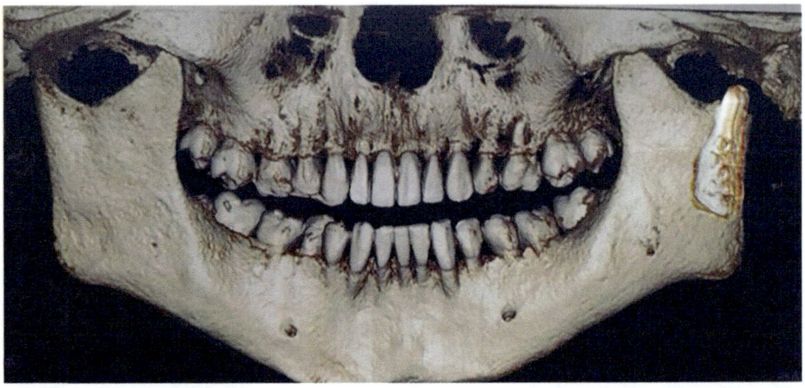

Fig. 22.11 Reconstructed computer tomographic image of the mandible showing vertical ramal rehabilitation using DARSN TMJ prosthesis to restore joint form and function

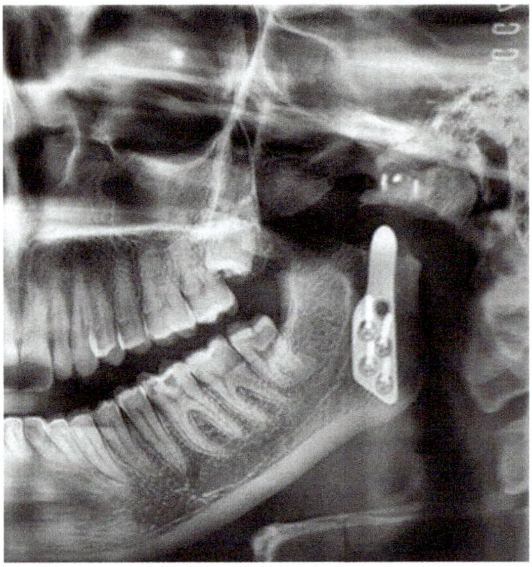

Fig. 22.12 Panoramic imaging of the mandible showing vertical ramal rehabilitation using alloplastic prosthesis to restore joint form and function

22.9 Alloplastic Prosthesis in Young/Growing Patient

Mercuri LG et al. have investigated the alloplastic TJR with favorable functional, esthetic, and occlusal outcomes in a growing patients where previous autogenous reconstruction have failed. Several studies in literature have evaluated the effects of autogenous grafts to reconstruct TMJ in growing patients with unfavorable outcomes such as unpredictable growth, graft failure, and donor site morbidity. TMJ TJR using alloplastic device has been considered lately by researchers among growing children in case of failed autogenous grafts, recurrent ankylosis unresponsive to other treatment modalities, and loss of vertical height of the mandible due to pathology or trauma. This requires several stages of treatment planning and careful execution. Further studies are required to fully understand the "long-term outcome" of using alloplastic TJR in growing patients [29–31].

22.10 Prophylactic Anti-biotics for Dental Procedures

As per the American Society of Orthopedics guidelines, prophylactic anti-biotics should be given to a patient who would require invasive dental procedures for two years after prosthesis insertion [11]. Various regimens are available currently that should be considered before undertaking dental procedures which may result in transient bacteremia in such patients (Table 22.6). It has been observed that the oral bacteria are known to cause infections in the alloplastic hip/knee joints after the patient had undergone an oral surgical procedure, where usually the presence of staphylococcus species was evident. Mercuri LG opined that the microbial bio-film is a source of alloplastic prosthesis failure which involves several interactions between the micro-organisms, host-factor, and alloplastic device [31–35].

Table 22.6 Antibiotic Prophylaxis Recommendations for dental treatment in total joint replacement patients

German Society of Orthopedics and Traumatology	Modified from American Academy of Orthopedic Surgeons
Amoxicillin-clavulanate 2 gm, per oral (or) Clindamycin 600 mg, per oral Shortly before the procedure and four hours after dental treatment	Amoxicillin, 2 gm, per oral (or) Cephalexin, 2 gm, per oral (or) Cephradine, 2 gm, per oral One hour prior to the procedure

Table 22.7 Definition of peri-prosthetic joint infection by Musculoskeletal Infection Society (MSIS)

1	Presence of sinus tract communicating with the prosthesis
2	A pathogen isolated by culture from two or more separate tissue or fluid samples from the affected prosthetic joint
3	Four of the following criteria (a) Elevated serum ESR and serum CRP concentration. (b) Elevated (synovial*) WBC count. (c) Elevated (synovial*) polymorphonuclear percentage. (d) Presence of purulence in the affected joint. (e) Isolation of micro-organisms in one culture of peri-prosthetic tissue/fluid. (f) > than five neutrophils/high power field in five different high power fields observed in a sample for histological analysis of peri-prosthetic tissue at ×400 magnification.

ESR: Erythrocyte Sedimentation Rate; CRP: C-reactive protein; WBC: White Blood Cell; *: use of synovial data is not relevant to TMJ TJR, instead peripheral WBC count and polymorphonuclear percentage may be considered

22.11 Identification of Risk Factors for Infection

Surgical site infections (SSIs) can pose a serious concern as it can lead to failure of the surgery. Fitzgerald Jr. et al. classified peri-prosthetic joint infection in orthopedics as acute post-operative, late deep, and late hematological infections. In 2011, universally accepted criteria to identify peri-prosthetic joint infection was given by Musculoskeletal Infection Society (MSIS) (Table 22.7). There are several patient related, surgery related, and post-operative risk factors that can cause failure of the alloplastic prosthesis. There are specified protocols for the management of early and late infections in the patients who have undergone TJR [35, 36, 37].

22.12 Pre-operative Factors

There are several pre-operative considerations which can enhance the success of the alloplastic TMJ TJR. This include administration of prophylactic anti-biotics which is a pre-requisite. The patient should be instructed to shave the hair in the vicinity of the incision. Ear should be examined to rule out any pathology or infection and it should be blocked with a snuggly fitting cotton plug to prevent any exchange of fluids intra-operatively. Before initiating the surgery, the nasoendo-tracheal tube should be secured in place using a suture and isolated from the surgical field to prevent displacement as it can pose a potential source of contamination. Sustained asepsis of the oral cavity and the skin throughout the surgery remains important. Oral cavity and the TJR surgical site should be stringently kept separate to avoid any contamination of the alloplastic joint with the oral fluids, during the course of the surgery. Contamination of the alloplastic material with oral fluids may progress to formation of a bio-film and may lead to device failure [36].

22.13 Intra-operative Factors

The incision should be placed accurately to facilitate adequate exposure. During layered dissection, parotid gland tissue is encountered which should be retracted as injury in this region can cause contamination of surrounding hard and soft tissue along with the device components with saliva which may lead to future and SSI. It is essential that the parotid capsule remains intact throughout TMJ TJR. It is also observed that the time taken to implant the alloplastic device can be a significant determinant of SSI. This greatly depends on the operator's familiarity with the procedure and proficiency that aid to minimize the duration of the surgery to place the implant. Adequate irrigation and hemostasis should be maintained throughout the intra-operative phase [36].

22.14 Post-operative Factors

In the immediate post-operative phase, pressure dressing should be placed to keep the dead spaces obliterated in order to minimize edema and to maintain post-operative hemostasis. Superficial infections such as stitch abscess and seroma should be managed aggressively before the organisms could progress to deeper tissues. The duration of hospital stay in the post-operative period should be minimized to prevent any nosocomial infections [36].

Wolford LM et al. classified infections after TMJ TJR as acute and chronic based on the onset of infection, if the infection occurs within 5 days it is considered as acute and chronic if it occurs after 30 days in the post-operative period. Counseling and informing the patient is an essential factor in managing SSI in TMJ TJRs [38, 39].

22.15 Complications

Any surgical procedure is not constantly free from complications. It is the onus of the operating surgeon to identify as well as manage the intra-operative and post-operative complications to circumvent failure of the alloplastic prosthesis (Table 22.8). Intra-operatively hemorrhage may occur due to the damage to the maxillary artery, retromandibular vein, superficial temporal vessels, masseteric vessels or pterygoid venous plexus. Vigilant surgical technique is the best way to avoid any vascular damage. At most instances a firm pressure controls a pre-auricular bleeders apart from other local measures. Occasionally, ligation of the external carotid artery may be required. Facial nerve palsy is a feared complication which can be avoided by careful assessment and surgical technique during incision placement and dissection. SSIs can occur if proper aseptic conditions are not maintained peri-operatively. Rarely dislocation of the alloplastic prosthesis may occur [11, 36, 37].

Table 22.8 Complications during TMJ TJR Surgery

Intra-Operative Complications
Hemorrhage—Internal maxillary/meningeal/facial artery
Injury to facial/auriculotemporal nerve
Post-Operative Complications
Infection via drain
Surgical site infections (SSIs)
Facial nerve palsy—Transient/ permanent
Myofascial pain syndrome
Hardware failure
Screw loosening
Allergy to the components of prosthesis (rare)
Dislocation of the alloplastic prosthesis

Several clinical studies have highlighted that alloplastic TMJ TJR is an effective option to reconstruct TMJ that cannot be salvaged, with satisfactory long-term results. TMJ TJRs have shown significant improvement in pain, mean MIO, JF, DI, nutritional status, and overall QoL in the post-operative period when compared to the pre-operative phase with satisfactory restoration of form and function [40–42].

22.16 Recommended Sterilization Protocol for the Prosthesis and Its Components

Various sterilization protocols have been summarized in Table 22.9 [43, 44]. These can/may be modified as per the local/regional/institutional guidelines on sterilization. The metal condylar component including screws can be sterilized using standard moist heat sterilization method just before use. UHMWPE material can be sterilized using Gamma/Ethylene Oxide (EtO) [44]. All the sterilized components should be stored in a broad spectrum antibiotic solution and not exposed to air in the operation theater from the time of unpacking to in vivo fixation.

Table 22.9 Sterilization method of various TMJ alloplastic prosthesis

Alloplastic prosthesis	Method of sterilization
Zheng J et al. [42]	Glenoid fossa prosthesis: Ethylene oxide gas sterilization Mandibular components: Steaming sterilization
TMJ concepts	Components packed in double Tyvek/film pouches Sterilization done using an ethylene oxide gas cycle Screws: Steam sterilization [wrapped/unwrapped pre-vacuum steam sterilization], 15 minutes for 133–135 °C
Biomet micro-fixation	Mandibular and fossa components: Sterilization is done by gamma radiation exposure to minimum of 25 KGy Screws are wrapped with an FDA cleared sterilization wrap prior to steam sterilization in order to maintain sterility
DARSN TMJ prosthesis	The metal condylar component including screws is sterilized using standard moist heat sterilization method. UHMWPE material undergoes gamma/EtO sterilization. The sterilized components should be stored in a broad spectrum antibiotic solution and not exposed to air in the operation theater from the time of unpacking to in vivo fixation
Melbourne prosthesis (OMX solutions TMJ Total joint replacement system)	Total joint replacement system fossa and condyle component sterilization method is ethylene oxide (EtO). The screws are steam sterilized.

22.17 Conclusion

Alloplastic TMJ TJR is a suitable method when the joint and surrounding structures cannot be salvaged. A thorough clinical, radiographic, and laboratory work-up followed by formulating a customized treatment plan for an individual patient along with a strict aseptic surgical procedure enhances the success rate of the TJR surgery. The alloplastic total joint replacement may offer an effective option to reconstruct the TMJ in an adult patient with documented benefits, provided a wise and scientific approach to case selection and appropriate treatment plan is followed.

References

1. Mercuri LG. Temporomandibular joint Total joint replacement –TMJ TJR. Springer. 2015. https://doi.org/10.1007/978-3-319-21389-7_4.
2. Guarda-Nardini L, Manfredini D, Ferronato G. Temporomandibular joint total replacement prosthesis: current knowledge and considerations for the future. Int J Oral Maxillofac Surg. 2008 Feb;37(2):103–10.
3. Wolford LM, et al. TMJ concepts/Techmedica custom-made TMJ Total joint prosthesis: 5-year follow-up study. Int J Oral Maxillofac Surg. 2003;32(3):268–74.
4. Ferreira JN, Ko CC, Myers S, Swift J, Fricton JR. Evaluation of surgically retrieved temporomandibular joint alloplastic implants: pilot study. J Oral Maxillofac Surg. 2008;66(6):1112–24.
5. Leandro LF, Ono HY, Loureiro CC, Marinho K, Guevara HA. A ten-year experience and follow-up of three hundred patients fitted with the Biomet/Lorenz microfixation TMJ replacement system. Int J Oral Maxillofac Surg. 2013;42(8):1007–13.
6. Bhargava D, Neelakandan RS, Sharma Y, Dalsingh V, Beena S, Gurjar P. Predictability and Feasibility of Total Alloplastic Temporomandibular Joint Reconstruction using DARSN TM Joint Prosthesis for patients in Indian subcontinent-A prospective clinical study. J Stomatol Oral Maxillofac Surg. 2020;121(1):2–8. https://doi.org/10.1016/j.jormas.2019.06.005.
7. Quinn PD. Color atlas of temporomandibular joint surgery. 3rd ed. St. Louis: Mosby; 1998.
8. Total prosthetic replacement of the temporomandibular joint: NICE interventional procedure guidance 500. London: NICE; 2014.
9. Sidebottom AJ; UK TMJ Replacement surgeons; British Association of Oral and Maxillofacial Surgeons. Guidelines for the replacement of temporomandibular joints in the United Kingdom. Br J Oral Maxillofac Surg 2008;46(2):146–147.
10. Yoda T, Ogi N, Yoshitake H, Kawakami T, Takagi R, Murakami K, Kurita K. Clinical guidelines for total temporomandibular joint replacement. Jap Dent Sci Rev. 2020;56(1):77–83.
11. Langdon J, Patel M, Ord R, Brennan P. Operative Oral and maxillofacial surgery. 2nd ed. London: Hodder Arnold; 2014.
12. Elledge R, Mercuri LG, Attard A, Green J, Speculand B. Review of emerging temporomandibular joint total joint replacement systems. Br J Oral Maxillofac Surg. 2019; https://doi.org/10.1016/j.bjoms.2019.08.009.

13. Mercuri LG, Edibam NR, Giobbie-Hurder A. Fourteen year follow up of a patient fitted total TMJ reconstruction system. J Oral Maxillofac Surg. 2007;65(6):1140–8.
14. Wolford LM, Mercuri LG, Schneiderman ED, Movahed R, Allen W. Twenty-year follow-up study on a patient-fitted temporomandibular joint prosthesis: the Techmedica/TMJ concepts device J. Oral Maxillofac Surg. 2015;73:952–60.
15. Sanovich R, Mehta U, Abramowicz S, Widmer C, Dolwick MF. Total alloplastic temporomandibular joint reconstruction using Biomet stock prostheses: the University of Florida experience. Int J Oral Maxillofac Surg. 2014;43(9):1091–5.
16. Westermark A. Reconstruction of the temporomandibular joint. up to 8 years follow-up of patients with Biomet total joint prostheses. Int J Oral Maxillofac Surg. 2010;39:951–5.
17. Elledge R, Attard A, Green J, Lowe D, Rogers SN, Sidebottom AJ, Speculand B. UK temporomandibular joint replacement database: a report on one-year outcomes. Br J Oral Maxillofac Surg. 2017;55(9):927–93.
18. Mercuri LG, Wolford LM, Sanders B, et al. Long-term follow-up of the CAD/CAM patient-fitted total temporomandibular joint reconstruction system. J Oral Maxillofac Surg. 2002;60:1440–5.
19. Perez DE, Wolford LM, Schneiderman E, Movahed R, Bourland C, Gutierrez EP. Does unilateral temporomandibular Total joint reconstruction result in contralateral joint pain and dysfunction? J Oral Maxillofac Surg. 2016;74(8):1539–47.
20. Bhargava D, Neelakandan DRS, Dalsingh V, Sharma Y. Total alloplastic temporomandibular joint: proposal for a Total titanium condylar prosthesis with UHMWPE joint fossa design (DARSN TM joint prosthesis). Acta Scientific Orthop. 2018;1(1):22–7.
21. Schuurhuis JM, Dijkstra, et al. Groningen temporomandibular total joint prosthesis: an 8 year follow up on function and pain. J Cranio-Maxillo-Facial Surg. 2012;40:815e–20e.
22. van JP L, et al. Groningen temporomandibular joint prosthesis. Development and first clinical application. Int J Oral Maxillofac Surg. 2002;31:44–52.
23. Bhargava D, Neelakandan RS, Dalsingh V, Sharma Y, Beena S. A Likert Type psychometric scale to assess the temporomandibular joint (TMJ) function for evaluation of quality of life (QoL) following Total joint replacement surgeries. Sch J Appl Med Sci. 2018; https://doi.org/10.21276/sjams.2018.6.10.76.
24. Bhargava D, Neelakandan RS, Dalsingh V, Sharma Y, Pandey A, Pandey A, Beena S, Koneru G. A three dimensional (3D) musculoskeletal finite element analysis of DARSN temporomandibular joint (TMJ) prosthesis for total unilateral alloplastic joint replacement. J Stomatol Oral Maxillofac Surg. 2019;120(6):517–22. https://doi.org/10.1016/j.jormas.2019.04.001.
25. Ackland AC, Robinson D, Redhead M, et al. A personalized 3D-printed prosthetic joint replacement for the human temporomandibular joint: from implant design to implantation. J Mech Behav Biomed Mat. 2017;69:404–11.
26. Zou L, Zhao J, He D. Preliminary clinical study of standard Chinese alloplastic temporomandibular joint prosthesis. J Cranio Maxillofac Surg. 2019;47:602e–6e.
27. Bhargava D, Neelakandan RS, Sharma Y, Beena S, Gurjar P. Partial thickness temporalis rotation for alloplastic temporomandibular joint - how I do it. J Stomatol Oral Maxillofac Surg. 2019;120(4):355–57. https://doi.org/10.1016/j.jormas.2019.01.001.
28. Perler BA, Vander Kolk CA, Dufresne CR, Williams GM. Can infected prosthetic grafts be salvaged with rotational muscle flaps? Surgery. 1991;110(1):30–4.
29. Mercuri LG, Swift JQ. Considerations for the use of alloplastic temporomandibular joint replacement in the growing patient. J Oral Maxillofac Surg. 2009;67:1979–90.
30. Ellis E, Carlson DS. Histological comparison of the costochondral, sternoclavicular and temporomandibular joints during growth in the Macaca mulatta. J Oral Maxillofac Surg. 1986;44:312.
31. Saeed NR, Kent JN. A retrospective study of the costochondral graft in TMJ reconstruction. Int J Oral Maxillofac Surg. 2003;32:606.
32. Mercuri LG. Prophylaxis after Total joint replacement. Re to editor. J Oral Maxillofac Surg. https://doi.org/10.1016/j.joms.2009.12.042.
33. Freidlander AH. Staphylococcus species bacteria on Oral cavity: a potential risk for prosthetic hips and knee. Re to editor. J Oral Maxillofac Surg. https://doi.org/10.1016/j.joms.2009.09.043.
34. Mercuri LG. Microbial biofilms: a potential source for alloplastic device failure. J Oral Maxillofac Surg. 2006;64:1303–9.
35. Mercuri LG. Avoiding and managing temporomandibular total joint replacement surgical site infections. J Oral Maxillofac Surg. 2012;70:2280–9.
36. Mercuri LG. Temporomandibular joint replacement periprosthetic infections: a review of early diagnostic testing options. Int J Oral Maxillofac Surg. 2014;43:1236–42.
37. Wolford LM, Rodrigues DB, McPhillips A. Management of the infected temporomandibular joint total joint prosthesis. J Oral Maxillofac Surg. 2010;68(11):2810–23.
38. Mercuri LG. Prevention and detection of prosthetic temporomandibular joint infections-update. Int J Oral Maxillofac Surg. 2019;48(2):217–24.
39. Giannakopoulos HE, Sinn DP, Quinn PD. Biomet microfixation temporomandibular joint replacement system: a 3-year follow-up study of patients treated during 1995 to 2005. J Oral Maxillofac Surg. 2012;70(4):787–94.
40. Westermark A. Reconstruction of the temporomandibular joint. up to 8 years follow-up of patients with Biomet total joint prostheses. Int J Oral Maxillofac Surg. 2010;39:951–5.
41. Neelakandan RS, Raja AV, Krishnan AM. Total alloplastic temporomandibular joint reconstruction for

management of TMJ ankylosis. J Maxillofac Oral Surg. 2013;13(4):575–82.
42. Zheng J, Chen X, Jiang W, et al. An innovative total temporomandibular joint prosthesis with customized design and 3D printing additive fabrication: a prospective clinical study. J Transl Med. 2019;17(4) https://doi.org/10.1186/s12967-018-1759-1.
43. TMJ Concepts. Sterile Implant. Product Insert.
44. Affatato S, Bersaglia G, Emiliani D, Foltran I, Taddei P, Reggiani M, Ferrieri P, Toni A. The performance of gamma- and EtO-sterilised UHMWPE acetabular cups tested under severe simulator conditions. Part 2: wear particle characteristics with isolation protocols. Biomaterials. 2003;24(22):4045–55.

Syndromes Affecting Temporomandibular Joint

23

Shubhangi Mhaske and Suhani Ghai

23.1 Introduction

The clinicians dealing with the maxillofacial region routinely face challenges in tackling problems related to congenital anomalies or syndromic patients. Syndromes associated with temporomandibular joint (TMJ) are usually genetically inherited as an autosomal dominant trait, but sporadic cases with genetic mutations are also a major cause. TMJ disorders are mostly seen as bilateral conditions. Some anomalies are observed in very early stage right from the embryonic stage from the 20th day till 12th week of gestation. The cases should be preferably diagnosed in pre-natal stage or at birth and treatment is prioritised and directed on airway stabilisation followed by baby feeding. The affected child may require treatment for loss of hearing, occasionally vision and obvious compromised jaw function. Musculoskeletal disorders may develop or may be acquired later in life as a result of lifestyle disorder or due to psychological triggers

Developmental disorders resulting in recognisable morphologic abnormalities are recently been termed as "dysmorphology", as described by David Smith [1]. Maxillofacial specialists are nowadays confronted more frequently with congenital anomalies. There are remarkable advances during the past few decades in the clinical genetics of congenital malformations which are having an increase in medical attention for the diagnosis of various syndromes.

A syndrome is usually defined as "a group of signs and symptoms or a set of symptoms usually three or more, which occur together, characteristic of a morbid condition" or described as "the aggregate of signs and symptoms associated with any morbid process and constituting together a picture of the disease". Syndromes being a multisystem disease are difficult to classify in a specific pattern and can be of varied aetiology and clinical presentation [2].

The aetiological factors for the occurrence of syndromes are not definite. Frequently it occurs due to genetic influence or genetic disposition. Racial predominance is also known to be a causative factor. Offspring of an affected individual usually have likelihood of acquiring the disorder if inherited. A syndrome may become progressive with more severe deformities in the succeeding generations. Immune dysfunction or an abnormal immune response, dysfunction of certain glands, and vascular anomalies may also result in form of a syndrome. Diagnosis of a syndrome is a challenging task due to extreme variability in the clinical presentation or expression [2].

S. Mhaske (✉)
Oral Pathology and Microbiology, People's College of Dental Sciences and Research Centre, People's University, Bhopal, Madhya Pradesh, India

S. Ghai
Dharamshila Narayana Superspeciality Hospital, New Delhi, India

D. Bhargava (ed.), *Temporomandibular Joint Disorders*,
https://doi.org/10.1007/978-981-16-2754-5_23

23.2 Syndromes Associated with Craniofacial Anomalies of Genetic Origin

Genetic information in humans is carried by 23 pairs of chromosomes {46}, known as autosomes which carry information regarding the structure and body functions of which one pair {2} is known as the sex chromosome, which determines the sex of an individual (XY in male and XX in female) [3].

The genetics of craniofacial malformations is very complicated to understand due to the overlapping of the presenting features and the difficulties in interpretation with corelations to the huge database of human genome. Several thousand distinct syndromic entities have been identified, and most of them have not been encountered by the average specialist due to their rarity. In addition, the human genome is thought to contain about 80,000 genes. There are several unusual syndromes that are yet to be identified [3]. Genetically derived disorders can be considered into three major groups (Table 23.1).

23.2.1 Chromosomal Disorders

Sex-linked inheritance is when the X chromosome carries the abnormal gene, the disorder is said to be X-linked (X-linked recessive, X-linked dominant) and when a Y chromosome carries it, the condition is said to be a Y-linked disorder, for e.g., Hypohidrotic ectodermal dysplasia.

23.2.2 Single Gene [Monogenic] Disorders

This category of disorders is caused by mutations in a single gene, which refers to a primary error in the DNA code. They are inherited according to Mendelian rules, with sub-divisions based on the chromosome on which an irregular [mutant] gene is located and the type of the trait. The inheritance is known as autosomal when an abnormal gene is situated on the autosome, and the trait is said to be X-linked when such a gene is situated on the X chromosome. These traits may either be "dominant" or "recessive" (autosomal dominant or recessive, and X-linked dominant or recessive).

Autosomal dominant inheritance has the following characteristics

- At least one parent of any affected person is also affected.
- Both male and female are likely to be affected and are capable of transmitting the disease.
- Transmission is generally seen [father to son/daughter and mother to son/daughter] with no skipping of generation.
- Affected individual characteristically transmit the trait to half of their offsprings.

These general rules however are modified by

- **Penetrance:** Carrier of abnormal genes may be mildly affected to be entirely indistinguishable from normal individual. A gene is said to

Table 23.1 Genetically derived-disorders in the craniofacial region

Craniofacial malformation syndromes with autosomal dominant inheritance	Craniofacial syndromes with recessive inheritance	X-linked Inheritance Syndromes	Multi-factorial disorders
1. Blepharophimosis syndrome 2. Waardenburg syndrome 3. Treacher-Collin syndrome 4. Van der Woude syndrome 5. Oculo-dento-digital syndrome 6. Cranio-stenosis syndromes like Crouzon syndrome, Apert syndrome	1. Cryptophthalmos syndrome 2. Oro-facial digital syndrome 3. Roberts syndrome 4. Carpenter syndrome	1. Albinism–deafness syndrome 2. Aarskog syndrome 3. Focal dermal hypoplasia 4. X-linked hydrocephaly 5. Lowe syndrome. 6. Mucopolysaccharide II, hunter syndrome 7. Oro-facial digital syndrome	1. Sturge–weber syndrome 2. Moebius syndrome 3. Frontonasal dysplasia syndrome 4. Goldenhar syndrome

be "penetrant", if it is expressed in a given carrier.

- **Expressivity**: A parent who is slightly impaired may have a child who is seriously affected or vice versa. There is variation in the expression.
- **New mutation:** An individual who does not carry a gene for a particular inherited condition may rarely have an affected infant.

Autosomal recessive inheritance has the following characteristics:

- The trait usually appears only in siblings and not in their parents.
- Consanguinity is generally seen among the parents of the affected individual.
- Male and female tend to be equally affected.
- Affected individuals will generally have normal children but all of the children will be carrier of the condition.

23.2.3 Multi-Factorial Disorders

Multi-factorial disorders involve interaction between both genetic factors and environmental factors like trauma, neoplastic disease, toxic drugs, metabolic factors, and infections.

23.3 TMJ and Associated Syndromic Conditions

The syndromes associated with TMJ should be better understood with the craniofacial anomalies which may be inherited or transmitted by genetic or/and non-genetic factors. This chapter focuses on commonly documented syndromes affecting the TMJ irrespective of aetiologic classification. As discussed earlier the syndromes affecting TMJ may be having a combination of signs and symptoms making the diagnosis difficult. The key in diagnosing TMJ or jaw abnormality is to find the primary jaw pathology and look for evidences of syndromic findings affecting the skin, organ abnormalities, and extra-facial skeletal involvement.

Conditions affecting the jaws such as micrognathia, macrognathia, facial hemi-hypertrophy, facial hemi-atrophy may also affect TMJ due to direct or indirect syndromic manifestations owing to genetic or non-genetic causes. TMJ disorders (TMD) mostly form a group of degenerative musculoskeletal conditions combined with morphological and functional deformities. TMJ and muscle disorders are a category of conditions that cause pain and weakness in the jaw joint and the muscles that regulate it. To optimise function while minimising damage to the surrounding structures, the movement of the mandible requires coordination between both the joints [4–6]. TMDs have shown a consistent finding that the greatest majority affected are females. The ratio of affected women to men for TMD is 8:1 [7–9]. There are several syndromes in the head and neck affecting the TMJ which will be discussed in this chapter [10, 11].

23.4 TMJ Syndrome (Referred in occasional literature for TMD)

23.4.1 Introduction

TMD is a term guided by a cascade of circumstances afflicting the oro-facial region associated with TMJ, masticatory muscles, and peri-articular structures. TMJ syndrome was first described by Costen in 1936 as a muscular-skeletal pain-disease caused by hypertonia of the masticatory muscles and is projected into various regions of the head and neck. A primary dysfunctional aetiology as well as a secondary aetiology based on other diseases, particularly of the ear, nose, and throat region may be encountered. A process of exclusion is necessary in the diagnostic process. The signs and symptoms can range from a generalised headache and facial pain to a more localised or even neuralgic pain. Feeling of pressure or unusual sounds in the ear are common otogenic symptoms [12].

TMDs can be classified broadly in two categories:

1. TMD secondary to myofascial pain and dysfunction (MPD) also known as myofascial pain dysfunction syndrome (MPDS).
2. TMD secondary to true articular disease.

23.4.2 Aetiology

The major cause to MPDS is muscular hyperactivity which leads to severe pain in the TMJ region. The muscular dysfunction is secondary to malocclusion of variable degree and duration. In the recent years, the importance of psychological factors has been recognised which support the manifestations such as personality disorders, stress, and anxiety which may be associated with jaw clenching, night grinding of teeth/bruxism, and increased sensitivity. Disc displacement is the most common cause for TMD of articular origin. Other associated diseases such as degenerative joint disorders, rheumatoid arthritis, infection, neoplasia, ankylosis, and congenital anomalies may be seen.

23.4.3 Clinical Features

The primary clinical manifestations in MPD are pain, tenderness, and spasm of the masticatory muscles. It comprises of the majority of TMD cases. Pain is experienced by the patient with no visible destructive alterations to the joint on radiographic evaluation. In a stressed and nervous person, it is often associated with bruxism and daytime jaw clenching. The incidence of signs and symptoms in TMD is higher among general population (20%–75%) than the proportion of the population who report for the treatment (2%–4%). It is four times as common in females (8%–15%) as compared to males (3%–10%), and the affected age range varies from the second to fourth decade. It is of interest that the peak of TMD symptom development is at its highest in the second to fourth decade, which coincides with the child bearing years known to cause stress and anxiety [13–16].

There are four cardinal signs and symptoms of MPDS

1. Pain
2. Tenderness of muscle
3. Popping or clicking noise in the TMJ
4. Limitation of unilateral or bilateral jaw motion, with or without deviation on opening

There is characteristic peri-auricular pain which may be unilateral or bilateral in MPD and gets aggravated during periods of increased stress. Limited mouth opening due to pain or possible disc displacement may be a presenting feature. TMD may act as a trigger in patients prone to headaches. Some other symptoms associated with TMD are ear ache, dizziness, neck stiffness, and shoulder pain. Differential diagnoses include migraine headache, cluster headache, post herpetic neuralgia, trigeminal neuralgia (TN), and middle ear infections. With the current understanding of the TMJ Disorders, the concept of the pre-existing "TMJ Syndrome" is now diversified into various subsets of problems with clarity in the treatment of these entities.

23.5 Ehlers–Danlos Syndrome (EDS)

23.5.1 Introduction

The Ehlers–Danlos syndrome (EDS) is a group of hereditary disorders that affect collagen and connective tissue structures of the body in a generalised form. Several sub-types have been identified. Tissue fragility, skin hyper-extensibility, and joint hypermobility are all common characteristics in all cases. EDS creates unique restrictions in the treatment of patients with TMJ involvement. Although it is not a common cause of TMJ disorders, EDS can produce serious complications in patients receiving conventional TMJ therapy, and thus should be recognised in diagnostic procedures so that treatment planning can be modified accordingly [17].

23.5.2 Aetiology

The ability to distinguish EDS from more than 200 other heritable connective tissue disorders has been made possible owing to genetic testing. Collagen structurally and functionally is altered in all forms of EDS. Excessive mandibular translation has been linked to pharyngeal collapse, which is linked to sleep apnoea.

23.5.3 Clinical Features

Mouth opening, clicking, crepitation, and permanent jaw locking are all symptoms of hypermobile joints. Many EDS patients indicated that as they got older, their joint hypermobility decreased [18]. Muscle spasms induced by tension, jaw clenching, ischaemia, osteoclastic and compression degeneration, and/or neurological input to the trigeminal nerve, which is a possible TMD contributory source of migraines, are thought to induce the classic TMD headache [19].

23.6 Goldenhar Syndrome [Oculo-Auriculo-Vertebral Syndrome/Hemifacial Microsomia (HM)]

23.6.1 Introduction

Goldenhar syndrome was first reported by Canton in 1861 [20]. HM primarily affects the oral, auricular, and mandibular development. The abnormalities may be mild to severe with hardly noticeable facial asymmetry to very prominent facial defects with more or less severe abnormalities of skeleton and internal organs. Muscle spasms induced by tension, jaw clenching, ischaemia, osteoclastic and compression degeneration, and/or neurological feedback to the trigeminal nerve, which is a possible TMD contributory source of migraines, have all been suggested as causes for the classic TMD headache [18].

23.6.2 Aetiology

It may have multi-factorial causes.

- There is a genetic component and is often familial, with autosomal dominant or recessive inheritance [20].
- Aneuploidy in chromosome X, translocation t[9;12] [p23;q12.2], inversion inv9[p11;q13], inv14[p11.2;q22.3], mosaicism of trisomy 7, 9, and 22 have all been discovered [21].
- During the formation of the first and second pharyngeal arches, which are responsible for the growth of craniofacial structures, abnormal vascularisation occurs in the fourth week of pregnancy [21]. During the first trimester of pregnancy, there is a developmental issue with the branchial arch. Like other birth defects, it is believed to be influenced by environmental factors such as exposure to alcohol, certain medications, diseases, infections, or poor diet.
- Diabetic mother, multiple pregnancies especially in twins, higher occurrence with in vitro fertilisation [21].

23.6.3 Clinical Features

Asymmetrical and unilateral hypoplasia of mandibular ramus and condyle is seen. It might even present as an absence of ramus and condyle on the affected side. At least 35% with agenesis of the mandibular ramus have associated macrostomia or pseudo-macrostomia which is lateral facial cleft, of mild degree. The maxillary temporal and malar bones on the more severely affected side are reduced in size and flattened. Occlusal plane canting and malocclusion are common. Bifid tongue, facial asymmetry, hemifacial microsomia, cleft lip and palate, dacryocystitis, atresia of the external auditory canal, pre-auricular appendages, auricular dysplasia with/without hearing loss, pre-auricular fistulas, middle and inner ear defects, anotia, and microtia are all manifestations of abnormalities of the first and second pharyngeal arches.

23.7 Treacher Collins Syndrome (Mandibulofacial Dysostosis, Bauru Type)

23.7.1 Introduction

Treacher Collins syndrome is a congenital autosomal dominant craniofacial disorder characterised by mandibulo-maxillary and malar hypoplasia and peri-orbital abnormalities. It is derived from first and second branchial arch, first described by Edward Treacher Collins, a British ophthalmologist in 1900. In 1949, Franceschetti and Klein proposed the term "mandibulofacial dysostosis" (Franceschetti–Klein syndrome). There is malformation of the ossicles and hypoplasia up to middle ear and patients have conductive hearing loss [22].

23.7.2 Aetiology

The failure or incomplete migration of neural crest cells to the facial region caused malformation in structures formed from the first and second branchial arches. TCOF1, POLR1D, and POLR1C genes are all known to have mutations. Bad ribosome biogenesis and consequent neural crest cell insufficiency are caused by mutations in the TCOF1 gene on chromosome 5q31.3-q33.3, which codes for the Treacle protein.

23.7.3 Clinical Features

Underdevelopment of zygomatic bone and lateral aspect of orbit is seen, resulting in midfacial deformity. The convex facial profile, macrostomia, micrognathia, and retrognathia of the mandible with a steep mandibular angle with TMJ involvement give rise to a fish or bird like facies. Other features include brachycephaly with bi-temporal narrowing, airway obstruction, atresia of external ear canal, microtia, coloboma of the lower lid, and pre-auricular hair displacement.

23.8 Hallermann–Streiff Syndrome

Hallermann–Streiff syndrome is a rare congenital disorder characterised by skull and facial bone defects. The vast majority of cases tend to be intermittent in nature (occurring in individuals with no history of the condition in the family).

Sparse hair, ocular anomalies, dental defects, degenerative skin changes, and proportionately short stature are all characteristic features. Brachycephaly with frontal bossing is present, as is Micrognathia, which leads to TMJ anomaly, a narrow strongly arched palate, and a small, pinched, tapering beaked nose. Clouding of the lens is one of the most common ocular anomalies.

The appearance of natal teeth and/or their absence and malformation and misalignment of teeth are both examples of dental defects. In around 80% of those who are affected, hypotrichosis is also present. Other symptoms include facial skin atrophy and/or clavicular and rib hypoplasia. In certain cases, intellectual disability is present [23].

23.9 Crouzon Syndrome (Craniofacial Dysostosis)

23.9.1 Introduction

Crouzon syndrome is an autosomal dominant condition, characterised by cranial synostosis, ocular proptosis, and hypoplastic maxilla. This syndrome was first reported by Louis Edouard, Octave Crouzon in 1912. It is considered the most common craniosynostosis syndrome. Craniosynostosis denotes premature fusion of coronal sutures which results in the skull and facial deformities [24].

23.9.2 Aetiology

Crouzon syndrome is caused by a mutation in the FGFR 2 gene, which codes for the fibroblast growth factor protein. Growth factor receptor 2, present on chromosome locus 10q25-10q26 is responsible for the deformities observed. During embryonic development, this protein directs immature cells to become bone cells. Mutation in this gene causes the skull bones to fuse prematurely. In approximately 50% of cases, the mutation is de novo [25, 26].

23.9.3 Clinical Features

Clinically patient presents with an ovoid skull, brachycephalic head, and often presents a horizontal supraorbital groove. Premature closure of the sutures occurs and often the anterior fontanelle is open due to late closure. Other manifestation includes coronal craniosynostosis with other cranial sutures fusion, frontal bossing, and strabismus. The appearance is quite characteristic because of exophthalmos due to shallow orbit, hypertelorism, and underdevelopment of maxilla. Maxillary hypoplasia is responsible for the relative mandibular prognathism which is a consistent feature of this syndrome. TMJ may be involved bilaterally associated with pain. Condylar dislocation may be seen on both the sides. The upper lip is usually short with a parrot like nose. Intra-oral features include malocclusion, cleft lip, and palate with V shaped palate. Some of the occasional findings include peg shaped teeth and partial anodontia.

23.10 Apert's Syndrome (Acrocephalosyndactyly)

Apert's syndrome is transmitted by an autosomal dominant gene occurring sporadically with mutations found in the FGFR2 [fibroblast growth factor receptor 2] gene. Clinical features include ovoid skull, brachycephalic and often presents a horizontal supraorbital groove. Premature closure of the sutures occurs and often the anterior fontanelle is open due to late closure. Features of hand and feet include syndactyly. Osseous or cutaneous fusion of fingers is usually present. Intra-orally, a high palatal vault posterior palatal and uvular cleft can be evident. Dental malocclusion is always present. Other oral features include mandibular prognathism, malocclusion, and retarded eruption. TMJ may be affected secondarily due to mandibular prognathism as malocclusion may eventually lead to bilateral unbalanced stress on the condyle [11].

23.11 Sapho Syndrome

SAPHO stands for Synovitis, Acne, Pustulosis, Hyperostosis, and Osteitis. It encompasses a wide range of inflammatory bone diseases that are accompanied by skin changes. In 1987, the word SAPHO was coined to describe a range of inflammatory bone disorders that may or may not be linked to dermatologic pathology [27].

23.11.1 Clinical Features

Synovitis is the inflammation of the joint lining in SAPHO. It causes warmth, tenderness, discomfort, swelling, and stiffness in the joints involved (arthritis). Hyperostosis is the term for abnormally rapid bone development. The SAPHO syndrome hyperostosis is commonly found at the points of the bone where tendons join. The inflammation of the bone is referred to as osteitis [28].

23.12 Jacob Disease

Jacob disease is a rare disorder characterised by the development of a joint between an expanded mandibular coronoid process and the inner part of the zygomatic body. Aetiological factors include coronoid process enlargement and chronic TMJ disc displacement. It is characterised by TMJ dysfunction associated with restricted inter-incisal opening and progressive zygomatic asymmetry. The coronoid sample's histopathological diagnosis reveals cartilage-capped exostoses of articular fibrous cartilage [29].

23.13 McCune–Albright Syndrome

McCune–Albright syndrome is a genetic condition that affects the bones, skin, and endocrine system. It was first identified in 1937 by Donovan James McCune, an American paediatrician, and

Fuller Albright, an endocrinologist [30]. The pathogenesis is related to an activated mutation in G-protein. It is a mosaic disease arising from somatic activating mutations in GNAS, which encodes the α-subunit of the Gs, G-protein coupled receptor. In McCune–Albright syndrome, fibrous dysplasia causes deformity due to expansile lesions of the jaws which leads to TMJ involvement and condylar displacement.

23.14 Osteopathia Striata with Cranial Sclerosis

Osteopathia straita is a bone disorder characterised by swollen sclerotic craniofacial bones. It is autosomal dominant or X-linked dominant. The face has a square and broad profile. The mid-face, despite being dense and enlarged, lacks projection. The cranial foramina encroachment causes cranial nerve dysfunction. Hearing deficiency affects more than half of the patients [31].

Frontal bossing, hypertelorism, hearing loss, cleft palate, bifid uvula, and a thick cranial base are among the other cranio-maxillofacial characteristics. Some patients have been diagnosed with TMJ ankylosis. Ventricular septal defect, atrial septal defect, laryngeal tracheal malacia, polydactyly, and syndactyly are some of the other systemic findings. A common symptom of focal dermal hypoplasia is this disease [32].

23.15 Pierre Robin Syndrome

Pierre Robin anomalad is a congenital condition of facial abnormalities, a sequence that is a chain of certain developmental malformation one entailing the next. It was first described by Lannelongue and Menard in 1891. Presenting features of this syndrome include micrognathia, retrognathia, glossoptosis, and cleft palate. Autosomal recessive inheritance has been documented, with an X-linked variant. According to recent research, genetic dysregulation of the SOX9 gene prevents the SOX9 protein from properly regulating facial structure growth [33].

23.16 Proteus Syndrome (Wiedemann Syndrome)

Proteus syndrome is a rare disorder characterised by bone, skin, and other tissue overgrowth. The disease causes organs and tissues to expand out of proportion to the rest of the body. This was first described by Rogers and Temtamy in 1976. It is caused due to tissue overgrowth involving all three embryonic lineages. It is a condition linked to PTEN on chromosome 10 while other researches pointed to chromosome 16. Clinical features include deformation of the skull associated with facial abnormalities, hemifacial hypertrophy, exostosis in left parietal region, severe degenerative changes and deformities on the affected side of TMJ, and asymptomatic condylar malformation maybe seen associated with deviation at mouth opening [34].

23.17 Beckwith–Wiedemann Syndrome

Beckwith–Wiedemann syndrome is a congenital overgrowth condition characterised by an elevated risk of childhood cancer and some congenital features. It is normally present at birth. It is caused by a mutation in the 11p15.5 region of chromosome 11, which results in overactivity of the IGF-2 gene [growth factor] and/or no active copy of CDKN1C [cell proliferation inhibitor gene]. Relevant features include macrosomia, and hemihyperplasia of face leads to TMJ involvement [35].

23.18 Hurler Syndrome

Hurler syndrome is an autosomal recessive disease also known as mucopolysaccharidosis Type I (MPS Type I) caused by a defect in the structural gene in the lysosomal enzyme that degrades lipose aminoglycans. The enzyme for MPS I is α-L-iduronidase on 4p16.3. Clinically patient presents with a large head with frontal bossing, hypertelorism, heavy lids, low nasal bridge, snub nose, long philtrum and open mouth, characteristic craniofacial dysmorphism and physical habitus, failure of growth after infancy, skeletal abnormalities at around the age of 6 months, dysostosis multiplex, and histochemical and biochemical evidence of intracellular lysosomal storage of GAGs [11].

23.19 Trismus-Pseudocampylodactyly Syndrome (Hecht-Beals Syndrome)

This syndrome was first described by Hecht and Beals in 1969. It is also known as congenital contractural arachnodactyly. This condition is inherited as autosomal dominant with variable expressivity. It is a connective tissue disease caused by a mutation in the FBN2 [Fibrillin-2] gene on chromosome 5q23, which shares phenotypic features with Marfan's syndrome [36].

The patient is normally proportioned, but stature is often reduced to between third and 25th centiles. Blepharochalasis is seen in older individuals and a quilted appearance of the cheeks. The coronoid process maybe enlarged or distorted, unilaterally or bilaterally and is often responsible for the inability to open the mouth widely because of their impingement on the zygomatic bone. The decreased opening maybe secondary to shortening of the muscles of mastication, which in turn causes elongation of the coronoid processes. Syndrome is associated with abnormalities of the extremities that result from shortness of various skeletal muscles or flexor tendons.

23.20 Klippel–Trénaunay Syndrome

Klippel–Trénaunay Syndrome also known as angio-osteohypertrophy syndrome is a rare congenital medical condition where the blood vessels and/or lymph vessels fail to form properly. It is possible that a translocation at t[8;14] [q22.3;q13] is involved. Hypertrophy of bony and soft tissues may cause local gigantism or shrinkage, most commonly in the lower body. TMJ may be involved with hypertrophy of condyle. Superficial thrombophlebitis may be present [11].

23.21 Other Less Common Syndromes

23.21.1 Carey-Fineman-Ziter Syndrome (CFZS)

CFZS is an autosomal recessive inherited disorder involving a combination of hypotonia with Moebius sequence and Pierre Robin anomalad and delay in growth. TMJ involvement in patients diagnosed with this syndrome was reported by Pasetti M et al. [37].

23.21.2 PASH Syndrome

Pyoderma gangrenosum, Acne, Suppurative hidradenitis (PASH) syndrome is an auto-inflammatory disorder. It can be associated with several disorders such as inflammatory bowel disease, inflammatory arthritis, and malignancy. Jeffrey J et al. reported a case of TMJ ankylosis in a patient diagnosed with PASH syndrome. TMJ ankylosis is commonly evident in syndromes that are associated with infections [38].

23.22 Goals of Treatment

The prognosis in some of the conditions is guarded, but disability may drastically be with early diagnosis and available advanced treatment modalities. Correction or reconstruction of existing deformities may be the focus of treatment. If there is a suspicion, the patient should be tested regularly during infancy and adolescence. Any signs of mental illness, premature sexual development, general disturbance in the growth and development should be closely monitored. Management of syndromes, in general, mandates a multidisciplinary approach.

References

1. Smith D. Smith's recognizable patterns of human malformation. 6th ed. Philadelphia: Elsevier Saunders; 2006. p. 954.
2. Ghom AG, Mhaske JS. Syndromes of the orofacial region. In: Textbook of Oral pathology. New Delhi, India: Jaypee Brothers Medical Publishers [P] Ltd; 2013.
3. https://www.who.int/genomics/gender/en/index1.html
4. Zarb GA, Carlsson GE. Temporomandibular disorders: osteoarthritis. J Orofac Pain. 1999;13(4):295–306.
5. Laskin DM, Greenfield W, Gale E. The President's conference on the examination, diagnosis, and Management of Temporomandibular Disorders. Chicago: American Dental Association; 1983.
6. Okeson JP. Treatment of temporomandibular joint disorders. In Management of temporomandibular disorders and occlusion. 5th ed. St. Louis: Mosby; 2003. p. 413–435.
7. Rugh JD, Solberg WK. Oral health status in the United States: temporomandibular disorders. J Dent Educ. 1985;49(6):398–406.
8. Sarnat BG, Laskin DM. The temporomandibular joint: a biological basis for clinical practice. In: 4th ed. Philadelphia: WB Saunders; 1992. p. 163–178.
9. McNeill C. Craniomandibular disorders: guidelines for evaluation, diagnosis and management. Chicago: Quintessence; 1990. p. 25–9.
10. Galea CJ, Dashow JE, Woerner JE. Congenital abnormalities of the temporomandibular joint. Oral Maxillofac Surg Clin North Am. 2018;30(1):71–82.
11. DeLuke DM. Syndromes of the head and neck. Atlas of the Oral & Maxillofacial Surgery Clinics. 2014;22
12. Wiegel W. Diagnosis and therapy of myo-arthropathy [Costen's syndrome]. Laryngorhinootologie. 1990;69(7):373–7.
13. Alkhudhairy MW, Al Ramel F, Al Jader G, Al Saegh L, Al Hadad A, Alalwan T, et al. A self-reported association between temporomandibular joint disorders, headaches, and stress. J Int Soc Prev Community Dent. 2018;8(4):371–80.
14. Stechman-Neto J, Porporatti AL. Porto de Toledo I, costa YM, Conti PCR, De Luca canto G, et al. effect of temporomandibular disorder therapy on otologic signs and symptoms: a systematic review. J Oral Rehabil. 2016;43(6):468–79.
15. Pedroni CR, De Oliveira AS, Guaratini MI. Prevalence study of signs and symptoms of temporomandibular disorders in university students. J Oral Rehabil. 2003;30(3):283–9.
16. LeResche L, Mancl L, Sherman JJ, Gandara B, Dworkin SF. Changes in temporomandibular pain and other symptoms across the menstrual cycle. Pain. 2003;106(3):253–61.
17. Castori M. C. Voermans N. neurological manifestations of Ehlers-Danlos syndrome[s]: a review. Iran. J Neurol. 2014;13(4):190–208.
18. Gorlin RJ, Cohen MM, Hennekam RC, Cohen MM, Hennekam RC. Syndromes of the head and neck. 4th ed. New York: Oxford University Press; 2001.
19. Abel MD, Carrasco LR. Ehlers-Danlos syndrome: classifications, oral manifestations, and dental considerations. Oral Surg Oral Med Oral Pathol Oral Radiol Endod. 2006;102(5):582–90.
20. Beleza-Meireles A, Hart R, Clayton-Smith J, Oliveira R, Reis CF, Venâncio M, et al. Oculo-auriculo-vertebral spectrum: clinical and molecular analysis of 51 patients. Eur J Med Genet. 2015;58(9):455–65.
21. Barisic I, Odak L, Loane M, Garne E, Wellesley D, Calzolari E, et al. Prevalence, prenatal diagnosis and clinical features of oculo-auriculo-vertebral spectrum: a registry-based study in Europe. Eur J Hum Genet. 2014;22(8):1026–33.
22. Posnick JC, Tiwana PS, Costello BJ. Treacher Collins syndrome: comprehensive evaluation and treatment. Oral Maxillofac Surg Clin North Am. 2004;16(4):503–23.
23. https://rarediseases.org/search/rdbdetail_abstract.html
24. Ciurea A, Toader C. Alexandru & Toader, Corneliu. Genetics of craniosynostosis: review of the literature. J Med Life. 2009:5–17.
25. Eswarakumar VP, Horowitz MC, Locklin R, Morriss-Kay GM, Lonai P. A gain-of-function mutation of Fgfr2c demonstrates the roles of this receptor variant in osteogenesis. Proc Natl Acad Sci U S A. 2004;101(34):12555–60.
26. Pal US, Gupta C, Chellappa AAL. Crouzon syndrome with primary optic nerve atrophy and normal brain functions: a case report. J Oral Biol Craniofac Res. 2012;2(2):116–8.
27. Rukavina I. SAPHO syndrome: a review. J Child Orthop. 2015;9(1):19–27.
28. Khanna L, El-khoury GY. SAPHO syndrome – a pictorial assay. Iowa Orthop J. 2012;32:189–95.
29. Capote A, Rodríguez FJ, Blasco A, Muñoz MF. Jacob's disease associated with temporomandibular joint dysfunction: a case report. Med Oral Patol Oral Cir Bucal. 2005;10(3):210–4.
30. Diaz A, Danon M, Crawford J. McCune-Albright syndrome and disorders due to activating mutations of GNAS1. J Pediatr Endocrinol Metab. 2007;20(8):853–80.
31. Whyte MP. Chapter 68 - hereditary disorders of the skeleton∗ chapter titles shaded in green indicate

chapters dedicated predominantly to pediatric endocrinology content. In: Jameson JL, De Groot LJ, de Kretser DM, Giudice LC, Grossman AB, Melmed S, et al., editors. Endocrinology: adult and Pediatric. 7th ed. Philadelphia: W.B. Saunders; 2016. p. 1173–1183.e4. [cited 2019 Oct 15]. Retrieved from: http://www.sciencedirect.com/science/article/pii/B9780323189071000688.
32. Ward LM, Rauch F, Travers R, Roy M, Montes J, Chabot G, et al. Osteopathia striata with cranial sclerosis: clinical, radiological, and bone histological findings in an adolescent girl. Am J Med Genet A. 2004;15:8–12.
33. Gangopadhyay N, Mendonca DA, Woo AS. Pierre Robin sequence. Semin Plast Surg. 2012;26(2):76–82.
34. Chakrabarti N, Chattopadhyay C, Bhuban M, Pal SK. Proteus syndrome: a rare cause of gigantic limb. Indian Dermatol Online J. 2014;5(2):193.
35. Shuman C, Beckwith JB, Weksberg R. Beckwith-Wiedemann syndrome. In: Adam MP, Ardinger HH, Pagon RA, Wallace SE, Bean LJ, Stephens K, et al., editors. GeneReviews®. Seattle, WA: University of Washington; 1993. [cited 2019 Oct 15]. Retrieved from http://www.ncbi.nlm.nih.gov/books/NBK1394/.
36. Viljoen D. Congenital contractural arachnodactyly [Beals syndrome]. J Med Genet. 1994;31(8):640–3.
37. Pasetti M, Mazzoleni F, Novelli G, Iascone M, Bozzetti A, Selicorni A. Temporomandibular joint ankylosis as part of the clinical spectrum of Carey–Fineman– Ziter syndrome? Am J Med Genet Part A. 2016;9999A:1–5.
38. Wargo JJ, Emmer BT. Systemic inflammation gone away: PASH syndrome and TMJ ankylosis. Am J Med. 2015;129(4):e1–3.

24 Paediatric Temporomandibular Joint Disorders

Parimala Tyagi, Rahul Hegde, and Nikita Agrawal

24.1 Introduction

Temporomandibular joint disorders (TMDs) in paediatric patient often go unnoticed. This impact is not only an unpleasant experience but poignant psychological aspect of a child. Dentist's aptitude can detect the early signs and symptoms of TMDs, facilitating agile resolution and forbid its progression. The potential inoperability of a child to commemorate the symptoms like location and nature of pain lead to a non-definitive history. Henceforth clinical examination plays a key role in the diagnosis. It includes palpation of masticatory musculature, temporomandibular joint (TMJ) and related structures. Comprehension of the condition provides adequate referral to appropriate health provider, reducing in frequency of consultation and investigations [1]. Recommendations for recognition and diagnosis of TMDs in infants, children and adolescents were given by Clinical Affairs Committee on Temporomandibular Joint Problems in Children in 1990 and was revised in 2019 [2, 3].

P. Tyagi (✉) · N. Agrawal
Department of Pediatric Dentistry, People's College of Dental Sciences and Research Centre, Bhopal, Madhya Pradesh, India

R. Hegde
D Y Patil College of Dental Sciences, Pune, Maharashtra, India

24.2 Epidemiology

Non-odontogenic origin of pain in orofacial region may be commonly associated with TMDs. The prevalence of TMD in paediatric patients varies widely in the scientific literature. This variation accounts on the diversity of the patient, diagnostic aids, examination tools and examiner's variability [3]. Contemporary lifestyle inclined to higher level of stress which brace in consequently developing various parafunctional habits such as clenching of teeth afflicting muscular circulation and accumulation of lactic acid, provoking pain receptors [4]. Additionally, variability could be because of treating children in their growing years. Numerous epidemiological studies in the last two decades suggested prevalence of TMD is more between 10–18 years of age followed by children of 5–7 years. Prevalence of signs and symptom in TMD varies in the age group of 6 to 22 years with 20–74% presenting with symptoms and 22–68% demostrating signs [5]. Prevalence of particular gender varies less in early childhood; however, in late adolescent female preponderance is documented [1]. The possible reason quoted was its association with the onset of puberty in girls [3]. TMD in the age group of 16–19 years, girls reported 32.5% prevalence when compared to boys with 9.7% prevalence [6].

D. Bhargava (ed.), *Temporomandibular Joint Disorders*,
https://doi.org/10.1007/978-981-16-2754-5_24

Contemporary protocol for "Diagnostic Criteria" (DC) in TMD was advocated to minimise the variability in the diagnosis [3]. Following this, paediatric researchers highlighted that around 11.9% prevalence of TMDs exists amongst adolescents [7]. Age wise prevalence according to DC was reported as 5–9% in 10–15-year-old whilst in another study it was 4.2% in the age group of 12–19 years [8, 9]. A meta-analysis on intra-articular TMDs revealed 16% prevalence of signs and 14% presented with temporomandibular joint (TMJ) sounds [10].

24.3 Aetiology

TMDs are multi-factorial in origin with unpredictability in its progression. The predisposing factors include macro-trauma (any external injury leading to soft tissue or bony injury to the joint), micro-trauma (due to para-functional habits like sleep bruxism), anatomical factors (skeletal or occlusal including skeletal anterior open bite, steep articular eminence, skeletal class II or III profile, posterior crossbite and deep bite), post-orthodontic treatment alterations, psychosocial factors (obsessive compulsive disorder, stress, anxiety etc.), systemic condition (rheumatoid, psoriatic or juvenile idiopathic arthritis; hormonal alterations and associated syndromes), genetic or congenital abnormalities (hemifacial microsomia, pharyngeal arch defects) [3, 11].

24.4 Diagnosis

Amalgamation of history, clinical examination, and TMJ imaging aids in arriving at a proper diagnosis for TMDs. Most common symptoms include headache, pain on mastication, ear pain, TMJ click/pop, locking and restricted joint movements [3, 5]. Whilst taking history, other common conditions should be ruled out like trigeminal neuralgia, otitis media, allergies, congestion in airway etc. [3]. In clinical examination, evaluating mandibular range of motion (ROM) for mandibular mobility which can be grossly noted by placing 3 fingers vertically between the upper and lower incisors. Normal value ranges from 35 to 45 mm. Besides this, evaluation of excursive mandibular movements (placement of lower jaw sideways) should also be done. It normally ranges from 8–10 mm. Any pain, discomfort, deviation, deflection or locking associated with mandibular movements should be noted (Refer Chap. 6).

24.4.1 Palpation of Muscles

Preliminary evaluation for tenderness should be noted by applying pressure on the temporalis and masseter muscle bilaterally on clenching. Detailed examination of various muscles is described in Chap. 6.

24.4.2 Palpation of TMJ

Joint may be palpated by placing the index finger in the pre-auricular area in front of the tragus and patient is instructed to execute the joint movements by opening and closing the mouth. This helps in evaluating the synchronised movement, presence of click or a pop and crepitus or grating sounds. Joint sounds are best heard using a stethoscope [1] (Refer Chap. 6).

24.4.3 TMJ Imaging

According to American Academy of Paediatric Dentistry (AAPD) 2019, the temporomandibular joint may be evaluated using following imaging modalities: panoramic radiographs, radiographs of the mandible in lateral oblique view, computed tomography (CT), cone-beam computed tomography (CBCT), magnetic resonance imaging (MRI) and ultrasonography (USG) [3] (Refer Chap. 7).

24.5 Embryology of TMJ

TMJ is the last joint to develop starting at the seventh week in utero. First evidence of TMJ appears as two mesenchymal blastemas in the region of future glenoid fossa. Condyle starts developing lateral and superior to Meckel's cartilage at tenth week in utero. From the condylar blastema, the mandibular condylar cartilage is derived, along with the lateral pterygoid muscle aponeurosis, disc and the capsule forming the lower joint compartment. The temporal blastema forms articular surface of the temporal bone and forms the upper compartment of the joint. Both condylar and temporal blastemas begin to grow and move towards each other by 10–12th week in utero. The disc develops by migration of the mesenchymal cells. Initially the disc is highly cellular which progressively becomes fibrous and at 14th week in utero a thin intermediate zone is formed with a thickened periphery. Postnatally, articular surface is covered by the fibrous connective tissue which is later converted to fibrocartilage. Remodelling leads to deepening of temporal fossa and increase in posterior slope of the articular tubercle [12] (Refer Chap. 3).

24.6 Classification

Kaneyama et al. classified developmental disturbances of the temporomandibular joint as [12, 13].

1. Hypoplasia or aplasia of the condyle
   - Congenital or primary hypoplasia or aplasia
   - Acquired or secondary hypoplasia or aplasia
2. Condylar hyperplasia
3. Bifid condyle

According to American Academy of Paediatric Dentistry (AAPD) 2019, TMDs are classified as under by dividing them into two broad categories, TMJ disorders and masticatory muscles disorders: [3].

I. TMJ disorders
   (A) Joint pain:
      1. Arthralgia
      2. Arthritis
   (B) Joint disorders:
      1. Disc-condyle complex disorders (disc displacement with reduction, disc displacement with reduction with intermittent locking, disc displacement without reduction with limited mouth opening, disc displacement without reduction without limited mouth opening)
      2. Hypomobility disorders (ankylosis, fibrous adhesions)
      3. Hypermobility disorders (subluxation, luxation)
   (C) Joint diseases:
      1. Osteoarthritis (degenerative joint disease, condylysis/idiopathic condylar resorption, osteochondritis dissecans, osteonecrosis)
      2. Systemic arthritides (rheumatoid arthritis,idiopathic juvenile arthritis, spondyloarthropathies, psoriatic arthritis, infections arthritis, Reiter syndrome, and crystal induced disease)
      3. Neoplasms
      4. Condylar fractures

II. Masticatory muscle disorders:
   (A) Muscle pain limited to orofacial region (myalgia, myofascial pain with spreading, myofascial pain with referral, tendonitis, myositis, spasm)
   (B) Muscle pain due to systemic/central disorders (centrally mediated myalgia, fibromyalgia)
   (C) Movement disorders (dyskinesia, dystonia)
   (D) Others: contracture, hypertrophy, neoplasm

24.7 Congenital Hypoplasia/Aplasia

Congenital hypoplasia: Under or non-development of the condyle is usually found in association with various craniofacial abnormalities. It may be unilateral or bilateral underdevelopment usually resulting as a part of a systemic condition affecting the first and second branchial arches. Congenital condylar aplasia or hypoplasia may be divided into five subtypes: (1) Mandibulofacial dysostosis (Treacher Collins syndrome), (2) Hemifacial macrosomia (first and second branchial arch syndrome), (3) Oculoauriculovertebral syndrome (Goldenhar syndrome), (4) Oculomandibulodyscephaly (Hallermann–Streiff syndrome), and (5) Hurler's syndrome.

Mandibulofacial dysostosis (MFD) is a rare syndrome, with an autosomal dominant inheritance caused by aberrations during histodifferentiation morphogenesis at 12th week in utero. Gene involved is TCOF1 which encodes for Nucleolar Phosphoprotein Treacle. It is characterised by bilateral deformity, convex facial profile, hypoplastic zygoma, maxilla and mandible. Retruded chin results in a fish or a bird like morphological appearnace. The eyes appears to have a lateral downward sloping palpebral fissures and the external ear may be malformed, absent or malposed with impaired hearing [12]. As a part of the correction for the deformity, these patients require reconstruction of the ramus condyle unit, malar augmentation, oto-oculoplastic interventions, orthognathic with orthodontic interceptive and corrective procedures [11].

Hemifacial microsomia (HFM) is the second most common congenital deformity after cleft lip and palate affecting 1 in 5600 live births. It is characterised by asymmetric mandible with affected side appears to be short, premature contact of dentoalveolar arches on the affected side results in an open bite on the unaffected side. The chin is deviated and the hypoplastic muscles and the soft tissues results in a facial deformity. It also causes obstruction in the growth of maxilla resulting in a short maxilla on the affected side with an upward occlusal cant. HFM is classified as: Type I skeletal deformity with micrognathia (TMJ with well formed structures and the range of motion is normal), Type II skeletal deformity with malformed mandible and TMJ; further divided into II-A (hypoplasia of the TMJ is mild with acceptable movements); II-B (hypoplastic TMJ with medial, anterior and inferior displacement as compared to the normal side), Type III complete absence of the ramus and the TMJ along with hypoplastic or absence of muscles of mastication and the articular disc.

The soft tissue defects include hypoplasia of the muscles of mastication and facial expression, facial clefts, restricted soft palate movement and altered external ear anatomy which vary in degree from mild to severe [11, 13, 14]. Neuromuscular defects are present in 25% or more cases consisting of facial palsy, deviation of the soft palate, and facial nerve weakness. The severity of the anomalies in HM is described by OMENS classification which scores the involvement of the orbit, mandible, ears, nerves, and soft tissues [15, 16]. The patients with greater OMENS score should be evaluated for skeletal, renal and cardiac anomalies [11].

Oculoauriculovertebral syndrome (OAVS) is a variant of hemifacial microsomia characterised by asymmetric hypoplastic mandible and the deformity in the vertebra. It is a consequence of deletion of 5q, trisomy of 18 and duplication of 7q [12]. The shift in arterial supply during development of the branchial arches might sometime cause haematoma that can result in branchial dysplasia. Implicated aetiological factors may be unkonwn or may include ingestion of tobacco, primidone, retinoic acid, thalidomide or infection like rubella, influenza or maternal diabetes. The hallmarks are ear deformity (Fig. 24.1), epibulbar dermoids and underdeveloped maxillo-mandibular complex with associated vertebral defect [12, 17].

Oculomandibulodyscephaly is a rare congenital disorder characterised by bird like face, congenital cataract with micro-ophthalmia. It is caused by single gene mutation or any abnormality in elastin and glycoprotein metabolism [12]. According to François, cardinal signs include dicephaly, bird face appearance, dental abnormalities, hypotrichosis, skin atrophy, bilateral congenital cataract with micro-ophthalmia, open fontanelles, and dwarfism with frontal and parietal bossing. Oral manifestations include microstomia, microglossia with glossoptosis, hypoplastic mandible with forward displacement

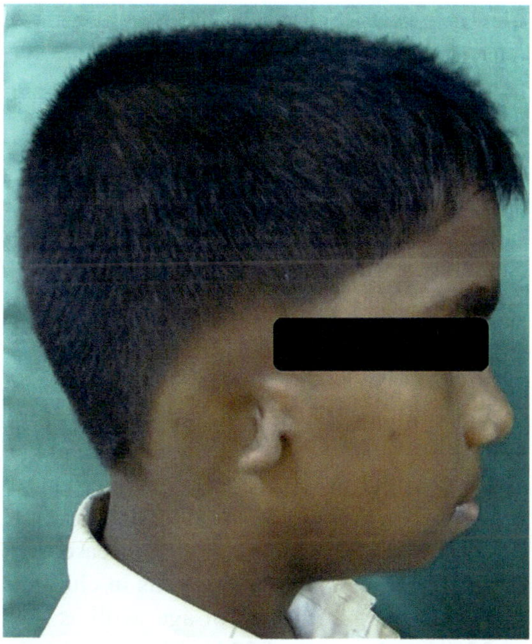

Fig. 24.1 Note the ear deformity in a patient diagnosed with characteristics of Goldenhar syndrome. (Image courtesy: Dr. Darpan Bhargava, India)

of the mandibuar condyle, high arched palate, open bite with class II molar relationship, tooth anomalies like oligodontia, supernumerary teeth and hypomineralised teeth leading to high caries risk [18–21].

Hurler's syndrome is a rare inborn defect in muco-polysaccharide metabolism called as mucopolysaccharidosis (MPS). It is characterised by mental and physical growth retardation, corneal defects, gargoyle like face, cat like back and limited growth of the mandible with restricted movements [12]. Its incidence is about in a range of 1:25,000 to 1:100,000 [22].

Maxillofacial manifestations include hypoplastic condyle causing trismus, wide maxilla and mandible because of macroglossia. Macroglossia occurs because of accumulation of degraded glycosaminoglycans (GAGs) in the tongue [12]. Radiographic presence of multiple rosettes in the developing dental follicle is characteristic of the disease [22, 23]. Although this condition is incurable, but with a multidisciplinary approach the quality of life may be improved [12].

24.8 Acquired Hypoplasia

Acquired or secondary hypoplasia may affect one or both the mandibular condyles. The factors affecting the growth of the condyle may include injury to the growing condyle, infection of the joint or the middle ear and childhood arthritis. The normal growth of the mandible depends significantly on the normal development and the function of mandibular condyles along with its associated soft tissues. In unilateral condylar hypoplasia, the sustained growth of the contralateral side causes deviation towards the affected side and results in a cross-bite. The ramus and the body of the mandible remain under-developed on the affected side. In cases with bilateral condylar hypoplasia, severe micrognathia would be evident with the crowding of the teeth. Anterior open bite may be a presenting feature [12, 24, 25].

24.9 Condylar Hyperplasia

Alterations in the growth pattern of the mandibular condyle during the normal growth period may result in condylar hyperplasia (CH). Condylar hyperplasia is characterized by the gradual enlargement of the mandibular condyle, usually a progressive unilateral enlargement of the mandible, facial asymmetry, and shifting of the midline of the chin to the unaffected side, with resultant cross-bite and malocclusion. Patients report at the age range of 10 to 30 years. The initiation of the hyperplastic process occurs in the growing condyle, with variable presentation of the deformity with age. The investigation of choice is technetium 99 m diphosphonate bone scan where increased uptake of the radionuclide is detected in the affected condyle [11, 26–28]. Depending on the age of initiation and the time of presentation the signs and symptoms may include unilateral condylar elongation, temporomandibular joint pain and dysfunction, facial asymmetry, chin deviation, mandibular prognathism, posterior crossbite and open bite, canting of the occlusal plane, masticatory dysfunction, and malocclusion.

Treatment: The treatment options include high condylectomy, compensatory orthodontics, surgical cosmetic camouflage and orthognathic surgery depending on the time of intervention, degree of facial asymmetry and the age of the patient [11, 27].

24.10 Bifid Mandibular Condyle

Bifid mandibular condyle is a rare condition characterized by a division of the mandibular condylar head. The etiology of bifid condyle is largely unknown, although various factors have been suggested as possible causes like endocrine disturbances, exposure to teratogens, nutritional deficiencies, infection, radiation or the obstructed blood supply during the development. Blackwood stated that the condylar cartilage during the early stages of development is divided by well-vascularized fibrous septa. He suggested that persistence of this type of septum in exaggerated form within the growing cartilage might lead to an error in development. But existence of such a septa is controversial. Gundlach et al. proposed that the bifid condyle is a form of embryopathy caused by a combination of a teratogenic agent and misdirection of muscle fibres, which then influences bone formation [29, 39] (Fig. 24.2a and b).

24.11 Common Acquired Abnormalities of Temporomandibular Joint in Children and Adolescents

24.11.1 Juvenile Idiopathic Arthritis

Juvenile idiopathic arthritis (JIA or Juvenile RA or Still disease) is a rheumatic disease of childhood that presents with no symptoms or very mild symptoms in most cases. Juvenile arthritis is a long-lasting, chronic disease. It is the most common form of arthritis in children. JIA starts before 16 years of age, with as high as 87% involvement of TMJ. TMJ may be the only joint involved with JIA. If a child's joints are swollen for 6 weeks in a row or longer, the suspicion of juvenile arthritis should be raised. The initial findings may be limited range of motion and asymmetry of the mandible from abnormal craniofacial growth. Bilateral TMJ involvement may result in progressive Class II

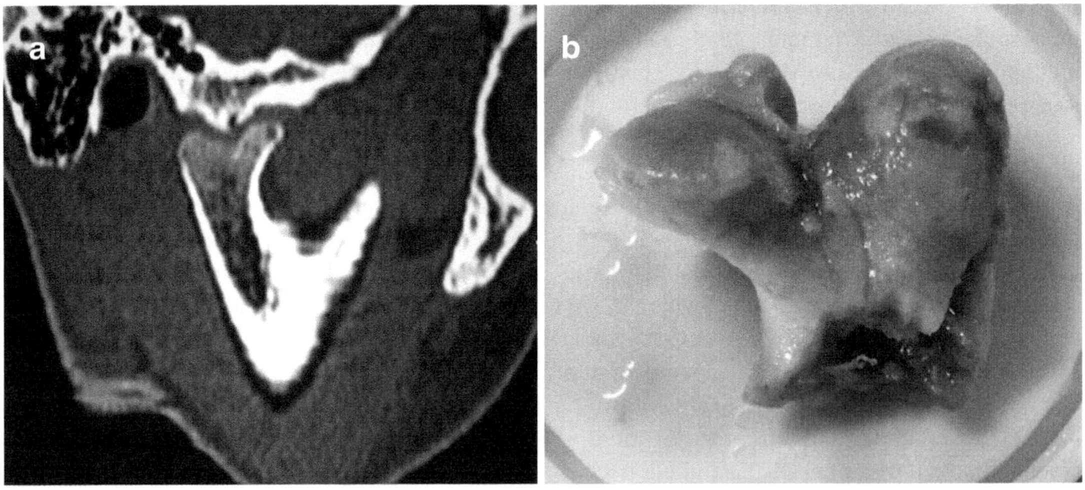

Fig. 24.2 (**a**) Computed tomography scan demonstrating a bifid mandibular condyle; (**b**) Resected condylectomy specimen of the bifid condyle. (Adapted with permission from Neelakandan R S and Darpan Bhargava. "Bifid hyperplastic mandibular condyle." Journal of maxillofacial and oral surgery vol. 12,4 (2013): 466–71. https://doi.org/10.1007/s12663-011-0257-2)

malocclusion and apertognathia due to loss of ramal height secondary to condylar destruction (bird face deformity) and ankylosis later. Further, the condition may interfere with proper oral hygiene, leading to dental caries (Refer Chap. 5).

24.11.2 Idiopathic Condylar Resorption

Idiopathic Condylar Resorption (ICR) is a condition characterized by progressive change in the shape and decrease in the volume of the mandibular condyle, which usually go unnoticed as the patient remains asymptomatic. The clinical features include a marked reduction in posterior facial height, progressive anterior open bite (with clockwise rotation of the mandible) and retrognathism.

ICR is also referred as "cheerleader syndrome". The aetiology of the condition is still unexplained but various systemic conditions (systemic lupus erythematosus, rheumatoid arthritis and neoplasia), altered vascularity to the condyle, external forces to the joint resultant to trauma and orthodontic or orthognathic treatment may be considered as triggering factors. ICR is highly prevalent in females with the age range of 15 to 35 years (rarely develops after 20 years of age) and commonly affect both the joints. Predisposition for ICR includes, female sex; age range from 10 to 20 years, with a strong predilection for teenagers in their pubertal growth phase; high occlusal plane angle and mandibular plane angle (dolicocephalic) facial morphology; and predominance of class II skeletal (retruded lower jaw) and occlusal relationships with or without open bite.

On radiographic examination the joint space appears to have increased and there is a decrease in volume of the affected condyle. In cases of active ICR, surgical removal of the hyperplastic synovial tissue should be performed which may be accompanied with the reconstruction of the condyle with a costochondral graft. In inactive cases or after cessation of the active phase of the condition, secondary skeletal correction surgery (sagittal split osteotomy) and orthodontic intervention may be required to correct the subsequent deformities [3, 5, 11, 41].

24.11.3 TMJ Ankylosis

Ankylosis is a Greek term meaning a "stiff joint". Temporomandibular joint ankylosis is defined as a union of mandibular condyle to the cranial base. This fusion may be osseous or fibrous, with partial or complete impediment of mandibular function [35]. The common causes for TMJ ankylosis in children are forceps delivery (uncommon now), trauma, or any accidental fall leading to joint hemarthrosis. Children with a history of fall or an injury to the chin or the mandible, with a complaint of a progressive reduction in the mouth opening should be evaluated thoroughly and followed up closely to intervene at an appropriate time. Other causes may include arthritis, and ear or joint infections. The implicated mechanism of congenital TMJ ankylosis is proposed to be because of an early fusion of embryonic mesenchyme, abnormal development of stapedial artery, hyper vitaminosis of vitamin A or loss of neural crest cells [36]. The abnormality in mouth opening at birth, should be diffentiated from a rare but documented condition, **Syngnathia** or fusion of the jaws (Fig. 24.3a, b and c). Maxillomandibular fusion (syngnathia) is a rare craniofacial anomaly which can be either fibrous (synechiae) or bony (synostosis) fusion of the jaws or fusion of mandible to zygoma, tuberosity, hard palate and temporal bone [40]. Clinical presentation in cases of ankylosis may show nil to limited mouth opening with a progessive facial deformity in childern as they grow. Other findings at the time of presentation may include facial asymmetry, malocclusion and compromised mastication leading to malnourishment [36]. The various surgical techniques documented for the treatment of TMJ ankylosis include gap arthroplasty with or without interposition (Fig. 24.4a–f), joint reconstruction using costochondral graft or alloplastic joints and distraction osteogenesis. These patients may require definitive corrective orthognathic, morphometric and orthodontic procedures for the correction of the established

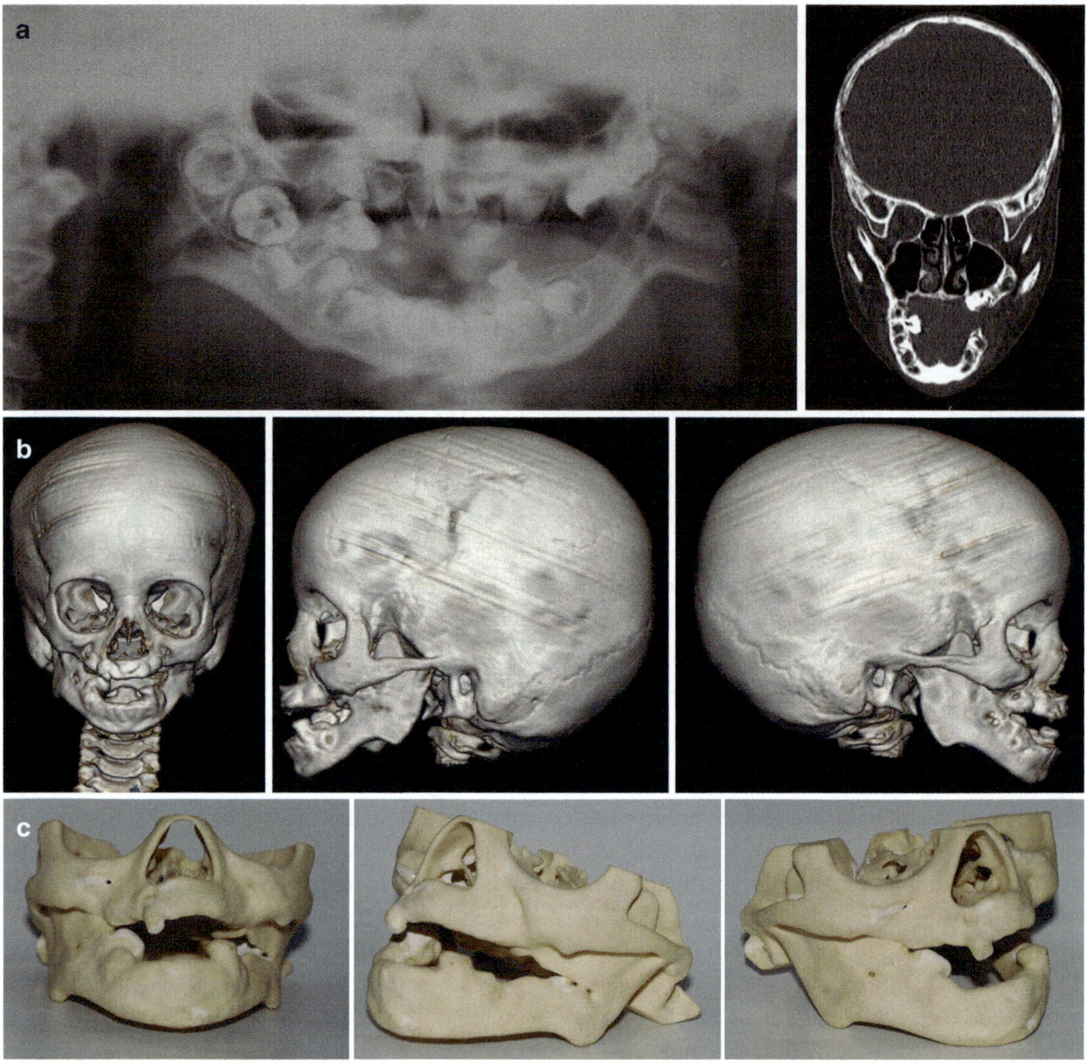

Fig. 24.3 Patient with congenital maxillomandibular syngnathia, reported at the age of 6 years (**a**) Orthopantomogram and a coronal section of a computed tomography scan; (**b**) 3D reconstructed images of the computed tomography scan; (**c**) Stereolithographic models of the patient. (Image courtesy: Dr. Darpan Bhargava, TMJ Consultancy, Bhopal, Madhya Pradesh, India)

secondary facial deformity and occlusal aberrancies [37, 38] (Refer Chap. 17).

24.12 Conclusion

Comprehensive history including documentation of pain, mandibular malfunctioning, any previous trauma or systemic ailment followed by detailed examination of the temporomandibular joint should be executed in pediatric patients reporting with the problems of the joint (Refer Chap. 6). The incidence of conditions involving condyle-disc conflict is reportedly increasing in younger age groups and should be considered as one of the important disorders that needs attention of the clinicians in adolescence. Evidence supports that the pain disorders including facial myalgia and disc derangement of

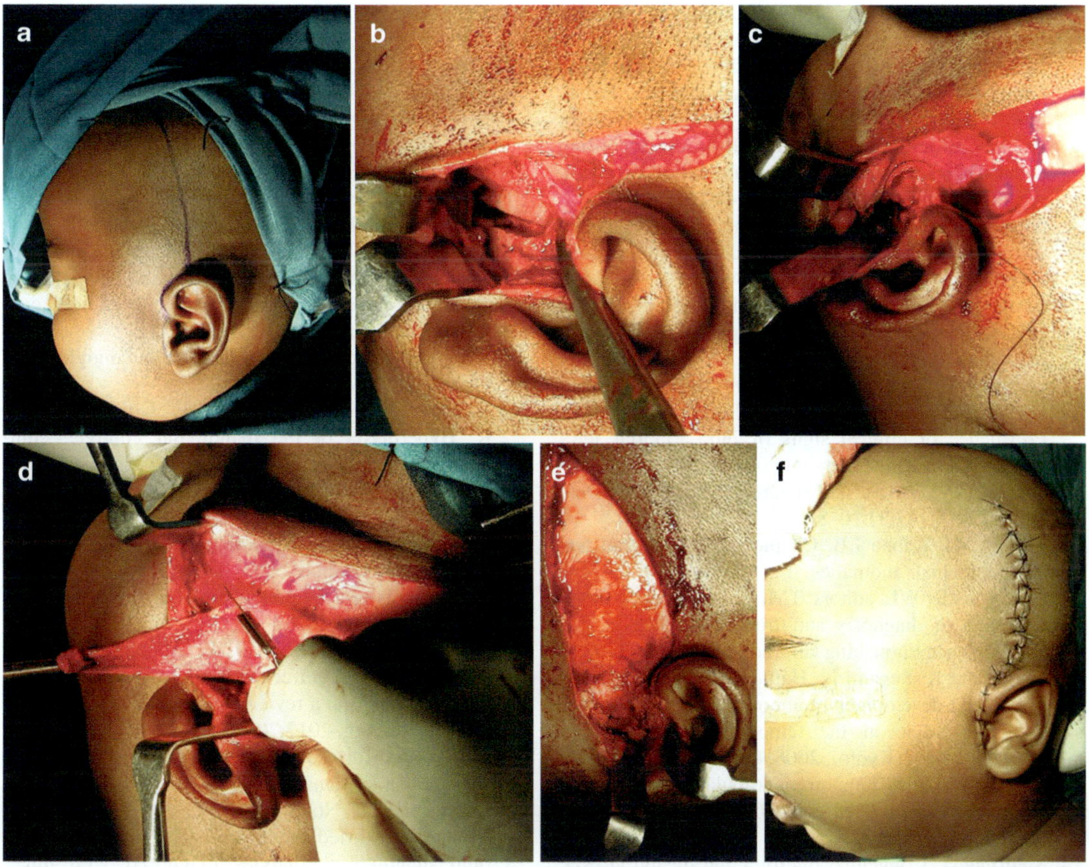

Fig. 24.4 Paediatric patient with temporomandibular joint ankylosis; (**a**) marking for a preauricular incision with temporal extension; (**b**) osteotomy for ankylosis release; (**c**) gap arthroplasty defect; (**d**) temporalis myofascial flap for interpositioning; (**e**) Gap arthroplasty defect interpositioned with temporalis myofascial flap; (**f**) closure of the surgical site. (Image courtesy: Dr. Darpan Bhargava, TMJ Consultancy, Bhopal, Madhya Pradesh, India)

the joint are associated with significant psychological or psychosocial disturbances in youngsters, coping with the modern lifestyle patterns. (Refer Chap. 15, for management of these disorders) Related factors like anxiety, depression and stress should be evaluated, especially in adolescents (Refer Chap. 8). Presentation of the TMDs and there management options surround with controversies thereby evidence based treatment protocols should be followed in order to avoid unfavourable consequences.

Acknowledgements Editor, Dr. Darpan Bhargava MDS, MOMS RCPS (Glasg.), PGDHM, Ph.D, Maxillofacial Surgery, TMJ Consultancy Services, Bhopal, Madhya Pradesh, India for providing the clinical data.

References

1. Howard JA. Temporomandibular joint disorders in children. Dent Clin N Am. 2013;57:99–127.
2. American Academy of Pediatric Dentistry. Guidelines for temporomandibular disorders in children and adolescents. Chicago, IL: American Academy of Pediatric Dentistry; 1990.
3. American Academy of Pediatric Dentistry. Acquired Temporomandibular Disorders in Infants, Children, and Adolescents, Pediatr Dent. 2019:379–86.
4. Minghelli B, Cardoso I, Porfírio M, Gonçalves R, Cascalheiro S, Barreto V, Soeiro A, Almeida L. Prevalence of temporomandibular disorder in children and adolescents from public schools in southern Portugal. N Am J Med Sci. 2014 Mar;6(3):126–32.
5. Okeson JP. Temporomandibular disorders in children. Pediatr Dent. 1989;11(4):325–9.

6. Nilsson IM, Drangholt M, List T. Impact of temporomandibular disorder pain in adolescents: differences by age and gender. J Orofac Pain. 2009;23(2):115–22.
7. Graue AM, Jokstad A, Assmus J, Skeie MS. Prevalence among adolescents in Bergen, Western Norway, of temporomandibular disorders according to the DC/ TMD criteria and examination protocol. Acta Odontol Scand. 2016;74(6):449–55.
8. Nilsson IM. Reliability, validity, incidence and impact of temporomandibular pain disorders in adolescents. Swed Dent J Suppl. 2007;183:7–86.
9. Bonjardim LR, Gavião MB, Carmagnani FG, Pereira LF, Castelo PM. Signs and symptoms of temporomandibular joint dysfunction in children with primary dentition. J Clin Pediatr Dent. 2003;28(1):53–8.
10. Da Silva CG, Pacheco-Pereira C, Porporatti AL, et al. Prevalence of clinical signs of intra-articular temporomandibular disorders in children and adolescents a systematic review and meta-analysis. J Am Dent Assoc. 2016;147(1):10–8.
11. Troulis MJ, Kaban LB. Chapter: 29 congenital and developmental anomalies. In: Laskin DM, Greene CS, Hylander WL, editors. TMDS: an evidence-based approach to diagnosis and treatment. Batavia, IL: Quintessence Publishing Co, Inc.; 2006. p. 762–98.
12. Kaneyama K, Segami N, Hatta T. Congenital deformities and developmental abnormalities of the mandibular condyle in the temporomandibular joint. CongenitAnom (Kyoto). 2008;48(3):118–25.
13. Dergin G. Aktop. Temporomandibular joint disorders in children and related comorbidities. J Arthritis S. 2014;3(1):1–4.
14. Meurman Y. Congenital microtia and meatal atresia; observations and aspects of treatment. AMA Arch Otolaryngol 1957;66:443–463.
15. Vento AR, LaBrie RA, Mulliken JB. OMENS classification of hemifacial microsomia. Cleft Palate J. 1989;28:68–76.
16. Mulliken JB, Ferraro NF, Vento AR. A retrospective analysis of growth of the constructed condyleramus in children with hemifacial microsomia. Cleft Palate J. 1989;26:312–7.
17. Subramaniam P, Girish Babu KL, Jayasurya S, Prahalad D. Dental management of a child with Goldenhar syndrome. Eur J Gen Dent. 2014;3:158–62.
18. Francois J. A new syndrome; dyscephalia with bird face and dental anomalies, nanism, hypotrichosis, cutaneous atrophy, microphthalmia, and congenital cataract. AMA Arch Ophthalmol 1958;60:842–862.
19. François J, Pierard J. The François dyscephalic syndrome and skin manifestations. Am J Ophthalmol 1971;71:1241–1250.
20. Gungor OE, Nur BZ, Yalcin H, Karayilmaz H, Mihci E. Comprehensive dental management in a Hallermann–Streiff syndrome patient with unusual radiographic appearance of teeth. Niger J Clin Pract. 2015;18(4):559–62.
21. Ohtsuki K, Ohnishi M, Watai Y, Yoshida M. Surgical correction of the mandible with genioplasty using a porous hydroxyapatite block graft for Hallermann-Streiff syndrome: a case report. Oral Medicine & Pathology. 2003;8(2):51–4.
22. Yoon JH, Lee HI, Jang JH, et al. Oral manifestation and root canal therapy of the patient with mucopolysaccharidosis. Restor Dent Endod. 2019;44(2): 1–12.
23. Sharma S, Sabharwal JR, Datta P, Sood S. Clinical manifestation of hurler syndrome in a 7 year old child. Contemp Clin Dent. 2012 Jan–Mar;3(1):86–9.
24. Shivhare P, Shankarnarayan L. Usha, Kumar M, Sowbhagya, MB. Condylar aplasia and hypoplasia: a rare case. Hindawi publishing corporation: case reports in. Dentistry. 2013:1–5.
25. Krogstad O. Aplasia of the mandibular condyle. Eur J Orthod. 1997;19(5):483–9.
26. Villanueva-Alcojol L, Monje F, González-García R. Hyperplasia of the mandibular condyle: clinical, histopathologic, and treatment considerations in a series of 36 patients. J Oral MaxillofacSurg. 2011;69:447–55.
27. Olate S, Netto HD, Chessa JR, Alister JP, Barbosa JA, Moraes M. Mandible condylar hyperplasia: a review of diagnosis and treatment protocol. Int J Clin Exp Med. 2013;6(9):727–37.
28. Raijmakers P, Karssemakers L, Tuinzing D. Female predominance and effect of gender on unilateral condylar hyperplasia: a review and meta-analysis. J Oral Maxillofac Surg. 2012;70:72–6.
29. Ferreres JB, Torres AS, Escoda CG. Bifid mandibular condyles: a systematic review. Med Oral Patol Oral Cir Bucal. 2018 Nov 1;23(6):672–80.
30. Tanner JM, Friedlander AH, Chang TI. Bilateral bifid mandibular condyles diagnosed with three-dimensional reconstruction. Dento Maxillofac Radiol. 2012;41(8):691–5.
31. Stoll ML, Cron RQ. Temporomandibular joint arthritis in juvenile idiopathic arthritis: the last frontier. Int J Clin Rheumatol. 2015;10(4):273–86.
32. Koos B, Twilt M, Kyank U, Fischer-Brandies H, Gassling V, Tzaribachev N. Reliability of clinical symptoms in diagnosing temporomandibular joint arthritis in juvenile idiopathic arthritis. J Rheumatol. 2014;41(9):1871–7.
33. Li LC, Scudds RA, Heck CS, Harth M. The efficacy of dexamethasone iontophoresis for the treatment of rheumatoid arthritic knees: a pilot study. Arthritis Care Res. 1996;9(2):126–32.
34. Pedersen TK, Carlaberta V. Functional and orthopaedic treatment in developing dentofacial growth deviation in juvenile idiopathic arthritis. Semin Orthod. 2015;21(2):134–9.
35. de Andrade LHR, Cavalcante MAA, Raymundo R, de Souza IPR. Temporomandibular joint ankylosis in children. J Dent Child. 2009;76:41–5.
36. Bello SD, Olokun BA, Olaitan AA, Ajike SO. Aetiology and presentation of ankylosis of the temporomandibular joint: report of 23 cases from Abuja, Nigeria. Br J Oral Maxillofac Surg. 2012;50:80–4.
37. Mabongo M. Temporomandibular joint ankylosis in children. J Dent Med Sci. 2013;12(5):35–41.

38. Cho JW, Park JH, Kim JW, Kim SJ. The sequential management of recurrent temporomandibular joint ankylosis in a growing child: a case report. Maxillofac Plast Reconstr Surg. 2016 Oct 5;38(1):39.
39. Neelakandan RS, Bhargava D. Bifid hyperplastic mandibular condyle. J Maxillofac Oral Surg. 2013;12(4):466–71. https://doi.org/10.1007/s12663-011-0257-2.
40. Kumar V, Rattan V, Rai S. Congenital Maxillo-mandibular Syngnathia: Review of Literature and Proposed New Classification System. J Maxillofac Oral Surg. 2021 Mar;20(1):19–36. https://doi.org/10.1007/s12663-019-01308-8.
41. Wolford LM. Idiopathic condylar resorption of the temporomandibular joint in teenage girls (cheerleaders syndrome). Proc (Bayl Univ Med Cent). 2001;14(3):246–52. https://doi.org/10.1080/08998280.2001.11927772.

Complications with Temporomandibular Joint Surgery

25

Vishal Bansal, Ankit Kapoor, and Saloni Gupta

25.1 Introduction

The complex anatomy of the temporomandibular joint (TMJ) owing to its close proximity to vital anatomical structures like facial nerve, maxillary artery, middle meningeal artery, parotid gland, external auditory meatus (EAM) and cranium explains the wide spectrum of structures surrounding this joint. The surgical procedures involving the TMJ that could give rise to complications are arthroscopy, open arthroplasty, tumor resections, open joint soft tissue procedures and total joint replacement. Various complications may arise at different stages of TMJ surgery, which may result in facial nerve injury, Frey's syndrome, haemorrhage from major vessels, damage to the ear, salivary gland complications, infection and failure of the alloplastic joint or material used (Table 25.1).

V. Bansal (✉) · A. Kapoor · S. Gupta
Department of Oral and Maxillofacial Surgery, Swami Vivekanand Subharti University, Meerut, Uttar Pradesh, India

Table 25.1 Complications in TMJ Surgery

Intra-operative complication	Post-operative complication
1. Inadequate exposure, dissection causing tissue damage 2. Nerve injury: Facial, mandibular, auriculotemporal 3. Haemorrhage 4. Damage to ear, middle cranial fossa 5. Salivary gland injury 6. Improper condylar positioning	1. Sialocele 2. Limited range of motion 3. Surgical site infection (SSI) 4. Malocclusion 5. Hardware failure 6. Allergic reaction to prosthesis 7. Reankylosis

25.2 Complications from Nerve Injury

25.2.1 Facial Nerve Injury

Facial nerve runs 1.5 cm below the inferior margin of the bony external auditory meatus (EAM). The temporal branch crosses the zygomatic arch at a minimum distance of 0.8 cm and a mean of 2.0 cm anterior to the bony EAM. Facial paralysis can be a distressing complication resulting from iatrogenic trauma during surgical intervention. The average reported incidence of facial nerve injury after open joint surgery is 37% with complete recovery within 6 weeks to 6 months [1].

D. Bhargava (ed.), *Temporomandibular Joint Disorders*,
https://doi.org/10.1007/978-981-16-2754-5_25

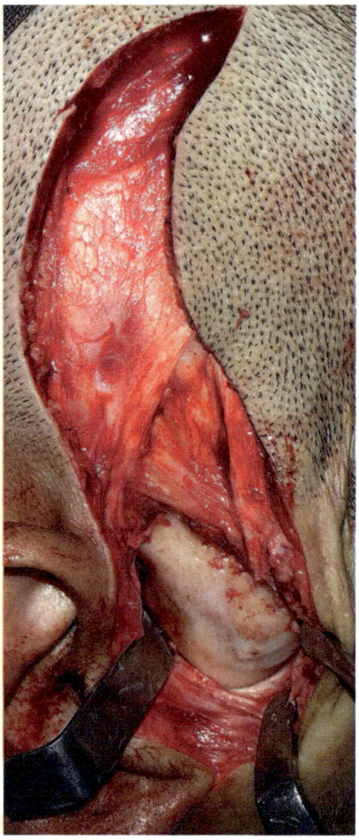

Fig. 25.1 Incision over the zygomatic arch and temporal region as described by Bramley

Excessive retraction causes compression and/or stretching of nerve fibres resulting in traction injury. The pre-auricular incision is given at 45-degree in an upward and forward direction through the superficial layer of temporalis fascia to enter internally containing fat and branches of facial nerve. At the level of zygomatic arch, temporal fascia tightly adheres to the periosteum and overlying superficial fascia. After crossing the zygomatic arch, temporal and zygomatic branches of facial nerve lie in the fusion of three layers. Bramley et al. advocated giving a subperiosteal incision over the zygomatic arch followed by blunt dissection in forward and downward direction to prevent the unseen and undamaged facial nerve filaments in the tightly adherent fusion of layers (Fig. 25.1). Later it was modified by Popowich by giving a vertical incision over the pre-auricular region for better retraction of flap, minimal traction injury to nerve and greater accessibility to the joint [2, 3].

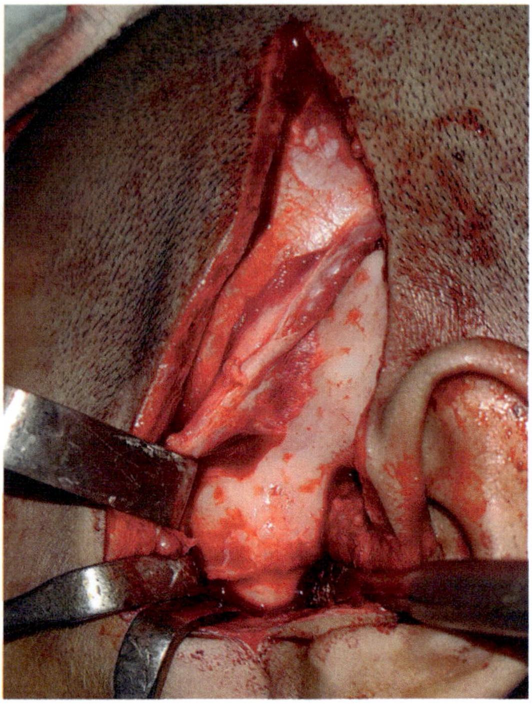

Fig. 25.2 Posteriorly extended full thickness temporal incision

Another approach to the TMJ could be a posteriorly extended full thickness temporal incision which aids in reflection of flap containing superficial, deep fascia, periosteum and branches of facial nerve (Fig. 25.2). In author's experience between the two approaches latter had reduced incidences of facial nerve injury owing to traction with added advantage of meticulous closure and complete coverage of hardware during total joint reconstruction. During open joint surgery instead of direct cauterization, use of bipolar cautery or passing a haemostatic suture around a bleeding point can prevent injury to branches of facial nerve [4].

Management of facial nerve injury depends upon patient factors like age, medical status, skin type, motivation for rehabilitation. Non-surgical conservative methods include physiotherapy, exercises and reassurance. Facial neuromuscular re-education using surface electromyogram (EMG) and biofeedback techniques have demonstrated improvements in facial movement in randomized trials. Botox and corrective makeup techniques have been reported in management. Surgical treatment options include primary nerve repair, facial reanimation using cross-face grafting, cable grafting, regional muscle transposition, free muscle flaps, hypoglossal-facial nerve transfer. Static facial procedures in permanent facial nerve injury include upper lid gold weight, brow lift and blepharoplasty [5, 6].

25.2.2 Inferior Alveolar Nerve Injury

A possible cause of inferior alveolar nerve injury during arthrocentesis and arthroscopy could be due to flow of the irrigating fluid on the medial aspect causing compression to the nerve. Close proximity of the nerve to medially extended ankylotic mass can also lead to injury of nerve during resection. Pre-operative three-dimensional (3D) imaging, stereo-lithographic model reconstruction and assessment followed by removal of ankylotic mass in piece of meal manner can minimize injury to nerve [1] (Figs. 25.3 and 25.4).

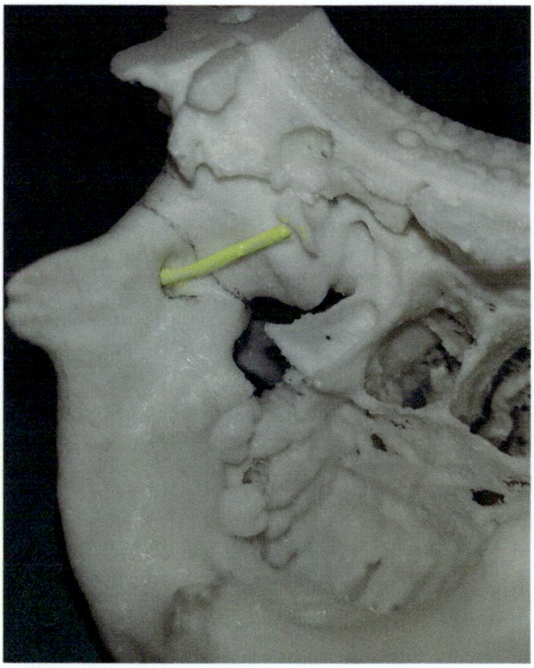

Fig. 25.3 Proximity of the inferior alveolar nerve to medially extended ankylotic mass

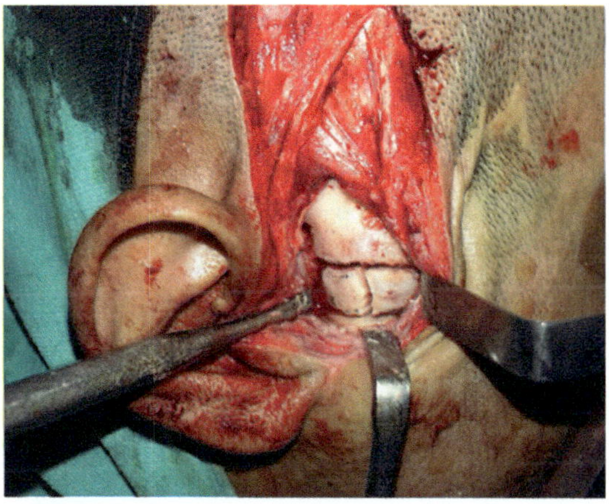

Fig. 25.4 Removal of ankylotic mass in piece-meal manner

25.2.3 Auriculotemporal Nerve Injury

The auriculotemporal branch of mandibular nerve passes immediately adjacent to the superficial vessels. After dividing from main trunk, the nerve traverses near anterior part of condylar neck. This region is highly prone to injury during surgical procedures such as condylectomy. It then courses over the lateral aspect of condyle to traverse in a postero-superior direction towards the EAM. Nerve injury at the upper pole commonly manifests as Frey's syndrome. The clinical syndrome associated with auriculotemporal nerve is auriculotemporal syndrome.

25.3 Auriculotemporal Syndrome (Frey's Syndrome)

Frey's syndrome is clinically manifested as gustatory sweating and flushing of skin in the preauricular area during mastication. The development is an aberrant process in which the post-ganglionic parasympathetic nerve fibres innervate the sweat glands and sub-cutaneous vascular plexus rather than the secretomotor cells of parotid gland. While performing TMJ surgery, dissection and flap elevation is undertaken directly over the auriculotemporal nerve, causing potential damage to the nerve. The nerve remains under the thin outer superficial fascia in the pre-helical area. To prevent nerve damage, the dissection plane should be kept just below the thin fascia keeping the nerve along with superficial temporal artery in the anterior flap [7].

In 1982, Dolwick and Kretzschmar studied the prevalence of various post-operative complications following TMJ surgery through pre-auricular and peri-meatal approaches. It was noted that all patients developed paresthesia over the distribution of auriculotemporal nerve. No incidence of gustatory sweating was reported.

The clinical presentation of Frey's syndrome is variable and its severity can be evaluated using Minor's starch iodine test. This test has remained the traditional method for evaluating gustatory sweating. After thoroughly cleaning and drying the area being considered, the skin is painted with a layer of 2% iodine solution and allowed to dry. A starch powder is then applied evenly over the site. The patient is asked to chew a piece of gum for several minutes. The patient will begin to sweat with the moistened starch reacting with the iodine to produce a dark blue discoloration on the skin surface. The clinical approach to both physical diagnosis and treatment of gustatory sweating is relatively simple [8].

A proposed conservative treatment for Frey's syndrome is using topical aluminium salts (up to 20%). If the condition is unresolved up to 1 month, intra-dermal injections of botulinum toxin are the preferred choice of treatment. Surgical management includes superficial musculo-aponeurotic system (SMAS) surgery, repositioning of temporo-parietal fascia flap, alloderm interposition [8, 9].

25.4 Trigeminocardiac Reflex

The trigeminocardiac reflex is characterized by inducing a cardiac depressor response via vagal stimulation. It is characterized by bradycardia, cardiac arrhythmias, ectopic beats, vomiting and bradycardia terminating in asystole. This is a simple vagus reflex or polysynaptic stimulation via central nervous system nuclei or excessive over-compensation by the parasympathetic system in an attempt to balance sudden sympathetic stimulation during surgical manipulation in the head and neck region [10, 11].

Increased intra-joint pressure during intra-articular injection and arthrocentesis may trigger sensory innervation of joint capsule. Stripping of periosteal innervation of zygomatic arch during exposure of TMJ, placement of sub-periosteal retractor over the medial aspect of the ascending mandibular ramus during resection of ankylotic mass and stretching of the temporalis muscle during coronoidectomy can lead to bradycardia. Management includes close monitoring, temporary cessation of procedure and administration of atropine [10].

25.5 Haemorrhage

The head and neck region have a rich vascular supply. The complication of massive haemorrhage during TMJ surgery is typically encountered intra-operatively. An expanding haematoma may progress and compromise the airway. During TJR surgery, bleeding can occur from maxillary artery, temporal artery, masseteric artery and facial artery and their associated veins. Stripping and dissecting masseter and the pterygoid muscles can lead to oozing of blood. Adequate knowledge of vascular anatomy and adherence to proper surgical technique with sufficient soft tissue retraction can minimize intra-operative bleeding [5, 12].

The superficial temporal and maxillary artery runs along the lateral and medial sides of the condylar neck, suggesting they are at increased risk during soft tissue procedures such as an elective arthroplasty of the TMJ. The clinically important artery that could be damaged during TMJ surgery is maxillary artery. It runs behind the condylar neck and at the level above the sigmoid notch. It can be prevented by retracting posterior and medial to the osteotomy cuts. If there is persistent bleeding from maxillary artery, it can be a serious complication as there is lack of accessibility to tie the vessel. The control of haemorrhage from the medial aspect of the TMJ can be troublesome and time-consuming during ankylosis surgery. A firm pressure for as long as necessary with the forefinger applied intra-orally and directed postero-laterally in the region of the maxillary tuberosity immediately controls bleeding by compressing muscle bed against the medial ramus [13]. Alternatively external carotid artery (ECA) exposure and embolization can be done immediately. Proper pre-operative evaluation can prevent this undue complication. If required, embolization of artery can be done pre-operatively by an interventional radiologist [14, 15].

25.5.1 Management of Haemorrhage

Close proximity of the vessels surrounding the ankylotic mass is best assessed and managed using CT/MRI angiogram and selective embolization. To prevent damage to the maxillary artery intra-operatively, surgeon should avoid violating the periosteum on the medial aspect of the joint which can be achieved with the use of condylar retractors or the use of a piezoelectric saw. Adjunctive therapy such as thrombin-soaked surgical pack, fibrin glue or use of other fibrin products to pack the area for sufficient time stops bleeding and minor ooze [5].

25.6 Injury to Ear and Middle Cranial Fossa

The TMJ is bounded by external auditory canal (EAC) posteriorly and middle cranial fossa superiorly. These structures are at a higher risk during TMJ surgeries even in the hands of experienced surgeons. The anatomy of EAC is complex and angled towards TMJ. The outer third cartilaginous wall of EAC is uninterrupted with auricular cartilage having a fibrous attachment to the bony meatus. The inner 2/3rd bony canal is composed of C-shaped tympanic part of temporal bone. Superior wall is composed of squamous and petrous part of temporal bone. The temporal bone consists of foramen of Huschke/foramen tympanicum. It normally closes in infancy but can persist in up to 18% population owing to incomplete ossification in the antero-inferior aspect of EAC. TMJ is located postero-medial to this foramen which can increase the risk of otologic complication during arthroscopy. It is also evident from the literature that Huguier's canal which is located in the inner extremity of petrotympanic fissure can potentially cause middle ear damage during TMJ surgery and arthroscopy. Studies suggested that surgical instruments should be directed towards the tubercle and away from the fossa. This avoids perforation and injury to the contents of the middle cranial fossa [16, 17].

Machado De Carvalho et al. reported that their patient developed cerebrospinal fluid (CSF) leak from the ear, soft tissue over the alloplastic joint blocking the entire EAC and deafness in the ipsilateral ear with extensive destruction involving the lateral base of skull, middle cranial fossa floor, middle and inner ear [18]. Other otologic complications such as infection, laceration, hypoacusis, otitis externa/media and mastoiditis can occur. It is prudent that the arthroscope is placed 10 mm anterior to the tragus along the cantho-tragal line and angled away from ear while the patient is lying in supine position with head turned at 90 degrees. A waterproof cotton pellet packing in the ear during TMJ surgery prevents accumulation of blood clots which is a common cause for ear infection.

Another cause of ear infection or hypoacusis is development of stenosis during post auricular approach which can be prevented by intra-operatively giving a sharp cut 4–5 mm above the bony canal which allows meticulous closure and placement of small antibiotic coated stent made by cutting the rounded side of rubber catheter into the external auditory canal for 7 days. It is suggested that these precautions limit the incidents of hypoacusis which if encountered is transient in nature and resolves within 3–6 months [19].

During eminectomy or eminoplasty care needs to be exercised as the medial part of the eminence represents very thin bone. Routine radiographs (OPG) represent pneumatization of temporal bone as asymptomatic radiolucent

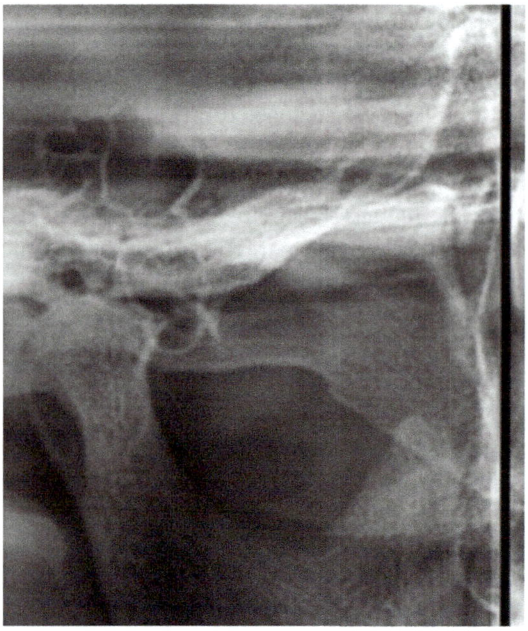

Fig. 25.5 Pneumatization of temporal bone

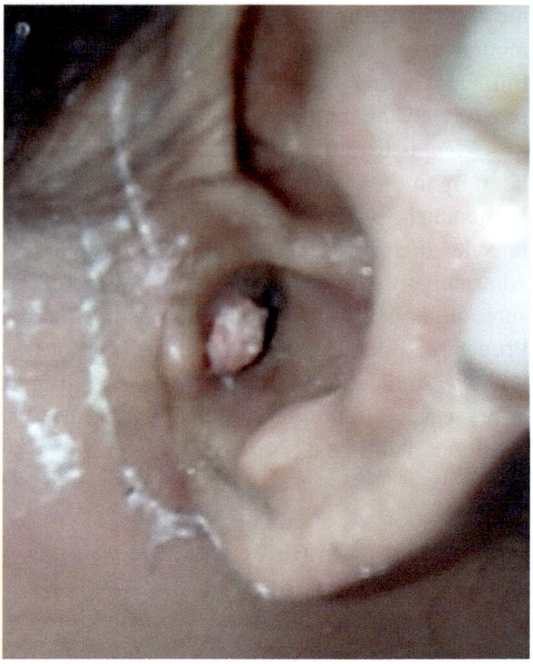

Fig. 25.6 Extrusion of polypoidal mass through aural fistula

defect (Fig. 25.5) whereas pathological condition may clinically manifest as swelling and radiographically as cortical destruction of zygoma. It should be evaluated pre-operatively via different imaging modalities like computed tomography (CT) or magnetic resonance imaging (MRI) to rule out pneumatization by air cells in the temporal bone or to consider the depth of bone reduction.

Perforation into the middle cranial fossa exposes the parietal lobe of the brain. If the dura is intact, no surgical intervention is required. If there is CSF leak or a larger defect is present, it should be sealed off with a bone graft or dural patch with a neurosurgical evaluation [5].

25.7 Aural-TMJ Communication or Fistula (Pre-auricular Sinus/Surgical Site Infection)

The occurrence of pre-auricular sinus may result after surgical site infection (SSI) or infected alloplastic implants. Clinically it can be manifested as polypoidal mass or discharge of synovial fluid from the ear during joint movement (Fig. 25.6). It may occur after resection of large ankylotic mass which extends posteriorly close to tympanic plate or infection of the hardware. Local debridement, closure with temporalis flap intra-operatively, packing of EAC with antibiotic impregnated gauze will resolve this complication.

25.8 Salivary Gland Complications

Parotid fistula or sialocele is an uncommon complication associated with TMJ surgeries. If the surgical plane is below the parotid-masseteric fascia, then an inadvertent iatrogenic injury or a direct injury to the gland can occur, exposing the rough surface of salivary tissue which secretes saliva into the surrounding tissues. This salivary leak might present as a persistent salivary fistula or sialocele (Fig. 25.7) [18]. Conservative management includes reduced intake of salty and sour food to avoid parasympathetic action to the gland. Common method of management includes pressure dressing over the affected region.

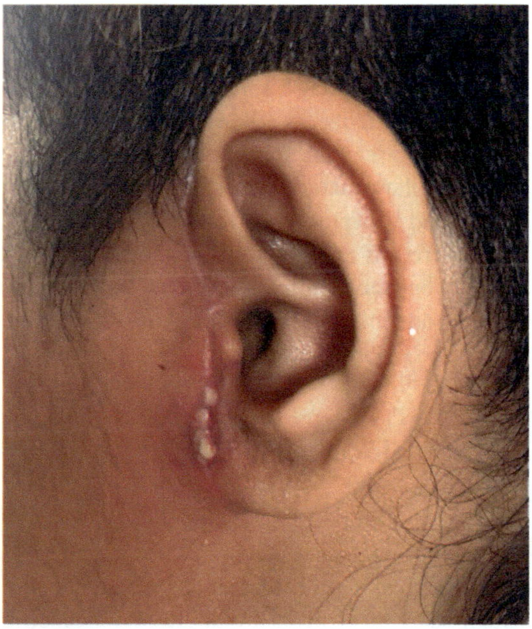

Fig. 25.7 Salivary fistulae

Adjuvant nasogastric tube feed can be advised to avoid gustatory stimulation [20].

Irrigation followed by application of tetracycline has proved to heal the sialocele since tetracycline causes localized fibrosis, healing the salivary leak. If complication persists, scopolamine patch application or intra-glandular hypertrophic saline or Botox injection could be chosen as treatment modality. In patients where these measures proved unsuccessful, irradiation of gland can induce fibrosis is found effective but it is less commonly used [21].

25.9 Heterotrophic Bone Formation, Reankylosis

Re-ankylosis of TMJ is one of the most exasperating situations for surgeons as well as the patient. It can be attributed to narrow posterior cut, incomplete removal of medial ankylotic mass or prejudiced debridement of loose bony fragments (Fig. 25.8). Wide posterior cut, complete removal of pathological bony mass, interposition with sufficient thickness of soft tissue like buccal fat pad or abdominal fat which obliterates the dead space, placement of drain tube for initial 48 to 72 hours to prevent formation of haematoma and aggressive physiotherapy for minimum 18 months are definitive means for preventing re-ankylosis. Administration of low dose of radiation (10 cGy) (experimental, rarely indicated in practice) and indomethacin has shown to reduce the chances of heterotrophic calcifications [22–24].

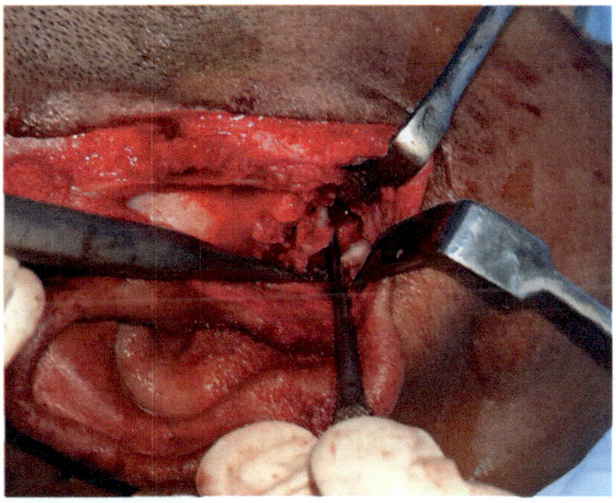

Fig. 25.8 Medial ankylotic mass and loose bony fragments

25.10 Infection of Alloplastic Joint

Placement of alloplastic joint is subjected to a plethora of infective agents either from the local site like saliva contamination from oral cavity or haematogenous spread from distant infections or improper sterilization protocol during operative handling of the prosthesis. Host factors like immune-compromised state, multiple previous surgeries and decreased surgical site vascularity also contribute to the development of infective condition around the prosthesis. To prevent contamination from the oral cavity, it is advised to change the drape, gloves, including suction tip, isolating the oral cavity by benzoin and loban which creates a water tight seal to prevent any small salivary leaks [25].

Acute infections developed within a week can be treated surgically by scrubbing of the prosthesis with sterile toothbrush and betadine to remove the adherent bio-film, placement of irrigating catheters medial to the prosthesis and one on the lateral side as well as a Penrose drain placed through the sub-mandibular incision. Management of chronic infected prosthesis involved removal of prosthesis, peripherally inserted central catheter (PICC) line placement, and appropriate administration of IV antibiotics for 6 weeks followed by oral antibiotics for an additional 1 month. A second surgery can be performed for re-insertion of the prosthesis [26–28].

25.11 Malposition of the Prosthesis

Satisfactory maintenance of occlusion and placement of condyle in a correct anatomic position in the glenoid fossa are two primary prerequisites for suitable post-operative functioning of the joint. Repeated inspection for occlusion before placing all the screws, fixation of the fossa component to sufficient bone and evaluation of condylar position helps prevent any functional derangement. These problems are commonly associated with stock prosthesis which can be overcome by custom-made prosthesis with 3D virtual planning [5].

25.12 Loosening of Prosthesis

The prosthesis is generally stable with 6 to 8 screws, but the fossa component may get displaced if the screws turn out to be loose due to porous or thin underlying bone, infection or trauma to the site. It is desirable that 3-point stabilization is achieved in stock prosthesis or custom fabricated prosthesis to achieve minimal to nil micro movements [5].

25.13 Instrument Breakage

It can rarely occur during arthroscopic surgery. Common causes for breakage of instrument are loss of structural integrity, excessive force and bending of instruments. Surgeon should be ready for retrieval of broken instrument arthroscopically or if required by open exploration of TMJ.

25.14 Allergic Reaction

Allergic reactions are rarely encountered with reported incidents of allergic reaction to the metallic components (chromium, cobalt, nickel) of the implant material. Localized eczema, erythema and vesicles on overlying skin can be encountered. If an implant material or prosthesis needs to be placed in the joint cavity, it is advised that pre-operatively metal allergy test should be performed by an allergist [5].

25.15 Malocclusion

Post-operative open bite or inability to achieve satisfactory occlusion is associated with bilateral coronoidectomy in TMJ ankylosis management which can be corrected by aggressive isometric and isotonic exercises and placement of guiding elastics for few days. Malocclusion can be associated with improper fit of alloplastic joint. This can be achieved by securing the occlusion intra-operatively, re-assuring during every step of surgery, good reconstructive arthroplasty or submissive gap arthroplasty [5, 29].

25.16 Miscellaneous

Other relatively less common complications include cervico-mediastinal abscess, pneumomediastinum and sub-cutaneous emphysema following TMJ surgeries [18].

25.17 Conclusion

The surgeon should have adequate knowledge regarding the anatomy and proper pre-operative planning should be done in order to avoid or to minimize complications. Inspite of careful planning and execution, complications may be inevitable. It is essential for the surgeon to possess the skills to identify and manage the complications for uneventful recovery when required.

References

1. Valerand WA, Dolwick MF. Complications of TMJ surgery. Oral Maxillofac Surg Clin North Am. 1990;2:481–99.
2. Bansal V, Mowar A, Dubey P, Bhatnagar A, Bansal A. Coronoid process and residual ankylotic mass as an autograft in the management of ankylosis of the temporomandibular joint in young adolescent patients: a retrospective clinical investigation. Br J Oral Maxillofac Surg. 2016;54(3):280–5.
3. Popowich L, Crane RM Jr. Modified preauricular access to the temporomandibular apparatus: experience with twenty-eight cases. Oral Surg Oral Med Oral Pathol. 1982;54(3):257–62.
4. Emam H, Jatana C, Ness GM. Facial nerve injury. Complications of Temporomandibular Joint Surgery. Cham: Springer; 2017. p. 57–74.
5. Hoffman D, Puig L. Complications of TMJ surgery. Oral Maxillofac Surg Clin N Am. 2015;27:109–24.
6. Moin A, Shetty AD, et al. Facial nerve injury in temporomandibular joint approaches. Ann Maxillofac Surg. 2018;8:51–5.
7. Kryshtalskyj B, Weinberg S. An assessment for auriculotemporal syndrome following temporomandibular joint surgery through the preauricular approach. J Oral Maxillofac Surg. 1989;47(1):3–6.
8. Minor V. EinneuesVerfahrenzu der klinischenUntersuchung der Schweissabsonderung. J Neurol. 1928;101(1):302–8.
9. Clayman MA, Clayman SM, Seagle MB. A review of the surgical and medical treatment of Frey syndrome. Ann Plast Surg. 2006;57(5):581–4.
10. Morey TE, Bjoraker DG. Asystole during temporomandibular joint arthrotomy. Anesthesiology. 1996;85(6):1488–91.
11. Bhargava D, Thomas S, Chakravorty N, Dutt A. Trigeminocardiac reflex: a reappraisal with relevance to maxillofacial surgery. J Maxillofac Oral Surg. https://doi.org/10.1007/s12663-013-0541-4.
12. Granquist EJ, Quinn PD. Massive Hemorrhage. Complications of Temporomandibular Joint Surgery. Cham: Springer; 2017. p. 99–110.
13. Kumar S, Bansal V, Agarwal R. An effective intraoperative method to control bleeding from vessels medial to the temporomandibular joint. J Maxillofac Oral Surg. 2009;8(4):371.
14. Talebzadeh N, Rosenstein TP, Pogrel MA. Anatomy of the structures medial to the temporomandibular joint. Oral Surg Oral Med Oral Pathol Oral Radiol Endod. 1999;88(6):674–8.
15. Cuccia AM, Caradonna C, Caradonna D, Anastasi G, Milardi D, Favaloro A, De Pietro A, Angileri TM, Caradonna L, Cutroneo G. The arterial blood supply of the temporomandibular joint: an anatomical study and clinical implications. Imaging Sci Dent. 2013;43(1):37–44.
16. Sugisaki M, Ikai A, Tanabe H. Dangerous angles and depths for middle ear and middle cranial Fossa injury during arthroscopy of the temporomandibular joint. J Oral Maxillofac Surg. 1995;53:803–10.
17. Surgical complications of TMJ SURGERY.
18. MachadoDe Carvalho G, et al. Surgical disaster in temporomandibular joint: case report. Rev Esp Cir Oral Maxilofac. 2012; https://doi.org/10.1016/j.maxilo.2012.06.006
19. Bansal V, Kumar S, Mowar A, Yadav A, Khare G. The post-auricular approach for gap arthroplasty–a clinical investigation. J Cranio-Maxillofac Surg. 2012;40(6):500–5.
20. Nageris B, Feinmesser R. Complications of parotidectomy: surgical techniques of repair. Oper Tech Otolaryngol Head Neck Surg. 1996;7(4):374–6.
21. Srinidhi D, Singh M, Rangaswamy S, Choudry S. Parotid sialocele and fistulae: current treatment options. Int J Contemp Dent. 2011;2(1):9–12.
22. Bansal V, Bansal A, Mowar A, Gupta S. Ultrasonography for the volumetric analysis of the buccal fat pad as an interposition material for the management of ankylosis of the temporomandibular joint in adolescent patients. Br J Oral Maxillofac Surg. 2015;53(9):820–5.
23. Jensen AW, Viozzi CF, Foote RL. Long-term results of radiation prophylaxis for heterotopic ossification in the temporomandibular joint. J Oral Maxillofac Surg. 2010;68(5):1100–5.
24. Bhatt K, Pandey S, Bhutia O, Roychoudhury A. Use of indomethacin as an adjuvant to surgery for recurrent temporomandibular joint ankylosis in adults. Natl J Maxillofac Surg. 2014;5(2):198–201.
25. Haug RH, Picard U, Matejczyk M, et al. The infected prosthetic total temporomandibular joint replacement: report of two cases. J Oral Maxillofac Surg. 1989;47:1210–4.
26. Mercuri LG. Microbial biofilms: a potential source for alloplastic device failure. J Oral Maxillofac Surg. 2006;64(8):1303–9.
27. Wolford LM, Rodrigues DB, McPhillips A. Management of the infected temporomandibular joint total joint prosthesis. J Oral Maxillofac Surg. 2010;68(11):2810–23.
28. Mercuri LG, Psutka D. Peri-operative, post-operative and prophylactic use of antibiotics in alloplastic total temporomandibular joint surgery: a survey and preliminary guidelines. J Oral Maxillofac Surg. https://doi.org/10.1016/j.joms.2011.01.006.
29. Bansal V, Dubey P, Bansal A, Gupta S. Submissive Osteoarthrectomy in temporomandibular joint AnkylosisSubharti experience. Am J Oral Maxillofac Surg. 2014;1:14–21.

Role of Distraction Osteogenesis in Restoration of Ramus-Condyle Unit

26

R. Manikandhan, Ganesh Koneru, and Darpan Bhargava

26.1 Introduction

Temporomandibular joint (TMJ) reconstruction is a challenging surgical procedure performed for the patients where the condyle is either absent, cannot be salvaged or is deformed. The various methods for reconstruction including autogenous and alloplastic materials have been discussed in detail previously. The evolution of TMJ reconstruction from a simple gap arthroplasty (with or without interposition) to alloplastic total joint prosthesis, along with distraction osteogenesis (DO) generating neo-condyle from posterior ramus has refined reconstruction and gained universal popularity in recent times.

It is best to reconstruct or regenerate the TMJ to near natural either with distraction or tissue engineering which functions like a normal joint and is able to bear the masticatory load. DO is a commonly used technique to lengthen long bones in the field of orthopaedic surgery that follows Ilizarov's principles. In recent times, this technique has gained popularity in the maxillofacial skeleton for reconstructing mandibular and maxillary deficiencies or defects [1–6]. One must consider patient's age and assess overall health for reconstruction as younger patients are more likely to need multiple revision surgeries throughout their lifetime to maintain adequate form and function [7].

Transport distraction osteogenesis (TDO) can be employed to reconstruct TMJ by accomplishing neo-condyle regeneration. It has an advantage of developing fibro-cartilaginous capping between the transported bone segment and glenoid fossa. Reconstruction of condyle using TDO was first reported by Stucki-McCormick in patients with ankylosis. One can also consider using an osteoplastic bone flap harvested from the ramus to reconstruct the ramus-condyle unit (RCU) without distraction in cases where vertical defect is small with adequate ramal bone [8–10].

R. Manikandhan
Department of Oral and Maxillofacial Surgery, Meenakshi Ammal Dental College and Hospital, Chennai, Tamil Nadu, India

Craniofacial Surgery, Meenakshi Ammal Dental College and Hospital, Chennai, Tamil Nadu, India

G. Koneru
Department of Oral and Maxillofacial Surgery, Sibar Institute of Dental Sciences, Guntur, Andhra Pradesh, India

D. Bhargava (✉)
TMJ Consultancy Services, Bhopal, Madhya Pradesh, India

Oral and Maxillofacial Surgery, People's College of Dental Sciences and Research Centre, People's University, Bhopal, Madhya Pradesh, India
e-mail: drdarpanbhargava@gmail.com

D. Bhargava (ed.), *Temporomandibular Joint Disorders*,
https://doi.org/10.1007/978-981-16-2754-5_26

26.2 History of TDO

The surgical technique of distraction osteogenesis, as described by Ilizarov in 1951, has long been used in the reconstruction of defects of the long bones. The first clinical application of distraction osteogenesis for craniomaxillofacial deformities in the human mandible was reported in 1992 by McCarthy et al. Stucki-McCormick was the first to report the use of distraction osteogenesis for the re-establishment of the condyle in two cases (1997), that included bony ankylosis and degenerative joint disease after tumor resection [11, 12].

26.3 Pre-surgical Evaluation and Planning

A thorough clinical and radiographic evaluation of the TMJ and the adjacent structures is required. Clinically, the size of the expected defect and health of the remaining mandibular bone are the factors to be considered. This can be assessed by using a computed tomography (CT) and its three-dimensional (3D) recontructed images. The reconstruction is expected to compensate for the deficiencies from only condylar stump regeneration to the entire ramus condylar component in both vertical and horizontal combinations. A stereo-lithographic model can be constructed on which the model surgery may be planned and the distractor can be adapted which can further be executed in a patient intra-operatively.

26.4 Imaging Modalities

Clinical, photographic and orthopantomogram (OPG) records are mandatory for all patients at regular intervals in the post-operative period. Cone beam computed tomography (CBCT) aids to evaluate the quality and morphology of the bone in ramus. It also helps in preparation of surgical guides for precise positioning of cuts, distractor placement and planing on a stereo-lithographic model for adaptation of distractor plates prior to placement. This approach reduces operating time and improves efficiency and thus the, patient outcome. Ultrasound (USG) examination may be used post-operatively to assess the healing of the callus [5].

26.5 Surgical Procedure for TDO to Restore RCU

The procedure should be performed under general anaesthesia (GA) followed by securing the airway using naso-endotracheal intubation. Following strict aseptic precautions, Risdon's incision is usually preferred to expose the ramus and condylar region. A layered dissection is carried out followed by periosteal stripping. The periosteum should be kept intact on the medial side to maintain the soft tissue cover as it is the source of blood supply to the transport segment for distraction.

A reverse L shaped osteotomy should be performed in the ramus extending from the sigmoid notch to around 1 cm above inferior mandibular border. The osteotomy cut should not be extended to the angle region. The vertical osteotomy cut in the ramus should be parallel to the vector desired to direct the transport disc towards the glenoid fossa. The superior end of the transport disc should be rounded to mimic the condylar head. The vector of distraction and the sliding guidance of the vertical ramus osteotomy for the transport segment may be pre-operatively determined to advance the distracted bone superiorly right into the antero-posterior midpoint of planned glenotemporal preparation or pre-existing fossa.

The device should be placed parallel to the vertical osteotomy cut and fixed using screws similar to miniplate fixation used to stabilize a fractured mandible (Fig. 26.1). After fixation, osteotomy should be carried out to mobilize the transport segment. Confirmation should be done intra-operatively to check unrestricted movement by activating the device for 1–2 mm. A small stab

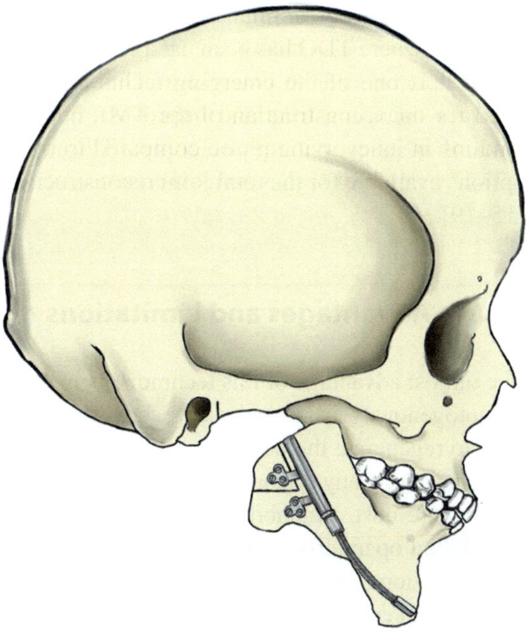

Fig. 26.1 Distraction device fixation following the bone osteotomy

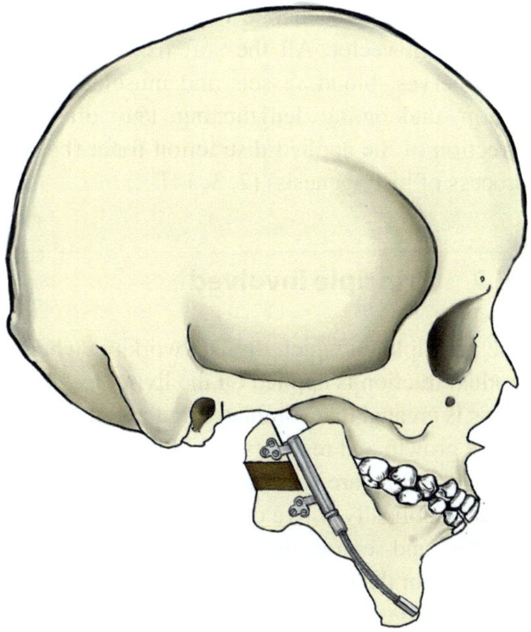

Fig. 26.2 Neocondyle following bone transport distraction osteogenesis

incision is placed for making an exit port for the activation arm of the device in the retromandibular or angle region. Once the device is placed and fixed, the incision is closed in layers using 3–0 polyglactin and 4–0 nylon sutures. Post-operative analgesics and anti-biotics should be administered as per the institutional protocols.

After the latency period of 5–7 days, activation of the distractor device should be initiated. Activation should be performed at the optimum rate of 1 mm daily. It can be fractionated as 0.5 mm in the morning and 0.5 mm in the evening or as 0.25 mm every six hours for four times in a day. It is preferred to activate the distractor device daily at a fixed time of the day. Ilizarov has proposed that, greater the distraction frequency there are better outcomes with 1 mm daily activation being the most favourable till the desired length of the RCU is obtained and the transport disc is in a close contact with the articular surface. The distractor should be left in situ for consolidation of the distracted callus for 8–12 weeks (Fig. 26.2).

Patient should be advised to consume a soft diet and physiotherapy to maintain the mouth opening during the post-operative period. The distractor is removed under GA when the mature bone is evident radiographically after the consolidation period [8–10, 13].

26.6 Distraction Histiogenesis

Histology of the distracted bone from studies has revealed that in early stages, the distraction gap is filled with soft callus which is gradually replaced by mature bone almost indistinguishable from the normal bone at around 24 weeks after distraction. The neo-condyle formed with distraction is considered unique as the resultant head formed will have fibro-cartilaginous cover, considering it acts as the advancing front of the transport disc during the active transport distraction osteogenesis process. Histologically, the regenerate will have features which are a combination of endochondral and intra-membranous ossifications.

The distraction regenerate is always parallel to the tension vector. All the soft tissues such as skin, nerves, blood vessels and muscles in the region undergoing lengthening and grow in direction of the applied distraction force (by the process of histiogenesis) [2, 3, 14].

26.7 Principle Involved

The principle on which the DO works is when a gradual traction is applied on the living tissues, a stress is created that stimulates and maintains the active growth and regeneration of the tissues. All the tissues that are stretched slowly and steadily are metabolically active due to increase in intracellular and extracellular synthesis which is essential for the maintenance of blood supply and coping with the functional loading. In DO, gradual traction is applied to the soft callus before it can ossify. The stretched callus has the ossification potential and converts into bone when left for consolidation.

The biologic and clinical principles important to obtain appropriate bone formation without the undue stretch of the distraction callus should include the following:

1. **At the time of surgical procedure:** Maximum preservation of the periosteal blood supply and soft tissues. The transport distraction disc osteotomy should be well planned and executed, to meet the resultant vector demand.
2. **Period of latency:** 5 to 7 days. Stable fixation to prevent micro-motion at the osteotomy site.
3. **Period of active Distraction:** Depends on the size of the defect.
4. **Distraction rate and rhythm**: The ideal activation rate should not exceed 1 mm/day. It can be modified depending on the characteristics of bone formation, when necessary. Rhythm (number of activations in a day) can be fractionated but rate (total activation per day) should be kept constant for the patient.
5. **Period of consolidation**: 8 to 12 weeks.
6. **Normal physiologic function of the mandible**: It helps in promoting rapid ossification of the neo-condyle [3].

There are several animal and human studies in literature where TDO has been used to restore the RCU. It is one of the emerging techniques utilized for the reconstruction of the TMJ, but still remains in its evolving phase compared to other options available for the total joint reconstruction [15–19].

26.8 Advantages and Limitations

The utmost advantage of this technique being that an autogenously harvested native bone block is used to regenerate the bone to cover the defective area preventing any donor site morbidity. The limitations are cost, availability of distractor device and skilled operator(s), who are well versed with the distraction of the facial bones. An essential factor is patient compliance as the distractor will have to be present in the oro-facial region for a long period causing physical and social inconvenience with a requirement of device activation daily during the distraction phase. A second surgery is required for the device removal. Infection, sialocele and iatrogenic nerve damage may occur at the local site [13]. All the possibilities of post-operative complications should be informed to the patient, along with a thorough patient counselling for the procedure.

26.9 Goals of Treatment

DO is an emerging technique in the field of maxillofacial surgery to regenerate the condyle. The treatment plan should involve meticulous planning in case selection, informing patients of the benefits and possible risks and complications. Adequate pre-operative work-up and executing the surgery with appropriate post-operative care yields the desired results. Compromise at any of the above steps may result in an undesirable outcome. Although no reconstruction can meet the requirements of function, form, and aesthetics equally, the ideal reconstruction should be able to (1) adapt to changes in the occlusal environment, (2) adapt to changes in the condyle/fossae relationship, (3) provide strength and durability to withstand wear, (4) provide frictionless function, (5) be non-inflammatory or non-allergic, (6) heal itself after periods of functional wear or breakdown, (7) reduce discomfort and pain and (8) appear aesthetically pleasing to the patient [7].

References

1. Ilizarov GA. The tension-stress effect on the genesis and growth of tissues. Part I. The influence of stability of fixation and soft-tissue preservation. Clin Orthop Relat Res. 1989;238:249–81.
2. Ilizarov GA. The tension-stress effect on the genesis and growth of tissues. Part II. The influence of the rate and frequency of distraction. Clin Orthop Relat Res. 1989;239:263–85.
3. Ilizarov GA. Clinical application of the tension-stress effect for limb lengthening. Clin Orthop Relat Res. 1990;250:8–26.
4. Andrade N, Gandhewar T, Kalra R. Development and evolution of distraction devices: use of indigenous appliances for distraction osteogenesis: an overview. Ann Maxillofac Surg. 2011;1(1):58–65.
5. Neelakandan RS, Bhargava D. Transport distraction osteogenesis for maxillomandibular reconstruction: current concepts and applications. J Maxillofac Oral Surg. 2012;11(3):291–9.
6. Sharma R, Manikandhan R, Sneha P, Parameswaran A. Neocondyle distraction osteogenesis in the management of temporomandibular joint ankylosis. Report of five cases with review of literature. Indian J Dent Res. 2017;28(3):269–74.
7. Spagnoli DB, Gollehon SG. Distraction osteogenesis in reconstruction of the mandible and temporomandibular joint. Oral Maxfax Surg Clin N Am. 2006;18(3):383–98.
8. Alwala AM, Kasireddy SK, Nalamolu B, Malyala SK. Transport distraction osteogenesis in reconstruction of condyle: use of a 3D model for vector planning. J Maxillofac Oral Surg. 2017;17(3):276–80.
9. Stucki McCormick SU. Reconstruction of mandibular condyle using transport distraction osteogenesis. J Craniofac Surg. 1997;8(1):48–52.
10. Stucki McCormick SU, Fox RM, Mizrahi RD. Reconstruction of a neocondyle using transport distraction osteogenesis. Semin Orthod. 1999;5:59–63.
11. McCarthy J, et al. Lengthening the human mandible by gradual distraction. Plast Recons Surg. 1992;89(1):1–8.
12. Stucki-McCormick SU, Winick R, Winick A. Distraction osteogenesis for the reconstruction of the temporomandibular joint. N Y State Dent J. 1998;64(3):36–41.
13. Sharma R, Manikandhan R, Sneha P, Parameswaran A, Kumar JN, Sailer HF. Neocondyle distraction osteogenesis in the management of temporomandibular joint ankylosis: report of five cases with review of literature. Indian J Dent Res. 2017 May–Jun;28(3):269–74.
14. Naveenkumar J, Anantanarayanan P, Sneha P. Role of bilateral mandibular distraction for asymmetry due to unilateral ankylosis. Int J Oral Maxillofac Surg. 2016 Dec;45(12):1671–2.
15. Schwartz H, Robert R. Distraction osteogenesis for temporomandibular joint reconstruction. J Oral Maxillofac Surg. 2008;66:718–23. https://doi.org/10.1016/j.joms.2007.11.016.
16. Bansal V, Singh S, Garg N, Dubey P. Transport distraction osteogenesis as a method of reconstruction of the temporomandibular joint following gap arthroplasty for post-traumatic ankylosis in children: a clinical and radiological prospective assessment of outcome. Int J Oral Maxillofac Surg. 2014;43(2):227–36.
17. Gabbay JS, Heller JB, Song YY, Wasson KL, Harrington H, Bradley JP. Temporomandibular joint bony ankylosis: comparison of treatment with transport distraction osteogenesis or the Matthews device arthroplasty. J Craniofac Surg. 2006 May;17(3):516–22.
18. Kohli S, et al. The autogenous graft versus transport distraction osteogenesis for reconstruction of the ramus–condyle unit: a prospective comparative study. Int J Oral Maxillofac Surg. 2017;46(9):1106–17.
19. Yoon HJ, Kim HG. Intraoral mandibular distraction osteogenesis in facial asymmetry patients with unilateral temporomandibular joint bony ankylosis. Int J Oral Maxillofac Surg. 2002;31(5):544–8.

Fibreoptic Intubation for Patients Undergoing Temporomandibular Joint Surgery

27

Rajkumar Ahirwal and Darpan Bhargava

27.1 Introduction

Airway maintenance is an essential aspect of general anaesthesia (GA) for any surgical procedure. Temporomandibular joint (TMJ) surgery poses a challenge, considering the difficult intubation as visualising the vocal cords directly may be difficult in cases with reduced mouth opening. The difficulty in intubation is attributed to several factors in patients diagnosed with joint ankylosis, as the craniomandibular fusion has associated skeletal and soft tissue deformity that includes mandibular hypoplasia, narrowed pharyngeal passage caused by decreased mandibular space along with pseudomacroglossia (in cases of microgenia) usually leading to obstructive sleep apnoea and compromised airway. All these factors make the conventional intubation options including naso/orotracheal intubation less useful in such patients. There is no single standard intubation technique for patients undergoing surgery for the jaw joint with restricted mouth opening [1, 2].

There are several intubation techniques documented which prove to be useful in securing airway for the patients requiring TMJ surgery, these include blind awake nasal intubation, fibreoptic laryngoscope assisted intubation, retrograde endotracheal intubation and very rarely tracheostomy [1].

27.2 Aetiology for Difficult Intubation

Patients requiring any form of TMJ surgery usually report at an advanced phase of the disease process after the onset of the disease. As there is progression of the clinical symptoms causing reduced mouth opening in majority of the patient population which may lead to difficulty in intubation with altered airway anatomy as noted in cases with temporomandibular joint ankylosis. Hence it is difficult or at times impossible to intubate such patients using regular techniques. Upward thrusting of the jaw to perform the airway manoeuvre is almost impossible in patients with an established diagnosis of TMJ ankylosis [1–3].

R. Ahirwal
Department of Anaesthesiology and Critical Care, Gandhi Medical College and Associated Hospitals, Bhopal, Madhya Pradesh, India

D. Bhargava (✉)
TMJ Consultancy Services, Bhopal, Madhya Pradesh, India

Oral and Maxillofacial Surgery, People's College of Dental Sciences and Research Centre, People's University, Bhopal, Madhya Pradesh, India
e-mail: drdarpanbhargava@gmail.com

D. Bhargava (ed.), *Temporomandibular Joint Disorders*,
https://doi.org/10.1007/978-981-16-2754-5_27

27.3 Intubation Techniques for TMJ Surgery with Restricted Mouth Opening

Fibreoptic intubation is the gold standard in patients having TMJ ankylosis and reduced mouth opening due to other pathologies associated with the joint. The possible constraints to universally adopt this technique are the financial factor involved, technique sensitivity, unavailability of various tube and scope diameters as desired. There is a possibility of unwarranted bleeding during the manoeuvre posing difficulty in intubation while using the fibroscope [1].

Blind nasal intubation was a regular practice before the fiberoptic era for cases with reduced mouth opening. Blind awake intubation can be performed to secure airway in patients with TMJ pathologies which has adequate success outcome provided the anaesthesiologist is well trained for the procedure. It is atraumatic, cost effective when done with adequate pre-operative work-up by the operating team to achieve an uneventful outcome [1, 4]. The major limitation with this technique remains exploration and a ready backup of alternative intubation technique in case of futile blind intubation. Considering limitations of other techniques, fiberoptic bronchoscope should form a part of the difficult airway cart, which must be available in operation theatres.

The intubation technique in paediatric patients undergoing TMJ surgery requires utmost care owing to the factors like growing mandible and other facial bones with less mouth opening and most commonly uncooperativeness for the procedure. In such patients it is a real challenge for the anaesthesiologist to secure and maintain airway, as TMJ pathology specially ankylosis is common in paediatric age group [4].

27.4 Procedure for Fibreoptic Intubation (Figs. 27.1, 27.2, 27.3, 27.4 and 27.5)

1. The light source of the bronchoscope should be checked and focused on the gauze piece followed by defogging with 70% isopropyl alcohol.
2. Anaesthetic (lignocaine) jelly should be applied on to the entire length of the scope which facilitates the scope introduction and passage of endotracheal tube.
3. Fibreoptic intubation should be started upon achieving the adequate sedation level. The patient should be pre-operatively prepared adequately. Preperation of the nasal mucosa should be done with packing the nostrils with xylometazoline and lignocaine soaked gauge. Nebulization with 2% lignocaine is an alternative technique for anaesthetising the upper airway and may be combined with superior laryngeal and trans-tracheal local anesthetic blocks.
4. Topical anaesthesia using 'spray as you go (local anesthetic solution through the fibroscope)' for lower airway while advancing the bronchoscope is also advocated, until epiglottis is visualised.
5. The bronchoscope tip should be turned inferiorly to visualise the glottis in case the posterior pharyngeal wall is encountered while advancement.
6. Bronchoscope should be manipulated under the epiglottis to visualise the vocal cords in case there is any obstruction due to epiglottis.
7. The scope should then be advanced close to the larynx followed by application of local anaesthesia onto the glottis and between the vocal cords through fibre-scope.
8. Avoiding excessive force on the bronchoscope reduces the risk of laryngeal trauma and the bronchoscope tip damage.
9. As the scope enters the trachea, the endotracheal tube is advanced over the scope and is secured in position. The carina is identified, and the endotracheal tube is positioned short of it to facilitate uniform bilateral ventilation.
10. The scope is carefully withdrawn leaving the endotracheal tube in position for administering general anaesthesia [3].
11. The outside diameter of the bronchoscope determines the size of the endotracheal tube that can be used for the patient. Hence a proper pre-anaesthetic patient evaluation is necessary to facilitate smooth intubation in these cases.

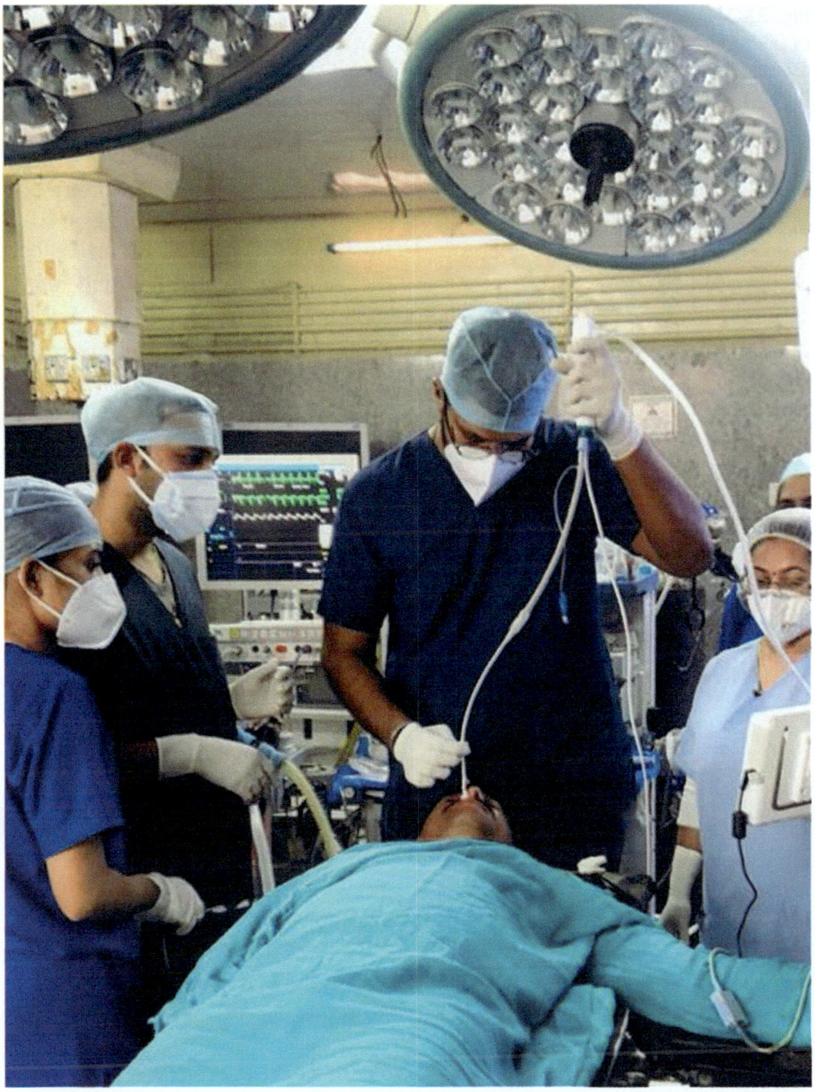

Fig. 27.1 Positioning of the fiberscope at the nasal aperture before introduction of the scope in the nasal cavity

Fig. 27.2 Introduction of fiberoptic scope assisted endotracheal tube

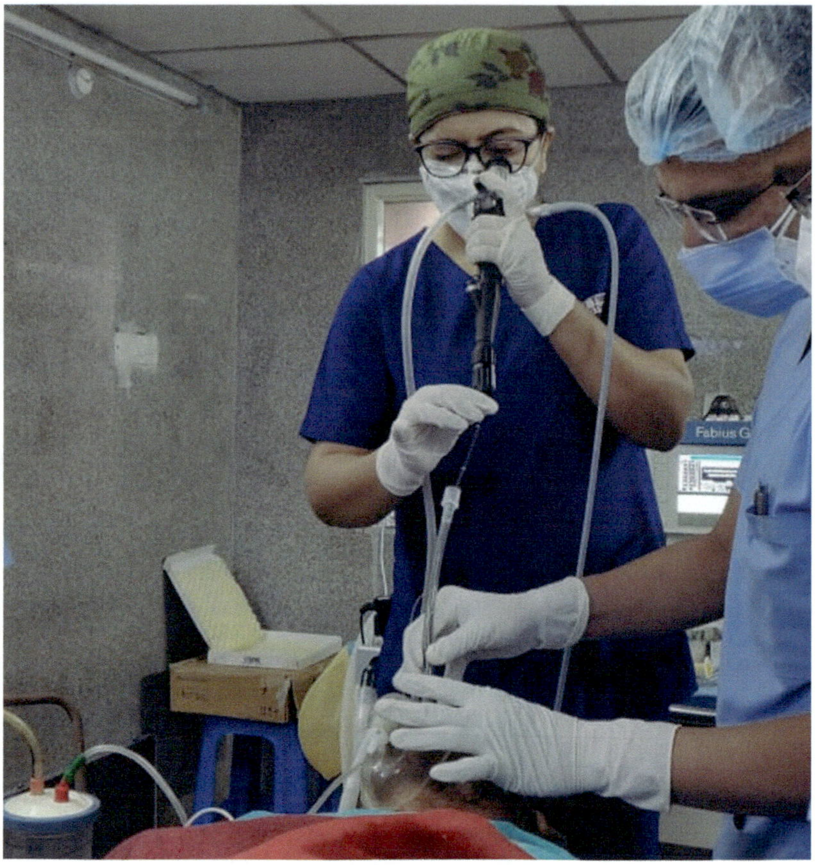

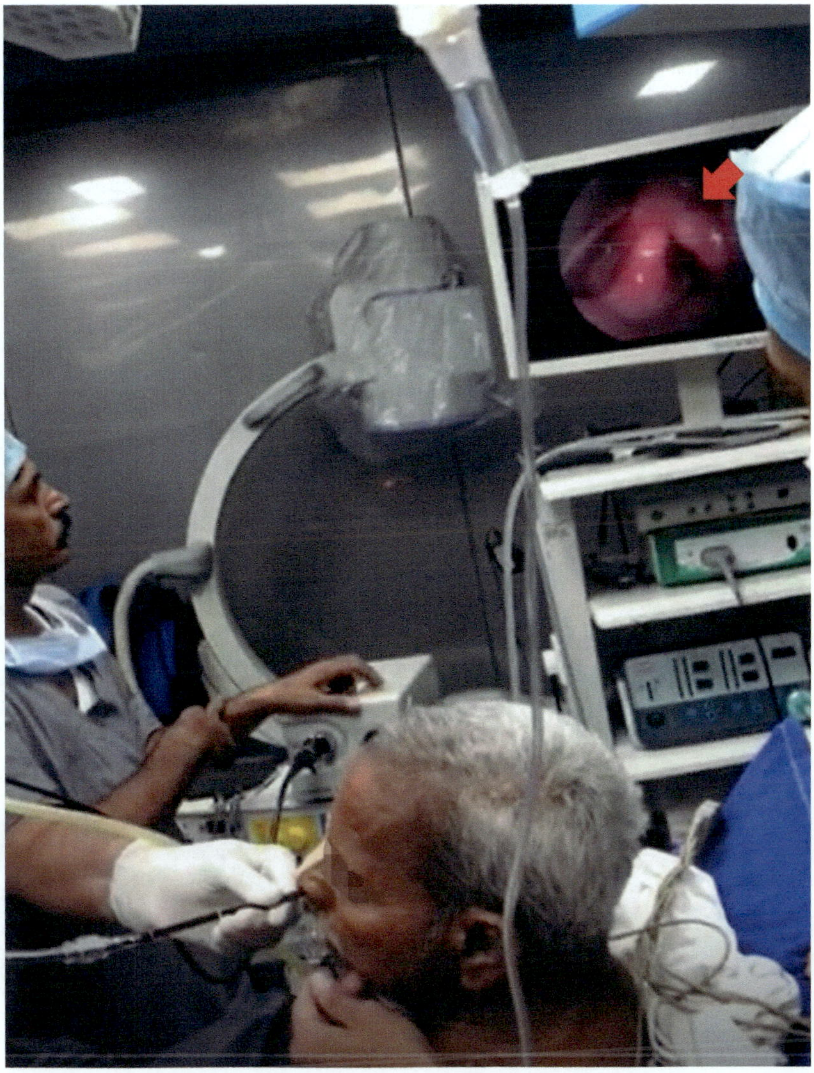

Fig. 27.3 Vocal cords (indicated by an arrow) as visualised using a fiberoptic scope

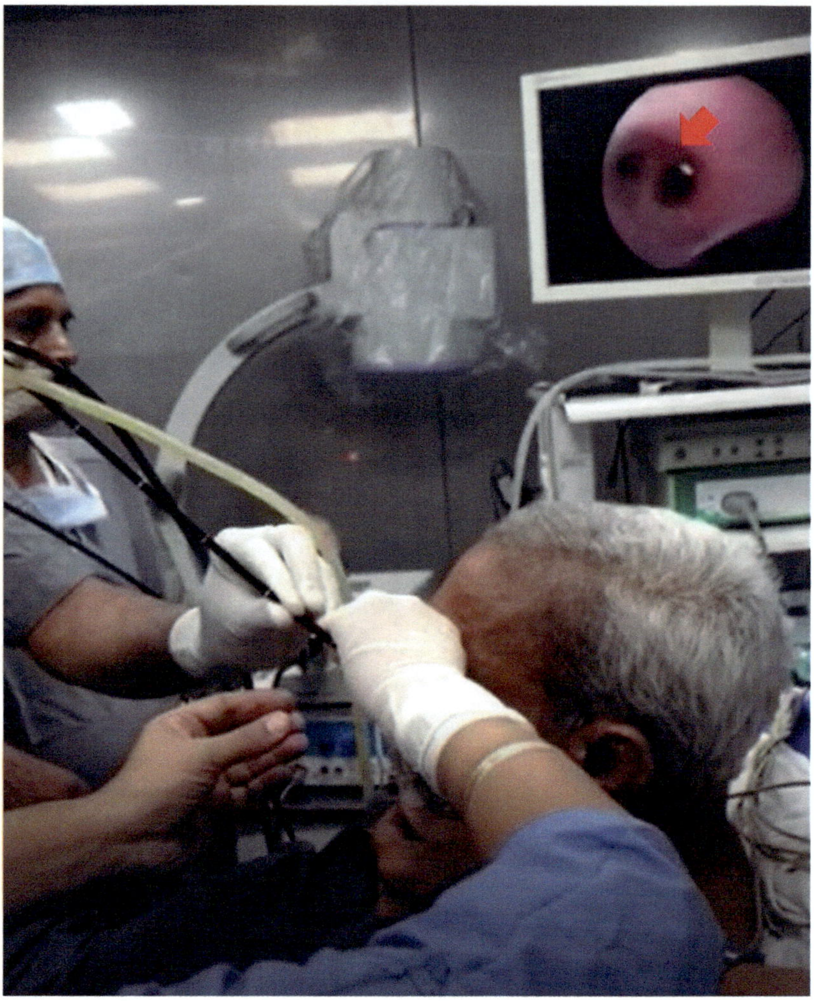

Fig. 27.4 Scope assisted view of carina and bifurcation of the trachea (indicated by an arrow)

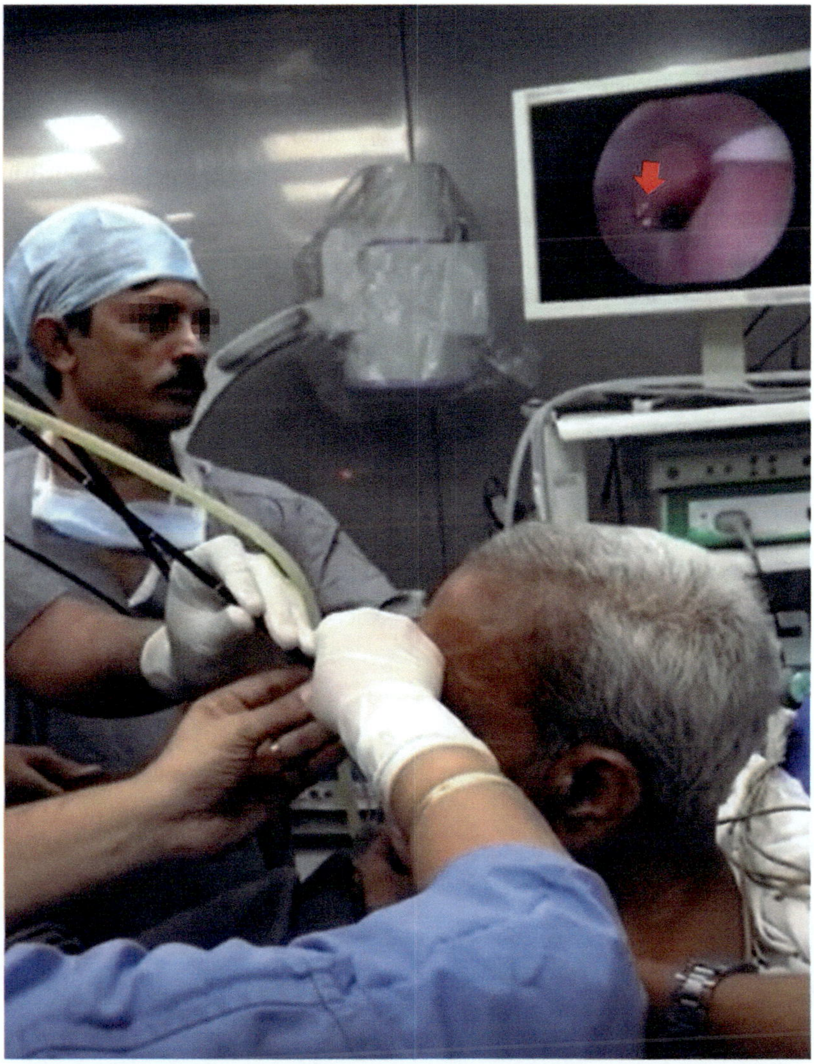

Fig. 27.5 Final position of the endotracheal tube (indicated by an arrow), for uniform bilateral ventilation

27.5 Conclusion

The anaesthesiologist and the operating surgeon should assess and discuss every single patient pre-operatively to decide on the type of intubation to secure and maintain the airway based on the type and duration of the surgery. The anaesthesiologist should be aware of the consequences and complications that can happen with such alternative intubation techniques as they are technique sensitive and require additional training. Appropriate assessment, planning followed by execution for securing airway in such patients can prevent unwarranted complications.

References

1. Sankar D, Krishnan R, Veerabahu M, Vikraman BP, Nathan JA. Retrospective evaluation of airway management with blind awake intubation in temporomandibular joint ankylosis patients: a review of 48 cases. Ann Maxillofac Surg. 2016;6(1):54–7.
2. Goel A, Dave N, Shah H, Muneshwar P. The troublesome triumvirate: temporomandibular joint ankylosis, Pierre Robin syndrome and severe obstructive sleep apnoea. Indian J Anaesth. 2020;64:800–3.
3. Gupta K, Jain M, Gupta PK, Rastogi B, Saxena SK, Manngo A. Dexmedetomidine premedication for fiberoptic intubation in patients of temporomandibular joint ankylosis: a randomized clinical trial. Saudi J Anaesth. 2012;6(3):219–23.
4. Asghar A, Shamim F, Aman A. Fiberoptic intubation in a paediatric patient with severe temporomandibular joint (TMJ) ankylosis. J Col Physic Surg Pak. 2012;22(12):783–5.

GPSR Compliance

The European Union's (EU) General Product Safety Regulation (GPSR) is a set of rules that requires consumer products to be safe and our obligations to ensure this.

If you have any concerns about our products, you can contact us on ProductSafety@springernature.com

In case Publisher is established outside the EU, the EU authorized representative is:

Springer Nature Customer Service Center GmbH
Europaplatz 3
69115 Heidelberg, Germany

Batch number: 10731383

Printed by Printforce, the Netherlands